Step-Up to Medicine

Second Edition

Step-Up to Medicine

Second Edition

STEVEN S. AGABEGI, MD
Resident
Department of Orthopaedic Surgery
University of Cincinnati
Cincinnati, Ohio

ELIZABETH D. AGABEGI, MD
Resident
Department of Ophthalmology
University of Cincinnati
Cincinnati, Ohio

Wolters Kluwer | Lippincott Williams & Wilkins
Health
Philadelphia · Baltimore · New York · London
Buenos Aires · Hong Kong · Sydney · Tokyo

Publisher: Betty Sun
Senior Managing Editor: Stacey L. Sebring
Marketing Manager: Jennifer Kuklinski
Production Editor: Beth Martz
Design Coordinator: Holly Reid McLaughlin
Compositor: International Typesetting and Composition

Second Edition

Copyright © 2005, 2008 Lippincott Williams & Wilkins, a Wolters Kluwer business.

351 West Camden Street   530 Walnut Street
Baltimore, MD 21201   Philadelphia, PA 19106

First Edition, Copyright © 2005 Lippincott Williams & Wilkins

The publisher is not responsible (as a matter of product liability, negligence, or otherwise) for any injury resulting from any material contained herein. This publication contains information relating to general principles of medical care that should not be construed as specific instructions for individual patients. Manufacturers' product information and package inserts should be reviewed for current information, including contraindications, dosages, and precautions.

Printed in the United States of America

Library of Congress Cataloging-in-Publication Data

Agabegi, Steven S.
  Step-up to medicine / Steven S. Agabegi, Elizabeth D. Agabegi.—2nd ed.
      p. ; cm. —(Step up series)
  Includes bibliographical references and index.
  ISBN-13: 978-0-7817-7153-5
  ISBN-10: 0-7817-7153-6
  1. Internal medicine—Outlines, syllabi, etc. 2. Clinical clerkship—Outlines, syllabi, etc. 3. Physicians—Licenses—United States—Examinations—Study guides. I. Agabegi, Elizabeth D. II. Title. III. Series.
  [DNLM: 1. Clinical Medicine—Outlines. 2. Clinical Medicine—Problems and Exercises. W 18.2 A259s 2008]
  RC59.A35 2008
  616—dc22

                                                                                    2007047325

Care has been taken to confirm the accuracy of the information presented and to describe generally accepted practices. However, the authors, editors, and publisher are not responsible for errors or omissions or for any consequences from application of the information in this book and make no warranty, expressed or implied, with respect to the currency, completeness, or accuracy of the contents of the publication. Application of this information in a particular situation remains the professional responsibility of the practitioner.

  The authors, editors, and publisher have exerted every effort to ensure that drug selection and dosage set forth in this text are in accordance with current recommendations and practice at the time of publication. However, in view of ongoing research, changes in government regulations, and the constant flow of information relating to drug therapy and drug reactions, the reader is urged to check the package insert for each drug for any change in indications and dosage and for added warnings and precautions. This is particularly important when the recommended agent is a new or infrequently employed drug.

  Some drugs and medical devices presented in this publication have Food and Drug Administration (FDA) clearance for limited use in restricted research settings. It is the responsibility of health care providers to ascertain the FDA status of each drug or device planned for use in their clinical practice.

  The publishers have made every effort to trace copyright holders for borrowed material. If they have inadvertently overlooked any, they will be pleased to make the necessary arrangements at the first opportunity.

  To purchase additional copies of this book, call our customer service department at **(800) 638-3030** or fax orders to **(301) 223-2320**. International customers should call **(301) 223-2300**. Visit Lippincott Williams & Wilkins on the Internet: at LWW.com. Lippincott Williams & Wilkins customer service representatives are available from 8:30 am to 6 pm, EST.

10 9 8 7 6 5 4 3

B. Adenomatous polyps—benign lesions, but have significant malignant potential; precursors of adenocarcinoma
   1. Can be one of three types of adenoma
      a. Tubular (most common; up to 60% to 80% of cases)—smallest risk of malignancy
      b. Tubulovillous—intermediate risk of malignancy
      c. Villous—greatest risk of malignancy
   2. Can determine malignant potential by the following:
      a. Size—the larger the polyp, the greater the malignant potential
      b. Histologic type
      c. Atypia of cells
      d. Shape—sessile (flat, more likely to be malignant) versus pedunculated (on a stalk)

C. Treatment: complete removal of polyp

Diverticulosis

A. General characteristics
   1. Caused by **increased intraluminal pressure**—inner layer of colon bulges through focal area of weakness in colon wall (usually an area of blood vessel penetration)
   2. Risk factors
      a. **Low-fiber diets:** Constipation causes intraluminal pressures to increase.
      b. Positive family history
   3. Prevalence increases with age.
   4. **The most common location is the sigmoid colon.** However, diverticula may occur anywhere in the colon.

B. Clinical features
   1. Usually asymptomatic and discovered incidentally on barium enema or colonoscopy done for another reason
   2. Vague LLQ discomfort, bloating, constipation/diarrhea may be present
   3. Only 10% to 20% become symptomatic (i.e., develop complications—see below).

C. Diagnosis
   1. Barium enema is the test of choice.
   2. Abdominal x-rays are usually normal and are not diagnostic for diverticulosis.

D. Treatment
   1. High-fiber foods (such as bran) to increase stool bulk
   2. Psyllium (if the patient cannot tolerate bran)

E. Complications
   1. Painless rectal bleeding (up to 40% of patients)
      a. Bleeding is usually clinically insignificant and stops spontaneously. No further treatment is necessary in these patients.
      b. Bleeding can be severe in about 5% of patients. In many cases, the bleeding stops spontaneously. Colonoscopy may be performed to locate site of bleeding

- Most polyps are found in the rectosigmoid region.
- Most patients are asymptomatic.
- In symptomatic patients, rectal bleeding is the most common symptom.

Diverticulosis (pouches in the colon wall) should be distinguished from diverticulitis, which refers to inflammation or infection of the diverticula and is a complication of diverticulosis.

- Complications of **diverticulosis** include painless rectal bleeding and diverticulitis.
- Complications of **diverticulitis** include bowel obstruction, abscess, and fistulas.

Box 3-2 **Complications of Diverticulitis**

- Abscess formation (can be drained either percutaneously under CT guidance or surgically)
- Colovesical fistula—accounts for 50% of fistulas secondary to diverticulitis; 50% close spontaneously
- Obstruction—due to chronic inflammation and thickening of bowel wall
- **Free colonic perforation—uncommon but catastrophic (leads to peritonitis)**

DISEASES OF THE GASTROINTESTINAL SYSTEM

- Diverticulitis recurs in about 30% of patients treated medically, usually within the first 5 years.
- Lower GI bleeding is very rare in diverticulitis, but common in diverticulosis.

- Diverticulosis—barium enema is test of choice
- Diverticulitis—CT scan is test of choice (barium enema and colonoscopy contraindicated)

As many as 25% of patients with bleeding arteriovenous malformations have aortic stenosis. However, no cause-and-effect relationship has been proven.

- Acute mesenteric ischemia is much more common than chronic mesenteric ischemia.
- Patients with acute mesenteric ischemia often have preexisting heart disease (e.g., congestive heart failure, coronary artery disease).

Differences in presentation of types of acute mesenteric ischemia

- Embolic—symptoms are more sudden and painful than other causes
- Arterial thrombosis—symptoms are more gradual and less severe than embolic causes
- Nonocclusive ischemia—typically occurs in critically ill patients
- Venous thrombosis—symptoms may be present for several days or even weeks, with gradual worsening

(mesenteric angiography in certain cases). If bleeding is persistent and/or recurrent, surgery may be needed (segmental colectomy).

2. **Diverticulitis** (15% to 25% of patients)

   a. Occurs when feces become impacted in the diverticulum, leading to erosion and microperforation

   b. Clinical features: fever, LLQ pain, leukocytosis
      - Other possible features: alteration in bowel habits (constipation or diarrhea), vomiting, and sometimes a painful mass on rectal examination if inflammation is near the rectum

   c. Diagnostic tests
      - **CT scan (abdomen and pelvis) with oral and IV contrast is the test of choice;** it may reveal a swollen, edematous bowel wall or an abscess.
      - Abdominal radiographs help in excluding other potential causes of LLQ pain, and can rule out ileus or obstruction (indicated by air-fluid levels, distention), and perforation (indicated by free air).
      - **Barium enema and colonoscopy are contraindicated in acute diverticulitis due to the risk of perforation.**

   d. Treatment of diverticulitis
      - Initial episode—Use IV antibiotics, bowel rest (NPO), IV fluids. Mild episodes can be treated on outpatient basis if patient is reliable and has few or no comorbid conditions. If symptoms persist after 3 to 4 days, surgery may be necessary.
      - Second and subsequent episodes—Surgery is recommended (resection of involved segment) once acute inflammation resolves.
      - Low-residue diet (e.g., no nuts, seeds)

Angiodysplasia of the Colon (Arteriovenous Malformations, Vascular Ectasia)

- Tortuous, dilated veins in submucosa of the colon (usually proximal) wall
- A common cause of lower GI bleeding in patients over age 60
- Bleeding is usually low grade, but 15% of patients may have massive hemorrhage if veins rupture.
- Diagnosed by colonoscopy (preferred over angiography)
- In about 90% of patients, bleeding stops spontaneously.
- It can frequently be treated by colonoscopic coagulation of the lesion. If bleeding persists, a right hemicolectomy should be considered.

Acute Mesenteric Ischemia

A. Introduction

1. Results from a compromised blood supply, usually to the superior mesenteric vessels

2. There are four types (three are due to arterial disease, one due to venous disease):

   a. **Arterial embolism** (50% of cases): Almost all emboli are of a cardiac origin (e.g., atrial fibrillation, MI, valvular disease).

   b. **Arterial thrombosis** (25% of cases)
      - Most of these patients have atherosclerotic disease (e.g., coronary artery disease [CAD], PVD, stroke) at other sites.
      - Acute occlusion occurs over preexisting atherosclerotic disease. The acute event may be due to a decrease in cardiac output (e.g., resulting from MI, CHF) or plaque rupture.
      - Collateral circulation has usually developed.

   c. **Nonocclusive mesenteric ischemia** (20% of cases)
      - Splanchnic vasoconstriction secondary to low cardiac output
      - Typically seen in critically ill elderly patients

   d. **Venous thrombosis** (<10% of cases)

- Many predisposing factors—e.g., infection, hypercoagulable states, oral contraceptives, portal HTN, malignancy, pancreatitis
3. The overall mortality rate for all types is about 60% to 70%. If bowel infarction has occurred, the mortality rate can exceed 90%. *overall bad prognosis.*

B. Clinical features

1. Classic presentation is acute onset of **severe abdominal pain disproportionate to physical findings.** Pain is due to ischemia and possibly infarction of intestines, analogous to MI in CAD.
   a. The abdominal examination may appear benign even when there is severe ischemia. This can lead to a delay in diagnosis.
   b. The acuteness and the severity of pain vary depending on the type of acute mesenteric ischemia (see Quick Hit).
2. Anorexia, vomiting
3. GI bleeding (mild)
4. Peritonitis, sepsis, and shock may be present in advanced disease.

- Signs of intestinal infarction include hypotension, tachypnea, lactic acidosis, fever, and altered mental status (eventually leading to shock).
- Check the lactate level if acute mesenteric ischemia is suspected.

C. Diagnosis

1. **Mesenteric angiography** is the definitive diagnostic test.
2. Obtain a plain film of the abdomen to exclude other causes of abdominal pain.
3. "Thumbprinting" on barium enema due to thickened edematous mucosal folds

D. Treatment

1. Supportive measures: IV fluids and broad-spectrum antibiotics
2. Direct intra-arterial infusion of papaverine (vasodilator) into the superior mesenteric system during arteriography is the therapy of choice for all arterial causes of acute mesenteric ischemia. This relieves the occlusion and vasospasm.
3. Direct intra-arterial infusion of thrombolytics or embolectomy may be indicated in some patients with embolic acute mesenteric ischemia.
4. Heparin anticoagulation is the treatment of choice for venous thrombosis.
5. Surgery (resection of nonviable bowel) may be needed in all types of acute mesenteric ischemia if signs of peritonitis develop.

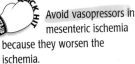

Avoid vasopressors in mesenteric ischemia because they worsen the ischemia.

Chronic Mesenteric Ischemia

- Caused by **atherosclerotic occlusive disease** of main mesenteric vessels (celiac artery, superior and inferior mesenteric arteries)
- Abdominal angina—dull pain, typically **postprandial** (when there is increased demand for splanchnic blood flow); analogous to anginal pain of CAD
- Significant **weight loss** may occur due to abdominal angina.
- Mesenteric arteriography confirms the diagnosis.
- Surgical revascularization is definitive treatment and leads to pain relief in 90% of cases.

Patients with Ogilvie's syndrome are usually ill and commonly have a history of recent surgery or medical illness.

Ogilvie's Syndrome

- An unusual problem in which signs, symptoms, and radiographic evidence of large bowel obstruction are present, but **there is no mechanical obstruction.**
- Common causes include recent surgery or trauma, serious medical illnesses (e.g., sepsis, malignancy), and medications (e.g., narcotics, psychotropic drugs, anticholinergics).
- The diagnosis cannot be confirmed until mechanical obstruction of the colon is excluded.
- Treatment consists of stopping any offending agent (e.g., narcotics) and supportive measures (IV fluids, electrolyte repletion).
- Decompression with gentle enemas or nasogastric suction may be helpful. Colonoscopic decompression is usually successful if the above measures fail.
- Surgical decompression with cecostomy or colostomy is a last resort.

Whenever there is colonic distention and when the colon diameter exceeds 10 cm, bowel is at risk of impending rupture leading to peritonitis and even death; **decompress immediately.**

Pseudomembranous Colitis

A. General characteristics

1. This is also referred to as **antibiotic-associated colitis** because many patients do not have grossly visible pseudomembranes.
2. Antibiotic treatment kills organisms that normally inhibit growth of *Clostridium difficile*, leading to overgrowth of *C. difficile* and toxin production.
3. Almost all antibiotics have been associated, but the most frequently implicated antibiotics are clindamycin, ampicillin, and cephalosporins.
4. Symptoms usually begin during first week of antibiotic therapy. However, up to 6 weeks may elapse after stopping antibiotics before clinical findings become apparent.
5. Disease severity varies widely.

Complications of severe pseudomembranous colitis (may require surgery):
- Toxic megacolon
- Colonic perforation
- Anasarca, electrolyte disturbances

B. Clinical features

1. Profuse watery diarrhea (usually no blood or mucus) *7/8 per day.*
2. Crampy abdominal pain
3. **Toxic megacolon** (in severe cases) with risk of perforation

C. Diagnosis

1. Demonstration of *C. difficile* toxins in stool is diagnostic, but results take at least 24 hours (95% sensitivity).
2. Flexible sigmoidoscopy is most rapid test and is diagnostic, but because of discomfort/expense, it is infrequently used (usually reserved for special situations).
3. Abdominal radiograph (to rule out toxic megacolon and perforation)
4. Leukocytosis (very common)

D. Treatment

1. Discontinue the offending antibiotic, if possible. *↦ or breast-feeding.*
2. Metronidazole is drug of choice (cannot be used in infants or pregnant patients)
3. Oral vancomycin used if patient is resistant to metronidazole or cannot tolerate it.
4. Regardless of choice of antibiotic, recurrence may occur within 2 to 8 weeks after stopping the antibiotic. This occurs in 15% to 35% of successfully treated patients.
5. Cholestyramine may be used as an adjuvant treatment to improve diarrhea.

Cholestyramine also used for itching.

Colonic Volvulus

A. General characteristics

1. Defined as twisting of a loop of intestine about its mesenteric attachment site
2. May result in obstruction or vascular compromise (with potential for necrosis and/or perforation if untreated)
3. The **most common site is the sigmoid colon** (75% of all cases).
4. Cecal volvulus accounts for 25% of all cases.
5. Risk factors
   a. Chronic illness, age, institutionalization, and CNS disease increase risk of sigmoid volvulus.
   b. Cecal volvulus is due to congenital lack of fixation of the right colon and tends to occur in younger patients.
   c. Chronic constipation, laxative abuse, antimotility drugs
   d. Prior abdominal surgery

B. Clinical features

1. Acute onset of colicky abdominal pain
2. Obstipation, abdominal distention
3. Anorexia, nausea, vomiting

C. Diagnosis

1. Plain abdominal films
   a. Sigmoid volvulus—*Omega loop sign* (or bent inner-tube shape) indicates a dilated sigmoid colon.
   b. Cecal volvulus (distention of cecum and small bowel)—*Coffee bean sign* indicates a large air-fluid level in RLQ.
2. Sigmoidoscopy—preferred diagnostic and therapeutic test for **sigmoid volvulus** (not for cecal volvulus); leads to successful treatment (untwisting and decompression) in many cases
3. Barium enema—reveals the narrowing of the colon at the point where it is twisted ("*bird's beak*")

D. Treatment

1. Sigmoid volvulus: Nonoperative reduction (decompression via sigmoidoscopy) is successful in >70% of cases. The recurrence rate is high, so elective sigmoid colon resection is recommended.
2. Cecal volvulus: Emergent surgery is indicated.

> **QUICK HIT**
> Do not perform a barium enema if strangulation is suspected!

DISEASES OF THE LIVER

Cirrhosis

A. General characteristics

1. Cirrhosis is chronic liver disease characterized by fibrosis, disruption of the liver architecture, and widespread nodules in the liver. The fibrous tissue replaces damaged or dead hepatocytes.
2. The distortion of liver anatomy causes two major events.
   a. Decreased blood flow through the liver with subsequent hypertension in portal circulation (**portal hypertension**)—This has widespread manifestations, including ascites, peripheral edema, splenomegaly, and varicosity of veins "back stream" in the circulation (e.g., gastric/esophageal varices, hemorrhoids).
   b. Hepatocellular failure that leads to impairment of biochemical functions, such as decreased albumin synthesis and decreased clotting factor synthesis
3. Assessment of hepatic functional reserve
   a. **Child's classification** (see Table 3-1) estimates hepatic reserve in liver failure. It is used to measure disease severity and is a predictor of morbidity and mortality.
   b. Child's class C indicates most severe disease, and Child's class A indicates milder disease.

hypoalbuminemia—Muehrcke's nails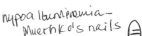

> **QUICK HIT**
> **Cirrhosis**
> • The most common causes of cirrhosis are alcoholic liver disease and chronic viral infection (especially hepatitis C).
> • **Liver biopsy** is the gold standard for diagnosis of cirrhosis.
> *see fibrosis*

B. Causes

1. **Alcoholic liver disease—most common cause**
   a. Refers to a range of conditions from fatty liver (reversible, due to acute ingestion) to cirrhosis (irreversible)
   b. Fifteen percent to 20% of heavy drinkers develop alcoholic cirrhosis.
2. **Chronic hepatitis B and C infections—next most common causes**
3. Drugs (e.g., acetaminophen toxicity, methotrexate)
4. Autoimmune hepatitis *→ seen in young women*
5. Primary biliary cirrhosis (PBC), secondary biliary cirrhosis
6. Inherited metabolic diseases (e.g., hemochromatosis, Wilson's disease)
7. Hepatic congestion secondary to right-sided heart failure, constrictive pericarditis
8. α_1-Antitrypsin (AAT) deficiency
9. Hepatic veno-occlusive disease—can occur after bone marrow transplantation
10. Nonalcoholic steatohepatitis (NASH)— *have to do a liver biopsy to make the diagnosis*

C. Clinical features

1. Some patients have no overt clinical findings, especially early in the disease.
2. Patients may have signs or symptoms suggestive of one or more of the complications of cirrhosis (see Complications section).

TABLE 3-1	Child's Classification to Assess Severity of Liver Disease		
	A	**B**	**C**
Ascites	None	Controlled	Uncontrolled
Bilirubin	<2.0	2.0–2.5	>3.0
Encephalopathy	None	Minimal	Severe
Nutritional status	Excellent	Good	Poor
Albumin	>3.5	3.0–3.5	<3.0

QUICK HIT

Classic signs of chronic liver disease:
• Ascites
• Varices
• Gynecomastia, testicular atrophy
• Palmar erythema, spider angiomas on skin
• Hemorrhoids
• Caput medusae

D. Complications

1. Portal HTN
   a. Clinical features are listed before. **Bleeding** (hematemesis, melena, hematochezia) secondary to esophagogastric varices is the most life-threatening complication of portal HTN (see below).
   b. Diagnose based on above features. Paracentesis can help in diagnosis.
   c. Treat the specific complication. Use transjugular intrahepatic portal-systemic shunt (TIPS) to lower portal pressure.

2. Varices
   a. Esophageal/gastric
      • Clinical features include massive hematemesis, melena, and exacerbation of hepatic encephalopathy.
      • Esophageal varices account for 90% of varices, and gastric varices for 10%.
      • Initial treatment is hemodynamic stabilization (give fluids to maintain BP). See Box 3-4 for methods aimed at stopping bleeding.
      • Perform **emergent upper GI endoscopy** (once patient is stabilized) for diagnosis if the patient presents with hematemesis.
      • Give β-blockers as long-term therapy to prevent rebleeding. *ex Propranalol.*
   b. Rectal hemorrhoids
   c. *Caput medusae* (distention of abdominal wall veins)

3. Ascites
   a. Accumulation of fluid into the peritoneal cavity due to **portal HTN** (increased hydrostatic pressure) and **hypoalbuminemia** (reduced oncotic pressure)
   b. Clinical features: abdominal distention, shifting dullness, and fluid wave.
   c. Abdominal ultrasound can detect as little as 30 mL of fluid.
   d. Diagnostic **paracentesis** determines whether ascites is due to portal HTN or another process.
      • Indications include new-onset ascites, worsening ascites, and suspected spontaneous bacterial peritonitis (see below).
      • Examine cell count, ascites albumin, Gram stain, and culture to rule out infection (e.g., spontaneous bacterial peritonitis). *only 1 bacteria*

Box 3-3 Differential Diagnosis of Ascites

• Cirrhosis, portal HTN
• CHF
• Chronic renal disease
• Massive fluid overload
• Tuberculous peritonitis
• Malignancy
• Hypoalbuminemia
• Peripheral vasodilation secondary to endotoxin-induced release of nitrous oxide, which leads to increased renin secretion (and thus secondary hyperaldosteronism)
• Impaired liver inactivation of aldosterone

Box 3-4   Treatment of Bleeding Esophageal Varices

- **Variceal ligation/banding**
  - Initial endoscopic treatment of choice
  - Effective control of active bleeding
  - Lower rate of rebleeding than sclerotherapy
- **Endoscopic sclerotherapy**
  - Sclerosing substance is injected into varices during endoscopy.
  - This controls acute bleeding in 80% to 90% of cases.
  - Up to 50% of patients may have rebleeding.
- **IV vasopressin**
  - This is an alternative to octreotide, but is less popular due to the risk of complications.
  - Vasoconstriction of mesenteric vessels reduces portal pressure.
  - Nitroglycerin is given to prevent side effects of vasopressin (coronary vasoconstriction/MI, decreased cardiac output, HTN).
- **IV octreotide infusion**
  - Now replacing vasopressin as first-line therapy; causes splanchnic vasoconstriction and reduces portal pressure.
  - Fewer side effects than vasopressin
- **Other options** include esophageal balloon tamponade (Sengstaken-Blakemore tube is a temporary measure), repeat sclerotherapy, transjugular intrahepatic portosystemic shunt (TIPS), surgical shunts, and liver transplantation.

- Measure the **serum ascites albumin gradient**. If it is >1.1 g/dL, portal HTN is very likely. If <1.1 g/dL, portal HTN is unlikely, and other causes must be considered.
- e. Treatment
  - Bed rest, a low-sodium diet, and diuretics (furosemide and spironolactone) *40mg* *100mg* *to effectively treat 2° hyperaldosteronism.*
  - Perform therapeutic paracentesis if tense ascites, shortness of breath, or early satiety is present.
  - Peritoneovenous shunt or TIPS to reduce portal HTN

4. Hepatic encephalopathy
  - a. Toxic metabolites (there are many, but **ammonia** *(base)* is believed to be most important) that are normally detoxified or removed by the liver accumulate and reach the brain.
  - b. Occurs in 50% of all cases of cirrhosis, with varying severity
  - c. Precipitants include alkalosis, hypokalemia (e.g., due to diuretics), sedating drugs (narcotics, sleeping medications), GI bleeding, systemic infection, and hypovolemia.
  - d. Clinical features
    - Decreased mental function, confusion, poor concentration, even stupor or coma
    - *Asterixis* ("flapping tremor")—Have the patient extend the arms and dorsiflex the hands. (However, this is not a specific sign.)
    - Rigidity, hyperreflexia
    - *Fetor hepaticus*—musty odor of breath *due to dimethylsulfide*
  - e. Treatment
    - Lactulose prevents absorption of ammonia. Metabolism of lactulose by bacteria in colon favors formation of NH_4^+, which is poorly absorbed from GI tract, thereby promoting excretion of ammonia.
    - Neomycin (antibiotic): kills bowel flora, so decreases ammonia production by intestinal bacteria
    - Diet: Limit protein to 30 to 40 mg/day.

5. **Hepatorenal syndrome**—indicates end-stage liver disease
  - a. Progressive renal failure in advanced liver disease, secondary to renal hypoperfusion resulting from vasoconstriction of renal vessels

QUICK HIT

Ascites can be managed by salt restriction and diuretics in most cases.

QUICK HIT

Monitoring patients with cirrhosis
- Order periodic laboratory values every 3 to 4 months (CBC, renal function tests, electrolytes, LFTs, and coagulation tests).
- Perform an endoscopy to determine the presence of esophageal varices.
- If hepatocellular carcinoma is suspected, perform a CT-guided biopsy for diagnosis.

GI bleeding.
could cause marked
inc. in

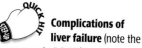

Complications of liver failure (note the mnemonic **AC, 9H**)
- **A**scites
- **C**oagulopathy
- **H**ypoalbuminemia
- Portal **H**ypertension
- **H**yperammonemia
- **H**epatic encephalopathy
- **H**epatorenal syndrome
- **H**ypoglycemia
- **H**yperbilirubinemia/jaundice
- **H**yperestrinism
- **H**epatocellular carcinoma

SBP: Look for fever and/or change in mental status in a patient with known ascites.

Signs of acute liver failure (any of the following may be present):
- Coagulopathy
- Jaundice
- Hypoglycemia (liver stores glycogen)
- Hepatic encephalopathy
- Infection
- Elevated LFT values
- Any complication associated with cirrhosis

b. Often precipitated by infection or diuretics

c. This is a functional renal failure—Kidneys are normal in terms of morphology, and no specific causes of renal dysfunction are evident. This condition does not respond to volume expansion.

d. Clinical features: azotemia, oliguria, hyponatremia, hypotension, low urine sodium (<10 mEq/L)

e. Treatment: Liver transplantation is only cure. In general, the prognosis is very poor, and the condition is usually fatal without liver transplantation.

6. Spontaneous bacterial peritonitis (SBP)—infected ascitic fluid; occurs in up to 20% of patients hospitalized for ascites
   a. Usually occurs in patients with ascites caused by chronic liver disease; associated with high mortality rate (20% to 30%)
   b. Has a high recurrence rate (up to 70% in first year)
   c. Etiologic agents
      - *Escherichia coli* (most common)
      - *Klebsiella*
      - *Streptococcus pneumoniae*
   d. Clinical features: abdominal pain, fever, vomiting, rebound tenderness. SBP may lead to sepsis.
   e. Diagnosis is established by paracentesis and examination of ascitic fluid for WBCs (especially PMNs), Gram stain with culture, and sensitivities.
      - WBC > 500, PMN > 250
      - Positive ascites culture; culture-negative spontaneous bacterial peritonitis is common as well
   f. Treatment
      - Broad-spectrum antibiotic therapy: Give specific antibiotic once organism is identified.
      - Clinical improvement should be seen in 24 to 48 hours. Repeat paracentesis in 2 to 3 days to document a decrease in ascitic fluid PMN (<250).

7. Hyperestrinism
   a. *Spider angiomas*—dilated cutaneous arterioles with central red spot and reddish extensions that radiate outward like a spider's web
   b. Palmar erythema
   c. Gynecomastia
   d. Testicular atrophy

8. Coagulopathy occurs secondary to decreased synthesis of clotting factors.
   a. Prolonged PT; PTT may be prolonged with severe disease.
   b. Vitamin K ineffective because it cannot be used by diseased liver.
   c. Treat coagulopathy with fresh frozen plasma.

9. Hepatocellular carcinoma (HCC)—present in 10% to 25% of patients with cirrhosis

E. Treatment
1. Treat underlying cause—e.g., abstinence from alcohol, interferons for hepatitis B and C
2. Once cirrhosis develops, aim treatment at managing any complications that arise, as described above. The most serious complications are variceal bleeding, ascites, and hepatic encephalopathy.
3. Liver transplantation is the only hope for a cure. Abstinence from alcohol for more than 6 months is required before a patient is eligible for transplantation.

Wilson's Disease

A. General characteristics
1. An autosomal recessive disease of **copper metabolism**
2. Normally excess copper is excreted by the liver, but the livers of patients with Wilson's disease cannot do so because there is usually a **deficiency of ceruloplasmin**, a copper-binding protein that is necessary for copper excretion.

3. Therefore, copper accumulates in liver cells. As hepatocytes die, copper leaks into plasma and accumulates in various organs, including kidney, cornea, and brain.
4. The disease is most often apparent during childhood/adolescence (after age 5), and the majority of cases present between ages 5 and 35.

B. Clinical features
1. Clinical features are due to copper deposition in various organs.
2. Liver disease (most common initial manifestation): Manifestations vary and may include acute hepatitis, cirrhosis, and fulminant hepatic failure.
3. *Kayser-Fleischer rings* (yellowish rings in cornea) are caused by copper deposition in cornea; they do not interfere with vision (see Color Figure 3-1).
4. CNS findings are due to copper deposition in the CNS.
   a. Extrapyramidal signs—parkinsonian symptoms (resting tremor, rigidity, bradykinesia), chorea, drooling, incoordination due to copper deposition in basal ganglia
   b. Psychiatric disturbances—depression, neuroses, personality changes, psychosis
5. Renal involvement—aminoaciduria, nephrocalcinosis

C. Diagnosis
1. Diagnosis is made by determining the following (patients may have many or only a few of these findings):
   a. Hepatic disease—elevated aminotransferases; impaired synthesis of coagulation factors and albumin
   b. Decreased serum ceruloplasmin levels, although ranges within normal do not exclude the diagnosis
   c. Liver biopsy—significantly elevated copper concentration
2. If diagnosed, first-degree relatives must be screened as well.

D. Treatment
1. Chelating agents—e.g., D-penicillamine, which removes and detoxifies the excess copper deposits
2. Zinc
   • Prevents uptake of dietary copper
   • Given alone (presymptomatic or pregnant patients) or in conjunction with chelating agents (to symptomatic patients)
3. Liver transplantation (if unresponsive to therapy or fulminant liver failure)
4. Monitor patient's copper levels, urinary copper excretion, ceruloplasmin, and liver function; physical examination for signs of liver or neurologic disease; psychological health

Hemochromatosis

A. General characteristics
1. An autosomal recessive disease of iron absorption
2. Excessive iron absorption in the intestine leads to increased accumulation of iron (as ferritin and hemosiderin) in various organs. Over many years, fibrosis in involved organs occurs secondary to hydroxyl free radicals that are generated by the excess iron.
3. Affected organs
   a. Liver (primary organ)
   b. Pancreas
   c. Heart
   d. Joints
   e. Skin
   f. Thyroid, gonads, hypothalamus
4. This is an inherited disease, so screen the patient's siblings. Early diagnosis and treatment before development of complications (primarily cirrhosis, but also heart disease and diabetes) improves survival.

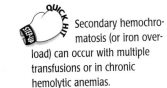

Secondary hemochromatosis (or iron overload) can occur with multiple transfusions or in chronic hemolytic anemias.

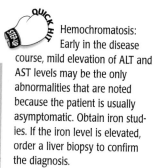

Hemochromatosis: Early in the disease course, mild elevation of ALT and AST levels may be the only abnormalities that are noted because the patient is usually asymptomatic. Obtain iron studies. If the iron level is elevated, order a liver biopsy to confirm the diagnosis.

B. Clinical features

1. Most patients are asymptomatic initially.
2. Findings may include signs of liver disease, fatigue, arthritis, impotence/amenorrhea, abdominal pain, and cardiac arrhythmias.

C. Complications

1. Cirrhosis
   a. Cirrhosis increases the risk of hepatocellular carcinoma by 200-fold.
   b. The presence of liver disease is a primary factor in determining the prognosis.
2. Cardiomyopathy—CHF, arrhythmias
3. Diabetes mellitus—due to iron deposition in the pancreas
4. Arthritis—most common sites are the second and third metacarpophalangeal joints, hips, and knees
5. Hypogonadism—impotence, amenorrhea, loss of libido
6. Hypothyroidism
7. Hyperpigmentation of skin (resembles suntan, "bronzelike")

D. Diagnosis

1. Markedly elevated serum iron and serum ferritin
2. Elevated iron saturation (transferrin saturation)
3. Decreased total iron-binding capacity (TIBC)
4. **Liver biopsy (determines hepatic iron concentration) required for diagnosis.**
5. Genetic testing for chromosomal abnormalities

E. Treatment

1. **Perform repeated phlebotomies**—this is the treatment of choice and improves survival dramatically if initiated early in the course of the disease.
2. Treat any complications (e.g., CHF, diabetes, hypothyroidism, arthritis).
3. Consider liver transplantation in advanced cases.

Hepatocellular Adenoma

- Benign liver tumor, most often seen in young women (15 to 40 years of age). Oral contraceptive use, female sex, and anabolic steroid use are the main risk factors.
- Patient may be asymptomatic; hepatocellular adenoma may be discovered incidentally on abdominal imaging studies. RUQ pain or fullness may be present.
- Malignant potential is very low (<1%). However, the adenoma may rupture, leading to hemoperitoneum and hemorrhage.
- Diagnosis made by CT scan, ultrasound, or hepatic arteriography (most accurate but invasive).
- Treatment: Discontinue oral contraceptives; surgically resect tumors >5 cm that do not regress after stopping oral contraceptives (otherwise there is a risk of rupture).

Cavernous Hemangiomas

- Vascular tumors that are usually small and asymptomatic. They are the **most common type of benign liver tumor.**
- As the size of the tumor increases (e.g., due to pregnancy or use of oral contraceptives), the symptoms increase and include RUQ pain or mass.
- Complications (uncommon unless tumor is very large) include rupture with hemorrhage, obstructive jaundice, coagulopathy, CHF secondary to a large AV shunt, and gastric outlet obstruction.
- Diagnose with ultrasound or CT scan with IV contrast. Biopsy contraindicated because of risk of rupture and hemorrhage.
- Most cases do not require treatment. Consider resection if the patient is symptomatic or if there is a high risk of rupture (as with large tumors).

Focal Nodular Hyperplasia

- This benign liver tumor without malignant potential occurs in women of reproductive age. There is **no association** with oral contraceptives
- It is usually asymptomatic. Hepatomegaly may be present. Treatment not necessary in most cases.

Hepatocellular Carcinoma (Malignant Hepatoma)

A. General characteristics

1. HCC accounts for more than 80% of primary liver cancers and, although rare in the United States, accounts for most deaths due to cancers worldwide. High-risk areas include Africa and Asia.
2. There are two pathologic types.
   a. Nonfibrolamellar (most common)
   - Usually associated with hepatitis B or C and cirrhosis
   - Usually unresectable with very short survival time (months)
   b. Fibrolamellar
   - Usually **not** associated with hepatitis B or C or cirrhosis
   - More often resectable; relatively longer survival time
   - Seen most commonly in adolescents and young adults

The most common malignant liver tumors are hepatocellular carcinomas and cholangiocarcinomas. The most common benign liver tumor is the hemangioma.

B. Risk factors

1. **Cirrhosis**, especially in association with alcohol or hepatitis B or C; HCC develops in 10% of cirrhotic patients
2. Chemical carcinogens: e.g., aflatoxin, vinyl chloride, Thorotrast
3. AAT deficiency
4. Hemochromatosis, Wilson's disease
5. Schistosomiasis
6. Hepatic adenoma (10% risk of malignant transformation)
7. Cigarette smoking
8. Glycogen storage disease (type 1)

Prognosis of HCC
- If unresectable: less than 1 year
- If resectable: 25% of patients are alive at 5 years

C. Clinical features

1. Abdominal pain (painful hepatomegaly)
2. Weight loss, anorexia, fatigue
3. Signs and symptoms of chronic liver disease—portal HTN, ascites, jaundice, splenomegaly
4. Paraneoplastic syndromes—erythrocytosis, thrombocytosis, hypercalcemia, carcinoid syndrome, hypertrophic pulmonary osteodystrophy, hypoglycemia, high cholesterol

Hepatocellular carcinoma is likely in a patient with cirrhosis who has a palpable liver mass and elevated AFP level.

D. Diagnosis

1. Liver biopsy—required for definitive diagnosis
2. Laboratory tests—hepatitis B and C serology, LFTs, coagulation tests
3. Imaging studies—ultrasound, CT scan (chest, abdomen, pelvis); MRI or MRA if surgery is an option (they provide more detail about the anatomy of the tumor)
4. Tumor marker elevation (AFP) is useful as a screening tool. AFP level may be elevated in 40% to 70% of patients with HCC, and is also helpful in monitoring response to therapy.

E. Treatment

1. Liver resection (in the 10% of patients who have resectable tumors)
2. Liver transplantation if diagnosis is made early

Nonalcoholic Steatohepatitis (NASH)

- Histology of the liver is identical to that in patients with alcoholic liver disease, but these patients do not have a history of alcohol use!

- Associated with obesity, hyperlipidemia, diabetes mellitus (some patients have none of these)
- Usually asymptomatic and a benign course (but cirrhosis develops in 10% to 15%)
- Typically discovered on routine laboratory tests (mild elevation in ALT and AST)
- Treatment is not clearly established.

Gilbert's Syndrome

- Occurs in up to 7% of the population—autosomal dominant condition in which there is decreased activity of hepatic uridine diphosphate glucuronyl transferase activity
- Common cause of isolated elevation of unconjugated bilirubin
- Exacerbated by fasting (crash diets), fever, alcohol, and infection
- Asymptomatic in most cases, but occasionally mild jaundice may be present
- Liver biopsy results are normal, and usually no treatment is necessary.

Hemobilia

- Refers to blood draining into the duodenum via the common bile duct (CBD). The source of bleeding can be anywhere along the biliary tract, the liver, or the ampullary region.
- Causes—trauma (most common), papillary thyroid carcinoma, surgery (e.g., cholecystectomy, CBD exploration), tumors, infection
- Clinical features include GI bleeding (melena, hematemesis), jaundice, and RUQ pain.
- Arteriogram is diagnostic. Upper GI endoscopy shows blood coming out of ampulla of Vater.
- Treatment—resuscitation (may require transfusion). If bleeding is severe, surgery is necessary (options include ligation of hepatic arteries or arteriogram with embolization of vessel).

Liver Cysts

Polycystic Liver Cysts

- Autosomal dominant, usually associated with polycystic kidney disease. Polycystic kidney disease often results in renal failure and is the main determinant of prognosis, whereas liver cysts **rarely** lead to hepatic fibrosis and liver failure.
- Usually asymptomatic; some patients have abdominal pain and upper abdominal mass
- Treatment unnecessary in most cases

Hydatid Liver Cysts

- Caused by infection from the tapeworm *Echinococcus granulosus* or, less commonly, *Echinococcus multilocularis*. Cysts most commonly occur in the right lobe of the liver.
- Small cysts are asymptomatic; larger cysts may cause RUQ pain and rupture into the peritoneal cavity, causing fatal anaphylactic shock.
- Treatment is surgical resection (caution to avoid spilling contents of the cyst into the peritoneal cavity). Mebendazole is given after surgery.

Liver Abscess

Pyogenic Liver Abscess

- Most common cause is biliary tract obstruction—Obstruction of bile flow allows bacterial proliferation. Other causes include GI infection (e.g., diverticulitis, appendicitis), with spread via portal venous system, and penetrating liver trauma (e.g., gunshot wound, surgery).
- Causative organisms include *Escherichia coli*, *Klebsiella*, *Proteus*, *Enterococcus*, and anaerobes.

- Clinical features include fever, malaise, anorexia, weight loss, nausea, vomiting, RUQ pain, and jaundice. Patients appear quite ill.
- Diagnosed by ultrasound or CT scan; elevated LFTs
- Fatal if untreated. Treatment (IV antibiotics and percutaneous drainage of abscess) reduces mortality to about 5% to 20%. Surgical drainage is sometimes necessary.

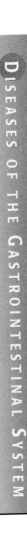

The most common location for liver abscess (both pyogenic and amebic) is the right lobe.

Amebic Liver Abscess

- Most common in men (9:1), particularly homosexual men. Transmitted through fecal–oral contact
- Caused by intestinal amebiasis (*Entamoeba histolytica*)—The amebae reach the liver via the hepatic portal vein.
- Clinical features—fever, RUQ pain, nausea/vomiting, hepatomegaly, diarrhea
- Serologic testing (immunoglobulin G enzyme immunoassay) establishes diagnosis. LFTs are often elevated. The *E. histolytica* stool antigen test (detects protozoa in stool) is not sensitive. Imaging studies (ultrasound, CT) identify the abscess, but it is difficult to distinguish from a pyogenic abscess.
- IV metronidazole is effective treatment in most cases. Therapeutic aspiration of the abscess (image-guided percutaneous aspiration) may be necessary if the abscess is large (high risk of rupture), or if there is no response to medical therapy.

Pyogenic and amebic abscesses are potentially life threatening if not detected early.

Budd-Chiari Syndrome

A. General characteristics
1. Liver disease caused by occlusion of hepatic venous outflow, which leads to hepatic congestion and subsequent microvascular ischemia
2. The course is variable, but most cases are indolent, with gradual development of portal HTN and progressive deterioration of liver function.
3. Rarely, disease is severe and leads to acute liver failure, which may be fatal without immediate therapy.

B. Causes—hypercoagulable states, myeloproliferative disorders (e.g., polycythemia vera), pregnancy, chronic inflammatory diseases, infection, various cancers, trauma. Condition is idiopathic in up to 40% of cases.

C. Clinical features (resemble those of cirrhosis)—hepatomegaly, ascites, abdominal pain (RUQ), jaundice, variceal bleeding

D. Diagnosis—hepatic venography; serum ascites albumin gradient >1.1 g/dL

E. Treatment
1. Medical therapy is usually unsatisfactory (e.g., anticoagulation, thrombolytics, diuretics)
2. Surgery is eventually necessary in most cases (balloon angioplasty with stent placement in inferior vena cava, portocaval shunts).
3. Liver transplantation if cirrhosis is present

Jaundice

A. General characteristics
1. Yellow coloration of skin, mucous membranes, and sclerae due to overproduction or underclearance of bilirubin
2. Clinical jaundice usually becomes evident when total bilirubin is >2 mg/dL.
3. Conjugated versus unconjugated bilirubin
   a. Conjugated (direct)
      - Loosely bound to albumin and therefore water soluble

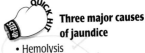

Three major causes of jaundice
- Hemolysis
- Liver disease
- Biliary obstruction

Box 3-5 Bilirubin Metabolism

- Eighty percent of bilirubin is derived from hemoglobin (RBC breakdown). The rest comes from myoglobin breakdown and liver enzymes.
- Hemoglobin is converted to bilirubin in the spleen. This unconjugated bilirubin circulates in plasma, bound to albumin. This bilirubin–albumin complex is not water soluble; therefore, it is not excreted in urine. In the liver, it dissociates from albumin, and the bilirubin is conjugated and excreted into the intestine, where bacteria act on it to produce urobilinogen and urobilin.
- Therefore, unconjugated hyperbilirubinemia results when there is a defect before hepatic uptake. Conjugated hyperbilirubinemia results when there is a defect after hepatic uptake.

- When present in excess, it is excreted in urine. Therefore, **dark urine is only seen with conjugated bilirubin!**
- Nontoxic
  b. Unconjugated (indirect)
  - Tightly bound to albumin and therefore not water soluble
  - Cannot be excreted in urine even if blood levels are high
  - Toxic—Unbound form can cross blood-brain barrier and cause neurologic deficits.

QUICK HIT

Dark urine and pale stools signal a diagnosis of conjugated hyperbilirubinemia.

B. Causes

1. **Conjugated hyperbilirubinemia—urine positive for bilirubin**
   a. Decreased intrahepatic excretion of bilirubin
   - Hepatocellular disease (viral or alcoholic hepatitis, cirrhosis)
   - Inherited disorders (**Dubin-Johnson syndrome, Rotor's syndrome**)
   - Drug-induced (oral contraceptives)
   - PBC
   - PSC
   b. Extrahepatic biliary obstruction
   - Gallstones
   - Carcinoma of head of pancreas
   - Cholangiocarcinoma
   - Periampullary tumors
   - Extrahepatic biliary atresia
2. **Unconjugated hyperbilirubinemia—urine negative for bilirubin**
   a. Excess production of bilirubin—hemolytic anemias
   b. Reduced hepatic uptake of bilirubin or impaired conjugation
   - **Gilbert's syndrome**
   - Drugs (e.g., sulfonamides, penicillin, rifampin, radiocontrast agents)
   - **Crigler-Najjar syndrome**, types I and II
   - Physiologic jaundice of the newborn (immaturity of conjugating system)
   - Diffuse liver disease (hepatitis, cirrhosis)

Box 3-6 Cholestasis

- This refers to blockage of bile flow (whether intrahepatic or extrahepatic) with a resultant increase in conjugated bilirubin levels.
- Clinical findings
  - Jaundice, gray stools, dark urine
  - Pruritus (bile salt deposition in skin)
  - Elevated serum alkaline phosphatase
  - Elevated serum cholesterol (impaired excretion)
  - Skin xanthomas (local accumulation of cholesterol)
  - Malabsorption of fats and fat-soluble vitamins

F I G U R E
3-1 Evaluation of jaundice

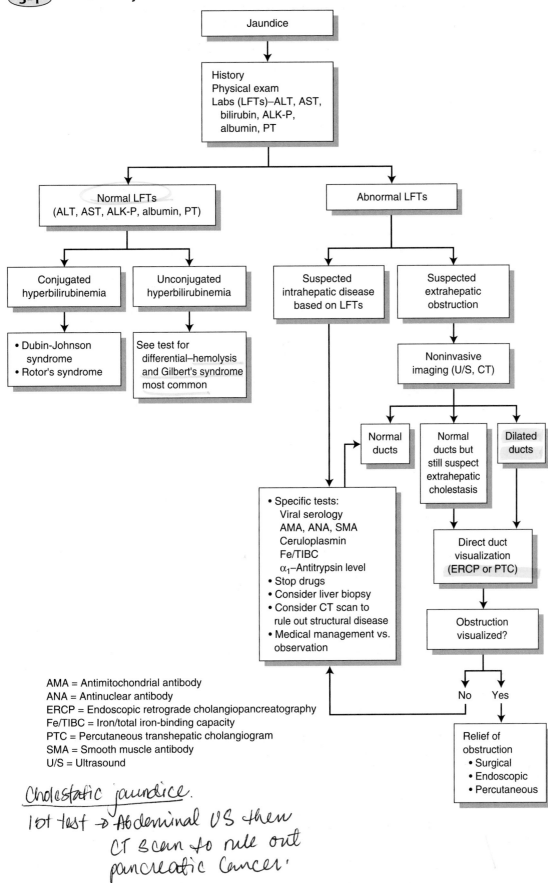

AMA = Antimitochondrial antibody
ANA = Antinuclear antibody
ERCP = Endoscopic retrograde cholangiopancreatography
Fe/TIBC = Iron/total iron-binding capacity
PTC = Percutaneous transhepatic cholangiogram
SMA = Smooth muscle antibody
U/S = Ultrasound

Cholestatic jaundice.
1st test → Abdominal US then
CT scan to rule out
pancreatic cancer.

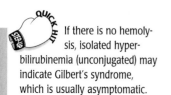

If there is no hemolysis, isolated hyperbilirubinemia (unconjugated) may indicate Gilbert's syndrome, which is usually asymptomatic.

- ALT is primarily found in the liver.
- AST is found in many tissues (e.g., skeletal muscle, heart, kidney, brain).

- In alcoholic hepatitis, the AST level is almost never >500, and the ALT level is almost never >300.
- The higher the AST–ALT ratio, the greater the likelihood that alcohol is contributing to the abnormal LFTs.

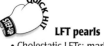

LFT pearls
- Cholestatic LFTs: markedly elevated alkaline phosphatase and GGT; ALT and AST slightly elevated
- Hepatocellular necrosis or inflammation: normal or slightly elevated alkaline phosphatase; markedly elevated ALT and AST

C. Diagnosis

1. Serum levels of total conjugated and unconjugated bilirubin
2. If unconjugated hyperbilirubinemia, CBC, reticulocyte count, haptoglobin, LDH, peripheral smear (may aid in diagnosis of hemolysis as the cause of jaundice)
3. If conjugated hyperbilirubinemia, LFTs may point to the cause
4. Ultrasound (or CT scan) to assess biliary tract for obstruction or anatomic changes
5. Additional tests (e.g., endoscopic retrograde cholangiopancreatography [ERCP], percutaneous transhepatic cholangiography [PTC])—depending on the findings of the above tests
6. Liver biopsy may be indicated in some cases to determine cause of hepatocellular injury

D. Treatment: Treat the underlying cause.

Liver Function Tests (LFTs)

A. Aminotransferases [alanine aminotransferase (ALT) and aspartate aminotransferase (AST)]

1. ALT is more sensitive and specific than AST for liver damage.
2. ALT and AST usually have a similar increase. The exception is in alcoholic hepatitis, in which the AST–ALT ratio may be >2:1.
3. If ALT and AST levels are **mildly elevated** (low hundreds), think of chronic viral hepatitis or acute alcoholic hepatitis.
4. If ALT and AST levels are **moderately elevated** (high hundreds to thousands), think of acute viral hepatitis.
5. If ALT and AST levels are **severely elevated** (>10,000), extensive hepatic necrosis has occurred. Typical cases are:
   a. Ischemia, shock liver (prolonged hypotension or circulatory collapse)
   b. Acetaminophen toxicity
   c. Severe viral hepatitis
6. Note that liver transaminases are often normal or even low in patients with cirrhosis (without any active cell necrosis) or metastatic liver disease, because the number of healthy functioning hepatocytes is markedly reduced.
7. The following can cause an elevation in ALT or AST levels in asymptomatic patients (note the mnemonic):
   a. Autoimmune hepatitis
   b. Hepatitis **B**
   c. Hepatitis **C**
   d. Drugs or toxins
   e. Ethanol
   f. Fatty liver (triglyceridemia)
   g. Growths (tumors)
   h. Hemodynamic disorders (e.g., CHF)
   i. Iron (hemochromatosis), copper (Wilson's disease), or AAT deficiency

B. Alkaline phosphatase (ALK-P): Not specific to liver—also found in bone, gut, and placenta

1. ALK-P is elevated when there is obstruction to bile flow (e.g., cholestasis) in any part of the biliary tree. Normal levels make cholestasis unlikely.
2. If levels are **very high** (10-fold increase), think of extrahepatic biliary tract obstruction or intrahepatic cholestasis (e.g., PBC or drug-induced cirrhosis).
3. If levels are **elevated**, measure the GGT (Gamma-glutamyl-transferase) level to make sure the elevation is hepatic in origin (rather than bone or intestinal). If the GGT level is also elevated, this strongly suggests a hepatic origin. If the GGT level is normal but ALK-P is elevated, consider pregnancy or bone disease.

C. Bilirubin (see Jaundice section)

D. GGT is often used to confirm that the ALK-P elevation is of hepatic origin.

E. Albumin—decreased in chronic liver disease, nephrotic syndrome, malnutrition, and inflammatory states (e.g., burns, sepsis, trauma)

F. Prothrombin time (PT)
1. The liver synthesizes clotting factors I, II, V, VII, IX, X, XII, and XIII, the function of which is reflected by PT.
2. PT is not prolonged until most of the liver's synthetic capacity is lost, which corresponds to advanced liver disease.

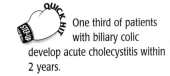

Cholestasis refers to obstruction of bile flow from any cause. If LFTs reveal cholestasis, obtain an abdominal or RUQ ultrasound.

DISEASES OF THE GALLBLADDER AND BILIARY TRACT

Cholelithiasis

A. General characteristics
1. Cholelithiasis refers to stones in the gallbladder (i.e., gallstones).
2. There are three types of stones.
   a. Cholesterol stones (yellow to green)—associated with the following:
      - Obesity, diabetes, hyperlipidemia
      - Multiple pregnancies, oral contraceptive use
      - Crohn's disease, ileal resection
      - Advanced age
      - Native American ancestry
      - Cirrhosis
      - Cystic fibrosis
   b. Pigment stones
      - Black stones are usually found in the gallbladder and are associated with either **hemolysis** (e.g., sickle cell disease, thalassemia, hereditary spherocytosis, artificial cardiac valves) or **alcoholic cirrhosis**.
      - Brown stones are usually found in bile ducts and are associated with biliary tract infection.
   c. Mixed stones have components of both cholesterol and pigment stones and account for the majority of stones.

B. Clinical features
1. Most cases are asymptomatic.
2. Biliary colic is due to temporary obstruction of cystic duct by a gallstone. Pain occurs as the gallbladder contracts against this obstruction.
   a. Pain is typically located in the RUQ or epigastrium and may be mild, moderate, or severe.
   b. Patients classically report pain after eating and at night.
   c. *Boas' sign*—referred right subscapular pain of biliary colic

One third of patients with biliary colic develop acute cholecystitis within 2 years.

C. Complications
1. Cholecystitis (chronic or acute) with prolonged obstruction of cystic duct
2. Choledocholithiasis with its associated complications—see below
3. Gallstone ileus
4. Malignancy

D. Diagnosis
1. RUQ ultrasound has high sensitivity and specificity (>95%) for stones >2 mm.
2. CT scan and MRI are alternatives.

Pain in acute cholecystitis is secondary to gallbladder wall inflammation, whereas the pain of biliary colic is secondary to the contraction of the gallbladder against the obstructed cystic duct. Also, the pain of acute cholecystitis persists for several days, whereas the pain of biliary colic lasts only a few hours.

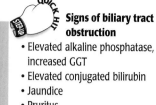

Signs of biliary tract obstruction
- Elevated alkaline phosphatase, increased GGT
- Elevated conjugated bilirubin
- Jaundice
- Pruritus
- Clay-colored stools
- Dark urine

Complications of cholecystitis
- Gangrenous cholecystitis
- Perforation of gallbladder
- Emphysematous cholecystitis
- Cholecystenteric fistula with gallstone ileus
- Empyema of gallbladder

Gallstone ileus
- Gallstone enters bowel lumen via cholecystenteric fistula–gets "stuck" in terminal ileum and causes obstruction
- Accounts for 1% to 2% of bowel obstructions

E. Treatment
1. No treatment if the patient is asymptomatic
2. Elective cholecystectomy for patients with recurrent bouts of biliary colic

Acute Cholecystitis

A. General characteristics
1. Obstruction of the cystic duct (**not** infection) induces acute inflammation of the gallbladder wall.
2. Chronic cholecystitis may develop with recurrent bouts of acute cholecystitis.
3. Ten percent of patients with gallstones develop acute cholecystitis.

B. Clinical features
1. Symptoms
   a. Pain is always present and is located in RUQ or epigastrium; it may radiate to the right shoulder or scapula.
   b. Nausea and vomiting, anorexia
2. Signs
   a. RUQ tenderness, rebound tenderness in RUQ
   b. *Murphy's sign* is pathognomonic—inspiratory arrest during deep palpation of the RUQ; not present in many cases
   c. Hypoactive bowel sounds
   d. Low-grade fever, leukocytosis

C. Diagnosis
1. RUQ ultrasound is the test of choice.
   a. High sensitivity and specificity
   b. Findings include thickened gallbladder wall, pericholecystic fluid, distended gallbladder, and presence of stone(s).
2. CT scan is as accurate as ultrasound but is more sensitive in identifying complications of acute cholecystitis (e.g., perforation, abscess, pancreatitis).
3. Radionuclide scan (hepatoiminodiacetic acid [HIDA])
   a. Used when ultrasound is inconclusive. Its sensitivity and specificity parallel that of ultrasound. If HIDA scan is normal, acute cholecystitis can be ruled out.
   b. A positive HIDA scan means the gallbladder is not visualized.
   c. If gallbladder is not visualized 4 hours after injection, diagnosis of acute cholecystitis is confirmed.

D. Treatment
1. Conservative measures: hydration with IV fluids, bowel rest (NPO), IV antibiotics, analgesics
2. Surgery—Cholecystectomy is indicated in most patients with symptomatic gallstones. Early cholecystectomy is preferred (first 24 to 48 hours).

Acalculous Cholecystitis

- Acute cholecystitis without stones obstructing the cystic duct (up to 10% of patients with acute cholecystitis)
- Usually idiopathic and seen in patients with severe underlying illness; possibly associated with dehydration, ischemia, burns, severe trauma, and a postoperative state
- Signs and symptoms are the same as for acute cholecystitis.
- Diagnosis may be difficult because patients with this condition are often severely ill and have other medical problems, so clinical features are less apparent.
- Emergent cholecystectomy is the treatment of choice. For patients who are too ill for surgery, perform percutaneous drainage of the gallbladder with cholecystostomy.

TABLE 3-2 Cholelithiasis Versus Choledocholithiasis

	Cholelithiasis	Choledocholithiasis
Abnormality	Stone in gallbladder	Stone in CBD
Clinical features	Asymptomatic; biliary colic	Asymptomatic, RUQ/epigastric pain, jaundice
Complications	Cholecystitis, choledocholithiasis, gallstone ileus, malignancy	Cholangitis, obstructive jaundice, acute pancreatitis, biliary cirrhosis
Diagnosis	RUQ ultrasound is highly sensitive	ERCP is test of choice; RUQ ultrasound is not sensitive
Treatment	No treatment in most cases; elective cholecystectomy if biliary colic is severe or recurrent	Removal of stone via ERCP and sphincterotomy

Choledocholithiasis

A. General characteristics
1. Refers to gallstones in the common bile duct (CBD)
2. Primary versus secondary stones
   a. Primary stones originate in the CBD (usually pigmented stones).
   b. Secondary stones originate in the gallbladder and then pass into the CBD (usually cholesterol or mixed stones). These account for 95% of all cases.

B. Clinical features
1. Patients may be asymptomatic for years.
2. Symptoms, when present, include RUQ or epigastric pain and jaundice.

C. Diagnosis
1. Laboratory tests: Total and direct bilirubin levels are elevated, as well as ALK-P.
2. RUQ ultrasound is usually the initial study, but is not a sensitive study for choledocholithiasis. It detects CBD in only 50% of cases, so it cannot be used to rule out this diagnosis.
3. ERCP is gold standard (sensitivity and specificity of 95%) and should follow ultrasound. ERCP is diagnostic and therapeutic (see below).
4. PTC is an alternative to ERCP.

D. Treatment
1. ERCP with sphincterotomy and stone extraction with stent placement (successful in 90% of patients)
2. Laparoscopic choledocholithotomy (in select cases)

Cholangitis

A. General characteristics
1. Infection of biliary tract secondary to obstruction, which leads to biliary stasis and bacterial overgrowth
   a. Choledocholithiasis accounts for 60% of cases.
   b. Other causes include pancreatic and biliary neoplasm, postoperative strictures, invasive procedures such as ERCP or PTC, and choledochal cysts.
2. Cholangitis is potentially life-threatening and requires emergency treatment.

B. Clinical features
1. *Charcot's triad*: RUQ pain, jaundice, and fever—this classic triad is present in only 50% to 70% of cases

Complications of CBD stones
- Cholangitis
- Obstructive jaundice
- Acute pancreatitis
- Biliary colic
- Biliary cirrhosis

Patients with CBD stones may be asymptomatic for years. However, unlike patients with cholelithiasis, in which biliary colic may lead to acute cholecystitis, the **onset of symptoms** in **choledocholithiasis** can signal the development of **life-threatening** complications such as cholangitis and acute pancreatitis.

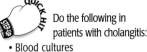

Do the following in patients with cholangitis:
- Blood cultures
- IV fluids
- IV antibiotics after blood cultures obtained
- Decompress CBD when patient stable

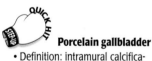

QUICK HIT

Reynolds' pentad is a highly toxic state that requires emergency treatment. **It can be rapidly fatal.**

QUICK HIT

RUQ ultrasound is very accurate in detecting gallstones and biliary tract dilatation, but not very accurate in detecting CBD stones.

QUICK HIT

Hepatic abscess is the most serious and dreaded complication of acute cholangitis—**it has a high mortality rate.**

QUICK HIT

Porcelain gallbladder
• Definition: intramural calcification of the gallbladder wall
• Prophylactic cholecystectomy is recommended because approximately 50% of patients with porcelain gallbladder will eventually develop cancer of the gallbladder.

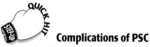

QUICK HIT

Complications of PSC
• Cholangiocarcinoma (in up to 20% to 30% of patients)
• Recurrent bouts of cholangitis (in about 15% of patients)
• Can progress to secondary biliary cirrhosis, portal HTN, and liver failure

2. *Reynolds' pentad*: Charcot's triad plus septic shock and altered mental status (CNS depression—e.g., coma, disorientation)
3. Patient is acutely ill, and abdominal symptoms may be lacking or may go unrecognized.

C. Diagnosis
1. RUQ ultrasound is the initial study.
2. Laboratory findings—hyperbilirubinemia, leukocytosis, mild elevation in serum transaminases
3. Cholangiography (PTC or ERCP)
   a. This is the definitive test, but it should not be performed during the acute phase of illness. Once cholangitis resolves, proceed with PTC or ERCP to identify the underlying problem and plan treatment.
   b. Perform PTC when the duct system is dilated (per ultrasound) and ERCP when the duct system is normal.

D. Treatment
1. IV antibiotics and IV fluids
   a. Close monitoring of hemodynamics, BP, and urine output is important.
   b. Most patients respond rapidly. Once the patient has been afebrile for 48 hours, cholangiography (PTC or ERCP) can be performed for evaluation of the underlying condition.
2. Decompress CBD via PTC (catheter drainage); ERCP (sphincterotomy), or laparotomy (T-tube insertion) once the patient is stabilized, or emergently if the condition does not respond to antibiotics.

Carcinoma of the Gallbladder

• Most are adenocarcinomas and typically occur in the elderly.
• Associated with gallstones in most cases; other risk factors include cholecystenteric fistula and porcelain gallbladder
• Clinical features are nonspecific and suggest extrahepatic bile duct obstruction: jaundice, biliary colic, weight loss, anorexia, and RUQ mass. Palpable gallbladder is a sign of advanced disease.
• Difficult to remove with surgery: cholecystectomy versus radical cholecystectomy (with wedge resection of liver and lymph node dissection) depending on depth of invasion
• Prognosis is dismal—more than 90% of patients die of advanced disease within 1 year of diagnosis. Disease often goes undetected until it is advanced.

Primary Sclerosing Cholangitis (PSC)

A. General characteristics
1. A chronic idiopathic progressive disease of intrahepatic and/or extrahepatic bile ducts characterized by thickening of bile duct walls and narrowing of their lumens; leads to cirrhosis, portal hypertension, and liver failure
2. There is a strong association with UC (less so with Crohn's disease). UC is present in 50% to 70% of patients with PSC; often the UC may dominate the clinical picture. (Note: The course of PSC is unaffected by a colectomy done for UC.)

B. Clinical features
1. Signs and symptoms begin insidiously.
2. Chronic cholestasis findings, including jaundice and pruritus; all patients eventually present with chronic obstructive jaundice
3. Other symptoms: fatigue, malaise, weight loss

C. Diagnosis
1. ERCP and PTC are diagnostic studies of choice: see multiple areas of bead-like stricturing and bead-like dilatations of intrahepatic and extrahepatic ducts.
2. Laboratory tests show cholestatic LFTs.

D. Treatment
1. There is no curative treatment other than liver transplantation.
2. When a dominant stricture causes cholestasis, ERCP with stent placement for biliary drainage and bile duct dilatation may relieve symptoms.
3. Use cholestyramine for symptomatic relief (to decrease pruritus).

Primary Biliary Cirrhosis (PBC)

A. General characteristics
1. PBC is a chronic and progressive cholestatic liver disease characterized by **destruction of intrahepatic bile ducts** with portal inflammation and scarring.
2. It is a slowly progressive disease with a variable course. It may progress to cirrhosis and end-stage liver failure.
3. It is an **autoimmune disease** that is often associated with other autoimmune disorders.
4. It is most common in **middle-aged women.**

B. Clinical features
1. Fatigue
2. Pruritus (early in course of disease)
3. Jaundice (late in course of disease)
4. RUQ discomfort
5. Xanthomata and xanthelasmata
6. Osteoporosis
7. Portal HTN (with resultant sequelae)

C. Diagnosis
1. Laboratory findings
   a. Cholestatic LFTs (elevated ALK-P)
   b. **Positive antimitochondrial antibodies (AMAs) found in 90% to 95% of patients.** This is the hallmark of the disease (specificity of 98%). If serum is positive for AMAs, perform a liver biopsy to confirm diagnosis.
   c. Elevated cholesterol, HDL
   d. Elevated immunoglobulin M
2. Liver biopsy (percutaneous or laparoscopic) to confirm the diagnosis
3. Abdominal ultrasound or CT scan to rule out biliary obstruction

D. Treatment
1. Treatment is symptomatic for pruritus (cholestyramine) and osteoporosis (calcium, bisphosphonates, vitamin D).
2. Ursodeoxycholic acid (a hydrophilic bile acid) has been shown to slow progression of the disease.
3. Liver transplantation is the only curative treatment available.

Cholangiocarcinoma

A. General characteristics
1. Tumor of intrahepatic or extrahepatic bile ducts: most are adenocarcinomas
2. Mean age of diagnosis is in the seventh decade
3. Located in three regions: proximal third of the CBD (most common, also called Klatskin's tumor), distal extrahepatic (best chance of resectability), intrahepatic (least common)
4. Prognosis is dismal—survival is less than 1 year after diagnosis
5. Risk factors
   a. PSC is the major risk factor in the United States.
   b. Other risk factors include UC, choledochal cysts, and *Clonorchis sinensis* infestation (in Hong Kong).

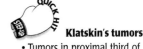

Etiology of secondary biliary cirrhosis. This disease occurs in response to chronic biliary obstruction from the following:
- Long-standing mechanical obstruction
- Sclerosing cholangitis
- Cystic fibrosis
- Biliary atresia

Klatskin's tumors
- Tumors in proximal third of CBD—involve the junction of right and left hepatic ducts
- Very poor prognosis because they are unresectable

B. Clinical features

1. Obstructive jaundice and associated symptoms: dark urine, clay-colored stools, and pruritus
2. Weight loss

C. Diagnosis

1. Cholangiography (PTC or ERCP) for diagnosis and assessment of resectability
2. If the patient has an unresectable tumor (more likely the case with proximal than distal bile duct tumors), stent placement is an option during either PTC or ERCP and may relieve biliary obstruction.

D. Treatment

1. Most patients do not have resectable tumors at diagnosis.
2. The survival rate is low despite aggressive chemotherapy, stenting, or biliary drainage.

Choledochal Cysts

- Cystic dilatations of biliary tree involving either the extrahepatic or intrahepatic ducts, or both; more common in women (4:1)
- Clinical features: epigastric pain, jaundice, fever, and RUQ mass
- Complications: cholangiocarcinoma (most feared complication—risk is about 20% over 20 years), hepatic abscess, recurrent cholangitis/pancreatitis, rupture, biliary obstruction, cirrhosis, and portal HTN
- Ultrasound is the best noninvasive test, and ERCP is definitive for diagnosis.
- Treatment is surgery: complete resection of the cyst with a biliary-enteric anastomosis to restore continuity of biliary system with bowels

Bile Duct Stricture

- Most common cause is iatrogenic injury (e.g., prior biliary surgery such as cholecystectomy, liver transplantation); other causes include recurring choledocholithiasis, chronic pancreatitis, and PSC.
- Clinical features are those of obstructive jaundice.
- Complications can be life-threatening: secondary biliary cirrhosis, liver abscess, and ascending cholangitis.
- Treatment involves endoscopic stenting (preferred), or surgical bypass if obstruction is complete or if endoscopic therapy fails.

Biliary Dyskinesia

- Motor dysfunction of the sphincter of Oddi, which leads to recurrent episodes of biliary colic without any evidence of gallstones on diagnostic studies such as ultrasound, CT scan, and ERCP
- Diagnosis is made by HIDA scan. Once the gallbladder is filled with labeled radionuclide, give cholecystokinin (CCK) intravenously, then determine the ejection fraction of the gallbladder. If the ejection fraction is low, dyskinesia is likely.
- Treatment options include laparoscopic cholecystectomy and endoscopic sphincterotomy.

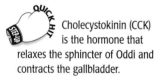
Cholecystokinin (CCK) is the hormone that relaxes the sphincter of Oddi and contracts the gallbladder.

DISEASES OF THE APPENDIX

Acute Appendicitis

A. General characteristics

1. Pathogenesis
   a. The lumen of the appendix is obstructed by hyperplasia of lymphoid tissue (60% of cases), a fecalith (35% of cases), a foreign body, or other rare causes (parasite or carcinoid tumor [5% of cases]).

b. Obstruction leads to stasis (of fluid and mucus), which promotes bacterial growth, leading to inflammation.

c. Distention of the appendix can compromise blood supply. The resulting ischemia can lead to infarction or necrosis if untreated. Necrosis can result in appendiceal perforation, and ultimately peritonitis.

2. Peak incidence is in the teens to mid-20s. Prognosis is far worse in infants and elderly patients (higher rate of perforation).

B. Clinical features

1. Symptoms
    a. Abdominal pain—Classically starts in the epigastrium, moves toward umbilicus, and then to the RLQ. With distention of the appendix, the parietal peritoneum may become irritated, leading to sharp pain.
    b. Anorexia always present. Appendicitis is unlikely if patient is hungry.
    c. Nausea and vomiting (typically follow pain)

2. Signs
    a. Tenderness in RLQ (maximal tenderness at *McBurney's point*: two thirds of the distance from the umbilicus to the right anterior superior iliac spine)
    b. Rebound tenderness, guarding, diminished bowel sounds
    c. Low-grade fever (may spike if perforation occurs)
    d. *Rovsing's sign*: Deep palpation in LLQ causes referred pain in RLQ
    e. *Psoas sign*: RLQ pain when right thigh is extended as patient lies on left side
    f. *Obturator sign*: Pain in RLQ when flexed right thigh is internally rotated when patient is supine

C. Diagnosis

1. Acute appendicitis is a clinical diagnosis.
2. Laboratory findings (mild leukocytosis) are only supportive.
3. Imaging studies may be helpful if diagnosis uncertain or in atypical presentations.
    a. CT scan (sensitivity 98% to 100%)—lowers the false-positive rate significantly
    b. Ultrasound (sensitivity of 90%)

D. Treatment is an appendectomy (usually laparoscopic). Up to 20% of patients who are diagnosed with acute appendicitis are found to have a normal appendix during surgery. Because the illness is potentially life-threatening, this is an acceptable risk even during pregnancy.

Carcinoid Tumors and Carcinoid Syndrome

- Carcinoid tumors originate from **neuroendocrine cells** and secrete **serotonin**.
- The most common site for these tumors is the appendix, but they can be found in a variety of locations (e.g., small bowel, rectum, bronchus, kidney, pancreas).

DISEASES OF THE PANCREAS

Acute Pancreatitis

A. General characteristics

1. There is inflammation of the pancreas resulting from prematurely activated pancreatic digestive enzymes that invoke pancreatic tissue autodigestion.
2. Most patients with acute pancreatitis have mild to moderate disease, but up to 25% have severe disease.

B. Causes

1. Alcohol abuse (40%)
2. Gallstones (40%)—The gallstone passes into the bile duct and blocks the ampulla of Vater.

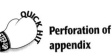

Perforation of appendix
- Complicates 20% of cases
- Risk factors: delay in treatment (>24 hours) and extremes of age
- Signs of appendiceal rupture (high fever, tachycardia, marked leukocytosis, peritoneal signs, toxic appearance)

Acute appendicitis is a clinical diagnosis. Laboratory findings (mild leukocytosis) are only supportive. Radiographs or other imaging studies are unnecessary unless the diagnosis is uncertain or the presentation is atypical.

Carcinoid syndrome develops in 10% of patients with carcinoid tumors.
- Excess serotonin secretion can lead to **carcinoid syndrome,** which is manifested by cutaneous flushing, diarrhea, sweating, wheezing, abdominal pain, and heart valve dysfunction.
- Risk factors of metastasis increase with the size of the tumor. Metastases are rare with appendiceal tumors. Ileal tumors have the greatest likelihood of malignancy.
- Surgical resection is the treatment of choice.

D I S E A S E S   O F   T H E   G A S T R O I N T E S T I N A L   S Y S T E M

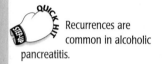

Most cases of acute pancreatitis are due to alcohol or gallstones (70% to 80%).

Recurrences are common in alcoholic pancreatitis.

The diagnosis of acute pancreatitis is usually made based on clinical presentation. Laboratory studies are supportive, and CT scan is confirmatory.

The level of either amylase or lipase does not reliably predict the severity of disease.

Hypocalcemia that results from acute pancreatitis is due to fat saponification: fat necrosis binds calcium.

3. Post-ERCP—Pancreatitis occurs in up to 10% of patients undergoing ERCP.
4. Viral infections (e.g., mumps, Coxsackievirus B)
5. Drugs: Sulfonamides, thiazide diuretics, furosemide, estrogens, HIV medications and many other drugs have been implicated.
6. Postoperative complications (high mortality rate)
7. Scorpion bites
8. Pancreas divisum (controversial)
9. Pancreatic cancer
10. Hypertriglyceridemia, hypercalcemia
11. Uremia
12. Blunt abdominal trauma (most common cause of pancreatitis in children)

C. Clinical features

1. Symptoms
   a. Abdominal pain, usually in the epigastric region
      • May radiate to back (50% of patients)
      • Often steady, dull, and severe; worse when supine and after meals
   b. Nausea and vomiting, anorexia
2. Signs
   a. Low-grade fever, tachycardia, hypotension, leukocytosis
   b. Epigastric tenderness, abdominal distention
   c. Decreased or absent bowel sounds indicate partial ileus.
   d. The following signs are seen with hemorrhagic pancreatitis as blood tracks along fascial planes:
      • *Grey Turner's sign* (flank ecchymoses)
      • *Cullen's sign* (periumbilical ecchymoses)
      • *Fox's sign* (ecchymosis of inguinal ligament)

D. Diagnosis

1. Laboratory studies
   a. Serum amylase is the most common test, but many conditions cause hyperamylasemia (nonspecific) and its absence does not rule out acute pancreatitis (nonsensitive). However, if levels are more than five times the upper limit of normal, there is a high specificity for acute pancreatitis.
   b. Serum lipase—more specific for pancreatitis than amylase
   c. LFTs—to identify cause (gallstone pancreatitis)
   d. Hyperglycemia, hypoxemia, and leukocytosis may also be present.
   e. Order the following for assessment of prognosis (see Table 3-3—Ranson's criteria): glucose, calcium, hematocrit, BUN, arterial blood gas (Pao$_2$, base deficit), LDH, AST, WBC count.
2. Abdominal radiograph
   a. Has a limited role in the diagnosis of acute pancreatitis.
   b. More helpful in ruling out other diagnoses, such as intestinal perforation (free air). The presence of calcifications can suggest chronic pancreatitis.
   c. In some cases one may see a sentinel loop (area of air-filled bowel usually in LUQ, which is a sign of localized ileus) or a colon cut-off sign (air-filled segment of transverse colon abruptly ending or "cutting off" at the region of pancreatic inflammation).
3. Abdominal ultrasound
   a. Can help in identifying cause of pancreatitis (e.g., gallstones)
   b. Useful for following up pseudocysts or abscesses
4. CT scan of the abdomen
   a. Most accurate test for diagnosis of acute pancreatitis and for identifying complications of the disease
   b. Indicated in patients with severe acute pancreatitis
5. ERCP (indications):
   a. Severe gallstone pancreatitis with biliary obstruction
   b. To identify uncommon causes of acute pancreatitis if disease is recurrent

E. Complications

1. Pancreatic necrosis (may be sterile or infected)
   a. Sterile pancreatic necrosis—Infection may develop, but half of all cases resolve spontaneously.
   b. Infected pancreatic necrosis—has high mortality rate (results in multiple organ failure in 50% of cases); surgical débridement and antibiotics indicated
   c. The only way to distinguish sterile from infected necrosis is via CT-guided percutaneous aspiration with Gram stain/culture of the aspirate.
2. Pancreatic pseudocyst
   a. Encapsulated fluid collection that appears 2 to 3 weeks after an acute attack—unlike a true cyst, it lacks an epithelial lining
   b. Complications of untreated pseudocysts include rupture, infection, gastric outlet obstruction, fistula, hemorrhage into cyst, and pancreatic ascites. It may impinge on adjacent abdominal organs (e.g., duodenum, stomach, transverse colon) if large enough; or if located in the head of the pancreas, it may cause compression of the CBD.
   c. Diagnosis: CT scan is the study of choice.
   d. Treatment
      • Cysts <5 cm: observation
      • Cysts >5 cm: drain either percutaneously or surgically
3. Hemorrhagic pancreatitis
   a. Characterized by Cullen's sign, Grey Turner's sign, and Fox's sign
   b. CT scan with IV contrast is the study of choice.
4. Adult respiratory distress syndrome—a life-threatening complication with high mortality rate
5. Pancreatic ascites/pleural effusion—The most common cause is inflammation of peritoneal surfaces.
6. Ascending cholangitis—due to gallstone in ampulla of Vater, leading to infection of biliary tract; see section on cholangitis
7. Pancreatic abscess (rare)—develops over 4 to 6 weeks and is less life-threatening than infected pancreatic necrosis

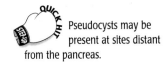

QUICK HIT
Pseudocysts may be present at sites distant from the pancreas.

F. Treatment

1. Bowel rest (NPO)—goal is to rest the pancreas
2. IV fluids—Patients may have severe intravascular volume depletion.
3. Pain control, but be cautious in giving narcotics.
4. Nasogastric tube if severe nausea/vomiting or ileus present; routine use is controversial

G. Prognosis

1. Ranson's criteria are used to determine prognosis and mortality rates.
2. Patients with more than three or four Ranson's criteria should be monitored in an ICU setting.

TABLE 3-3 Ranson's Criteria

Admission Criteria (GA LAW)	Initial 48 Hours Criteria (C HOBBS)	Mortality
Glucose >200 mg/dL	**C**alcium <8 mg/dL Decrease in **H**ematocrit >10%	<3 criteria—1%
Age >55 years	Pao$_2$ <60 mm Hg	3–4 criteria—15%
LDH >350	**B**UN increase >8 mg/dL	5–6 criteria—40%
AST >250	**B**ase deficit >4 mg/dL	>7 criteria—100%
WBC >16,000	Fluid **s**equestration >6 L	

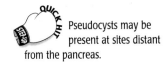

DISEASES OF THE GASTROINTESTINAL SYSTEM

The combination of chronic epigastric pain and calcifications on plain abdominal films is diagnostic for chronic pancreatitis. The classic triad of steatorrhea, diabetes mellitus, and pancreatic calcification on plain films or CT scan is also diagnostic.

Chronic Pancreatitis

A. General characteristics

1. Persistent or continuing inflammation of the pancreas, with fibrotic tissue replacing pancreatic parenchyma, and alteration of pancreatic ducts (areas of stricture/dilation); eventually results in irreversible destruction of the pancreas
2. The endocrine and exocrine functions of the pancreas are impaired.
3. Causes
   a. **Chronic alcoholism is the most common cause (>80% of cases).**
   b. Other causes include hereditary pancreatitis, tropical pancreatitis, and idiopathic chronic pancreatitis.

B. Clinical features

1. Severe pain in the epigastrium; recurrent or persistent abdominal pain
   a. Often accompanied by **nausea and vomiting**
   b. May be aggravated by a drinking episode, or by eating
   c. Radiates to the back (in 50% of cases)
2. Weight loss, due to malabsorption, alcohol abuse, and diabetes; steatorrhea secondary to malabsorption

C. Diagnosis

1. CT scan (see Figure 3-2) is the initial study of choice. It may show calcifications not seen on plain films. Mild to moderate cases may not be detectable, so a normal CT scan does not necessarily rule out chronic pancreatitis.
2. Abdominal radiograph: The presence of pancreatic calcifications is 95% specific, but is found in only 30% of cases.
3. ERCP is gold standard, but is not done routinely because it is invasive.
4. Laboratory studies are not helpful in diagnosis. Serum amylase and lipase levels are not elevated in chronic pancreatitis.

D. Complications

1. Narcotic addiction—probably the most common complication
2. Diabetes mellitus/impaired glucose tolerance
   a. Caused by progressive loss of islets of Langerhans
   b. Eventually appears in up to 70% of patients
3. Malabsorption/steatorrhea
   a. Caused by pancreatic exocrine insufficiency—occurs when pancreatic enzyme secretion decreases significantly
   b. A late manifestation of chronic pancreatitis
4. Pseudocyst formation
5. Pancreatic ductal dilation
6. CBD obstruction (may occur secondary to fibrosis in head of gland)
7. Vitamin B_{12} malabsorption
8. Effusions (e.g., pleural, pericardial, peritoneal)
9. Pancreatic carcinoma—Patients with chronic pancreatitis have an increased risk.

E. Treatment

1. Nonoperative management
   a. Narcotic analgesics for pain
   b. Bowel rest (NPO)
   c. Pancreatic enzymes and H_2 blockers (give simultaneously)
      • Pancreatic enzymes inhibit CCK release and thus decrease pancreatic secretions after meals.
      • H_2 blockers inhibit gastric acid secretion, preventing degradation of the pancreatic enzyme supplements by gastric acid.
   d. Insulin—may be necessary due to severe pancreatic endocrine insufficiency
   e. Alcohol abstinence
   f. Frequent, small-volume, low-fat meals—may improve abdominal pain

FIGURE
3-2 — A. CT scan of chronic pancreatitis. Note the area of calcification (small arrow) and a pseudocyst (large arrow) in the head of the pancreas. B. Typical findings on ERCP in chronic pancreatitis. Note the areas of stricture (large arrow) and duct dilatation (small arrow) throughout the pancreatic duct. This creates a "chain of lakes" appearance.

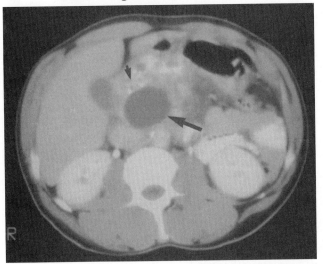

A

B

(From Humes DH, DuPont HL, Gardner LB, et al. Kelley's Textbook of Internal Medicine. 4th Ed. Philadelphia: Lippincott Williams & Wilkins, 2000:958, Figures 117.9 and 117.10, respectively.)

2. Surgery—main goal is relief of incapacitating abdominal pain
   a. Pancreaticojejunostomy (pancreatic duct drainage procedure to decompress the dilated pancreatic duct)—most common procedure
   b. Pancreatic resection (distal pancreatectomy, Whipple's procedure)

Pancreatic Cancer

A. General characteristics

1. Most common in elderly patients (75% of patients are >60 years old); rare before age 40; more common in African Americans
2. Anatomic location
   a. Pancreatic head (75% of cases)
   b. Pancreatic body (20% of cases)
   c. Pancreatic tail (5% to 10% of cases)

3. Risk factors
   a. **Cigarette smoking** (most clearly established risk)
   b. Chronic pancreatitis
   c. Diabetes
   d. Heavy alcohol use
   e. Exposure to chemicals—benzidine and β-naphthylamine
4. The prognosis is dismal: most patients die within months of diagnosis.

B. Clinical features
1. Abdominal pain (90% of patients)—may be a vague and dull ache
2. Jaundice
   a. Most common with carcinoma of head of pancreas—less than 10% of patients with cancer involving body and tail of pancreas have jaundice
   b. Indicates obstruction of intrapancreatic CBD and is a sign of advanced disease
3. Weight loss (common due to decreased food intake and malabsorption); anorexia
4. Recent onset of glucose intolerance, but the diabetes is mild
5. Depression, weakness, fatigue
6. Migratory thrombophlebitis—develops in 10% of cases
7. *Courvoisier's sign* (palpable gallbladder)—present in 30% of patients with cancer involving head of pancreas; presents without pain

C. Diagnosis
1. ERCP is the most sensitive test for diagnosing pancreatic cancer. It can also distinguish cancer of the head of the pancreas from tumors of the CBD, duodenum, ampulla, and lymphomas, which have a more favorable prognosis.
2. CT scan is the preferred test for diagnosis and assessment of disease spread.
3. Tumor markers
   a. CA 19-9 (sensitivity of 83% and specificity of 82%)
   b. CEA (sensitivity of 56% and specificity of 75%)

D. Treatment
1. Surgical resection (Whipple's procedure) is the only hope for a cure; however, only a minority of tumors are resectable (roughly 10%). **The prognosis is grim even after resection, with a 5-year survival rate of 10%.**
2. If the tumor is unresectable and biliary obstruction is present, perform PTC or ERCP with stent placement across the obstruction for palliation.

GASTROINTESTINAL BLEEDING

A. General characteristics
1. Upper GI bleeding refers to a source of bleeding above the ligament of Treitz in the duodenum.
2. Lower GI bleeding is classically defined as bleeding below the ligament of Treitz.

B. Causes
1. Upper GI bleeding
   a. PUD—duodenal ulcer (25% of cases), gastric ulcer (20% of cases), gastritis (25% of cases)
   b. Reflux esophagitis
   c. Esophageal varices (10% of cases)—venous bleeding
   d. Gastric varices
   e. Gastric erosions, duodenitis
   f. Mallory-Weiss tear
   g. Hemobilia
   h. Dieulafoy's vascular malformation—submucosal dilated arterial lesions that can cause massive GI bleeding

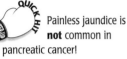

Painless jaundice is **not** common in pancreatic cancer!

The early clinical findings of pancreatic cancer are very vague and nonspecific. By the time a diagnosis is made, most patients have an incurable level of advanced disease.

Aortoenteric fistula is a rare but lethal cause of GI bleeding. The classic presentation is a patient with a history (sometimes distant) of aortic graft surgery who has a small GI bleed involving the duodenum before massive, fatal hemorrhage hours to weeks later. Perform endoscopy or surgery during this small window of opportunity to prevent death.

> **Box 3-7 Tests to Order in Patients With GI Bleeding**
>
> - Hematemesis—An upper GI endoscopy is the initial test.
> - Hematochezia—First rule out an anorectal cause (e.g., hemorrhoids). Colonoscopy should be the initial test because colon cancer is the main concern in patients over age 50.
> - Melena—Upper endoscopy is usually the initial test because the most likely bleeding site is in the upper GI tract. Order a colonoscopy if no bleeding site is identified from the endoscopy.
> - Occult blood—Colonoscopy is the initial test in most cases (colon cancer is the main concern). Order an upper endoscopy if no bleeding site is identified from the colonoscopy.

     i. Aortoenteric fistulas—after aortic surgery (ask about prior aortic aneurysm/graft)

     j. Neoplasm—bleeding is not rapid—usually not an emergency

  2. Lower GI bleeding

     a. Diverticulosis (40% of cases)—most common source of GI bleeding in patients under age 60; usually painless

     b. Angiodysplasia (40% of cases)—most common source in patients over age 60

     c. IBD (UC, Crohn's disease)

     d. Colorectal carcinoma

     e. Colorectal adenomatous polyps

     f. Ischemic colitis

     g. Hemorrhoids, anal fissures

     h. Small intestinal bleeding—diagnosed by excluding upper GI and colonic bleeding

 A lower GI bleed (or positive occult blood test of stool) in patients over 40 is colon cancer until proven otherwise. ·

C. Clinical features

  1. Type of bleeding:

     a. Hematemesis—vomiting blood; suggests upper GI bleeding

     b. "Coffee grounds" emesis—suggests upper GI bleeding as well as a **lower rate of bleeding** (enough time for vomitus to transform into "coffee grounds")

     c. Melena—black, tarry, liquid, foul-smelling stool

       • Caused by degradation of hemoglobin by bacteria in the colon; presence of melena indicates that blood has remained in GI tract for several hours

       • The further the bleeding site is from the rectum, the more likely melena will occur.

       • **Note that dark stools can also result from bismuth, iron, spinach, charcoal, and licorice.**

       • Melena suggests upper GI bleeding (esophagus, stomach or duodenum). Occasionally, the jejunum or ileum is the source. It is unusual for melena to be caused by a colonic lesion, but if it is, the ascending colon is the most likely site.

     d. Hematochezia—bright red blood per rectum

       • This usually represents a lower GI source (typically **left colon** or **rectum**). Consider diverticulosis, arteriovenous malformations, hemorrhoids, and colon cancers.

 About 80% of episodes of upper GI bleeding stop spontaneously and only need supportive therapy.

• Bleeding from the small bowel may manifest as melena or hematochezia.
• Colonic sources of bleeding present with either occult blood in the stool or hematochezia.

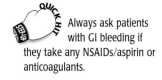 Always ask patients with GI bleeding if they take any NSAIDs/aspirin or anticoagulants.

> **Box 3-8 Factors That Increase Mortality in GI Bleeding**
>
> - Age >65 years
> - Severity of initial bleed
> - Extensive comorbid illnesses
> - Onset or recurrence of bleeding while hospitalized for another condition
> - Need for emergency surgery
> - Significant transfusion requirements
> - Diagnosis (esophageal varices have a 30% mortality rate)
> - Endoscopic stigmata of recent hemorrhage

Hematemesis and melena are the most common presentations of acute upper GI bleed, and patients may have both symptoms. Occasionally, a brisk upper GI bleed presents as hematochezia.

An elevated PT may be indicative of liver dysfunction, vitamin K deficiency, a consumptive coagulopathy, or warfarin therapy.

If you suspect lower GI bleeding, still exclude upper GI bleeding before attempting to localize the site of the lower GI bleed.

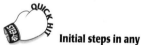

Initial steps in any patient with GI bleeding
- Vital signs: Decreased BP, tachycardia, or postural changes in BP or HR are signs of significant hemorrhage. However, vital signs may also be normal when significant hemorrhage is present.
- Resuscitation is the first step (e.g., IV fluids, transfusion).
- Perform rectal examination (Hemoccult test).

- It may result from an upper GI source that is bleeding very briskly (so that blood does not remain in colon to turn into melena—see above). This often indicates heavy bleeding, and patient often has some degree of hemodynamic instability. An upper GI source is present in about 5% to 10% of patients with hematochezia.
  e. Occult blood in stool—source of bleeding may be anywhere along GI tract
2. Signs of volume depletion (depending on rate and severity of blood loss)
3. Symptoms and signs of anemia (e.g., fatigue, pallor, exertional dyspnea)

D. Diagnosis
1. Laboratory tests
   a. Stool guaiac for occult blood
   b. Hemoglobin/hematocrit level (may not be decreased in acute bleeds): A hemoglobin level >7 to 8 g/dL is generally acceptable in young, healthy patients without active bleeding. However, most elderly patients (especially those with cardiac disease) should have a hemoglobin level >10 g/dL.
   c. A low mean corpuscular volume is suggestive of iron deficiency anemia (chronic blood loss).
   d. Coagulation profile (platelet count, PT, PTT, INR)
   e. LFTs, renal function
   f. The BUN–creatinine ratio is elevated with upper GI bleeding. This is suggestive of upper GI bleeding if patient has no renal insufficiency.
2. Upper endoscopy
   a. Most accurate diagnostic test in evaluation of upper GI bleeding
   b. Both diagnostic and potentially therapeutic (coagulate bleeding vessel)
3. Nasogastric tube
   a. This is often the initial procedure for determining whether GI bleeding is from an upper or lower GI source.
   b. Use the nasogastric tube to empty the stomach to prevent aspiration.
   c. False-negative findings are possible if upper GI bleeding is intermittent or from a lesion in the duodenum.
   d. Evaluation of aspirate
      - Bile but no blood—upper GI bleeding unlikely; source is probably distal to ligament of Treitz
      - Bright red blood or "coffee grounds" appearance—upper GI bleeding
      - Nonbloody aspirate (clear gastric fluid)—upper GI bleeding unlikely, but cannot be ruled out definitively (source may possibly be in the duodenum)
4. Anoscopy or proctosigmoidoscopy can exclude an anal/rectal source. Perform this if there is no obvious bleeding from hemorrhoids.
5. Colonoscopy identifies the site of the lower GI bleed in >70% of cases, and can also be therapeutic (see below).
6. A bleeding scan (radionuclide scanning) reveals bleeding even with a low rate of blood loss. It does not localize the lesion; it only identifies continued bleeding. Its role is controversial, but it may help determine whether arteriography is needed.
7. Arteriography definitively locates the point of bleeding.
   a. Mostly used in patients with lower GI bleeding
   b. Should be performed during active bleeding
   c. Potentially therapeutic (embolization or intra-arterial vasopressin infusion)
8. Exploratory laparotomy—last resort

E. Treatment
1. If patient is hemodynamically unstable, resuscitation is always top priority. Remember the ABCs. Once the patient is stabilized, obtain a diagnosis.
   a. Supplemental oxygen

b. Place two large-bore IV lines. Give IV fluids or blood if patient is volume depleted.

c. Draw blood for hemoglobin and hematocrit, PT, PTT, and platelet count. Monitor hemoglobin every 4 to 8 hours until the patient is hemoglobin stable for at least 24 hours.

d. Type and crossmatch adequate blood (PRBCs). Transfuse as the clinical condition demands (e.g., shock, patients with cardiopulmonary disease).

2. Treatment depends on the cause/source of the bleed.

a. Upper GI bleeding
   - EGD with coagulation of the bleeding vessel. If bleeding continues, repeat endoscopic therapy or proceed with surgical intervention (ligation of bleeding vessel).

b. Lower GI bleeding
   - Colonoscopy—polyp excision, injection, laser, cautery
   - Arteriographic vasoconstrictor infusion
   - Surgical resection of involved area—last resort

3. Indications for surgery

a. Hemodynamically unstable patients who have not responded to IV fluid, transfusion, endoscopic intervention, or correction of coagulopathies

b. Severe initial bleed or recurrence of bleed after endoscopic treatment

c. Continued bleeding for more than 24 hours

d. Visible vessel at base of ulcer (30% to 50% chance of rebleed)

e. Ongoing transfusion requirement (5 units within first 4 to 6 hours)

FIGURE 3-3 Evaluation of occult GI bleeding

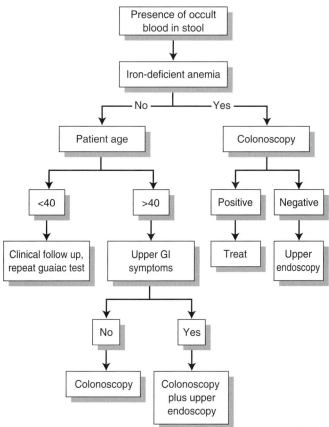

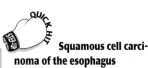

Squamous cell carcinoma of the esophagus
- Twenty percent survival rate at 1 year
- Five percent to 10% survival rate at 5 years

Barrett's esophagus is a complication of longstanding acid reflux disease in which there is columnar metaplasia of the squamous epithelium. Patients with Barrett's esophagus are at increased risk of developing adenocarcinoma of the esophagus.

DISEASES OF THE ESOPHAGUS

Esophageal Cancer

A. General characteristics

1. There are two pathologic types. In the past, squamous cell carcinoma (SCC) accounted for up to 90% of cases. However, the incidence of adenocarcinoma has increased dramatically in United States, and it now accounts for up to 50% of new cases.
   a. Squamous cell carcinoma (SCC)
      - Incidence is higher in African American men than in other groups.
      - Most common locations are the upper-thoracic and mid-thoracic esophagus. About one-third may be in distal 10 cm of esophagus.
      - Risk factors are **alcohol and tobacco use**, diet (nitrosamines, betel nuts, chronic ingestion of hot foods and beverages such as tea), human papillomavirus, achalasia, Plummer-Vinson syndrome, caustic ingestion, and nasopharyngeal carcinoma.
   b. Adenocarcinoma
      - More common in Caucasians and men (5:1 over women)
      - Most common in distal third of the esophagus/gastroesophageal junction (in 80% of cases)
      - Risk factors: **GERD and Barrett's esophagus** are main risk factors; alcohol and tobacco may not be as important as in SCC
2. **The prognosis is very poor:** 5-year survival rate is about 5% to 15% for both types.
3. Staging
   a. Stage I—tumor invades lamina propria or submucosa; nodes negative
   b. Stage IIa—tumor invades muscularis propria or adventitia; nodes negative
   c. Stage IIb—tumor invades up to muscularis propria; positive regional nodes
   d. Stage III—tumor invades adventitia (positive regional nodes) **or** tumor invades adjacent structures (positive or negative nodes)
   e. Stage IV—distant metastasis

B. Clinical features

1. Dysphagia—most common symptom (initially solids only, then progression to liquids)
2. Weight loss—second most common symptom
3. Anorexia
4. Odynophagia (pain with swallowing)—a late finding that suggests extraesophageal involvement (mediastinal invasion)
5. Hematemesis, hoarseness of voice (recurrent laryngeal nerve involvement)
6. Aspiration pneumonia, respiratory symptoms due to involvement of tracheobronchial tree
7. Tracheoesophageal or bronchoesophageal fistula
8. Chest pain

C. Diagnosis

1. Barium swallow useful in evaluation of dysphagia. A presumptive diagnosis can be made.
2. Upper endoscopy with biopsy and brush cytology is required for definitive diagnosis. It confirms the diagnosis in 95% of cases.
3. Transesophageal ultrasound helps determine the depth of penetration of the tumor and is the most reliable test for staging local cancer.
4. Full metastatic workup (e.g., CT scan of chest/abdomen, CXR, bone scan)

D. Treatment

1. Palliation is the goal in most patients because the disease is usually advanced at presentation.
2. Surgery (esophagectomy) may be curative for patients with disease in stage 0, 1, or 2A.

3. Chemotherapy plus radiation before surgery has been shown to prolong survival more than surgery alone.

Achalasia

A. General characteristics
1. Acquired motor disorder of esophageal smooth muscle in which the lower esophageal sphincter (LES) fails to completely relax with swallowing, and abnormal peristalsis of esophageal body replaces normal peristalsis of the esophageal body
2. Absolute criteria for diagnosis
   a. Incomplete relaxation of the LES
   b. Aperistalsis of esophagus

B. Causes
1. The majority in the United States are idiopathic.
2. In the United States, adenocarcinoma of proximal stomach is second most common cause.
3. Worldwide, Chagas' disease is an important cause

C. Clinical features
1. Dysphagia (odynophagia is less common)
   a. Equal difficulty swallowing solids and liquids (in contrast to esophageal cancer, in which dysphagia for solids is greater than for liquids)
   b. Patients tend to eat slowly and drink lots of water to wash down food. Also, they may twist their body, extend their neck, or walk about the room in an effort to force food into the stomach.
   c. It is exacerbated by fast eating and by emotional stress.
2. Regurgitation
   a. Food gets "stuck" in the esophagus and then comes back up.
   b. Regurgitation may lead to aspiration.
3. Chest pain
4. Weight loss
5. Recurrent pulmonary complications secondary to aspiration, which may cause lung abscess, bronchiectasis, or hemoptysis

D. Diagnosis
1. Barium swallow (see Figure 3-4)—"bird's beak"—beak-like narrowing of distal esophagus and a large, dilated esophagus proximal to the narrowing
2. Upper GI endoscopy—to rule out secondary causes of achalasia (gastric carcinoma) and retention esophagitis or esophageal cancer
3. Manometry—to confirm the diagnosis; reveals failure of LES relaxation and aperistalsis of esophageal body

E. Treatment
1. Instruct patient on adaptive measures: chew food to consistency of pea soup before swallowing; sleep with trunk elevated; avoid eating before sleep.
2. Medical therapy
   a. Antimuscarinic agents (dicyclomine)—usually unsatisfactory
   b. Sublingual nitroglycerin, long-acting nitrates, and calcium channel blockers
      • May improve swallowing in early stages of achalasia (before esophageal dilatation occurs)
      • Most useful in the short-term treatment of achalasia (before more definitive therapy)
3. Injection of botulinum toxin into the LES during endoscopy
   a. Blocks cholinergic activity in the LES
   b. Can be effective in up to 65% of cases; however, repeat procedure needs to be performed every 2 years

QUICK HIT

Patients with achalasia have a sevenfold increase in the risk of esophageal cancer (usually squamous cell)—it occurs in 10% of patients 15 to 25 years after the initial achalasia diagnosis. Often tumors go unnoticed (even when large) due to a dilated esophagus and chronic dysphagia. Therefore, perform surveillance esophagoscopy to detect the tumor at an early stage.

Next
When motility disorder is detected by barium studies do endoscopy to exclude mechanical causes of dysphagia like stricture or esophageal cancer.

QUICK HIT

There is no cure for achalasia. Treatment modalities (including surgery) are only palliative.

DISEASES OF THE GASTROINTESTINAL SYSTEM

FIGURE
3-4   Radiographs of achalasia (A) and diffuse esophageal spasm (B).

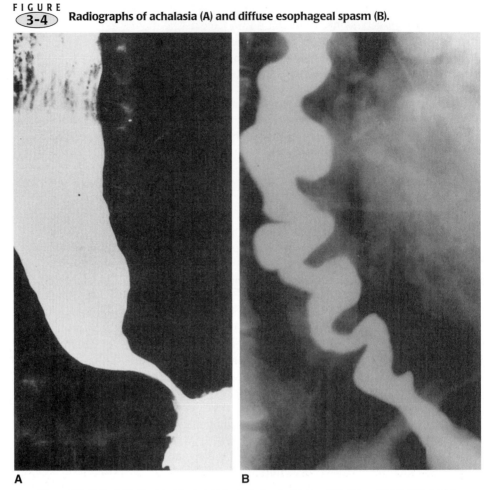

A   **B**

(From Humes DH, DuPont HL, Gardner LB, et al. Kelley's Textbook of Internal Medicine. 4th Ed. Philadelphia: Lippincott Williams & Wilkins, 2000:821, Figure 106.4.)

   4. Forceful dilatation—mechanical, pneumatic, or hydrostatic
      a. Pneumatic balloon dilatation is most effective.
      b. Lowers basal LES tone by disrupting the muscular ring
      c. Can be effective, but there is a 5% risk of perforation
   5. Surgical
      a. "Heller myotomy"—circular muscle layer of LES is incised
      b. Usually reserved for patients who do not respond to dilation therapy
   6. Early results are promising (80% to 90% of patients experience good to excellent palliation of dysphagia at 1 year).
   7. Long-term data are needed.

Diffuse Esophageal Spasm (DES)

A. General characteristics
   1. Nonperistaltic spontaneous contraction of the esophageal body—Several segments of the esophagus contract simultaneously and prevent appropriate advancement of food bolus.
   2. In contrast to achalasia, **sphincter function is normal** (normal LES pressure).

B. Clinical features
   1. There is **noncardiac chest pain** that mimics angina and may radiate to the jaw, arms, and back.
   2. Dysphagia is common; however, regurgitation of food is uncommon.

It can be difficult to distinguish the chest pain of diffuse esophageal spasm from cardiac chest pain. Therefore, many patients undergo a cardiac workup, including cardiac catheterization to rule out ischemic causes of chest pain, before an esophageal cause is investigated.

C. Diagnosis

1. Esophageal manometry is diagnostic—simultaneous, multiphasic, repetitive contractions that occur after a swallow; sphincter response is normal
2. Upper GI barium swallow ("corkscrew esophagus")—in 50%, which represents multiple simultaneous contractions

D. Treatment

1. In general there is no completely effective therapy—treatment failure rates are high.
2. Medical treatment involves nitrates and calcium channel blockers (decreases amplitude of contractions). Tricyclic antidepressants may provide symptomatic relief.
3. Esophagomyotomy is usually not performed, and its efficacy is controversial. Some support its use, whereas others only recommend it when a patient is incapacitated by symptoms.

Esophageal Hiatal Hernias

A. General characteristics: There are two types of hiatal hernias: sliding (type 1) and paraesophageal (type 2).

1. Sliding hiatal hernias (type 1) account for >90% of cases. Both the gastroesophageal junction and a portion of the stomach herniate into the thorax through the esophageal hiatus (so that the gastroesophageal junction is above the diaphragm). This is a common and benign finding that is associated with GERD.
2. Paraesophageal hiatal hernia accounts for <5% of cases. The stomach herniates into the thorax through the esophageal hiatus, but the gastroesophageal junction does not; it remains below the diaphragm. This uncommon hernia can become strangulated and should be repaired surgically.

B. Clinical features

1. The majority of cases are asymptomatic and are discovered incidentally.
2. Possible symptoms include heartburn, chest pain, and dysphagia.
3. Complications of sliding hiatal hernias include GERD (most common), reflux esophagitis (with risk of Barrett's esophagus/cancer), and aspiration.
4. Complications of paraesophageal hernias are potentially life-threatening and include obstruction, hemorrhage, incarceration, and strangulation.

C. Diagnosis: barium upper GI series and upper endoscopy

D. Treatment

1. Type 1 hernias are treated medically (with antacids, small meals, and elevation of the head after meals); 15% of cases may require surgery (Nissen's fundoplication) if there is no response to medical therapy or if there is evidence of esophagitis.
2. Type 2 hernias treated with elective surgery due to risk of above complications.

Mallory-Weiss Syndrome

- This is a mucosal tear at (or just below) the gastroesophageal junction as a result of forceful vomiting or retching. It usually occurs after repeated episodes of vomiting, but it may occur after one episode.
- It is most commonly associated with binge drinking in alcoholics, but any disorder that causes vomiting can induce the mucosal tear.
- Hematemesis is always present—it varies from streaks of blood in vomitus to massive bright red blood.
- Upper endoscopy is diagnostic.
- Most cases (90%) stop bleeding without any treatment.
- Treatment is surgery (oversewing the tear) or angiographic embolization if bleeding continues, but this is rarely necessary. Acid suppression is used to promote healing.

QUICK HIT

- Paraesophageal hernias tend to enlarge with time, and the entire stomach may ultimately move into the thorax.
- Type 3 hernias (combination of type 1 and 2) are treated as type 2 hernias (surgically).

QUICK HIT

If a patient with GERD also has a hiatal hernia, the hernia often worsens the symptoms of GERD.

QUICK HIT

During forceful vomiting, the marked increase in intra-abdominal pressure is transmitted to the esophagus. This can lead to two conditions, depending on the severity and location of the tear.

- If the tear is mucosal and at the gastroesophageal junction, it is referred to as **Mallory-Weiss syndrome.**
- If a tear is transmural (causing esophageal perforation), it is referred to as **Boerhaave's syndrome.**

Plummer-Vinson Syndrome (Upper Esophageal Webs)

- Key features: upper esophageal web (causes dysphagia), iron deficiency anemia, *koilonychia* (spoon-shaped fingernails), and atrophic oral mucosa
- Ten percent of patients develop SCC of the oral cavity, hypopharynx, or esophagus; therefore, this is considered a premalignant lesion.
- Treatment: esophageal dilatation; correct nutritional deficiency

Schatzki's Ring (Distal Esophageal Webs)

- A circumferential ring in the lower esophagus that is always accompanied by a sliding hiatal hernia.
- It is usually asymptomatic, but mild to moderate dysphagia may be present.
- If the patient is symptomatic (but has no reflux), consider esophageal dilatation. If the patient has reflux, consider antireflux surgery.
- Usually due to ingestion of alkali, acids, bleach, or detergents (e.g., in suicide attempts)
- Ingesting alkali is more dangerous than ingesting acid because it may lead to liquefactive necrosis of the esophagus with full-thickness perforation. Acid ingestion does not cause full-thickness damage (only causes necrosis of esophageal mucosa).
- Complications: stricture formation and risk of esophageal cancer
- Treatment is esophagectomy if full-thickness necrosis has occurred. Patient should avoid vomiting, gastric lavage, and all oral intake (can compound the original injury). Give the patient steroids and antibiotics as well. Perform bougienage for esophageal stricture.

Esophageal Diverticula

- Most esophageal diverticula are caused by an **underlying motility disorder** of the esophagus.
- **Zenker's diverticulum** is most common type; found in upper third of the esophagus.

FIGURE
3-5   **Causes of dysphagia**

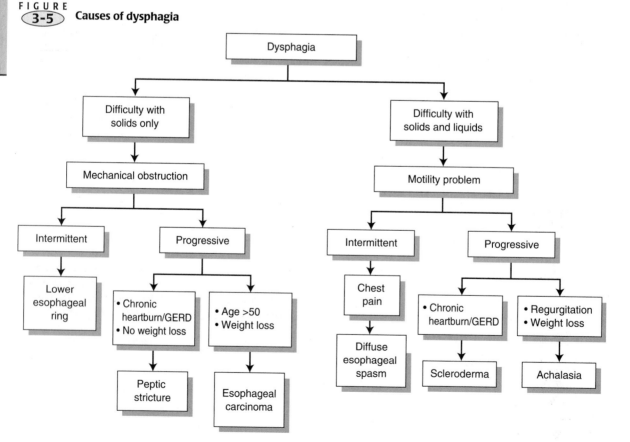

- Failure of the cricopharyngeal muscle to relax during swallowing leads to increased intraluminal pressure. This causes outpouching of mucosa through an area of weakness in the pharyngeal constrictors. *by pulsion mechanism.*
- Clinical features include dysphagia, regurgitation, halitosis (bad breath), weight loss, and chronic cough.
- It is typically seen in patients >50 years old.
- **Traction diverticula** is located in the midpoint of the esophagus near the tracheal bifurcation. It is due to traction from contiguous mediastinal inflammation and adenopathy (pulmonary tuberculosis). Tuberculosis causes hilar node scarring, which causes retraction of esophagus. It is usually asymptomatic and does not require treatment.
- **Epiphrenic diverticula** is found in lower third of esophagus. It is usually associated with spastic esophageal dysmotility or achalasia. Symptoms of dysphagia are more often related to the underlying motility disorder, unless the diverticulum is very large.
- Barium swallow is the best diagnostic test for diverticula.
- Treatment of Zenker's diverticula is surgery. Cricopharyngeal myotomy has excellent results. Treatment of epiphrenic diverticula is esophagomyotomy. Diverticulectomy is of secondary importance in both cases.

An underlying motility disorder is the cause of both proximal (**Zenker's**) and distal (**epiphrenic**) esophageal **diverticula.** Surgical treatment is aimed at correcting the motility disorder (i.e., myotomy). Diverticulectomy is of secondary importance.

Zenker's diverticulum
Complications – tracheal compression, ulcer → bleeding, regurg, pulm. aspiration

Esophageal Perforation

- Etiology: blunt trauma, medical tubes and instruments, forceful vomiting (**Boerhaave's syndrome**) that is associated with alcoholic binges and bulimia
- Clinical features: pain (severe retrosternal/chest/shoulder pain), tachycardia, hypotension, tachypnea, dyspnea, fever, *Hamman's sign* ("mediastinal crunch" produced by the heart beating against air-filled tissues), pneumothorax, or pleural effusion
- Contrast esophagram is definitive diagnostic study (soluble Gastrografin swallow preferred)
- CXR usually shows air in the mediastinum.
- If the patient is stable and the perforation is small (draining into lumen), medical management is appropriate: IV fluids, NPO, antibiotics, and H₂ blockers.
- If patient is ill and the perforation is large (or if there is communication into pleural cavity), surgery should be performed within 24 hours of presentation (success rate is higher).

If gastric/esophageal contents leak into the mediastinum or pleura, infection and septic sequelae may result.

The time interval between esophageal perforation and surgery is the most important factor in determining survival. **If surgery is delayed beyond 24 hours, the mortality rate and the likelihood of fistulization increase.**

DISEASES OF THE STOMACH

Peptic Ulcer Disease (PUD)

A. Causes
1. Most common causes
   a. *Helicobacter pylori* infection
   b. NSAIDs—inhibit prostaglandin production, which leads to impaired mucosal defenses
   c. Acid hypersecretory states, such as Zollinger-Ellison syndrome
2. Other causes
   a. Smoking—ulcers twice as likely in cigarette smokers as in nonsmokers
   b. Alcohol and coffee—may exacerbate symptoms, but causal relationship as yet unproven
   c. Other potential but unproven causes include emotional stress, personality type ("type A"), and dietary factors

B. Clinical features
1. Epigastric pain
   a. Aching or gnawing in nature

Most cases of peptic ulcer disease are due to *H. pylori* infection and NSAID use. It can be difficult to determine the cause in a patient with *H. pylori* infection who also uses NSAIDs. Both may be responsible. Therefore, if in doubt, test for *H. pylori*.

TABLE 3-4 Duodenal Versus Gastric Ulcers		
	Duodenal Ulcers	**Gastric Ulcers**
Pathogenesis	Caused by an increase in offensive factors (higher rates of basal and stimulated gastric acid secretion)	Caused by a decrease in defensive factors (gastric acid level is normal/low unless ulcer is pyloric or prepyloric)
Helicobacter pylori infection	70% to 90% of patients	60% to 70% of patients
Malignant potential	Low (malignancy is very rare)	High (5% to 10% are malignant)—should undergo biopsy to rule out malignancy
Location	Majority are 1–2 cm distal to pylorus (usually on posterior wall)	Type I (most common, 70%): on lesser curvature Type II: gastric and duodenal ulcer Type III: prepyloric (within 2 cm of pylorus) Type IV: near esophagogastric junction
Age distribution	Occurs in younger patients (<40)	Occurs in older patients (>40)
Associated blood type	Type O	Type A
Risk factors	NSAIDs	Smoking
Other	Eating usually relieves pain. Nocturnal pain is more common than in gastric ulcers.	Eating does not usually relieve pain. Complication rates are higher than those of duodenal ulcers. There is a higher recurrence rate with medical therapy alone.

b. **Nocturnal symptoms and the effect of food on symptoms are variable** (see Table 3-4).
2. May be complicated by upper GI bleeding
3. Other symptoms: nausea/vomiting, early satiety, and weight loss

C. Diagnosis
1. Endoscopy
   a. Most accurate test in diagnosing ulcers
   b. Essential in diagnosis of gastric ulcers because biopsy is necessary to rule out malignancy—duodenal ulcers do not require biopsy
   c. Preferred when severe or acute bleeding is present (can perform electrocautery of bleeding ulcers)
   d. Can obtain endoscopic biopsy for diagnosis of *H. pylori*
2. Barium swallow
   a. Sometimes used initially but is less reliable than endoscopy
   b. Double-contrast techniques preferred due to improved accuracy
3. Laboratory test—for diagnosis of *H. pylori* infection
   a. Biopsy: histologic evaluation of endoscopic biopsy is gold standard.
   b. Urease detection via urea breath test is the most convenient test (sensitivity and specificity >95%). It documents active infection and helps to assess the results of antibiotic therapy.
   c. Serology (lower specificity)—The presence of antibodies to *H. pylori* does not necessarily indicate current infection—antibodies to *H. pylori* can remain elevated for months or even years after eradication of infection (90% sensitive).
4. Serum gastrin measurement—if considering Zollinger-Ellison syndrome as a diagnosis

QUICK HIT

If a peptic ulcer is uncomplicated, a barium study or endoscopy is not needed initially. Initiate empiric therapy. However, if you suspect any of the complications of peptic ulcer disease, order confirmatory studies.

D. Treatment · · ·

1. Medical
   a. Supportive (patient directives)
      - Discontinue aspirin/NSAIDs.
      - Restrict alcohol use but do not restrict any foods.
      - Stop smoking, decrease emotional stress.
      - Avoid eating before bedtime (eating stimulates nocturnal gastric acid levels); decrease coffee intake (although no strong link has been established with ulcer disease).
   b. Acid suppression
      - H_2 blockers—accelerate healing of ulcers
      - Proton pump inhibitors (PPIs)—most effective antisecretory agents (although expensive)
      - Antacids—somewhat outdated for primary therapy and more appropriately used for adjunctive therapy/symptomatic relief
   c. Eradicate *H. pylori* with triple or quadruple therapy (see Table 3-5). Once infection is cleared, the rate of recurrence is very low.
   d. Cytoprotection
      - Sucralfate—facilitates ulcer healing; must be taken frequently, is costly, and can cause GI upset
      - Misoprostol—reduces risk for ulcer formation associated with NSAID therapy; is costly and can cause GI upset (common side effect)
   e. Treatment regimens
      - If *H. pylori* test is positive, begin eradication therapy with either triple or quadruple therapy (see Table 3-5). Also begin acid-suppression with antacids, an H_2 blocker, or a PPI.
      - If the patient has an active NSAID-induced ulcer, stop NSAID use (may switch to acetaminophen). Also begin with either a PPI or misoprostol. Continue for 4 to 8 weeks, depending on severity. Treat the *H. pylori* infection as above if present.
2. Surgical
   a. Rarely needed electively
   b. Required for the complications of PUD (bleeding, perforation, gastric outlet obstruction) (see Table 3-6 and Figure 3-6)

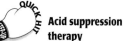

Acid suppression therapy
- H_2 blockers
- Ranitidine
- Famotidine
- Nizatidine
- Cimetidine) CYP 450 blocker
- Proton pump inhibitors
- Esomeprazole
- Omeprazole
- Lansoprazole
- Pantoprazole
- Rabeprazole

Complications of PUD
bleeding
Perforation
obstruction.

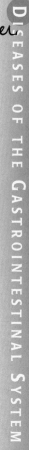

Acute Gastritis

- Acute gastritis refers to inflammation of the gastric mucosa.
- There are multiple causes: NSAIDs/aspirin; *H. pylori* infection; alcohol, heavy cigarette smoking, or caffeine; extreme physiologic stress (e.g., shock, sepsis, burns)
- It can either be asymptomatic or cause epigastric pain. The relationship between eating and pain is not consistent (i.e., food may either aggravate or relieve the pain).
- If epigastric pain is low or moderate and is not associated with worrisome symptoms/findings, empiric therapy with acid suppression is appropriate. Stop NSAIDs.

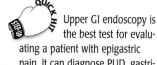

Upper GI endoscopy is the best test for evaluating a patient with epigastric pain. It can diagnose PUD, gastritis, and esophagitis. It can also rule out cancers of the esophagus and stomach, and H. pylori infection with biopsy.

TABLE 3-5 *Helicobacter pylori* Eradication

	Regimen	Advantage	Disadvantage
Triple therapy	PPI plus two antibiotics	Twice daily dosing	More expensive than bismuth-based triple therapy
Quadruple therapy	PPI, bismuth subsalicylate, and two antibiotics	Half the time as triple therapy (a 1-week program as opposed to 2 weeks for triple therapy), yet reaps similar eradication results	Expense of PPI

DISEASES OF THE GASTROINTESTINAL SYSTEM

TABLE 3-6 Complications of Peptic Ulcer Disease

	Clinical Findings	Diagnostic Studies	Management	Other
Perforation	Acute, severe abdominal pain, signs of peritonitis, hemodynamic instability	Upright CXR **(free air under diaphragm)**, CT scan is the most sensitive test for perforation (detects free abdominal air)	Emergency surgery to close perforation and perform definitive ulcer operation (such as highly selective vagotomy or truncal vagotomy/pyloroplasty)	**Can progress to sepsis and death if untreated**
Gastric outlet obstruction	Nausea/vomiting (poorly digested food), epigastric fullness/early satiety, weight loss	Barium swallow and upper endoscopy; saline load test (empty stomach with a nasogastric tube, add 750 mL saline, aspirate after 30 min—test is positive if aspirate >400 mL) Surgery is eventually necessary in 75% of patients.	Initially, nasogastric suction; replace electrolyte/volume deficits; supplement nutrition if obstruction is longstanding	Most common with duodenal ulcers and type III gastric ulcers
GI bleeding	Bleeding may be slow (leading to anemic symptoms) or can be rapid and severe (leading to shock)	Stool guaiac, upper GI endoscopy (diagnostic and therapeutic)	Resuscitation; diagnose site of bleed via endoscopy and treat; perform surgery for acute bleeds that require transfusion of ≥ 6 units of blood	**Peptic ulcer disease is the most common cause of upper GI bleeding.**

- If there is no positive response after 4 to 8 weeks of treatment, consider a diagnostic workup. Include upper GI endoscopy and ultrasound (to rule out gallstones), and test for *H. pylori* infection.
- If *H. pylori* infection is confirmed, antibiotic therapy is indicated (see Table 3-5).

Chronic Gastritis

- The most common cause is *H. pylori* infection (over 80% of cases).
- Autoimmune gastritis leads to chronic atrophic gastritis with serum antiparietal and anti-intrinsic factor antibodies (and possible development of pernicious anemia).

FIGURE 3-6 **A. An AP chest radiograph in a patient with a perforated duodenal ulcer and acute abdomen. The curved arrows show free subdiaphragmatic air due to the perforated ulcer. The straight arrows show the diaphragms bilaterally. B. Chest radiograph (upright) showing bilateral subdiaphragmatic intraperitoneal air. Double arrows represent right and left hemidiaphragms. Note the bilateral subdiaphragmatic air (straight arrows). There is air in the gastric fundus as well as free air surrounding the gastric fundus.**

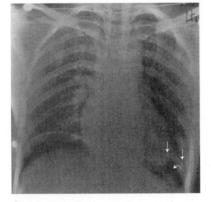

A

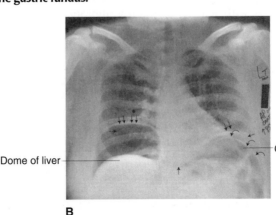

Dome of liver

Gastric fundus air

B

(From Erkonen WE, Smith WL. Radiology 101: The Basics and Fundamentals of Imaging. Philadelphia: Lippincott Williams & Wilkins, 1998:103, Figure 6-46, and 159, Figure 8-22, respectively.)

- Most patients with chronic gastritis due to *H. pylori* are asymptomatic and never develop complications. The condition may manifest as epigastric pain similar to PUD. Other associated symptoms such as nausea/vomiting, and anorexia are rare.
- Complications include PUD, gastric carcinoma, and mucosa-associated lymphoid tissue lymphoma.
- Upper GI endoscopy with biopsy is the test of choice for diagnosis of chronic gastritis. Other tests should be used to find the cause (usually *H. pylori*).
- If the patient is symptomatic, treatment involves *H. pylori* eradication with triple or quadruple therapy (see Table 3-5).

Gastric Cancer

A. General characteristics
1. The majority are adenocarcinomas.
2. Gastric cancer is rare in the United States (more common in Japan).
3. Morphology
   a. Ulcerative carcinoma—ulcer through all layers
   b. Polypoid carcinoma—solid mass projects into stomach lumen
   c. Superficial spreading—most favorable prognosis
   d. *Linitis plastica*—"leather bottle"—infiltrates early through all layers, stomach wall is thick and rigid, poor prognosis

linitis plastica – worse prognosis.

B. Risk factors
1. Severe atrophic gastritis, intestinal metaplasia, gastric dysplasia
2. Adenomatous gastric polyps, chronic atrophic gastritis
3. *H. pylori* infection—threefold to sixfold increase in risk
4. Postantrectomy—many cases reported after Billroth II anastomosis (15 to 20 years after surgery)
5. Pernicious anemia—threefold increase in risk
6. Ménétrier's disease—10% of these patients develop cancer
7. High intake of preserved foods (high salt, nitrates, nitrites—smoked fish)
8. Blood type A

H. pylori → gastric cancer

C. Clinical features
1. Abdominal pain and unexplained weight loss are most common symptoms
2. Reduced appetite, anorexia, dyspepsia, early satiety
3. Nausea and vomiting, anemia, melena, guaiac-positive stool

D. Diagnosis
1. Endoscopy with multiple biopsies—most accurate test
2. Barium upper GI series—less accurate, but can complement upper endoscopy/biopsy findings
3. Abdominal CT scan—for staging and to detect presence of metastases
4. FOBT

E. Treatment
1. Surgical resection with wide (>5 cm) margins (total or subtotal gastrectomy) with extended lymph node dissection
2. Chemotherapy may be appropriate in some cases.

Gastric Lymphoma

- A type of non-Hodgkin's lymphoma that arises in the stomach.
- Clinical features are similar to those of adenocarcinoma of the stomach (e.g., abdominal pain, weight loss, anorexia).
- Complications include bleeding, obstruction, and perforation (possibly presented as an emergency).
- EGD with biopsy is the standard for diagnosis (same as adenocarcinoma of stomach).
- Treatment depends on the stage of the disease and the presence of complications. Options include surgical resection, radiation, and chemotherapy.

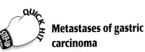

QUICK HIT

Metastases of gastric carcinoma
- **Krukenberg's tumor**—metastasis to the ovary
- **Blumer's shelf**—metastasis to the rectum (pelvic cul-de-sac)—can palpate on rectal examination
- **Sister Mary Joseph's node**—metastasis to the periumbilical lymph node
- **Virchow's node**—metastasis to the supraclavicular fossa nodes
- **Irish's node**—metastasis to the left axillary adenopathy

DISEASES OF THE SMALL INTESTINE

Small Bowel Obstruction (SBO)

A. General characteristics

1. There are three main points of differentiation to consider in SBO.
   a. Partial versus complete obstruction
      - With partial obstruction, patients are able to pass gas or have bowel movements, as opposed to complete obstruction.
      - However, patients with complete obstruction may occasionally be able to pass gas or stool because they may have residual stool or gas in the colon.
   b. Closed loop versus open loop obstruction
      - With closed loop obstruction, the lumen is occluded at two points by an adhesive band or hernia ring. This can compromise the blood supply, requiring emergent surgery.
   c. Proximal versus distal small bowel obstruction
      - Distal obstruction causes distention of proximal bowel segments, making diagnosis easier on plain radiograph.
2. Pathophysiology
   a. **Dehydration is a key event in SBO.** Intestinal distention causes reflex vomiting, increased intestinal secretion proximal to the point of obstruction, and decreased absorption. This leads to hypochloremia, hypokalemia, and metabolic alkalosis.
   b. The resulting hypovolemia leads to systemic findings such as tachycardia, hypotension, tachypnea, altered mental status, and oliguria.

B. Causes

1. Adhesions from previous abdominal surgery—most common cause in adults
2. Incarcerated hernias—second most common cause
3. Malignancy, intussusception, Crohn's disease, carcinomatosis, and superior mesenteric artery syndrome (compression of third portion of duodenum)

C. Clinical features

1. Cramping abdominal pain—If pain is continuous and severe, strangulation may be present.
2. Nausea, vomiting—may be feculent
3. Obstipation (absence of stool and flatus)
4. Abdominal distention

D. Diagnosis

1. Abdominal plain films—dilated loops of small bowel, air-fluid levels proximal to point of obstruction (on upright film), and minimal gas in colon (if complete SBO) (see Figure 3-7)
2. Barium enema—to rule out colonic obstruction if plain films do not distinguish small from large bowel obstruction; barium enema identifies site of obstruction
3. Upper GI series—with small bowel follow-through if above are not diagnostic

E. Treatment

1. Nonoperative management—appropriate if bowel obstruction is incomplete and there is no fever, tachycardia, peritoneal signs, or leukocytosis
2. IV fluids to establish adequate urine output; add potassium to fluids to correct hypokalemia (which is typically present)
3. Nasogastric tube to empty stomach (gastric decompression)
4. Antibiotics
5. Surgery is indicated for complete obstruction, for partial obstruction that is persistent and/or associated with constant pain, or if strangulation is suspected. Perform an exploratory laparotomy **with lysis of adhesions and resection of any necrotic bowel.**

SBO
- Proximal obstruction: frequent vomiting, severe pain, minimal abdominal distention
- Distal obstruction: less frequent vomiting and significant abdominal distention

Excessively high intraluminal pressure may compromise blood supply, leading to strangulation. This can lead to shock, gangrene, peritonitis, or perforation of bowel—all devastating complications.

Large bowel obstruction
- Causes: volvulus, adhesions, hernias, colon cancer (most common cause)
- Results in less fluid and electrolyte disorder than SBO
- See Figure 3-8 for radiographic findings

Manifestations of strangulated bowel in SBO include fever, severe and continuous pain, hematemesis, shock, gas in the bowel wall or portal vein, abdominal free air, peritoneal signs, and acidosis (increased lactic acid).

Paralytic Ileus

- Peristalsis is decreased or absent (no mechanical obstruction is present).
- Causes include medications (e.g., narcotics, drugs with anticholinergic effects), postoperative state (after abdominal surgery), spinal cord injury, shock, metabolic disorders (especially hypokalemia), and peritonitis.
- Abdominal plain films show a uniform distribution of gas in the small bowel, colon, and rectum (in contrast to small bowel or colonic obstruction).
- Failure to pass contrast medium beyond a fixed point is diagnostic.
- Treatment involves IV fluids, NPO, correction of electrolyte imbalances (especially hypokalemia), nasogastric suction if necessary, and placement of a long tube if ileus persists postoperatively.

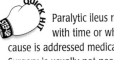

Paralytic ileus resolves with time or when the cause is addressed medically. Surgery is usually not needed.

FIGURE 3-7 **A.** An AP supine film of small bowel obstruction shows prominent valvulae conniventes. Air is confined to the small bowel, with no obvious air in the colon. Note surgical clips from previous surgery. **B.** An AP upright film in the same patient as shown in A. Note air fluid levels in the small bowel (arrow) with little or no distal bowel gas. **C.** An AP supine film of postoperative ileus. Note the presence of air throughout the entire GI tract.

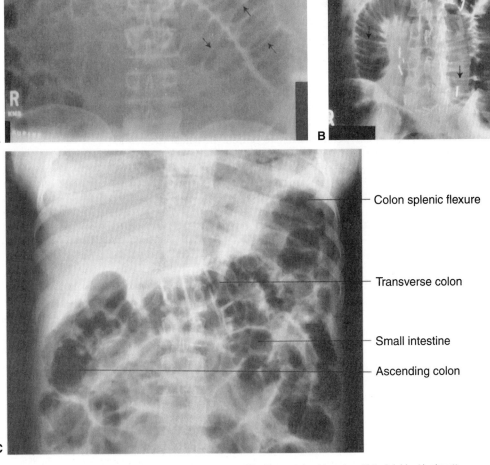

— Colon splenic flexure

— Transverse colon

— Small intestine

— Ascending colon

(From Erkonen WE, Smith WL. Radiology 101: The Basics and Fundamentals of Imaging. Philadelphia: Lippincott Williams & Wilkins, 1998:157, Figure 8-20A and C, and 156, Figure 8-19A.)

FIGURE
3-8 **A.** An AP supine film of large bowel obstruction. Note the dilated air-filled proximal colon with an absence of air in the distal colon. **B.** An AP upright film of large bowel obstruction. Note multiple colon air fluid levels (curved arrows).

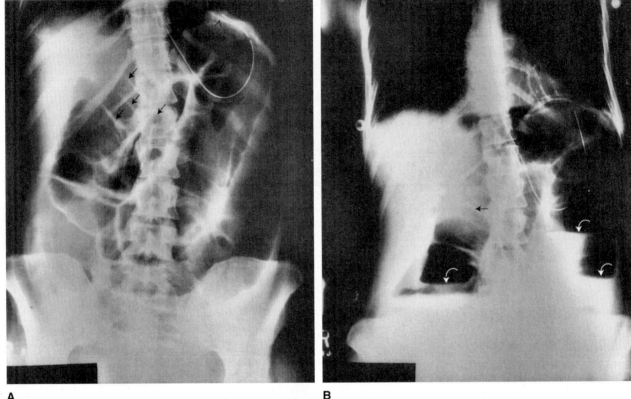

A   **B**

(From Erkonen WE, Smith WL. Radiology 101: The Basics and Fundamentals of Imaging. Philadelphia: Lippincott Williams & Wilkins, 1998:158, Figure 8-21A and B.)

Celiac Sprue

- Characterized by hypersensitivity to gluten (in wheat products)
- Results in weight loss, abdominal distention, bloating, diarrhea
- Biopsy in proximal small bowel reveals flattening of villi, which causes malabsorption.
- Strict adherence to a gluten-free diet is essential.

INFLAMMATORY BOWEL DISEASE (IBD)

Crohn's Disease ("Regional Enteritis")

A. General characteristics

1. Crohn's disease is a chronic transmural inflammatory disease that can affect any part of the GI tract (mouth to anus) but most commonly involves the small bowel (terminal ileum).
2. Distribution: There are three major patterns of disease.
   a. Forty percent of patients have disease in the terminal ileum and cecum.
   b. Thirty percent of patients have disease confined to the small intestine.
   c. Twenty-five percent of patients have disease confined to the colon.
   d. Rarely, other parts of GI tract may be involved (stomach, mouth, esophagus).
3. Pathology
   a. **Terminal ileum is the hallmark location,** but other sites of GI tract may also be involved.
   b. Skip lesions—discontinuous involvement

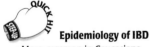

Epidemiology of IBD
- More common in Caucasians than other racial groups
- Particularly common in Jewish populations
- Mean age of onset is 15 to 35 years.

> ### Box 3-9 Extraintestinal Manifestations of Inflammatory Bowel Disease (IBD)
>
> - Eye lesions
>   - Episcleritis—parallels bowel's disease activity
>   - Anterior uveitis—independent course
> - Skin lesions
>   - Erythema nodosum—especially in Crohn's disease; parallels bowel disease activity
>   - Pyoderma gangrenosum—especially in UC; parallels bowel disease activity in 50% of cases
> - Arthritis—most common extraintestinal manifestation of IBD
>   - Migratory monoarticular arthritis—parallels bowel disease activity (coincides with exacerbation of colitis)
>   - Ankylosing spondylitis—Patients with UC have a 30 times greater incidence of ankylosing spondylitis than the general population; the course is independent of the colitis.
>   - Sacroiliitis—does not parallel bowel disease activity
> - Thromboembolic-hypercoagulable state—can lead to deep venous thrombosis (DVT), pulmonary embolism (PE), or a cardiovascular accident (CVA)
> - Idiopathic thrombocytopenic purpura
> - Osteoporosis
> - Gallstones in Crohn's disease (ileal involvement)
> - Sclerosing cholangitis in UC

   c. Fistulae
   d. Luminal strictures
   e. Noncaseating granulomas
   f. Transmural thickening and inflammation (full-thickness wall involvement)—results in narrowing of the lumen
   g. Mesenteric "fat creeping" onto the antimesenteric border of small bowel

B. Clinical features

1. Diarrhea (usually without blood)
2. Malabsorption and weight loss (common)
3. Abdominal pain (usually RLQ), nausea and vomiting
4. Fever, malaise
5. Extraintestinal manifestations in 15% to 20% of cases (uveitis, arthritis, ankylosing spondylitis, erythema nodosum, pyoderma gangrenosum, aphthous oral ulcers, cholelithiasis, and nephrolithiasis)

C. Diagnosis

1. Endoscopy (sigmoidoscopy or colonoscopy) with biopsy—typical findings are aphthous ulcers, cobblestone appearance, pseudopolyps, patchy (skip) lesions
2. Barium enema
3. Upper GI with small bowel follow-through

D. Complications

1. Fistulae—between colon and other segments of intestine (enteroenteral), bladder (enterovesical), vagina (enterovaginal), and skin (enterocutaneous)
2. Anorectal disease (in 30% of patients)—fissures, abscesses, perianal fistulas
3. SBO (in 20% to 30% of patients) is the most common indication for surgery. Initially, it is due to edema and spasm of bowel with intermittent signs of obstruction; later, scarring and thickening of bowel cause chronic narrowing of lumen.
4. Malignancy—increased risk of colonic and small bowel tumors (but less common than in UC)
5. Malabsorption of vitamin B_{12} and bile acids (both occur in terminal ileum)
6. Cholelithiasis may occur secondary to decreased bile acid absorption.
7. Nephrolithiasis—Increased colonic absorption of dietary oxalate can lead to calcium oxalate kidney stones.

 Crohn's disease has a chronic, indolent course characterized by unpredictable **flares and remissions.** The effectiveness of medical treatment decreases with advancing disease, and complications eventually develop, requiring surgery. There is no cure, and recurrence is common even after surgery.

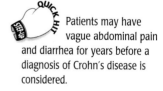 Patients may have vague abdominal pain and diarrhea for years before a diagnosis of Crohn's disease is considered.

8. Aphthous ulcers of lips, gingiva, and buccal mucosa (common)
9. Toxic megacolon—less common in Crohn's disease than in UC
10. Growth retardation
11. Narcotic abuse, psychosocial issues due to chronicity and often disabling nature of the disease

E. Treatment

1. Medical
   a. Sulfasalazine
      - This is useful if the colon is involved. 5-ASA (mesalamine) is the active compound and is released in the colon—it is more useful in UC than in Crohn's disease.
      - 5-ASA compounds block prostaglandin release and serve to reduce inflammation.
      - There are preparations of 5-ASA that are more useful in distal small bowel disease.
   b. Metronidazole—if no response to 5-ASA
   c. Systemic corticosteroids (prednisone)—for acute exacerbations and if no response to metronidazole
   d. Immunosuppressants (azathioprine, 6-mercaptopurine)—in conjunction with steroids if the patient does not respond to above agents
   e. Bile acid sequestrants (cholestyramine or colestipol)—for patients with terminal ileal disease who cannot absorb bile acids
   f. Antidiarrheal agents generally not a good choice (may cause ileus)
2. Surgical (eventually required in most patients)
   a. Reserve for complications of Crohn's disease
   b. Involves segmental resection of involved bowel
   c. Disease recurrence after surgery is high—up to 50% of patients experience disease recurrence at 10 years postoperatively.
   d. Indications for surgery include SBO, fistulae (especially between bowel and bladder, vagina), disabling disease, and perforation or abscess.
3. Nutritional supplementation and support—Parenteral nutrition is sometimes necessary.

Ulcerative Colitis (UC)

A. General characteristics

1. UC is a chronic inflammatory disease of the colon or rectal mucosa.
2. It may occur at any age (usually begins in adolescence or young adulthood).
3. Distribution: UC **involves the rectum in all cases** and can involve the colon either partially or entirely.
   a. Rectum alone (in 10% of cases)
   b. Rectum and left colon (in 40% of cases)
   c. Rectum, left colon, and right colon (in 30% of cases)
   d. Pancolitis (in 30% of cases)
   e. The small bowel is not usually involved in UC, but it may reach the distal ileum in a small percentage of patients ("backwash ileitis" in 10% of cases).
4. The course is unpredictable and variable and is characterized by periodic exacerbations and periods of complete remission. Less than 5% of patients have an initial attack without any recurrence.
5. Pathology
   a. Uninterrupted involvement of rectum and/or colon—**no skip lesions**
   b. Inflammation is not transmural (as it is in Crohn's disease). It is limited to the mucosa and submucosa.
   c. PMNs accumulate in the crypts of the colon (crypt abscesses).

B. Clinical features (wide range of presentation)

1. **Hematochezia (bloody diarrhea)**
2. **Abdominal pain**

3. Bowel movements are frequent but small
4. Fever, anorexia, and weight loss (severe cases)
5. Tenesmus (rectal dry heaves)
6. Extraintestinal symptoms (e.g., jaundice, uveitis, arthritis, skin lesions)—see Box 3-9

C. Diagnosis: Perform the following initial studies.

1. Stool cultures for *Clostridium difficile*, ova, and parasites—to rule out infectious diarrhea
2. Fecal leukocytes
3. WBCs can appear in UC, ischemic colitis, or infectious diarrhea.
4. Colonoscopy—to assess the extent of disease and the presence of any complications

D. Complications

1. Iron deficiency anemia
2. Hemorrhage
3. Electrolyte disturbances and dehydration secondary to diarrhea
4. Strictures, benign and malignant (usually malignant)
5. Colon cancer—The risk correlates with extent and duration of colitis. In distal proctitis there is no increased risk of colorectal cancer.
6. Sclerosing cholangitis (SC)—The course not parallel with bowel disease and is not prevented by colectomy.
7. Cholangiocarcinoma—Half of all bile duct cancers are associated with UC.
8. Toxic megacolon is the leading cause of death in UC and affects <5% of patients. It is associated with the risk of colonic perforation.
9. Growth retardation
10. Narcotic abuse
11. Psychosocial issues (e.g., depression) due to chronicity and often disabling nature of the disease

E. Treatment

1. Medical
   a. Systemic corticosteroids are used for acute exacerbations.
   b. Sulfasalazine is the mainstay of treatment.
      • It is effective in maintaining remissions. 5-ASA (mesalamine) is the active component.
      • 5-ASA enemas can be used for proctitis and distal colitis.
   c. Immunosuppressive agents in patients with refractory disease may prevent relapses but are not effective for acute attacks.
2. Surgical—often curative (unlike Crohn's disease) and involves total colectomy. Indications for surgery include:

QUICK HIT Patients with UC may have nonbloody diarrhea at first, with eventual progression to bloody diarrhea.

QUICK HIT Sulfasalazine is metabolized by bacteria to 5-ASA and sulfapyridine. 5-ASA is the effective moiety of the drug, and sulfapyridine causes the side effects.

→ N'l 4.5g after 5 hrs in urine

D-Xylose absorption is abnormal both in bacterial overgrowth & whipple's dc. However, w/ bacterial overgrowth, the test becomes n'l after antibiotic treatment.

TABLE 3-7	Crohn's Disease Versus Ulcerative Colitis	
	Crohn's Disease	**Ulcerative Colitis**
Involvement	Transmural—intestinal wall from mucosa to serosa	Mucosa and submucosa
	Discontinuous involvement (skip lesions)	Continuous involvement (no skip lesions)
Location	Terminal ileum (most common) Can involve any part of the GI tract (resection is not curative—recurrences occur)	Confined to colon and rectum Colectomy is curative
Complications	Fistulae and abscesses are more common than in UC because the entire wall is involved.	SC and colorectal cancer are more common than in Crohn's disease.

DISEASES OF THE GASTROINTESTINAL SYSTEM

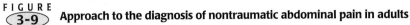

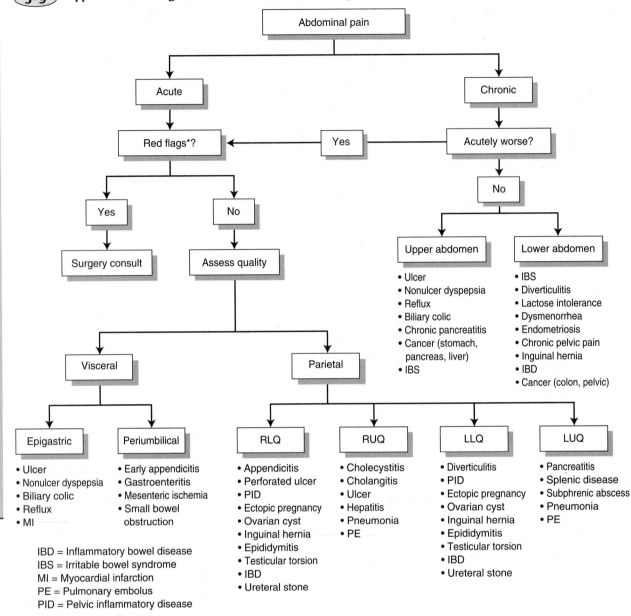

FIGURE 3-9 Approach to the diagnosis of nontraumatic abdominal pain in adults

IBD = Inflammatory bowel disease
IBS = Irritable bowel syndrome
MI = Myocardial infarction
PE = Pulmonary embolus
PID = Pelvic inflammatory disease

*"Red flags" include peritoneal signs such as
rigid abdomen, guarding, and rebound tenderness.

(Adapted from Sloane PD, Slatt LM, Ebell MH, et al. Essentials of Family Medicine. 4th Ed. Philadelphia: Lippincott Williams & Wilkins, 2002:245, Figure 16.2.)

a. Severe disease that is debilitating, refractory, and unresponsive to medical therapy
b. Toxic megacolon (risk of perforation), obstruction (due to stricture), severe hemorrhage, perforation
c. Fulminant exacerbation that does not respond to steroids
d. Evidence of colon cancer or increased risk of colon cancer
e. Growth failure or failure to thrive in children
f. Systemic complications

CHAPTER 4

Endocrine and Metabolic Diseases

DISEASES OF THE THYROID GLAND

Hyperthyroidism

A. Causes

1. **Graves' disease (diffuse toxic goiter)** is most common cause—80% of all cases
   a. An autoimmune disorder: A thyroid-stimulating immunoglobulin (Ig) G antibody binds to the TSH receptors on the surface of thyroid cells and triggers the synthesis of excess thyroid hormone.
   b. Commonly associated with other autoimmune disorders.
   c. A radioiodide scan would show diffuse uptake because every thyroid cell is hyperfunctioning.

2. **Plummer's disease (multinodular toxic goiter)**—15% of all cases
   a. Characterized by hyperfunctioning areas that produce high T_4 and T_3 levels, thereby decreasing TSH levels. As a result, the rest of the thyroid is not functioning (atrophy due to decreased TSH).
   b. Consequently, patchy uptake appears on the thyroid scan.
   c. It is more common in elderly patients.

3. Toxic thyroid adenoma (single nodule)—2% of all cases

4. Hashimoto's thyroiditis and subacute (granulomatous) thyroiditis (both can cause **transient** hyperthyroidism)

5. Other causes (rare)
   a. Postpartum thyroiditis (transient hyperthyroidism)
   b. Iodine-induced hyperthyroidism
   c. Excessive doses of levothyroxine (e.g., iatrogenic by health care provider or surreptitious self-administration)

B. Clinical features

1. Symptoms
   a. Nervousness, insomnia, irritability
   b. Hand tremor, hyperactivity, tremulousness
   c. Excessive sweating, heat intolerance
   d. Weight loss despite increased appetite
   e. Diarrhea, frequent defecation
   f. Palpitations (due to tachyarrhythmias)
   g. Muscle weakness

2. Signs
   a. Thyroid gland
      • Graves' disease: a diffusely enlarged (symmetric), nontender thyroid gland; **a bruit may be present**

QUICK HIT

Hyperthyroidism in the elderly

• In the elderly, classic symptoms of hyperthyroidism (e.g., nervousness, insomnia, hyperactivity) may be absent. The only manifestations may be weight loss, weakness, and/or atrial fibrillation.

• Consider hyperthyroidism before assuming that an elderly patient with unexplained weight loss has depression or occult malignancy.

or wt loss
Pt. w/ A. fib → always check TSH for hyperthyroidism.

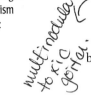

There are three signs of hyperthyroidism specific to Graves' disease:
• Exophthalmos
• Pretibial myxedema
• Thyroid bruit

• Subacute thyroiditis: an exquisitely tender, diffusely enlarged gland (with a viral illness)
• Plummer's disease and Hashimoto's thyroiditis (if multinodularity is present): thyroid gland is bumpy, irregular, and asymmetric
• Toxic adenoma: single nodule with an otherwise atrophic gland

multinodular toxic goiter.

b. Extrathyroidal
• Eyes: **Proptosis, due to edema of the extraocular muscles and retro-orbital tissue, is a hallmark of Graves' disease** (but not always present). Irritation and excessive tearing are common due to corneal exposure. Lid retraction may be the only sign in milder disease. (See Color Figure 4-1.) Lid lag may be present.
• Cardiovascular effects: arrhythmias (sinus tachycardia, atrial fibrillation, and premature ventricular contractions), elevated BP
• Skin changes: warm and moist, **pretibial myxedema** (edema over tibial surface due to dermal accumulation of mucopolysaccharides)
• Neurologic: brisk deep tendon reflexes, tremor

C. Diagnosis
1. Serum TSH level (low)—**initial test of choice**: If TSH is normal or high, hyperthyroidism is unlikely (TSH-induced hyperthyroidism is quite uncommon).
2. Next order thyroid hormone levels: T_4 level should be elevated. Consider a free T_4 assay.
3. Testing the T_3 level is usually unnecessary but may be helpful if TSH level is low and free T_4 is not elevated, because excess T_3 alone can cause hyperthyroidism.
4. Other tests (less commonly used but often tested)
   a. Radioactive T_3 uptake
   • Gives information regarding status of TBG (thyroid binding globulin)
   • Radioactive T_3 can bind either to TBG or to "resin" that has been given (binds to resin only if there is no "space" on TBG, as in hyperthyroidism when T_4 is bound to TBG). Consequently, you measure how much radioactive T_3 was taken up by the resin.
   • **The importance of this test is that it helps differentiate between elevations in thyroid hormones due to increased TBG from true hyperthyroidism (due to an actual increase in free T_4).**
   • **Consider** hyperthyroidism **when the thyroid gland is producing excess T_4.** In this case, all of the binding sites on TBG will be bound by T_4, so radioactive T_3 uptake will increase.
   • **Consider** pregnancy **when there is high TBG.** There are more binding sites for radioactive T_3, so radioactive T_3 uptake decreases. Therefore, high TBG production leads to low radioactive T_3 uptake.
   b. FTI (free thyroxine index)
   • FTI = (radioactive T_3 uptake × serum total T_4)/100
   • FTI = (patient's radioactive T_3 uptake/normal radioactive T_3 uptake) × total T_4
   • Normal FTI values are 4 to 11. FTI should not change (as T_4 decreases, radioactive T_3 uptake increases, and vice versa).
   • FTI is proportional to actual free T_4 concentration.

Thyroid hormones and TBG
• T_4 is converted to T_3 by deiodination outside of the thyroid.
• T_3 is more biologically active than T_4.
• Most of T_4 (and T_3) is reversibly bound to TBG and is inactive.
• Factors that increase TBG (and therefore total T_4) include pregnancy, liver disease, oral contraceptives, and aspirin.

↑TBG = ↑ total T_4
→ Pregnancy
→ liver dx
→ oral contraceptives
→ Aspirin.

D. Treatment types
1. Pharmacologic
   a. Thionamides—methimazole and propylthiouracil (PTU) inhibit thyroid hormone synthesis, and PTU also inhibits conversion of T_4 to T_3. Treatment with thionamides results in long-term remission in a minority of patients; a major serious side effect is agranulocytosis.
   b. β-blockers—for acute management of some symptoms such as palpitations, tremors, anxiety, tachycardia, sweating, and muscle weakness
   c. Sodium ipodate or iopanoic acid—lowers serum T_3 and T_4 levels and causes rapid improvement of hyperthyroidism; appropriate for acute management of severe hyperthyroidism that is not responding to conventional therapy

 ok in pregnancy

For all patients taking antithyroid medication, consider monitoring the leukocyte count on a regular basis (for agranulocytes).

2. Radioiodine 131 (^{131}I)
    a. Causes destruction of thyroid follicular cells
    b. Most common therapy in the United States for Graves' hyperthyroidism
    c. Main complication is hypothyroidism and occurs in majority of patients
    d. If the first dose does not control the hyperthyroidism within 6 to 12 months, then administer another dose.
    e. Contraindicated during pregnancy and breastfeeding due to risk of cretinism
3. Surgical—subtotal thyroidectomy
    a. Very effective, but only 1% of patients with hyperthyroidism are treated with surgery due to the following side effects: permanent hypothyroidism (30%), recurrence of hyperthyroidism (10%), recurrent laryngeal nerve palsy (1%), permanent hypoparathyroidism (1%)
    b. Often reserved for patients with very large goiters, those who are allergic to antithyroid drugs, or patients who prefer surgery over medication
    c. Watch for hypocalcemia after surgery that may not return to normal due to parathyroid inflammation or accidental removal.

E. Treatment

1. For immediate control of adrenergic symptoms of hyperthyroidism (of any cause): β-blocker (propranolol)
2. For nonpregnant patients with Graves' disease
    a. Start methimazole (in addition to the β-blocker).
    b. Taper β-blocker after 4 to 8 weeks (once methimazole starts to take effect).
    c. Continue methimazole for 1 to 2 years. Measure thyroid-stimulating IgG antibody at 12 months. If it is absent, then discontinue therapy. If relapse occurs, then resume methimazole for about 1 more year or consider radioiodine therapy.
3. For pregnant patients with Graves' disease
    a. Endocrinology consult is indicated before starting treatment
    b. PTU is preferred
4. Radioactive iodine ablation therapy
    a. Leads to hypothyroidism over time in many patients
    b. Consider therapy with ^{131}I for the following patients:
        • Elderly patients with Graves' disease
        • Patients with a solitary toxic nodule (will most likely only destroy the hyperactive one).
        • Patients with Graves' disease in whom therapy with antithyroid drugs fails (e.g., due to relapse, agranulocytosis)

Handwritten margin notes: Methimazole - Tapazole. 1st line treatment - drugs then radioactive iodine ablation and if nothing works than surgery.

Thyroid Storm

- **This is a life-threatening complication of thyrotoxicosis** characterized by an acute exacerbation of the manifestations of hyperthyroidism.
- There is usually a precipitating factor, such as infection, diabetic ketoacidosis (DKA), or stress (e.g., severe trauma, surgery, illness, childbirth).
- High mortality rate: up to 20% of patients enter a coma or die
- Clinical manifestations include marked fever, tachycardia, agitation or psychosis, confusion, and GI symptoms (e.g., nausea, vomiting, diarrhea).
- Provide supportive therapy with IV fluids, cooling blankets, and glucose. *b/c metabolism is revved up.*
- Give antithyroid agents (PTU every 2 hours). Follow with iodine to inhibit thyroid hormone release.
- Administer β-blockers for control of heart rate. Give dexamethasone to impair peripheral generation of T_3 from T_4 and to provide adrenal support.

QUICK HIT margin note: Thyroid cells are the only cells in the body that absorb iodine. Therefore, giving radioactive iodine destroys only thyroid cells.

*QUICK HIT margin note: The terms hyperthyroidism and thyrotoxicosis are interchangeable and refer to hyperfunctioning thyroid disease. **Thyroid storm is a medical emergency with life-threatening sequelae.***

Hypothyroidism

A. General characteristics

1. The onset of symptoms is usually insidious, and the condition may go undetected for years.

Box 4-1 Myxedema Coma

- A rare condition that presents with a depressed state of consciousness, profound hypothermia, and respiratory depression
- May develop after years of severe untreated hypothyroidism
- Precipitating factors are trauma, infection, cold exposure, and narcotics.
- **A medical emergency, with a high mortality rate (50% to 75%) even with treatment**
- Provide supportive therapy to maintain BP and respiration. Give IV thyroxine and hydrocortisone while carefully monitoring the hemodynamic state.

---

2. Sometimes a diagnosis is made solely on laboratory evidence in an asymptomatic patient.

B. Causes

1. Primary hypothyroidism is the failure of the thyroid to produce sufficient thyroid hormone. This accounts for about 95% of all cases.
   a. **Hashimoto's disease (chronic thyroiditis)**—most common cause of primary hypothyroidism
   b. Iatrogenic-second most common cause of primary hypothyroidism; results from prior treatments of hyperthyroidism, including:
      - Radioiodine therapy
      - Thyroidectomy
      - Medications (e.g., lithium)
2. Secondary hypothyroidism (due to pituitary disease; i.e., deficiency of TSH) and tertiary hypothyroidism (due to hypothalamic disease; i.e., deficiency of TRH) account for less than 5% of cases. **Both are associated with a low free T_4 and a low TSH level.**

C. Clinical features

1. Symptoms
   a. Fatigue, weakness, lethargy
   b. Heavy menstrual periods (menorrhagia), slight weight gain (10 to 30 lb)—patients are **not** typically obese
   c. Cold intolerance
   d. Constipation
   e. Slow mentation, inability to concentrate (mild at first, in later stages dementia can occur), dull expression
   f. Muscle weakness, arthralgias
   g. Depression
   h. Diminished hearing
2. Signs
   a. Dry skin, coarse hair; thickened, puffy features
   b. Hoarseness
   c. Nonpitting edema (edema due to glycosaminoglycan in interstitial tissues, not water and salt)
   d. Carpal tunnel syndrome
   e. Slow relaxation of deep tendon reflexes
   f. Loss of lateral portion of eyebrows
   g. Bradycardia
   h. Goiter (Hashimoto's disease-goiter is rubbery, nontender, and even nodular; subacute thyroiditis-goiter is very tender and enlarged, although not always symmetrically)

D. Diagnosis

1. **High TSH level-most sensitive indicator of hypothyroidism**
2. Low TSH level (secondary hypothyroidism)

QUICK HIT

Hashimoto's thyroiditis is associated with other autoimmune disorders (e.g., lupus, pernicious anemia).

QUICK HIT

TSH is primary test in screening for thyroid dysfunction. Also, order a lipid profile and a CBC.

Box 4-2   Subclinical Hypothyroidism

- Thyroid function is inadequate, but increased TSH production maintains T_4 level within the reference range of normalcy; therefore, TSH level is elevated and T_4 level is normal.
- Look for nonspecific or mild symptoms of hypothyroidism, as well as elevated serum LDL levels.
- Treat with thyroxine if patients develop a goiter, hypercholesterolemia, symptoms of hypothyroidism, or significantly elevated TSH level (>20 μU/mL).

---

3. Low free T_4 level (or free T_4 index) in patients with clinically overt hypothyroidism. Free T_4 may be normal in subclinical cases.
4. Increased antimicrosomal antibodies (Hashimoto's thyroiditis)
5. Other laboratory value abnormalities that may be present:
   a. Elevated LDL and decreased HDL levels
   b. Anemia—Mild normocytic anemia is the most common.

E. **Treatment:** levothyroxine (T_4)—treatment of choice
   1. Effect is evident in 2 to 4 weeks; highly effective in achieving euthyroid state
   2. Convenient once-daily morning dose
   3. Treatment is continued indefinitely.
   4. Monitor TSH level and clinical state periodically.

Thyroiditis

A. **Subacute (viral) thyroiditis** (subacute granulomatous thyroiditis)
   1. Causes—usually follows a viral illness
   2. Clinical features
      a. Prodromal phase of a few weeks (fever, flu-like illness)
      b. It can cause transient hyperthyroidism due to leakage of hormone from inflamed thyroid gland. This is followed by a euthyroid state and then a hypothyroid state (as hormones are depleted).
      c. **Painful**, tender thyroid gland (may be enlarged)
   3. Diagnosis
      a. **Radioiodine uptake is low** because thyroid follicular cells are damaged and cannot trap iodine.
      b. Low TSH level secondary to suppression by increased T_4 and T_3 levels; high erythrocyte sedimentation rate (ESR).
   4. Treatment
      a. Use NSAIDs and aspirin for mild symptoms; corticosteroids if the pain is more severe.
      b. Most patients have recovery of thyroid function within a few months to 1 year.

B. **Subacute lymphocytic thyroiditis** (painless thyroiditis, silent thyroiditis)
   1. A transient thyrotoxic phase of 2 to 5 months may be followed by a hypothyroid phase. The hypothyroid phase is usually self-limited and may be the only manifestation of this disease if the hyperthyroid phase is brief.
   2. Low radioactive iodine uptake—differentiates it from Graves' disease during thyrotoxic phase
   3. Similar to subacute (viral) thyroiditis, only without the pain or tenderness of the thyroid gland

C. **Chronic lymphocytic thyroiditis** (Hashimoto's thyroiditis, lymphocytic thyroiditis)
   1. Most common cause of autoimmune thyroid disorder; more common in women
   2. Causes
      a. Genetic component—Family history is common.
      b. Antithyroid antibodies are present in the majority of patients.
   3. Clinical manifestations

(handwritten margin notes): ① subacute granulomatous thyroiditis → ② subacute lymphocytic thyroiditis. inflammatory process.

Box 4-3 Thyroid-Associated Ophthalmopathy (TAO)

- TAO is an autoimmune attack on the periorbital connective tissue and extraocular muscles.
- Clinical findings include lid retraction ("thyroid stare"), proptosis, eyelid edema, lagophthalmos (inability to close eyelids completely), and diplopia.
- Patients may be hypothyroid, hyperthyroid (Graves' disease), or euthyroid when TAO presents. Most euthyroid patients will go on to develop thyroid dysfunction within 2 years of developing TAO.
- Treatment of thyroid dysfunction has little effect on the course of TAO. TAO is usually self-limited, but surgery may be required if disease is severe. Oral steroids may also be helpful.

    a. Goiter is the most common feature.
    b. Hypothyroidism is present in 20% of cases when first diagnosed and may occur later in disease.
  4. Diagnosis
    a. Thyroid function studies are normal (unless hypothyroidism is present).
    b. Antithyroid antibodies: antiperoxidase antibodies (present in 90% of patients), antithyroglobulin antibodies (present in 50%)
    c. Irregular distribution of ^{131}I on thyroid scan—not required for diagnosis
  5. Treatment—thyroid hormone (to achieve euthyroid state)

D. Fibrous thyroiditis (Riedel's thyroiditis)
  1. Fibrous tissue replaces thyroid tissue, leading to a firm thyroid.
  2. Surgery may be necessary if complications occur.
  3. Patient may be hypothyroid as well, in which case thyroid hormone should be prescribed.

Thyroid Nodules

A. General characteristics
  1. Cancer is found in 10% to 20% of nodules that are investigated.
  2. A solitary nodule can be either thyroid cancer or a benign adenoma. However, multinodular conditions may be leading, because only one of these nodules may be palpable.
  3. The most important function of the physical examination is the detection of the thyroid nodule, rather than the determination of its benign or malignant status.
  4. To be detectable on palpation, a nodule must be at least 1 cm in diameter.
  5. Malignancy is suggested by the following:
    a. If the nodule is fixed in place and no movement occurs on swallowing
    b. Unusually firm consistency or irregularity of the nodule
    c. If the nodule is solitary

Box 4-4 Fine-Needle Aspiration (FNA)

- A needle is inserted into the nodule, and cells are aspirated and then examined under a microscope.
- False-positive and false-negative rates approach 5%.
- **This is the only test that can reliably differentiate between benign and malignant nodules.**
  - Ultrasound differentiates between solid and cystic nodules, but either may be malignant.
  - On the thyroid scan, "cold" nodules are more likely to be malignant than "hot," but this is not reliable.
- FNA findings:
  - Probable cancer (15%): Most of these are really cancers. Surgery is indicated.
  - Indeterminate (19%): A thyroid scan should be performed, and if the lesion is "cold" by the scan, surgical resection is indicated because about 20% of these lesions are found to be malignant.
  - Benign (66%): Most of these are benign. Observe for 1 year, then follow up with an ultrasound.
  - Follicular neoplasm: Surgery is recommended because it is difficult to distinguish between benign and malignant follicular cells on histology.

d. History of radiation therapy to the neck
e. History of rapid development
f. Vocal cord paralysis (recurrent laryngeal nerve paralysis)
g. Cervical adenopathy
h. Elevated serum calcitonin

B. Diagnosis (see Figure 4-2)
1. Fine-needle aspiration (FNA) biopsy
   a. **Test of choice for initial evaluation of a thyroid nodule**
   b. Accuracy
      - FNA has a sensitivity of 95% and a specificity of 95%. Therefore, if FNA shows a benign nodule, the nodule is likely to be benign.
      - However, FNA biopsies have 5% false-negative results, so follow up with periodic FNA if thyroid nodularity persists. Benign lesions should continue to show consistently benign cytology.
      - FNA is reliable for all cancers (papillary, medullary, anaplastic) **except follicular.**
2. Thyroid scan (radioactive iodine) (see Figure 4-1)
   a. Thyroid scan plays a supplemental role. It is performed if the FNA biopsy is indeterminate.
   b. It gives graphic representations of the distribution of radioactive iodine in the gland—useful in identifying whether thyroid nodules show decreased ("cold") or increased ("hot") accumulation of radioactive iodine compared with normal paranodular tissue. Nodules are classified as "cold" (hypofunctional), "warm" (normally functioning), or "hot" (hyperfunctional).
   c. It should be limited to patients whose FNA biopsy results suggest neoplasm. (It is not cost effective to scan all patients with thyroid nodules.) When such lesions are "cold" on scan, thyroid lobectomy is recommended.
3. Thyroid ultrasound
   a. Differentiates a solid from a cystic nodule; most cancers are solid
   b. Can identify nodules 1 to 3 mm in diameter
   c. Cystic masses larger than 4 cm in diameter are not malignant.
   d. Cannot distinguish between benign and malignant thyroid nodules

Thyroid Cancer

A. General characteristics
1. Risk factors
   a. Head and neck radiation (during childhood)
   b. Gardner's syndrome and Cowden's syndrome for papillary cancer
   c. MEN type II for medullary cancer
2. Types
   a. Papillary carcinoma
      - Accounts for 70% to 80% of all thyroid cancers

> **QUICK HIT**
> In general, most patients with thyroid cancer do not die of thyroid cancer (although this depends on the type of thyroid cancer).

Box 4-5 Nodules

"Cold" Nodules	"Hot" Nodules
• Increased iodine uptake = hypofunctioning nodule	• Increased iodine uptake = hyperfunctioning nodule
• Significant risk of malignancy—Approximately 20% of cold nodules are malignant.	• Rarely associated with malignancy
• Of all nodules, 70% to 90% are cold, and most of these are benign. Therefore, scanning may indicate a greatly reduced risk of malignancy in a nodule that is warm or hot, but it does not yield much additional information in a nodule that is cold.	

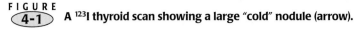

FIGURE 4-1 A ^{123}I thyroid scan showing a large "cold" nodule (arrow).

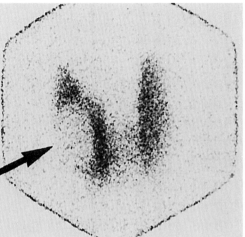

(From Fishman MC, Hoffman AR, Klausner RD, et al. Medicine. 5th Ed. Philadelphia: Lippincott Williams & Wilkins, 2004:185, Figure 22-1.)

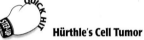

Hürthle's Cell Tumor
- A variant of follicular cancer but more aggressive
- Spread by lymphatics; does not take up iodine
- Treatment: total thyroidectomy

- Least aggressive thyroid cancer-slow growth and slow spreading
- Spreads via lymphatics in neck; frequently metastasizes to cervical lymph nodes (cervical lymphadenopathy); distant metastasis is rare
- Positive iodine uptake

b. Follicular carcinoma
- Accounts for 15% of all thyroid cancers; avidly absorbs iodine
- Prognosis is worse than for papillary cancer—it spreads early via a hematogenous route (brain, lung, bone, liver). Distant metastasis occurs in 20% of patients; lymph node involvement is uncommon.
- More malignant than papillary cancer, but these are also slow growing

FIGURE 4-2 Algorithm for the evaluation of a solitary thyroid nodule. Once a thyroid nodule is detected on physical examination, FNA is the initial study of choice. (FNA, fine-needle aspiration; U/S, ultrasound)

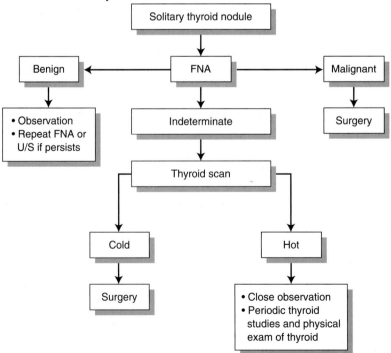

c. Medullary carcinoma
  - Accounts for 2% to 3% of all thyroid cancers
  - One-third sporadic, one-third familial, one-third associated with MEN II (always screen for pheochromocytoma) *↳ urine metanephrine*
  - Produces calcitonin
  - More malignant than follicular cancer but less so than anaplastic cancer–survival of approximately 10 years
d. Anaplastic carcinoma
  - Accounts for 5% of all thyroid cancers; mostly seen in (elderly patients)
  - Highly malignant
  - Prognosis (grim)—Death typically occurs within a few months. Mortality is usually due to invasion of adjacent organs (trachea, neck vessels). *locally spreading aggressive tumor*

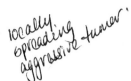

Papillary carcinoma is the most common type of thyroid cancer to develop after radiation exposure (accounts for 80% to 90% of postradiation cancers of the thyroid).

B. Diagnosis
1. Thyroid hormone level (frequently normal)
2. Calcitonin level (if medullary carcinoma)
3. Refer to section on thyroid nodules for diagnostic approach. *→ FNA*

C. Treatment
1. Papillary carcinoma
   a. Lobectomy with isthmusectomy
   b. Total thyroidectomy if tumor is >3 cm, tumor is bilateral, tumor is advanced, or distant metastases are present.
   c. Adjuvant treatment: TSH suppression therapy; radioiodine therapy for larger tumors
2. Follicular carcinoma—total thyroidectomy with postoperative iodine ablation
3. Medullary carcinoma—total thyroidectomy; radioiodine therapy usually unsuccessful
   No chemotherapy.
4. Anaplastic carcinoma—Chemotherapy and radiation may provide a modest improvement in survival.

DISEASES OF THE PITUITARY GLAND

Pituitary Adenomas

A. General characteristics
1. Pituitary adenomas account for about 10% of all intracranial neoplasms.
2. Almost all pituitary tumors are benign. They may grow in any direction causing "parasellar" signs and symptoms.
3. Size: microadenoma (diameter ≤10 mm); macroadenoma (diameter ≥11 mm)

B. Clinical features
1. Hormonal effects occur due to hypersecretion of one or more of the following hormones:
   a. Prolactin—see the following section on hyperprolactinemia
   b. GH—results in acromegaly (or gigantism if epiphyseal closure has not occurred) *– also diabetes–*
   c. ACTH—results in Cushing's disease
   d. TSH—results in hyperthyroidism
2. Hypopituitarism—compression of hypothalamic-pituitary stalk; GH deficiency and hypogonadotropic hypogonadism are the most common problems
3. Mass effects
   a. Headache
   b. Visual defects—Bitemporal hemianopsia (due to compression of optic chiasm) is the most common finding, but it depends on the size and symmetry of the tumor. *do a visual fields test on pts. complaining of chronic headache.*

C. Diagnosis
1. MRI is the imaging study of choice.
2. Pituitary hormone levels

D. Treatment
1. Transsphenoidal surgery is indicated in most patients (except patients with prolactinomas, for which medical management can be tried first).
2. Radiation therapy and medical therapy are adjuncts in most patients.

bromocriptine

Hyperprolactinemia

A. Causes
1. Prolactinoma
   a. Most common cause of hyperprolactinemia
   b. Most common type of pituitary adenoma (up to 40%)
2. Medications (e.g., psychiatric medications, H_2 blockers, metoclopramide, verapamil, estrogen)
3. Pregnancy
4. Renal failure
5. Suprasellar mass lesions (can compress hypothalamus or pituitary stalk)
6. Hypothyroidism
7. Idiopathic

> **QUICK HIT**
> High levels of prolactin inhibit secretion of GnRH. This leads to decreased secretion of LH and FSH, which in turn leads to decreased production of estrogen and testosterone.

B. Clinical features
1. Men
   a. Hypogonadism, decreased libido, infertility, impotence
   b. Galactorrhea or gynecomastia (uncommon)
   c. Parasellar signs and symptoms (visual field defects and headaches)
2. Women
   a. Premenopausal: menstrual irregularities, oligomenorrhea or amenorrhea, anovulation and infertility, decreased libido, dyspareunia, vaginal dryness, risk of osteoporosis, galactorrhea
   b. Postmenopausal: parasellar signs and symptoms (less common than in men)

> **QUICK HIT**
> Parasellar signs and symptoms (mass effects of the tumor) are more prevalent in men than in women. This is largely because the early symptoms in men (e.g., impotence) are often attributed to psychological causes and medical evaluation is delayed, allowing for larger tumor growth.

C. Diagnosis
1. Elevated serum prolactin level
2. Order a pregnancy test and TSH level, because both pregnancy and primary hypothyroidism are on the differential diagnosis for hyperprolactinemia.
3. CT scan or MRI to identify any mass lesions

D. Treatment
1. Treat the underlying cause (e.g., stop medication, treat hypothyroidism)
2. If prolactinoma is the cause and the patient is symptomatic, treat with bromocriptine, a dopamine agonist that secondarily diminishes production and release of prolactin. Continue treatment for approximately 2 years before attempting cessation. Cabergoline (dopamine agonist) may be better tolerated than bromocriptine.
3. Consider surgical intervention if symptoms progress despite bromocriptine. However, the recurrence rate after surgery is high.

> **QUICK HIT**
> Microadenomas (<10 mm diameter) tend to either remain the same size or regress with time. Only 10% to 20% continue to grow.

Acromegaly

A. General characteristics
1. Acromegaly is a broadening of the skeleton that results from excess secretion of pituitary GH after epiphyseal closure (if before epiphyseal closure, gigantism [excessive height] results).
2. It is almost always caused by a GH-secreting pituitary adenoma (represents 10% of pituitary adenomas).

B. Clinical features
1. Growth promotion
   a. Soft tissue and skeleton overgrowth

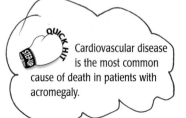

> **QUICK HIT**
> Cardiovascular disease is the most common cause of death in patients with acromegaly.

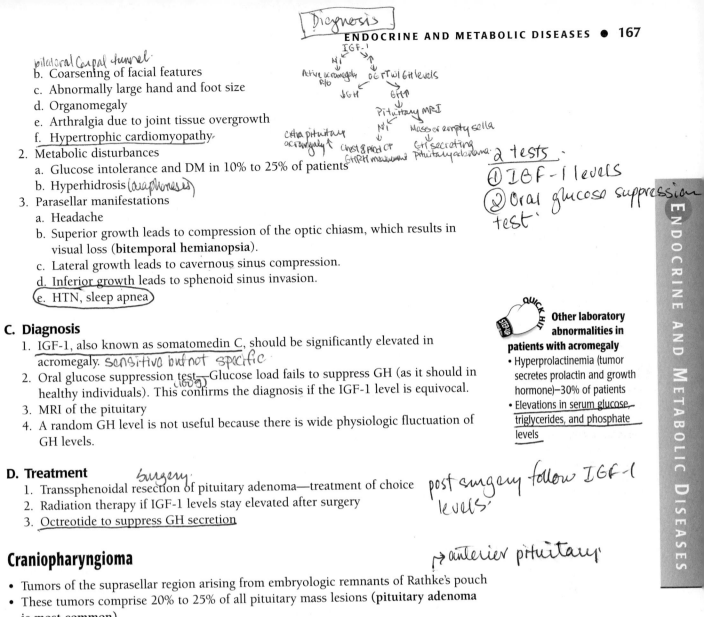

(handwritten) Diagnosis

b. Coarsening of facial features *(handwritten: bilateral carpal tunnel)*
c. Abnormally large hand and foot size
d. Organomegaly
e. Arthralgia due to joint tissue overgrowth
f. Hypertrophic cardiomyopathy
2. Metabolic disturbances
    a. Glucose intolerance and DM in 10% to 25% of patients
    b. Hyperhidrosis *(handwritten: diaphoresis)*
3. Parasellar manifestations
    a. Headache
    b. Superior growth leads to compression of the optic chiasm, which results in visual loss (**bitemporal hemianopsia**).
    c. Lateral growth leads to cavernous sinus compression.
    d. Inferior growth leads to sphenoid sinus invasion.
    e. HTN, sleep apnea

C. Diagnosis
1. IGF-1, also known as somatomedin C, should be significantly elevated in acromegaly. *(handwritten: sensitive but not specific)*
2. Oral glucose suppression test—Glucose load fails to suppress GH (as it should in healthy individuals). This confirms the diagnosis if the IGF-1 level is equivocal. *(handwritten: 100g)*
3. MRI of the pituitary
4. A random GH level is not useful because there is wide physiologic fluctuation of GH levels.

D. Treatment
(handwritten: surgery)
1. Transsphenoidal resection of pituitary adenoma—treatment of choice *(handwritten: post surgery follow IGF-1 levels)*
2. Radiation therapy if IGF-1 levels stay elevated after surgery
3. Octreotide to suppress GH secretion

QUICK HIT

Other laboratory abnormalities in patients with acromegaly
- Hyperprolactinemia (tumor secretes prolactin and growth hormone)–30% of patients
- Elevations in serum glucose, triglycerides, and phosphate levels

(handwritten right margin: 2 tests. ① IGF-1 levels ② Oral glucose suppression test)

Craniopharyngioma

(handwritten: anterior pituitary)

- Tumors of the suprasellar region arising from embryologic remnants of Rathke's pouch
- These tumors comprise 20% to 25% of all pituitary mass lesions (**pituitary adenoma is most common**).
- They result in visual field defects (bitemporal hemianopsia) due to compression of the optic chiasm, and may also cause headaches, papilledema, and changes in mentation.
- They are diagnosed by brain MRI.
- They may cause hyperprolactinemia, diabetes insipidus, or panhypopituitarism.
- Treatment is surgical excision (total or partial resection) with or without radiation therapy.

Hypopituitarism

A. General characteristics
1. All or some of the hormones released from the anterior pituitary may be absent.
2. Loss of hormones is unpredictable, but LH, FSH, and GH are usually lost before TSH and ACTH.
3. Clinical manifestations depend on which hormones are lost.

B. Causes
1. Hypothalamic or pituitary tumor is the most common cause.
2. Other causes: radiation therapy, Sheehan's syndrome, infiltrative processes (e.g., sarcoidosis, hemochromatosis), head trauma, cavernous sinus thrombosis, surgery

C. Clinical features
1. Reduced GH: growth failure (decreased muscle mass in adults)
2. Reduced prolactin: failure to lactate

3. Reduced ACTH: adrenal insufficiency
4. Reduced TSH: hypothyroidism
5. Reduced gonadotropins (LH and FSH): infertility, amenorrhea, loss of secondary sex characteristics, diminished libido
6. Reduced ADH (if hypothalamic lesion): diabetes insipidus
7. Reduced melanocyte-stimulating hormone: decreased skin and hair pigmentation

D. Diagnosis

1. Low levels of target hormones with low or normal levels of trophic hormones (it is the suppression of the trophic hormone that is important, although the absolute level may be in the normal reference range).
2. MRI of the brain (may miss microadenomas)

E. Treatment

1. Replacement of appropriate hormones
2. Women who want to conceive should be referred to an endocrinologist.

Diabetes Insipidus (DI)

A. General characteristics

1. Two forms
   a. Central DI is the most common form—due to low ADH secretion by posterior pituitary
   b. Nephrogenic DI—ADH secretion is normal but tubules cannot respond to ADH.
2. Causes
   a. Central DI
      • Idiopathic—50% of all cases
      • Trauma—surgery, head trauma
      • Other destructive processes involving the hypothalamus, including tumors, sarcoidosis, tuberculosis, syphilis, Hand-Schüller-Christian disease, eosinophilic granuloma, and encephalitis
   b. Nephrogenic DI—causes include hypokalemia, hypercalcemia, lithium, demeclocycline, and pyelonephritis; it may also be congenital.

B. Clinical features

1. Polyuria is a hallmark finding: 5 to 15 L daily; urine is colorless (because it is so dilute).
2. Thirst and polydipsia—Hydration is maintained if the patient is conscious and has access to water.
3. Hypernatremia is usually mild unless the patient has an impaired thirst drive.

C. Diagnosis

1. Urine—Low specific gravity and low osmolality indicate DI.
2. Plasma osmolality
   a. Normal: 250 to 290 mOsm/kg
   b. Primary polydipsia: 255 to 280 mOsm/kg
   c. DI: 280 to 310 mOsm/kg
3. A water deprivation test (dehydration test) is required to make the diagnosis (see Table 4-1).
   a. Procedure
      • Withhold fluids, and measure urine osmolality every hour.
      • When urine osmolality is stable (<30 mOsm/kg hourly increase for 3 hours), inject 2 g desmopressin subcutaneously. Measure urine osmolality 1 hour later.
   b. Response—see Table 4-1
4. ADH level (not the test of choice; takes a long time to get results)
   a. Low in central DI
   b. Normal or elevated in nephrogenic DI

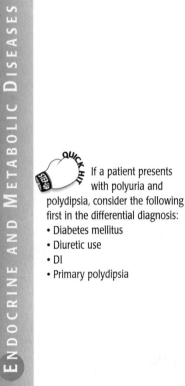

If a patient presents with polyuria and polydipsia, consider the following first in the differential diagnosis:
• Diabetes mellitus
• Diuretic use
• DI
• Primary polydipsia

• Primary polydipsia is usually seen in patients with psychiatric disturbances.
• If the patient is deprived of water, urine osmolality will increase appropriately.

TABLE 4-1 **Response to the Water Deprivation Test**

	Increase in Urine Osmolality Above 280 mOsm/kg With Dehydration	Further Response to ADH
Normal patients	+	−
Diabetes insipidus patients	−	+
Nephrogenic diabetes insipidus patients	−	−

Adapted from Step-Up, pg 144, Table 6-9.

D. Treatment
1. Central DI
   a. Desmopressin (DDAVP) is the primary therapy and can be given by nasal spray, orally, or by injection.
   b. Chlorpropamide increases ADH secretion and enhances the effect of ADH.
   c. Treat the underlying cause.
2. Nephrogenic DI—Treat with thiazide diuretics.
   a. These deplete the body of sodium, which leads to increased reabsorption of sodium and water in the proximal tubules.
   b. The reabsorption of sodium and water in the proximal tubules means that less water reaches the distal tubules, leading to decreased urine volume.

Syndrome of Inappropriate Secretion of Antidiuretic Hormone (SIADH)

A. General characteristics
1. Pathophysiology
   a. Excess ADH is secreted from the posterior pituitary or an ectopic source. Elevated levels lead to water retention and excretion of concentrated urine. This has two major effects: hyponatremia and volume expansion.
   b. **Despite volume expansion, edema is not seen in SIADH.** This is because natriuresis (excretion of excessive sodium in urine) occurs despite hyponatremia.
   c. Reasons for natriuresis
      • Volume expansion causes an increase in atrial natriuretic peptide (increases urine sodium excretion).
      • Volume expansion leads to a decrease in proximal tubular sodium absorption.
      • The renin-angiotensin-aldosterone system is inhibited.

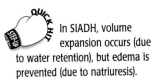

In SIADH, volume expansion occurs (due to water retention), but edema is prevented (due to natriuresis).

Hyponatremia pearls
• Hypovolemic hyponatremia–volume contracted
• Hypervolemic hyponatremia–volume expanded with edema
• SIADH–volume expanded without edema

B. Causes
1. Neoplasms (e.g., in lung, pancreas, prostate, bladder), lymphomas, leukemia
2. CNS disorders (e.g., stroke, head trauma, infection)
3. Pulmonary disorders (e.g., pneumonia, tuberculosis)
4. Ventilators with positive pressure
5. Medication (e.g., vincristine, selective serotonin reuptake inhibitors [SSRIs], chlorpropamide, oxytocin, morphine, desmopressin)
6. Postoperative state (e.g., as a result of anesthesia, pain)

C. Clinical features
1. Acute hyponatremia—Signs and symptoms are secondary to brain swelling (osmotic water shifts, leading to increased ICF volume), and are primarily neurologic.
   a. Lethargy, somnolence, weakness
   b. **Can lead to seizures, coma, or death if untreated**
2. Chronic hyponatremia
   a. May be asymptomatic

b. Anorexia, nausea, and vomiting

c. CNS symptoms are less common because chronic loss of sodium and potassium from brain cells decreases brain edema (due to secondary water shifts from ICF to ECF).

D. Diagnosis

1. **SIADH is a diagnosis of exclusion** (after other causes of hyponatremia have been ruled out). The following help in supporting the diagnosis:

   a. Hyponatremia and inappropriately concentrated urine; plasma osmolality <270 mmol/kg

   b. Low serum uric acid level

   c. Low BUN and creatinine

   d. Normal thyroid and adrenal function, as well as renal, cardiac, and liver function

   e. Measurement of plasma and urine ADH level

   f. Absence of significant hypervolemia

2. **Water-load test**—The patient drinks a water load, and urine output is measured hourly. If a large amount of water is excreted in the urine (>65% in 4 hours), consider SIADH a likely diagnosis.

E. Treatment

1. Correct the underlying cause, if known.

2. For asymptomatic patients

   a. Water restriction is usually sufficient.

   b. Use normal saline in combination with a loop diuretic if faster results are desired.

   c. Lithium carbonate or demeclocycline are other options (with side effects)—both inhibit the effect of ADH in the kidney.

3. For symptomatic patients

   a. Restrict water intake.

   b. Give isotonic saline. Hypertonic saline may occasionally be indicated in severe cases.

4. Do not raise the serum sodium concentration too quickly. Rapid flux of water into the ECF can result in **central pontine myelinolysis** (demyelination syndrome may result). A general guideline is that the rate of sodium replacement should not exceed 0.5 mEq/L per hour.

DISEASES OF THE PARATHYROID GLANDS

Hypoparathyroidism

A. Causes

1. Head and neck surgery account for the majority of cases—thyroidectomy, parathyroidectomy, radical surgery for head and neck malignancies.

2. Nonsurgical hypoparathyroidism is rare.

B. Clinical features

1. Cardiac arrhythmias

2. Rickets and osteomalacia

3. Increased neuromuscular irritability due to hypocalcemia

   a. Numbness/tingling—circumoral, fingers, toes

   b. Tetany
      • Hyperactive deep tendon reflexes
      • *Chvostek's sign*—Tapping the facial nerve elicits contraction of facial muscles.
      • *Trousseau's sign*—Inflating the BP cuff to a pressure higher than the patient's systolic BP for 3 minutes elicits carpal spasms.

   c. Grand mal seizures

4. Basal ganglia calcifications

5. **Prolonged QT interval** on ECG—Hypocalcemia should always be in the differential diagnosis of a prolonged QT interval.

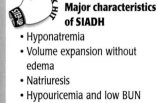

Major characteristics of SIADH
- Hyponatremia
- Volume expansion without edema
- Natriuresis
- Hypouricemia and low BUN
- Normal or reduced serum creatinine level because of dilution
- Normal thyroid and adrenal function

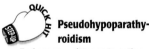

Pseudohypoparathyroidism
- End-organ resistance to action of PTH
- Laboratory value findings: hypocalcemia, hyperphosphatemia, high PTH, low urinary cAMP

C. Diagnosis
1. Low serum calcium
2. High serum phosphate
3. Serum PTH inappropriately low
4. Low urine cAMP

D. Treatment
1. IV calcium gluconate in severe cases, oral calcium in mild to moderate cases
2. Vitamin D supplementation (calcitriol)
3. Note that both vitamin D and calcium replacement can increase urinary calcium excretion, precipitating kidney stones. Therefore administer with caution to avoid hypercalciuria (the goal is to keep serum calcium at 8.0 to 8.5 mg/dL).

Primary Hyperparathyroidism

A. General characteristics
1. One or more glands produce inappropriately high amounts of PTH relative to the serum calcium level.
2. Most common cause of hypercalcemia

B. Causes
1. Adenoma (80% of cases)—majority involve only one gland
2. Hyperplasia (15% to 20% of cases)—all four glands usually affected
3. Carcinoma (<1% of cases)

C. Clinical features
1. "Stones"
   a. Nephrolithiasis
   b. Nephrocalcinosis
2. "Bones"
   a. Bone aches and pains
   b. **Osteitis fibrosa cystica ("brown tumors")**—predisposes patient to pathologic fractures
3. "Groans"
   a. Muscle pain and weakness
   b. Pancreatitis
   c. Peptic ulcer disease
   d. Gout
   e. Constipation
4. "Psychiatric overtones"—depression, fatigue, anorexia, sleep disturbances, anxiety, lethargy
5. Other symptoms:
   a. Polydipsia, polyuria
   b. HTN, shortened QT interval
   c. Weight loss

D. Diagnosis
1. Laboratory
   a. Calcium levels (hypercalcemia)—When calculating calcium levels, be aware of albumin levels. Calculate the ionized fraction or get an ionized calcium level.

Box 4-6   Secondary Hyperparathyroidism

- Characterized by an elevated concentration of PTH and a low or low-normal serum calcium level
- Caused by chronic renal failure (most common cause), as well as vitamin D deficiency and renal hypercalciuria
- Treatment depends on the cause: if vitamin D deficiency, give vitamin D; if renal failure, give calcitriol and oral calcium supplements plus dietary phosphorus restriction.

ENDOCRINE AND METABOLIC DISEASES

b. PTH levels
- Should be elevated relative to serum calcium level
- Note that in the presence of hypercalcemia, a normal PTH level is "abnormal" (i.e., high) because high calcium levels suppress PTH secretion.

c. Hypophosphatemia
d. Hypercalciuria
e. Urine cAMP is elevated
f. Chloride/phosphorus ratio of >33 is diagnostic of primary hyperparathyroidism (33-to-1 rule). Chloride is high secondary to renal bicarbonate wasting (direct effect of PTH).

2. Radiographs
a. Subperiosteal bone resorption (usually on radial aspect of second and third phalanges)
b. Osteopenia

E. Treatment

1. Surgery is the only definitive treatment, but not all patients require it. If the patient is over 50 years of age and is asymptomatic (with normal bone mass and renal function), surgery may not be needed.
a. Primary hyperparathyroidism due to hyperplasia—all four glands are removed. A small amount of parathyroid tissue is placed in forearm muscle to retain parathyroid function.
b. Primary hyperparathyroidism due to adenoma—Surgical removal of the adenoma is curative.
c. Primary hyperparathyroidism due to carcinoma—Remove the tumor, ipsilateral thyroid lobe, and all enlarged lymph nodes.

2. Medical—Encourage fluids. Give diuretics (furosemide) to enhance calcium excretion if hypercalcemia is severe. (Do not give thiazide diuretics!)

DISEASES OF THE ADRENAL GLANDS

Cushing's Syndrome

A. General characteristics

1. Cushing's **syndrome** results from excessive levels of glucocorticoids (cortisol is the principal glucocorticoid) due to any cause.
2. Cushing's **disease** results from pituitary Cushing's syndrome (pituitary adenoma).

B. Causes

1. Iatrogenic Cushing's syndrome is the most common cause, and is due to prescribed prednisone or other steroids. Androgen excess is absent (because the exogenous steroid suppresses androgen production by the adrenals).
2. ACTH-secreting adenoma of the pituitary (Cushing's disease) is the second most common cause and leads to bilateral adrenal hyperplasia. Androgen excess is common.
3. Adrenal adenomas and carcinomas (10% to 15%)
4. Ectopic ACTH production (10% to 15%)
a. ACTH-secreting tumor stimulates the cortisol release from the adrenal glands without the normal negative feedback loop (because the source of the ACTH is outside the pituitary gland).
b. More than two-thirds are small cell carcinomas of the lung. Bronchial carcinoid and thymoma may be the cause.

C. Clinical features

1. Changes in appearance: central obesity, hirsutism, moon facies, "buffalo hump," purple striae on abdomen, lanugo hair, acne, easy bruising
2. HTN

Relative indications for surgery in primary hyperparathyroidism
- Age <50 years
- Marked decrease in bone mass
- Nephrolithiasis, renal insufficiency
- Markedly elevated serum calcium level or episode of severe hypercalcemia
- Urine calcium >400 mg in 24 hours

Effects of cortisol (generally catabolic)
- Impaired collagen production, enhanced protein catabolism
- Anti-insulin effects (leading to glucose intolerance)
- Impaired immunity (has inhibitory effects on PMNs, T cells)
- Enhances catecholamine activity (HTN)

3. Decreased glucose tolerance (diabetes)
4. Hypogonadism—menstrual irregularity and infertility
5. Masculinization in females (androgen excess)—only seen in ACTH-dependent forms
6. Musculoskeletal—proximal muscle wasting and weakness (due to protein catabolism), osteoporosis, aseptic necrosis of femoral head may occur (especially with exogenous steroid use)
7. Psychiatric disturbances—depression, mania
8. Increased likelihood of infections (due to impaired immunity)

D. Diagnosis (see Figure 4-3)

1. Initial screening
   a. An overnight (low-dose) dexamethasone suppression test is the initial screening test. Give the patient 1 mg of dexamethasone at 11 PM. Measure the serum cortisol level at 8 AM.
      • If the serum cortisol is <5, Cushing's syndrome can be excluded (this test is very sensitive).
      • If the serum cortisol is >5 (and often >10), the patient has Cushing's syndrome. Order a high-dose dexamethasone suppression test to determine the cause (Cushing's disease versus adrenal tumor versus ectopic ACTH tumor).
   b. The 24-hour urinary free cortisol level is another excellent screening test; values greater than four times normal are rare except in Cushing's syndrome.
2. ACTH level—Once you establish a diagnosis of Cushing's syndrome, measure the ACTH level. If it is low, the cause of high cortisol levels is likely an adrenal tumor or hyperplasia, not a pituitary disease or an ectopic ACTH-producing tumor.
3. High-dose dexamethasone suppression test
   a. In Cushing's disease, the result is a decrease in cortisol levels (greater than 50% suppression occurs).
   b. If cortisol suppression does **not** occur and plasma ACTH levels are high, an ectopic ACTH-producing tumor is likely the diagnosis.
4. CRH stimulation test—CRH is administered intravenously.
   a. If ACTH/cortisol levels increase (deemed a "response"), then Cushing's disease is the diagnosis.
   b. If ACTH/cortisol levels do not increase (deemed "no response"), then patient has either ectopic ACTH secretion or an adrenal tumor.
5. Imaging tests (once hormonal studies have established the site of disease, e.g., pituitary or adrenal)—CT scan or MRI of the appropriate area

E. Treatment

1. Iatrogenic Cushing's syndrome: tapering of glucocorticoid
2. Pituitary Cushing's syndrome: surgery (transsphenoidal ablation of pituitary adenoma)—usually safe and effective
3. Adrenal adenoma or carcinoma: surgery (adrenalectomy)

Pheochromocytoma

A. General characteristics

1. Pheochromocytomas are rare tumors that produce, store, and secrete catecholamines. (Norepinephrine)
2. 90% found in adrenal medulla (10% extra-adrenal)
3. Curable if diagnosed and treated, but **may be fatal if undiagnosed**

B. Clinical features

1. HTN—BP is persistently high, with episodes of severe HTN (paroxysmal).
2. Severe pounding headache
3. Inappropriate severe sweating

Some signs and symptoms in patients with high cortisol (e.g., obesity, HTN, osteoporosis, DM) are nonspecific and less helpful in diagnosing the patient. On the other hand, easy bruising, typical striae, myopathy, and virilizing signs are more helpful in diagnosis.

Patients with **Cushing's disease** may have **hyperpigmentation** due to elevated ACTH levels, whereas patients with Cushing's syndrome due to other causes will not have hyperpigmentation.

Rule of 10s for pheochromocytoma tumors
• 10% are familial
• 10% are bilateral (suspect MEN type II)
• 10% are malignant
• 10% are multiple
• 10% occur in children
• 10% are extra-adrenal (more often malignant)—The most common site is the organ of Zuckerkandl, which is located at the aortic bifurcation.

If the following are all present, pheochromocytoma is the diagnosis until proven otherwise.
• Headache
• Profuse sweating
• Palpitations
• Apprehension or sense of impending doom

TABLE 4-2	Response to Diagnostic Tests in Cushing's Syndrome
Healthy patient	• Normal cortisol/normal ACTH • Suppression with low-dose dexamethasone • Suppression with high-dose dexamethasone • Mild increase with CRH test
Cushing's disease	• High cortisol/high ACTH • No suppression with low-dose dexamethasone • Suppression with high-dose dexamethasone • Great increase in cortisol with CRH test
Adrenal tumor	• High cortisol/low ACTH • No suppression with low-dose dexamethasone • No suppression with high-dose dexamethasone • No change after CRH test
Ectopic ACTH-producing tumor	• High cortisol/high ACTH • No suppression with low-dose dexamethasone • No suppression with high-dose dexamethasone • No change after CRH test

4. Palpitations, with sudden severe HTN
5. Anxiety
6. Feeling of impending doom
7. Laboratory findings: hyperglycemia, hyperlipidemia, hypokalemia

FIGURE
4-3 **Algorithm for the diagnosis of Cushing's syndrome and its cause. (ACTH, adrenocorticotropic hormone; DM, dexamethasone)**

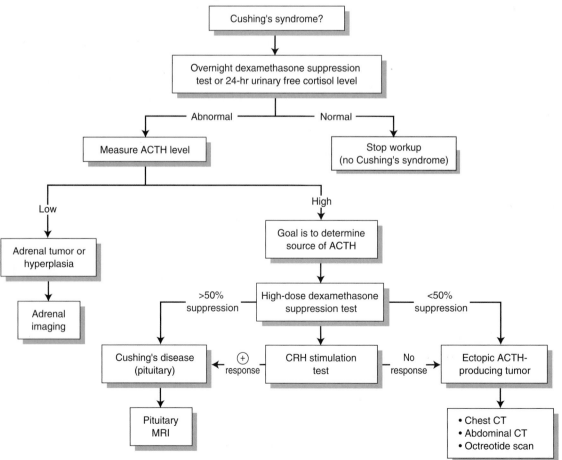

(Adapted from Humes DH, DuPont HL, Gardner LB, et al. Kelley's Textbook of Internal Medicine. 4th Ed. Philadelphia: Lippincott Williams & Wilkins, 2000:2725, Figure 407.3.)

C. Diagnosis

1. Urine screen—test for the presence of the following breakdown products of catecholamines:
   a. Metanephrine—best indicator
   b. Vanillylmandelic acid, normetanephrine
2. Urine/serum epinephrine and norepinephrine levels—If the epinephrine level is elevated, the tumor must be adrenal or near the adrenal gland (organ of Zuckerkandl) because nonadrenal tumors cannot methylate norepinephrine to epinephrine.
3. Tumor localization tests
   a. CT, MRI
   b. I- metaiodobenzylguanidine scan
      • When labeled with ^{131}I, it is taken up by the tumor
      • A norepinephrine analog that collects in pheochromocytomas
      • Identifies intra-adrenal as well as extra-adrenal pheochromocytomas
4. Inferior vena cava venous sampling—rarely indicated
   a. Sample patient's blood for catecholamines from each adrenal vein
   b. Only needed if biochemical and localizing procedures (CT, MRI, I-metaiodobenzylguanidine) are equivocal

D. Treatment

1. Surgical tumor resection with early ligation of venous drainage is the treatment of choice. Ligation lowers the possibility of catecholamine release/crisis by tying off drainage.
2. Medical—consists of β-blockers (phenoxybenzamine): standard medical treatment and preoperative preparation of pheochromocytoma

Primary Hyperaldosteronism

A. General characteristics

1. Excessive production of aldosterone by the adrenal glands independent of any regulation by the renin-angiotensin system
2. Excessive mineralocorticoids increase activity of the Na$^+$/K$^+$ pumps in the cortical collecting tubules
   a. Sodium retention, causing ECF volume expansion and HTN
   b. Potassium loss—results in hypokalemia

QUICK HIT

Always suspect hyperaldosteronism in a hypertensive patient with hypokalemia who is not on a diuretic.

Box 4-7 Multiple Endocrine Neoplasia (MEN) Syndrome

- Inherited condition: propensity to develop multiple endocrine tumors
- Autosomal dominant inheritance with incomplete penetrance
- Types
  - **MEN type I** (Wermer's syndrome)—"3 Ps"
    - **P**arathyroid hyperplasia (in 90% of patients with MEN I)
    - **P**ancreatic islet cell tumors (in two-thirds of patients with MEN I)—Zollinger-Ellison syndrome (50%), insulinoma (20%)
    - **P**ituitary tumors (in two-thirds of patients with MEN I)
  - **MEN type IIA** (Sipple's syndrome)—"MPH"
    - **M**edullary thyroid carcinoma (in 100% of patients with MEN IIA)
    - **P**heochromocytoma (in more than one-third of patients with MEN IIA)
    - **H**yperparathyroidism (in 50% of patients with MEN IIA)
  - **MEN type IIB**—"MMMP"
    - **M**ucosal neuromas (in 100% of patients with MEN IIB)—in the nasopharynx, oropharynx, larynx, and conjunctiva
    - **M**edullary thyroid carcinoma (in 85% of patients with MEN IIB)—more aggressive than in MEN IIA
    - **M**arfanoid body habitus (long/lanky)
    - **P**heochromocytoma

3. Excess aldosterone also increases the secretion of hydrogen ions into the lumen of the medullary collecting tubules; results in metabolic alkalosis.

B. Causes

1. Adrenal adenoma (in two-thirds of cases)—aldosterone producing adenoma (**Conn's syndrome**)
2. Adrenal hyperplasia (in one-third of cases)
3. Adrenal carcinoma (in <1% of cases)

C. Clinical features

1. HTN (most common clinical feature); may otherwise be asymptomatic
2. Headache, fatigue, weakness
3. Polydipsia, nocturnal polyuria (due to hypokalemia)
4. **Absence of peripheral edema**

D. Diagnosis

1. Ratio of the plasma aldosterone level to plasma renin—A screening test in primary hyperaldosteronism reveals inappropriately elevated levels of plasma aldosterone with coexistent decreased plasma renin activity. Therefore, if the plasma aldosterone-to-renin ratio is >30, evaluate further.
2. Saline infusion test—for definitive diagnosis
   a. Infusion of saline will decrease aldosterone levels in normal patients but not in those with primary aldosteronism.
   b. If aldosterone levels are <8.5 ng/dL after saline infusion, primary aldosteronism may be ruled out.
3. To diagnose cause of primary aldosteronism:
   a. Adrenal venous sampling for aldosterone levels—A high level of aldosterone on one side indicates an adenoma. High levels on both sides indicate bilateral hyperplasia.
   b. Renin–aldosterone stimulation test—Recumbency or upright positions are assumed, followed by measurement of serum aldosterone.
   c. Imaging tests
      • CT scan/MRI of adrenals—may demonstrate adenoma or hyperplasia anatomically
      • Iodocholesterol scanning—a functional approach to differentiating between adenoma and hyperplasia
      • Arteriography/venography (retrograde)

E. Treatment

1. For adenoma—Surgical resection (adrenalectomy) is often curative.
2. For bilateral hyperplasia
   a. Spironolactone inhibits action of aldosterone.
   b. Surgery is not indicated.

QUICK HIT

It is important to distinguish adenoma from hyperplasia because HTN associated with hyperplasia is **not** benefited by bilateral adrenalectomy, whereas HTN associated with adenoma is usually improved/cured by removal of the adenoma.

Box 4-8 Adrenal Crisis

• An acute and severely symptomatic stage of adrenal insufficiency that can include severe hypotension and cardiovascular collapse, abdominal pain (can mimic an acute abdomen), acute renal failure, and death.
• Any stress (e.g., trauma, infection, surgery) can precipitate an adrenal crisis.
• **Can be fatal if untreated.**
• Treatment
• IV fluids (several liters of normal saline with 5% dextrose)
• IV hydrocortisone
• Search for the underlying condition that precipitated the crisis and treat it.

Adrenal Insufficiency

A. Causes

1. Primary adrenal insufficiency (**Addison's disease**)
   a. Idiopathic (thought to be autoimmune disease) is the most common type in the industrialized world.
   b. Infectious diseases—These include tuberculosis (most common cause worldwide) and fungal infections. Causes also include cytomegalovirus, cryptococcus, toxoplasmosis, and pneumocystitis.
   c. Iatrogenic—for example, a bilateral adrenalectomy
   d. Metastatic disease—from lung or breast cancer
2. Secondary adrenal insufficiency
   a. Patients on long-term steroid therapy—**This is the most common cause of secondary adrenal insufficiency today.** When these patients develop a serious illness or undergo trauma, they cannot release an appropriate amount of cortisol because of chronic suppression of CRH and ACTH by the exogenous steroids. Therefore, symptoms of adrenal insufficiency result.
   b. Hypopituitarism (rare)—due to a variety of insults
3. Tertiary adrenal insufficiency—hypothalamic disease

B. Clinical features

1. Lack of cortisol
   a. GI symptoms—anorexia, nausea and vomiting, vague abdominal pain, weight loss
   b. Mental symptoms—lethargy, confusion, psychosis
   c. **Hypoglycemia**—cortisol is a gluconeogenic hormone
   d. **HTN** (especially orthostatic)
   e. **Hyperpigmentation**
      • This is a common finding in primary adrenal insufficiency; not seen in secondary adrenal insufficiency because in secondary adrenal insufficiency ACTH levels are low, not high.
      • Low cortisol stimulates ACTH and melanocyte-stimulating hormone secretion.
   f. Intolerance to physiologic stress is a feared complication.
2. Low aldosterone (only seen in primary adrenal insufficiency because aldosterone depends on the renin-angiotensin system, not ACTH). Results in:
   a. Sodium loss, causing hyponatremia and hypovolemia, which may lead to:
      • Hypotension, decreased cardiac output, and decreased renal perfusion
      • Weakness, shock, and syncope
   b. Hyperkalemia (due to retention of potassium)

C. Diagnosis (see Figure 4-4)

1. Decreased plasma cortisol level
2. Plasma ACTH level—if low, this implies a secondary adrenal insufficiency (ACTH-dependent cause)
3. Standard ACTH test
   a. This is a definitive test for primary adrenal insufficiency; give an IV infusion of ACTH, and measure plasma cortisol at the end of the infusion.
   b. In primary adrenal insufficiency, cortisol does not increase sufficiently.
   c. In secondary adrenal insufficiency, cortisol fails to respond to ACTH infusion, as in primary adrenal insufficiency (the adrenals are not used to being stimulated, so they do not respond right away). If the test is repeated for 4 or 5 days, the adrenals eventually respond normally.
4. Perform imaging tests (MRI of brain—pituitary/hypothalamus) if secondary or tertiary adrenal insufficiency is diagnosed.

D. Treatment

1. Primary adrenal insufficiency: daily oral glucocorticoid (hydrocortisone or prednisone) and daily fludrocortisone (mineralocorticoid)

The most common cause of Addison's disease worldwide is tuberculosis (autoimmune disease is the most common cause in the Western world). However, the most common cause of adrenal insufficiency overall (99% of all cases) is abrupt cessation of exogenous glucocorticoids.

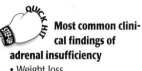
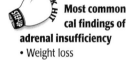
Most common clinical findings of adrenal insufficiency
• Weight loss
• Weakness
• Pigmentation
• Anorexia
• Nausea
• Postural HTN
• Abdominal pain

Hyperpigmentation and hyperkalemia appear in primary, not secondary, adrenal insufficiency.

ENDOCRINE AND METABOLIC DISEASES

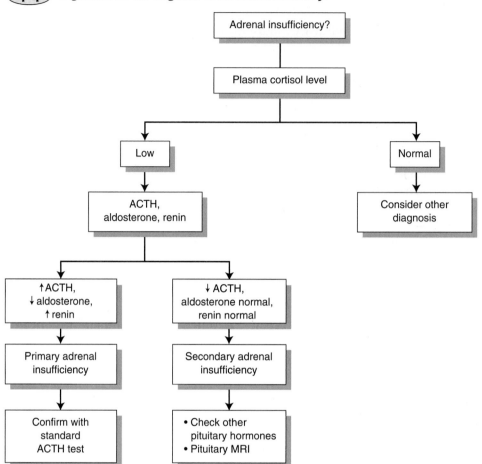

FIGURE
4-4 Algorithm for the diagnosis of adrenal insufficiency.

(Adapted from Humes DH, DuPont HL, Gardner LB, et al. Kelley's Textbook of Internal Medicine. 4th Ed. Philadelphia: Lippincott Williams & Wilkins, 2000:2730, Figure 407.5.)

2. Secondary adrenal insufficiency: same as in primary adrenal insufficiency, except that mineralocorticoid replacement is not necessary

Congenital Adrenal Hyperplasia (CAH)

A. General characteristics
1. Autosomal recessive disease
2. Ninety percent of cases are due to 21-hydroxylase deficiency (11-hydroxylase deficiency is the next most common cause).

B. Clinical features
1. Decreased cortisol and aldosterone production are the main events. Increased ACTH secretion (due to the lack of negative feedback) causes adrenal hyperplasia.
2. As precursors of cortisol and aldosterone build up, they are shunted toward the synthesis of androgens (e.g., DHEA, testosterone), causing virilization.
3. Virilizing features
   a. Female infants—born with **ambiguous external genitalia but normal female ovaries and uterus**
   b. Male infants—no genital abnormalities
4. Salt wasting form (more severe form of disease)
   a. Emesis, dehydration, hypotension, and shock—can develop in first 2 to 4 weeks of life

QUICK HIT

Congenital adrenal hyperplasia is a very treatable condition. Affected female patients will develop normally and will be fertile if treated early.

    b. **Hyponatremia and hyperkalemia**—due to lack of aldosterone

    c. Hypoglycemia—due to lack of cortisol

C. Diagnosis: High levels of **17-hydroxyprogesterone** in the serum

D. Treatment

  1. Medically—Use cortisol and mineralocorticoid; this shuts off the excess ACTH secretion (via negative feedback). Beware of undertreatment and overtreatment.

  2. Surgically—Early correction of female genital abnormalities is generally recommended.

DISEASES OF THE PANCREAS

Diabetes Mellitus (DM)

A. General characteristics

  1. Classification

    a. Type I IDDM—5% to 10% of all diabetic patients

      • This is characterized by a severe deficiency of insulin. **Patients require insulin to live.**

      • The onset is typically in youth (before age 20), but can occur at any age.

    b. Type II NIDDM—90% of all diabetic patients

      • Insulin levels are usually normal to high but may diminish over many years of having diabetes.

      • Insulin resistance (due to obesity) plays a major role.

      • It often goes undiagnosed for many years.

    c. Impaired glucose tolerance

      • Fasting glucose between 110 and 126 mg/dL or a 2-hour postprandial glucose between 140 and 200 mg/dL

      • 1% to 5% annual increase in risk of developing type II diabetes

      • Increased risk for cardiovascular disease

  2. Pathogenesis of type I diabetes

    a. An autoimmune disease—The immune system mediates the destruction of β cells.

    b. It develops in genetically susceptible individuals who are exposed to an environmental factor that triggers the autoimmune response; β-cell destruction ensues.

    c. Overt IDDM does not appear until about 90% of β cells are destroyed.

  3. Pathogenesis of type II diabetes

    a. Risk factors

      • Obesity (greatest risk factor)

      • Genetics

      • Age (insulin production decreases with age)

    b. Obesity (plays a major role)

      • Obesity is associated with increased plasma levels of free fatty acids, which make muscles more insulin resistant, reducing glucose uptake. **Therefore, obesity exacerbates insulin resistance.**

      • In the liver, free fatty acids increase the production of glucose.

Box 4-9 Dawn Phenomenon and Somogyi Effect

• Both cause morning hyperglycemia.

• The dawn phenomenon is probably due to an increase in the nocturnal secretion of growth hormone. This phenomenon is independent of the Somogyi effect.

• The Somogyi effect is a rebound response to nocturnal hypoglycemia—i.e., counterregulatory systems are activated in response to hypoglycemia, leading to morning hyperglycemia.

• If morning hyperglycemia is present, check a glucose level at 3:00 AM. If the glucose level is elevated, the patient has the dawn phenomenon and his or her evening insulin should be increased to provide additional coverage in the overnight hours. If the glucose level is low, the patient has the Somogyi effect and his or her evening insulin should be decreased to avoid nocturnal hypoglycemia.

> **Box 4-10 General Principles in Outpatient Management and Monitoring of All Diabetic Patients**
>
> - Monitor HbA_{1c} level every 3 months. Keeping $HbA_{1c} < 7.0$ is the objective (although difficult to achieve) because it is associated with a marked reduction in risk for microvascular complications.
> - All diabetic patients should monitor daily glycemic levels with home blood glucose determinations. Patients on insulin therapy should check blood glucose levels before meals and at bedtime. Monitoring blood glucose 90 to 120 minutes after meals enables the patient to control postprandial hyperglycemia and should be strongly encouraged.
> - Screen for microalbuminuria at least once per year in diabetic patients with no evidence of nephropathy.
> - Check BUN and creatinine level at least once per year.
> - Order eye screening yearly by an ophthalmologist to screen for diabetic retinopathy.
> - Check the feet at every visit. Refer high-risk patients to a foot care specialist (e.g., podiatrist). Patients should check their feet regularly.
> - Check cholesterol levels at least once per year.
> - Take BP at every visit.
> - Check for neuropathy every 6 months.

QUICK HIT

Hypertriglyceridemia with HDL depletion is the characteristic lipid profile of insulin resistance and poorly controlled diabetes.

c. Lack of compensation in type II diabetic patients
   - In normal individuals, the pancreas secretes more insulin in response to free fatty acids, thus neutralizing the excess glucose.
   - In type II diabetic patients, free fatty acids fail to stimulate pancreatic insulin secretion. Therefore, compensation does not occur and hyperglycemia develops; β cells become desensitized to glucose, leading to decreased insulin secretion.

B. Diagnosis

1. Testing recommendations
   a. Screen all adults over age 45 every 3 years.
   b. For those with risk factors for diabetes (obesity, family history, history of gestational diabetes), start screening earlier. Some recommend early screening for African Americans and Native Americans.
   c. Test anyone with signs or symptoms of diabetes.
2. Perform any one of the following tests on two separate days (see Table 4-4).
   a. Fasting plasma glucose—criteria for DM: glucose >126 mg/dL
      - Preferred test for screening
      - If between 100 and 126 mg/dL, perform a 75-g oral glucose tolerance test (although this is rarely done) or recheck fasting glucose
   b. Random plasma glucose—criteria for DM: glucose >200 mg/dL in a person with diabetic symptoms
   c. Two-hour postprandial plasma glucose level—criteria for DM: glucose >200 mg/dL after administration of the equivalent of a 75-g glucose load (more sensitive than fasting glucose level, but less convenient)

FIGURE 4-5 Progression of type I diabetes mellitus.

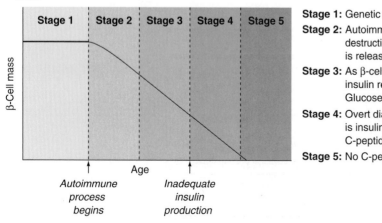

Stage 1: Genetic susceptibility

Stage 2: Autoimmune process of β-cell destruction begins. Normal insulin is released.

Stage 3: As β-cell destruction continues, insulin release is decreased. Glucose level is still normal.

Stage 4: Overt diabetes mellitus. Patient is insulin dependent at this point. C-peptide is still present.

Stage 5: No C-peptide present

TABLE 4-3 Comparison of Type I and II Diabetes Mellitus

	Type I	Type II
Onset	Sudden	Gradual
Age at onset	Any age (typically young)	Mostly in adults
Body habitus	Usually thin	Frequently obese
Ketosis	Common	Rare
Autoantibodies	Present in most cases	Absent
Endogenous insulin	Low or absent	Can be normal, decreased, or increased
Genetic factors	Concordance rate between identical twins is 50%.	Concordance rate between identical twins is 90%. Therefore, type II demonstrates a much stronger genetic component than type I.

C. Clinical presentation (see Table 4-5)

1. Type I
   a. Symptoms develop quickly over days to weeks.
   b. Sometimes symptoms appear after an illness.
   c. Patients often present with acute DKA.
2. Type II
   a. This is usually discovered on screening urinalysis or blood sugar measurement. Sometimes the diagnosis is made during evaluation for other diseases (e.g., heart, kidney, neurologic, infection).
   b. Symptomatic patients may present with polyuria, polydipsia, polyphagia, fatigue, blurred vision, weight loss, and/or candidal vaginitis.
   c. Patients who have not routinely sought medical attention may present with complications such as myocardial ischemia, stroke, intermittent claudication, impotence, peripheral neuropathy, proteinuria, or retinopathy.

D. Treatment

1. Insulin (see Table 4-6)
   a. Method of administration
      • Self-administered by SC injection in abdomen, buttocks, arm, leg
      • Given intravenously for emergency ketoacidosis
   b. Regimens
      • Most type I diabetic patients require 0.5 to 1.0 unit/kg per day to achieve acceptable glycemic control.
      • It is generally distributed as two-thirds of the daily dose in the morning (two-thirds of this dose will be NPH and one-third regular) and one-third of the daily dose in the evening (one-half to two-thirds of this dose will be NPH and one-third to one-third regular).
      • Start with a conservative dose and adjust the regimen according to the patient's glucose levels.
      • Many different regimens exist, and every patient has unique needs (see Table 4-6).

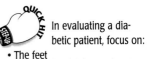

In evaluating a diabetic patient, focus on:
• The feet
• Vascular disease (CAD, PVD)
• Neurologic disease (neuropathies)
• Eyes (retinopathy)
• Renal disease
• Infectious disease

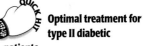

Optimal treatment for type II diabetic patients
• Glycemic control
• BP control—goal is <130/85 (the lower the better, as long as tolerated by the patient)
• Optimization of serum lipids—goals: LDL ≤ 100, triglyceride ≤ 150, HDL ≥ 40
• Smoking cessation
• Daily aspirin (if not contraindicated)

TABLE 4-4 Diagnostic Criteria for Diabetes Mellitus

Glucose Test	Impaired Glucose Tolerance (mg/dL)	Diabetes Mellitus (mg/dL)
Random plasma	—	>200 with diabetic symptoms
Fasting	110–126	>126 on two occasions
2-hr postprandial	140–200	>200

TABLE 4-5 Symptoms of Diabetes Mellitus

Symptom	Cause
Polyuria	Glucose in renal tubule causes osmotic retention of water, causing a diuresis
Polydipsia	A physiologic response to diuresis to maintain plasma volume
Fatigue	Mechanism unknown, but probably due to increased glucose in plasma
Weight loss	Due to loss of anabolic effects of insulin
Blurred vision	Swelling of lens due to osmosis (caused by increased glucose)
Fungal infections	Fungal infections of mouth and vagina common—*Candida albicans* thrives under increased glucose conditions
Numbness, tingling of hands and feet	Neuropathy Mononeuropathy: due to microscopic vasculitis leading to axonal ischemia Polyneuropathy: etiology is probably multifactorial

QUICK HIT

Insulin versus oral hypoglycemic agents in type II diabetes

- If the patient has severe hyperglycemia (fasting glucose >240 mg/dL), insulin typically is the agent of choice (whether type I or type II disease).
- Oral hypoglycemic agents are effective in type II disease with moderate hyperglycemia (fasting glucose between 140 and 240 mg/dL).

c. Intensive insulin therapy
  - This is appropriate for patients who are willing to monitor glucose levels multiple times per day and for pregnant diabetics.
  - With intensive insulin therapy, the risk for hypoglycemia is a serious concern.
  - Long-acting insulin is given once daily in the evening. Regular insulin is given 30 to 45 minutes before each meal, and should be adjusted according to preprandial home glucose measurements.
  - Alternatively, a continuous SC infusion of insulin can be given via an insulin pump. Preprandial boluses are given in addition to the basal infusion.
d. If the patient is unable/unwilling to carry out an intensive insulin program:
  - Give 70/30 units before breakfast and before the evening meal for basal coverage.
  - Give a short-acting insulin (regular) for prandial control if necessary.
  - Adjust doses according to fasting and 4 PM glucose determinations.
e. Inpatient management of diabetic patients (sliding scale)
  - An insulin sliding scale (SSI) of regular insulin doses given according to bedside finger-stick glucose determinations is helpful in controlling blood glucose levels in the hospital setting.
  - In general, SSI should be used in addition to a regimen of intermediate-acting insulin. If given alone, hyperglycemia usually results.
  - Monitor blood glucose four times per day: before meals and at bedtime.
  - If the home insulin dose is unclear, or if the patient anticipates greater requirements of insulin due to an illness, use the following approach to adjust appropriate insulin doses:
  - Take the total number of units of regular insulin that the patient required in 1 day (while on the sliding scale).
  - Add two-thirds of this to the prebreakfast dose and one-third before dinner. It should be given as 70/30 (i.e., 70% NPH/30% regular).
f. Modifying insulin doses
  - Physical activity—depending on the intensity of the activity, decrease insulin dosage 1 to 2 units per 20 to 30 minutes of activity.

Box 4-11 Monitoring Glucose Levels in DM

- HbA$_{1c}$ gives an estimate of the degree of glucose control over 2 to 3 months.
- The American Diabetes Association recommends a treatment goal of HbA$_{1c}$<7.0%. In general, HbA$_{1c}$ >10% is poor control, 8.5% to 10% is fair control, 7.0% to 8.5% is good control, and <7.0% is ideal.
- The American Diabetes Association recommends keeping fasting blood glucose level <130 mg/dL and peak postprandial blood glucose <180 mg/dL.

TABLE 4-6 Types of Insulin

Type	Onset	Duration	Comments
Human insulin lispro	15 min	4 hr	
Regular insulin	30–60 min	4–6 hr	Only type that can be given intravenously
NPH insulin/Lente insulin	2–4 hr	10–18 hr	Most widely used form of insulin
Ultralente insulin (long-lasting)	6–10 hr	18–24 hr	
70/30 mixture	30 min	10–16 hr	70% NPH, 30% regular
Glargine (Lantus)	3–4 hr	24 hr	Given at bedtime

- During illness, administer all of the routine insulin. Many episodes of DKA occur during episodes of illness.
- Stress and changes in diet require dosing adjustments.
- Patients undergoing surgery should get one-third to one-half of the usual daily insulin requirement that day, with frequent monitoring and adjustments as necessary.

2. Diet and exercise should ideally be the only interventions in most type II diabetic patients.
   a. Diet and exercise are especially effective in obese and sedentary patients (who constitute the majority of type II diabetic patients).
   b. Most patients, however, do not lose enough weight to control glucose levels through diet and exercise alone, and will require pharmacologic treatment.
3. Oral hypoglycemic drugs
   a. Use these in type II diabetic patients when conservative therapy (diet and exercise) fails.
   b. Start with one agent (metformin or sulfonylurea are common choices). If monotherapy fails, use two agents from different classes in combination. Each agent has advantages and disadvantages, so clinical judgment is required in selecting the initial agent.
   c. In patients with relatively mild disease, use of these drugs (alone or in combination) can bring glucose levels to normal, but patients with severe disease often do not respond adequately. Therefore, many type II diabetic patients eventually require insulin (see above).
   d. Do not give to patients who cannot eat (e.g., because of illness or surgery).
4. Islet cell transplantation offers definitive treatment for selected qualified patients.

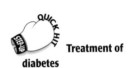

Treatment of diabetes
- Type I diabetic patients require insulin to live.
- Type II diabetic patients require exercise and diet (initial steps) as well as oral hypoglycemic drugs. The current emphasis is to treat aggressively and move quickly to insulin if needed to optimize HgA$_{1C}$.

FIGURE 4-6 A typical two-third to one-third insulin dosing regimen in a 72-kg patient.

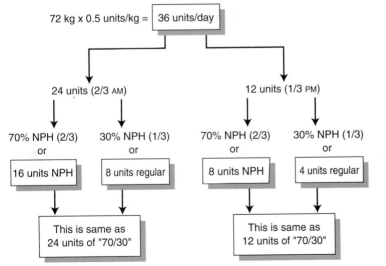

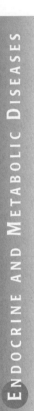

F I G U R E

4-7 Graphic depiction of three different insulin dosing regimens, illustrating time of injection (30 minutes before each meal) and insulin effect. Note that many different regimens exist and each patient has unique needs.

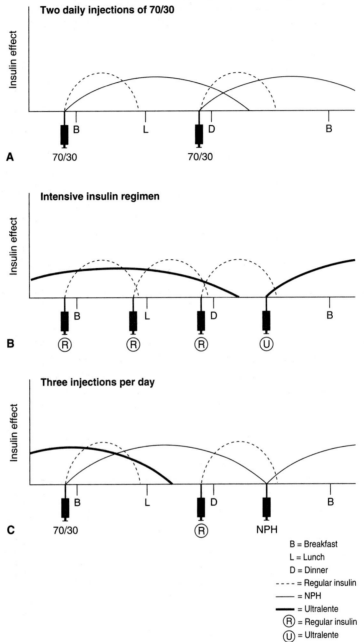

Two daily injections of 70/30

A

70/30   70/30

Intensive insulin regimen

B

Ⓡ   Ⓡ   Ⓡ   Ⓤ

Three injections per day

C

70/30   Ⓡ   NPH

B = Breakfast
L = Lunch
D = Dinner
- - - - = Regular insulin
——— = NPH
━━━ = Ultralente
Ⓡ = Regular insulin
Ⓤ = Ultralente

Box 4-12 **Example Order for Typical Insulin Sliding Scale (Regular Insulin)**

Blood glucose		Insulin dose
150–200	→	2 units
201–250	→	4 units
251–300	→	6 units
301–350	→	8 units
351–400	→	10 units
>400	→	Call house officer (who will usually give 10 to 14 units and adjust the SSI)

Chronic Complications of Diabetes Mellitus (see Figure 4-9)

A. Macrovascular complications

1. The main problem is accelerated atherosclerosis. The cause of this is not known, although glycation of lipoproteins and increased platelet adhesiveness/aggregation are thought to be two potential causes. In addition, the process of fibrinolysis may be impaired in diabetic patients.
2. The manifestations of atherosclerosis include the following:
   a. Coronary artery disease (CAD)
      • Risk of CAD is two to four times greater in diabetic than in nondiabetic persons.
      • **Most common cause of death in diabetic patients**
      • Silent myocardial infarctions are common.
   b. Peripheral vascular disease—in up to 60% of diabetic patients
   c. Cerebrovascular disease (strokes)

B. Microvascular complications—risk can be markedly reduced by achieving tight glucose control

1. **Diabetic nephropathy**—most important cause of ESRD
   a. Pathologic types
      • Nodular glomerular sclerosis (Kimmelstiel-Wilson syndrome)—hyaline deposition in **one** area of glomerulus—pathognomonic for DM
      • Diffuse glomerular sclerosis—hyaline deposition is global—also occurs in HTN
   b. Microalbuminuria/proteinuria
      • If microalbuminuria is present, strict glycemic control is critical (has been shown to limit progression from microalbuminuria to clinical proteinuria).
      • Without effective treatment, the albuminuria gradually worsens—HTN usually develops during the transition between microalbuminuria and progressive proteinuria. Persistent HTN and proteinuria cause a decrease in GFR, leading to renal insufficiency and eventually ESRD.

The risk of coronary events is greatly reduced if the patient can eliminate or reduce other major cardiovascular risk factors (smoking, HTN, hyperlipidemia, obesity).

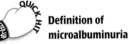

Definition of microalbuminuria
• 30 to 300 mg/day
• 20 to 200 g/min
• Albumin-creatinine ratio of 0.02 to 0.20

TABLE 4-7 Oral Hypoglycemic Drugs				
Medication	**Mechanism**	**Site of Action**	**Advantages**	**Major Side Effects**
Sulfonylureas (e.g., glyburide, glipizide, glimepiride)	Stimulate pancreas to produce more insulin	Pancreas	Effective Inexpensive	Hypoglycemia, weight gain
Metformin[a]	Enhances insulin sensitivity	Liver	May cause mild weight loss Does not cause hypoglycemia (insulin levels do not increase)	GI upset (diarrhea, nausea, abdominal pain), lactic acidosis, metallic taste
Acarbose	Reduces glucose absorption from the gut, thereby reducing calorie intake	GI tract	Low risk (does not have significant toxicity)	GI upset (diarrhea, abdominal cramping flatulence)
Thiazolidinediones (e.g., rosiglitazone, pioglitazone)	Reduce insulin resistance	Fat, muscle	Reduce insulin levels	Hepatotoxicity (monitor LFTs)

Note: Most oral hypoglycemic drugs are contraindicated in pregnancy (potentially teratogenic). Treat with insulin.
[a]Serum creatine ≥ 1.5 (≥ 1.4 in women) is a contraindication to metformin.

Box 4-13   Radiocontrast Agents in Diabetic Patients

- Patients with diabetes are particularly susceptible to developing radiocontrast-induced acute renal failure.
- If IV contrast is necessary, give generous hydration before administering the contrast agent to avoid precipitating acute renal failure.
- Hold metformin for 48 hours after radiocontrast is given to prevent renal damage, and make sure renal function has returned to baseline before resuming it.

- **HTN increases the risk of progression of diabetic nephropathy to ESRD. Control BP aggressively.**
- **Initiate ACE inhibitors immediately.**
- **Microalbuminuria is the screening test!** If you wait for the dipstick to be positive for protein, you have waited too long.
- It usually takes 1 to 5 years for microalbuminuria to advance to full-blown proteinuria. However, with proper treatment (i.e., using ACE inhibitors to control BP) this can be prolonged.
  c. Once diabetic nephropathy has progressed to the stage of proteinuria or early renal failure, glycemic control does not significantly influence its course. ACE inhibitors and dietary restriction of protein are recommended.
2. **Diabetic retinopathy**
   a. Prevalence is approximately 75% after 20 years of diabetes. **Annual screening of all diabetic patients by an ophthalmologist is recommended.**
   b. Background (nonproliferative) retinopathy accounts for the majority of cases.
   - Funduscopic examination shows hemorrhages, exudates, microaneurysms, and venous dilatation.
   - These patients are usually asymptomatic unless retinal edema or ischemia involves the central macula.
   - Edema of the macula is the leading cause of visual loss in diabetic patients.
   - HTN and fluid retention exacerbate this condition.
   c. Proliferative retinopathy
   - Key characteristics are new vessel formation (neovascularization) and scarring.
   - Two serious complications are vitreal hemorrhage and retinal detachment.
   - **Can lead to blindness**
3. **Diabetic neuropathy**
   a. Peripheral neuropathy (distal symmetric neuropathy)
   - Usually affects sensory nerves in a "stocking/glove pattern"—usually begins in feet, later involves hands. Numbness and paresthesias are common.
   - Loss of sensation leads to the following: ulcer formation (patients do not shift their weight) with subsequent ischemia of pressure point areas; *Charcot's joints*.
   - Painful diabetic neuropathy—hypersensitivity to light touch; severe "burning" pain (especially at night) that can be difficult to tolerate.
   b. CN complications—secondary to nerve infarction
   - Most often involves CN III, but may also involve CN VI and IV
   - Diabetic third nerve palsy: eye pain, diplopia, ptosis, inability to adduct the eye; **pupils are spared**

QUICK HIT

- Ocular problems in diabetic patients include cataracts, retinopathy, and glaucoma.
- Diabetic retinopathy is the leading cause of blindness in the United States.

ENDOCRINE AND METABOLIC DISEASES

FIGURE 4-8   Progression in diabetic nephropathy. Strict glycemic control has been shown to slow or prevent progression from microalbuminuria to proteinuria. This is the critical stage (marked by star)—once proteinuria develops, glycemic control does little to control the course and will eventually lead to ESRD. (ESRD, end-stage renal disease; GFR, glomerular filtration rate)

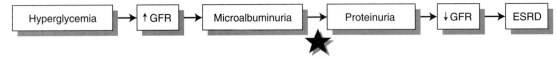

c. Mononeuropathies—secondary to nerve infarction
- Ulnar neuropathy, common peroneal neuropathy
- Diabetic lumbosacral plexopathy—severe, deep pain in the thigh; atrophy and weakness in thigh and hip muscles; recovery takes weeks to months
- Diabetic truncal neuropathy—pain in distribution of one of the intercostal nerves

d. Autonomic neuropathy
- Impotence in men (most common presentation)
- Neurogenic bladder—retention, incontinence
- Gastroparesis—chronic nausea and vomiting
- Constipation and diarrhea (alternating)
- Postural hypotension

4. **Diabetic foot**
   a. Caused by a combination of artery disease (ischemia) and nerve disease (neuropathy)—can lead to ulcers/infections and may require amputation
   b. With neuropathy, the patient does not feel pain, so repetitive injuries go unnoticed and ultimately lead to nonhealing.
   c. In addition, neuropathy may mask symptoms of PVD (claudication/rest pain). Also, calcific medial arterial disease is common and can cause erroneously high BP readings in lower extremities.

5. Increased susceptibility to infection
   a. This results from impaired WBC function, reduced blood supply, and neuropathy. Wound healing is impaired in diabetic patients, and this can be problematic postoperatively.
   b. Diabetic patients are at increased risk for the following infections: cellulitis, candidiasis, pneumonia, osteomyelitis, and polymicrobial foot ulcers.
   c. Infections of ischemic foot ulcers may lead to osteomyelitis and may require amputation.

QUICK HIT The Diabetes Control and Complications Trial showed that tight glucose control reduces the risk of microvascular disease by 50% to 60%. However, whether it can reduce the risk of macrovascular disease remains to be proven. It is the macrovascular complications that cause death in the majority of type II diabetic patients.

FIGURE 4-9 Chronic complications of diabetes mellitus.

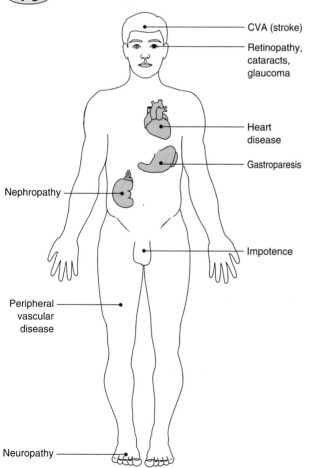

- CVA (stroke)
- Retinopathy, cataracts, glaucoma
- Heart disease
- Gastroparesis
- Nephropathy
- Impotence
- Peripheral vascular disease
- Neuropathy

C. Specific treatment of chronic diabetic complications

1. Macrovascular disease—Treatment involves reduction of risk factors (e.g., BP reduction, lipid-lowering agents, smoking cessation, exercise), a daily aspirin (if not contraindicated), and strict glycemic control.
2. Nephropathy—ACE inhibitors, benefits of which include:
   a. Slow progression of microalbuminuria to proteinuria
   b. Slow decline of GFR
3. Retinopathy—Treatment involves referral to an ophthalmologist and possible photocoagulation.
4. Neuropathy—Treatment is complex. Pharmacologic agents that may be helpful include NSAIDs, tricyclic antidepressants, and gabapentin. For gastroparesis, a promotility agent such as metoclopramide can be helpful, in addition to exercise and a low-fat diet.
5. Diabetic foot—The best treatment is prevention: regular foot care, **regular podiatrist visits**. Amputation is a last resort.

Acute Complications of Diabetes Mellitus

A. Diabetic ketoacidosis (DKA)

1. **General characteristics**
   a. DKA is an acute, life-threatening medical emergency that can occur in both type I and type II diabetic patients (more common in type I).
   b. Pathogenesis
      - This is secondary to insulin deficiency and glucagons excess, both of which contribute to accelerated severe hyperglycemia and accelerated ketogenesis.
      - Severe hyperglycemia leads to an osmotic diuresis, which causes dehydration and volume depletion.
   c. Consequences of DKA include hyperglycemia, ketonemia, metabolic acidosis, and volume depletion.
2. **Precipitating factors**
   a. Any type of stress or illness (e.g., infectious process, trauma, myocardial infarction, stroke, recent surgery, sepsis, GI bleeding)
   b. Inadequate administration of insulin
3. **Clinical features**
   a. Nausea and vomiting
   b. Kussmaul's respiration—rapid, deep breathing
   c. Abdominal pain (more common in children) that may mimic acute abdomen
   d. "Fruity" (acetone) breath odor
   e. Marked dehydration, orthostatic hypotension, tachycardia—Volume depletion is always present.
   f. Polydipsia, polyuria, polyphagia, weakness
   g. Altered consciousness, drowsiness, and frank coma may occur if not treated.
4. **Diagnosis**
   a. Hyperglycemia: serum glucose >250 mg/dL (in certain conditions, e.g., alcohol ingestion, the patient may be euglycemic)
   b. Metabolic acidosis
      - Blood pH <7.3 and serum HCO_3^- <15 mEq/L
      - Increased anion gap—due to production of ketones (acetoacetate and β-hydroxybutyrate)
   c. Ketonemia (serum positive for ketones) and ketonuria
      - Serum levels of acetoacetate, acetone, and β-hydroxybutyrate are greatly increased.
      - When DKA is accompanied by circulatory collapse, serum and urine may be falsely negative for ketones. This is because lactate production results in less acetoacetate and more β-hydroxybutyrate production, and acetoacetate is the only ketoacid that can be measured by nitroprusside agents.
   d. Ketonemia and acidosis are required for diagnosis of DKA.

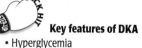

Key features of DKA

- Hyperglycemia
- Positive serum or urine ketones
- Metabolic acidosis

Differential diagnosis of DKA

- Alcoholic ketoacidosis
- Hyperosmolar hyperglycemic nonketotic syndrome (HHNS)
- Hypoglycemia (altered mental status, abdominal pain, and acidosis are possible)
- Sepsis
- Intoxication (e.g., methanol, ethanol, salicylates, isopropyl alcohol, paraldehyde, ethylene glycol)

If a patient presents with DKA:

- Take a history and perform a physical examination,
- Order laboratory tests: blood glucose, arterial blood gas, CBC, electrolytes, BUN, creatinine, and urinary analysis.
- Order ECG, CXR, and cultures.
- Initiate IV fluids.
- Give insulin and start potassium soon thereafter.
- Admit to the ICU or a very closely-monitored floor bed.

5. Other laboratory value abnormalities
   a. Hyperosmolarity
   b. Hyponatremia—Serum sodium decreases 1.6 mEq/L for every 100 mg/dL increase in glucose level because of the osmotic shift of fluid from the ICF to the ECF space. Total body sodium level is normal. This generally does not require treatment.
   c. Other electrolyte disturbances
      • Potassium—Because of the acidosis, hyperkalemia may be present initially, although total body potassium is low. As insulin is given, it causes a shift of potassium into cells, resulting in a hypokalemia, and this can happen very rapidly.
      • Phosphate and magnesium levels may also be low.
6. **Treatment**
   a. Insulin
      • Give insulin immediately after the diagnosis is established.
      • Give a priming dose of 0.1 units/kg of regular insulin (IV) followed by an infusion of 0.1 units/kg per hour. This is sufficient to replace the insulin deficit in most patients. **Be certain that the patient is not hypokalemic before giving insulin.**
      • Continue the insulin until the anion gap closes and metabolic acidosis is corrected, then begin to decrease the insulin. Give SC insulin when the patient starts eating again.
   b. Fluid replacement (normal saline)
      • Give fluids immediately after the diagnosis is established.
      • Add 5% glucose once the blood glucose reaches 250 mg/dL to prevent hypoglycemia.
   c. Replace potassium prophylactically with IV fluids.
      • Initiate within 1 to 2 hours of starting insulin.
      • Ensure adequate renal function (urine output) before administering these.
      • Monitor potassium, magnesium, and phosphate levels **very closely** and replace as necessary.
   d. HCO_3^- replacement is controversial and is not necessary in most cases.

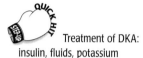

Treatment of DKA: insulin, fluids, potassium

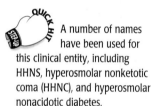

Complications of treatment of DKA
• Cerebral edema—if glucose levels decrease too rapidly
• Hyperchloremic nongap metabolic acidosis—due to rapid infusion of a large amount of saline

B. Hyperosmolar hyperglycemic nonketotic syndrome (HHNS)

1. **General characteristics**
   a. A state of severe hyperglycemia, hyperosmolarity, and dehydration typically seen in elderly type II diabetic patients.
   b. Pathogenesis
      • Low insulin levels lead to hyperglycemia. Severe hyperglycemia causes an osmotic diuresis, leading to dehydration.
      • Ketogenesis is minimal because a small amount of insulin is released to blunt counterregulatory hormone release (glucagons).
      • Ketosis and acidosis are typically absent or minimal.
      • Severe dehydration is due to continued hyperglycemic (osmotic) diuresis. The patient's inability to drink enough fluids (either due to lack of access in elderly/bedridden patients or to inadequate thirst drive) to keep up with urinary fluid losses exacerbates the condition.
   c. Precipitating events are similar to those of DKA.
2. **Clinical features**
   a. Thirst, oliguria
   b. Signs of extreme dehydration and volume depletion—hypotension, tachycardia
   c. CNS findings and focal neurologic signs are common (e.g., seizures)—secondary to hyperosmolarity.
   d. Lethargy and confusion may develop, leading to convulsions and coma.
3. **Diagnosis**
   a. Hyperglycemia: serum glucose >600 mg/dL
   b. Hyperosmolarity: serum osmolarity >320 mOsm/L

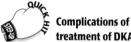

A number of names have been used for this clinical entity, including HHNS, hyperosmolar nonketotic coma (HHNC), and hyperosmolar nonacidotic diabetes.

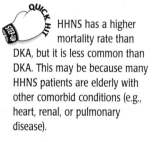

HHNS has a higher mortality rate than DKA, but it is less common than DKA. This may be because many HHNS patients are elderly with other comorbid conditions (e.g., heart, renal, or pulmonary disease).

TABLE 4-8 Diabetic Ketoacidosis Versus Hyperosmolar Hyperglycemic Nonketotic Syndrome

	DKA	HHNS
Pathophysiology	Insulin deficiency → hyperglycemia, ketosis, acidosis, dehydration	Insulin deficiency → hyperglycemia, hyperosmolarity, osmotic diuresis, profound dehydration
Laboratory findings	• Hyperglycemia (>250) • Metabolic acidosis (anion gap)—serum pH < 7.3 • Ketosis	• Hyperglycemia (>600 mg/dL) • Hyperosmolarity (>320 mOsm/L) • Serum pH >7.3 (no acidosis)
Treatment	Insulin, IV fluids, potassium	Aggressive IV fluids, low-dose insulin infusion
Mortality rate	5% to 10%	10% to 20%

QUICK HIT

Key features of HHNS
- Severe hyperosmolarity (>320 mOsm/L)
- Hyperglycemia (>600 mg/dL)
- Dehydration
- Acidosis and ketosis are absent (unlike in DKA)

c. Serum pH .7.3 (no acidosis); serum HCO_3^- >15
d. BUN is usually elevated. Prerenal azotemia is common.
4. **Treatment**
a. Fluid replacement is most important (normal saline): 1 L in the first hour, another liter in the next 2 hours. Most patients respond well. Switch to half normal saline once the patient stabilizes.
   - Glucose levels are lowered as the patient is rehydrated (but the patient still requires insulin).
   - When glucose levels reach 250 mg/dL, add 5% glucose ($D_5$1/2NS) as in DKA
   - Very rapid lowering of blood glucose can lead to cerebral edema in children (just as in DKA).
   - In patients with cardiac disease or renal insufficiency, avoid volume overload (can lead to CHF), but generous fluids are still needed.
b. Insulin: An initial bolus of 5 to 10 units intravenously, followed by a continuous low-dose infusion (2 to 4 units/hr) is usually appropriate.

Hypoglycemia

A. General characteristics
1. **The primary organ at risk in hypoglycemia is the brain**—the brain uses glucose as its main energy source (except when using ketone bodies during fasting).
2. Unlike other tissues, the brain cannot use free fatty acids as an energy source.
3. Hypoglycemia is really due to an imbalance between glucagon and insulin.
4. If there is no correlation between symptoms and low glucose levels (e.g., patient has symptoms when glucose levels are normal), an underlying disorder of glucose metabolism is unlikely (i.e., the patient does not have true hypoglycemia).

Box 4-14 Physiologic Responses to Hypoglycemia

- When glucose levels approach the low 80s, insulin levels decrease-this decrease is normally enough to prevent hypoglycemia.
- As glucose levels decrease further, glucagon levels increase (glucagon is the first line of defense against more severe hypoglycemia).
- Epinephrine is the next hormone to combat hypoglycemia. Cortisol and other catecholamines also play a role.
- As glucose levels decrease into the 50s and below, symptoms begin.

B. Causes

1. Drug-induced—Taking too much insulin is a common problem in diabetic patients attempting tight control of their disease.
2. Factitious hypoglycemia
   a. If the patient took insulin surreptitiously, there will be a high blood insulin level and a low blood C-peptide level (because exogenous insulin does not contain C-peptide).
   b. Patients taking exogenous insulin will also develop anti-insulin antibodies, which can be measured.
   c. If the patient took sulfonylurea, check urine or serum for levels of this drug.
3. Insulinoma
4. Ethanol ingestion—due to:
   a. Poor nutrition that leads to decreased glycogen (and loss of glycogenolysis)
   b. Metabolism of alcohol that lowers nicotinamide adenine dinucleotide levels and decreases gluconeogenesis
5. Postoperative complications after gastric surgery (due to rapid gastric emptying)
6. Reactive (idiopathic) hypoglycemia—symptoms occur 2 to 4 hours after a meal; rarely indicates a serious underlying disorder
7. Adrenal insufficiency
8. Liver failure
9. Critical illness

C. Clinical features

1. Symptoms occur at a blood glucose level of 40 to 50 mg/dL.
2. Elevated epinephrine levels cause sweating, tremors, increased BP and pulse, anxiety, and palpitations.
3. Neuroglycopenic symptoms—decreased glucose for the brain (CNS dysfunction), resulting in irritability, behavioral changes, weakness, drowsiness, headache, confusion, convulsions, coma, and even death

D. Diagnosis

1. Blood glucose level—Symptoms generally begin when levels drop below 50. However, there is no cutoff value to define hypoglycemia.
2. **Whipple's triad** is used to diagnose true hypoglycemia (i.e., hypoglycemia due to underlying disease). See the Insulinoma section (below).
3. Laboratory tests—for measurement of serum insulin, C-peptide, and glucose when symptoms occur (an overnight fast may be sufficient to produce symptoms)
4. 72-hour fast (24 hours is usually sufficient)—used to diagnose insulinoma (if suspected)

E. Treatment

1. Acute treatment of hypoglycemia
   a. If the patient can eat, give sugar-containing foods; if not, give 1/2 to 2 ampules of D50W intravenously.
   b. Repeat administration of D50W as necessary, but switch to D10W as clinical condition improves and glucose level is approximately >100 mg/dL.
2. Appropriate management of underlying cause (e.g., diabetes, insulinoma)
3. If reactive hypoglycemia is suspected, dietary interventions are appropriate.
4. If the patient is an alcoholic (or suspected alcoholic), give thiamine before administering glucose to avoid Wernicke's encephalopathy.

Insulinoma

A. General characteristics

1. Insulin-producing tumor arising from the β cells of the pancreas
2. Associated with MEN I syndrome
3. Usually benign (in up to 90% of cases)

If a patient presents with hypoglycemia of unknown cause, measure:
- Plasma insulin level
- C-peptide
- Anti-insulin antibodies
- Plasma and urine sulfonylurea levels

Hypoglycemic unawareness
- In diabetic patients, if severe neuropathy is present, the autonomic response (epinephrine) to hypoglycemia is not activated. This leads to neuroglycopenic symptoms.
- It is common for diabetic patients to become hypoglycemic with conventional therapy (insulin or oral hypoglycemics). With longstanding disease in which they lose their neurogenic symptom response to hypoglycemia, patients do not recognize the impending hypoglycemia and may even have a seizure or enter a coma.

ENDOCRINE AND METABOLIC DISEASES

TABLE 4-9 Laboratory Values in Hyperinsulinemic Hypoglycemia

Diagnosis	Insulin Level	Glucose Level	C-peptide Level	Proinsulin Level
Insulinoma	↑	↓	↑	↑
Surreptitious insulin	↑↑	↓	↓	↓
Sulfonylurea abuse	↑	↓	↑	Normal

The "Laboratory Value" spans Insulin Level, Glucose Level, C-peptide Level columns.

B. Clinical features: Hypoglycemia, which leads to:
 1. Sympathetic activation—diaphoresis, palpitations, tremors, high blood pressure, anxiety
 2. Neuroglycopenic symptoms—headache, visual disturbances, confusion, seizures, coma

C. Diagnosis
 1. 72-hour fast
    a. The patient becomes hypoglycemic. Normally, the insulin level should decrease as hypoglycemia develops.
    b. In persons with insulinoma, insulin does not respond appropriately to hypoglycemia. It may decrease or increase, or it may not change. Nevertheless, the insulin levels are still higher than they would be in a normal individual for any given glucose concentration.
 2. Whipple's triad
    a. Hypoglycemic symptoms brought on by fasting
    b. Blood glucose <50 mg/dL during symptomatic attack
    c. Glucose administration brings relief of symptoms

D. Treatment: Surgical resection of tumor (up to 80% to 90% cure rate)

Zollinger-Ellison Syndrome (ZES) (Gastrinoma)

- A pancreatic islet cell tumor that secretes high gastrin, which leads to profound gastric acid hypersecretion, resulting in ulcers.
- Up to 60% are malignant; 20% associated with MEN I (80% are sporadic); 90% located in the "gastrinoma triangle" (formed by the following points: cystic duct, junction of second and third portions of the duodenum, and neck of pancreas)
- Possible complications: GI hemorrhage, GI perforation, gastric outlet obstruction/stricture, and metastatic disease (liver is the most common site)
- Clinical features: peptic ulcers, diarrhea, weight loss, abdominal pain
- Secretin injection test is diagnostic test of choice. Normally, secretin inhibits gastrin secretion. In patients with ZES, gastrin levels increase substantially after being given secretin.
- Fasting gastrin level is elevated in patients with ZES
- Normal basal acid output is <10 mEq/hr; in patients with ZES: >15 mEq/hr
- Treatment consists of high-dose proton pump inhibitors
- All patients with ZES should undergo exploration to attempt curative resection (20% of patients are cured with complete resection). If there is widely metastatic or incurable gastrinoma, debulking surgery and chemotherapy are indicated.

Glucagonoma

- A glucagon-producing tumor located in the pancreas
- Clinical manifestations include **necrotizing migratory erythema** (usually below the waist), glossitis, stomatitis, DM (mild), and hyperglycemia (with low amino acid levels and high glucagon levels).
- Treatment is surgical resection.

Somatostatinoma

- A rare, malignant pancreatic tumor (metastases usually present by diagnosis)
- Poor prognosis
- Classic triad of gallstones, diabetes, and steatorrhea

VIPoma (Verner-Morrison or Watery Diarrhea, Hypokalemia, Achlorhydria Syndrome)

- A rare pancreatic tumor (>50% are malignant)
- Clinical features include watery diarrhea (leading to dehydration, hypokalemia, acidosis), achlorhydria (VIP inhibits gastric acid secretion), hyperglycemia, and hypercalcemia.
- Treatment is surgical resection.

Diseases of the Central and Peripheral Nervous Systems

CEREBROVASCULAR DISEASE (STROKE)

Ischemic Stroke (Cerebral Infarction)

A. General characteristics

1. Epidemiology
   a. Stroke, or cerebrovascular accident (CVA), is the third most common cause of death in the United States.
   b. It is the **leading cause of neurologic disability; third leading cause of death.**
2. Classes of ischemic stroke
   a. Transient ischemic attack (TIA)—see below
   b. Reversible ischemic neurologic deficit is the same as TIA except for the duration of symptoms. It lasts longer than 24 hours, but resolves in less than 2 weeks. This term is not commonly used.
   c. **Evolving stroke** is a stroke that is worsening.
   d. **Completed stroke** is one in which the maximal deficit has occurred.
3. TIAs
   a. A TIA is a neurologic deficit that lasts from a few minutes to no more than 24 hours (but usually lasts less than 30 minutes).
      • Stroke may be indistinguishable from a TIA at time of presentation: **duration of symptoms** is the determining difference.
      • Symptoms are transient with a TIA because reperfusion occurs, either because of collateral circulation or because of the breaking up of an embolus.
   b. **The blockage in blood flow does not last long enough to cause permanent infarction.**
   c. A TIA is usually embolic. However, transient hypotension in the presence of severe carotid stenosis (>75% occlusion) can lead to a TIA.
   d. **Once a patient has a TIA, there is a high risk of stroke in subsequent months.** The risk of a stroke in a patient with a history of TIA is about 10% per year. TIAs carry a **30% 5-year risk of stroke.** Therefore, cardiac risk factors should be closely investigated and, if possible, eliminated in a patient who has had a TIA.
4. Risk factors
   a. The most important risk factors are _age_ and **HTN**. Others include smoking, DM, hyperlipidemia, atrial fibrillation, coronary artery disease, family history of stroke, previous stroke/TIA, and carotid bruits.
   b. In younger patients, risk factors include oral contraceptive use, hypercoagulable states (e.g., protein C and S deficiencies, antiphospholipid antibody syndrome), vasoconstrictive drug use (e.g., cocaine, amphetamines), polycythemia vera, and sickle cell disease.

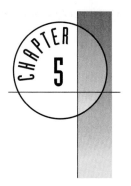

Types of strokes
• Ischemic strokes (85% of cases)
• Hemorrhagic strokes (15% of cases)

Box 5-1 **TIAs Can Involve Either the Carotid or the Vertebrobasilar System**

Carotid System
- Temporary loss of speech; paralysis or paresthesias of contralateral extremity; clumsiness of one limb
- Amaurosis fugax (an example of a TIA): transient, curtain-like loss of sight in ipsilateral eye due to microemboli to the retina

Vertebrobasilar System (i.e., Vertebrobasilar TIAs)
- Decreased perfusion of the posterior fossa
- Dizziness, double vision, vertigo, numbness of ipsilateral face and contralateral limbs, dysarthria, hoarseness, dysphagia, projectile vomiting, headaches, and drop attacks

---

B. Causes

1. **Embolic stroke** is the most common etiology of TIA/CVA. Possible origins of an embolus include:
   a. **Heart** (most common): typically due to embolization of mural thrombus in patients with atrial fibrillation
   b. Internal carotid artery
   c. Aorta
   d. Paradoxical: Emboli arise from blood clots in the peripheral veins, pass through septal defects (atrial septal defect, a patent foramen ovale, or a pulmonary AV fistula), and reach the brain.
2. Thrombotic stroke—Atherosclerotic lesions may be in the large arteries of the neck (carotid artery disease, which most commonly involves the bifurcation of the common carotid artery), or in medium-sized arteries in the brain (especially the middle cerebral artery [MCA]).
3. Lacunar stroke—**small vessel** thrombotic disease
   a. Causes approximately 20% of all strokes; usually affects subcortical structures (basal ganglia, thalamus, internal capsule, brainstem) and not the cerebral cortex
   b. Predisposing factor: A history of HTN is present in 80% to 90% of lacunar infarctions. Diabetes is another important risk factor.
   c. Narrowing of the arterial lumen is due to **thickening of vessel wall** (not by thrombosis).
   d. The arteries affected include small branches off of the MCA, the arteries that make up the circle of Willis, and the basilar and vertebral arteries.
   e. When these small vessels occlude, small infarcts result; when they heal, they are called lacunes.
4. Nonvascular causes—Examples include low cardiac output and anoxia (may cause global ischemia and infarction).

C. Clinical features

1. Thrombotic stroke—The onset of symptoms may be rapid or stepwise. **Classically the patient awakens from sleep with the neurologic deficits.**
2. Embolic stroke

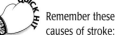

(handwritten margin notes): ⌐ Echo · Post stroke · → Echo → Carotid doppler · # hyperplasia 2° to the HTN insult · ⌐ during cardiac arrest ·

QUICK HIT — Remember these causes of stroke:
- Ischemia due to atherosclerosis
- Atrial fibrillation with clot emboli to brain
- Septic emboli from endocarditis

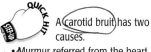

QUICK HIT — A carotid bruit has two causes.
- Murmur referred from the heart
- Turbulence in the internal carotid artery (serious stroke risk)

Box 5-2 **Subclavian Steal Syndrome**

- Caused by stenosis of subclavian artery proximal to origin of vertebral artery—exercise of left arm causes reversal of blood flow down the ipsilateral vertebral artery to fill the subclavian artery distal to the stenosis because it cannot supply adequate blood to left arm
- Leads to decreased cerebral blood flow (blood "stolen" from basilar system)
- Causes symptoms of vertebral basilar arterial insufficiency (see Box 5-1)
- BP in left arm is less than in right arm; decrease in pulse in left arm
- Upper extremity claudication
- Treatment: surgical bypass

FIGURE
5-1   **Etiology of stroke.**

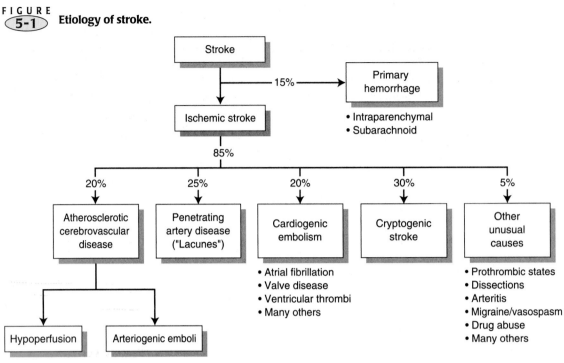

(Redrawn from Verstraete M, Fuster V, Topol EJ, eds. Cardiovascular Thrombosis–Thrombocardiology and Throm-boneurology. 2nd Ed. Philadelphia: Lippincott Williams & Wilkins, 1998:586, Figure 34-2.)

Completed stroke

a. The onset of symptoms is very rapid (within seconds), and deficits are maximal initially.
b. Clinical features depend on the artery that is occluded. The MCA is most commonly affected, and neurologic deficits seen in MCA involvement include:
   • Contralateral hemiparesis and hemisensory loss
   • Aphasia (if dominant hemisphere is involved)
   • Apraxia, contralateral body neglect, confusion (if nondominant hemisphere involved)

3. Lacunar stroke—Clinical features are focal and usually contralateral pure motor or pure sensory deficits. Lacunar stroke includes four major syndromes:
   a. Pure **motor** lacunar stroke—if lesion involves the **internal capsule**
   b. Pure **sensory** lacunar stroke—if lesion involves the **thalamus**
   c. Ataxic hemiparesis—incoordination ipsilaterally
   d. Clumsy hand dysarthria

*Basal ganglia
Thalamus
Internal Capsule
brainstem*

TABLE 5-1	Deficits Seen in Stroke
Distribution	**Location and/or Type of Deficiency**
Anterior cerebral artery	Contralateral *upper* lower extremity and face
Middle cerebral artery ✓	(Aphasia) contralateral hemiparesis
Vertebral/basilar	Ipsilateral: ataxia, diplopia, dysphagia, dysarthria, and vertigo *Cerebellar involvement* Contralateral: homonymous hemianopsia with basilar — PCA lesions
Lacunar Internal capsule Pons Thalamus PCA, posterior cerebral artery.	Pure motor hemiparesis Dysarthria, clumsy hand Pure sensory deficit

D. Diagnosis

1. CT scan (without contrast) of head
   a. This differentiates an ischemic from a hemorrhagic infarction and **is the first imaging study that you should obtain.** Contrast should not be used because a hemorrhagic CVA has not been excluded yet. Ischemic strokes appear as dark areas on the CT scan (hemorrhagic strokes appear white—see Figure 5-2).
   b. It may take 24 to 48 hours to see an infarct, but it is useful in excluding an intracerebral hemorrhage (ICH).
   c. Smaller infarcts may be missed.
2. MRI of brain—more sensitive than CT scan
   a. Identifies all infarcts, and does so earlier than CT scan
   b. Not preferred in an emergency setting because it takes longer to perform and is not suitable for potentially unstable patients
3. ECG—Acute MI or atrial fibrillation may be the cause of embolic strokes.
4. Carotid duplex scan estimates the degree of carotid stenosis, if present.
5. Magnetic resonance arteriogram (MRA) is the definitive test for identifying stenosis of vessels of the head and neck, or for aneurysms. Evaluates carotids, vertebrobasilar circulation, the circle of Willis, and the anterior, middle, and posterior cerebral arteries.

E. Complications

1. Progression of neurologic insult *(evolving stroke)*
2. Cerebral edema occurs within 1 to 2 days and can cause **mass effects** for up to 10 days. Hyperventilation and mannitol may be needed to lower intracranial pressure.
3. Hemorrhage into the infarction—rare
4. Seizures—fewer than 5% of patients

F. Treatment *(first 24 hrs - lay the pt. flat)*

1. Acute—Supportive treatment (airway protection, oxygen, IV fluids) is initiated. Early recognition of the cause of stroke is unreliable, and early treatment is critical. Therefore, choose therapies that have broad efficacy and safety.
   a. Thrombolytic therapy (t-PA)
      • If administered **within 3 hours** of the onset of an acute ischemic stroke, improved clinical outcome is seen at 3 months.
      • Do not give t-PA if the time of stroke is unknown, if more than 3 hours have passed, or if the patient has any of the following: uncontrolled HTN, bleeding disorder or is anticoagulated, or a history of recent trauma or surgery. These patients are at increased risk for hemorrhagic transformation.

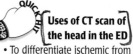

Uses of CT scan of the head in the ED

• To differentiate ischemic from hemorrhagic infarction
• Identifies 95% of SAHs (and all bleeds >1 cm)
• Identifies abscess, tumor
• Identifies subdural or epidural hematoma

best early study - MRI - Diffuse weighted image

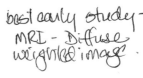

Screen all patients with a carotid duplex who have the following conditions:
• Carotid bruit
• Peripheral vascular disease
• Coronary artery disease

If a patient presents to the ED with findings suggestive of an acute stroke, order the following:
• Noncontrast CT scan of the brain
• ECG, chest radiograph
• CBC, platelet count
• PT, PTT
• Serum electrolytes
• Glucose level
• Bilateral carotid ultrasound
• Echocardiogram

Ischemic - dark nemorrhagic - white.

FIGURE 5-2 CT scan of a patient with a stroke from a nonhemorrhagic infarct (arrow).

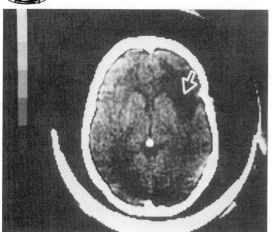

(From Fishman MC, Hoffman AR, Klausner RD, et al. Medicine. 5th Ed. Philadelphia: Lippincott Williams & Wilkins, 2004:593, Figure 64–7.)

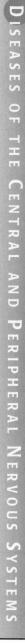

- If t-PA is given, there is risk of intracranial hemorrhage. Therefore, do not give aspirin for the first 24 hours, perform frequent neurologic checks (every hour), and carefully monitor BP. (Keep BP <185/110 mm Hg.)
  b. Aspirin is best if given within 24 hours of symptom onset. Do not give aspirin if the patient received thrombolytic therapy (due to an increased risk of ICH).
  c. Anticoagulants (heparin or warfarin) **have not been proven to have efficacy in acute stroke.** They are generally **not** given in the acute setting.
  d. Assess the patient's ability to protect his or her airway, keep NPO, and elevate the head of the bed 30° to prevent aspiration.

2. BP control—In general, do not give antihypertensive agents unless one of the following three conditions is present:
   a. The patient's BP is very high (systolic >220, diastolic >120, or mean arterial pressure >130 mm Hg).
   b. The patient has a significant medical indication for antihypertensive therapy. Examples include:
      - Acute MI
      - Aortic dissection
      - Severe heart failure
      - Hypertensive encephalopathy
   c. The patient is receiving thrombolytic therapy—Aggressive blood pressure control is necessary to reduce the likelihood of bleeding.

3. Prevention—Specific recommendations for the prevention of strokes depend on the underlying etiology of the stroke.
   a. Prevention of strokes due to atherosclerosis of the carotid arteries
      - Control of risk factors—HTN, DM, smoking, hypercholesterolemia, obesity
      - Aspirin
      - Surgery (carotid endarterectomy)
        - **Symptomatic patients:** Three major studies have established the benefit of carotid endarterectomy in symptomatic patients with carotid artery stenosis of >70% (The NASCET trial was the most influential.)
        - **Asymptomatic patients:** Four major studies have investigated the benefit of carotid endarterectomy in asymptomatic patients. Three found no benefit. One study (ACAS) found that in asymptomatic patients who have a carotid artery stenosis of >60%, the benefits of surgery are very small. **Therefore, in asymptomatic patients, reduction of atherosclerotic risk factors and use of aspirin are recommended.**

QUICK HIT If stroke is caused by emboli from a cardiac source, anticoagulation is the treatment.

QUICK HIT Treatment of strokes is prophylactic. Once a stroke has occurred, there is nothing that can be done to salvage the dead brain tissue. The goal is to prevent ischemic events in the future.

FIGURE 5-3 Effect of carotid endarterectomy in carotid stenosis.

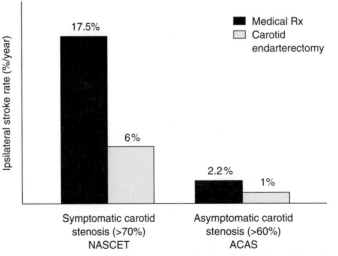

NASCET, North American Symptomatic Carotid Endarterectomy Trial; ACAS, Asymptomatic Carotid Atherosclerosis Study.
(Redrawn from Verstraete M, Fuster V, Topol EJ, eds. Cardiovascular Thrombosis–Thrombocardiology and Thromboneurology. 2nd Ed. Philadelphia: Lippincott Williams & Wilkins, 1998:590, Figure 34–4.)

b. Prevention of strokes due to embolic disease—anticoagulation (aspirin), reduction of atherosclerotic risk factors

c. Prevention of lacunar strokes—control of hypertension

Hemorrhagic Stroke

A. Intracerebral hemorrhage (ICH)

1. General characteristics
   a. ICH is associated with a high mortality rate (50% at 30 days). For those who survive, there is significant morbidity.
   b. Hematoma formation and enlargement may lead to local injury and increase in intracerebral pressure.

2. Causes
   a. HTN (**particularly a sudden increase in BP**) is the most common cause (50% to 60% of cases).
      - HTN causes a rupture of small vessels deep within the brain parenchyma. Chronic HTN causes degeneration of small arteries, leading to microaneurysms, which can rupture easily.
      - It is typically seen in older patients; risk increases with age.
   b. Ischemic stroke may convert to a hemorrhagic stroke.
   c. Other causes include amyloid angiopathy (10%), anticoagulant/antithrombolytic use (10%), brain tumors (5%), and AV malformations (5%).

3. Locations
   a. Basal ganglia (66%)
   b. Pons (10%)
   c. Cerebellum (10%)
   d. Other cortical areas

4. Clinical features
   a. Abrupt onset of a focal neurologic deficit that worsens steadily over 30 to 90 minutes   *usually in the morning.*
   b. Altered level of consciousness, stupor, or coma #
   c. Headache, vomiting
   d. Signs of increased intracranial pressure (ICP)- *papilledema.*

5. Diagnosis
   a. CT scan of the head diagnoses 95% of ICH (may miss very small bleeds) (see Figure 5-4).
   b. Coagulation panel and platelets—Check these to evaluate for bleeding diathesis.

6. Complications
   a. Increased ICP
   b. Seizures
   c. Rebleeding
   d. Vasospasm
   e. Hydrocephalus
   f. SIADH   *also caused by SCC or brain tumor.*

7. Treatment
   a. Admission to the ICU
   b. ABCs (airway, breathing, and circulation)—Airway management is important due to altered mental status and respiratory drives. Patients often require intubation.
   c. BP reduction
      - Elevated BP increases ICP and can cause further bleeding. However, hypotension can lower cerebral blood flow, worsening the neurologic deficits. Therefore, **BP reduction must be gradual so as to not induce hypotension.**
      - Treatment is indicated if systolic BP is >160 to 180 or diastolic BP is >105. Treatment for BP lower than these values is controversial.
      - Nitroprusside is often the agent of choice.
   d. Mannitol (osmotic agent) and diuretics can be given to reduce ICP. Use these agents only if ICP is elevated; do not give them prophylactically.

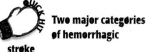

Two major categories of hemorrhagic stroke
- Intracerebral hemorrhage (ICH)–bleeding into brain parenchyma
- Subarachnoid hemorrhage (SAH)–bleeding into the CSF; outside brain parenchyma

Cocaine is one of the main causes of stroke in young patients. ICH, ischemic stroke, and SAH are all associated with cocaine use.

Pupillary findings in ICH and corresponding level of involvement
- Pinpoint pupils–pons
- Poorly reactive pupils–thalamus
- Dilated pupils–putamen

It is often difficult to distinguish ischemic stroke from an ICH on clinical grounds. The emergent treatment is initially the same until the diagnosis is certain. CT scan is the test that identifies ICH in the initial period.

DISEASES OF THE CENTRAL AND PERIPHERAL NERVOUS SYSTEMS

FIGURE
5-4
A. Spontaneous intracerebral hemorrhage in a hypertensive patient. **B.** On CT scan, ischemic stroke appears dark, whereas hemorrhagic stroke appears white.

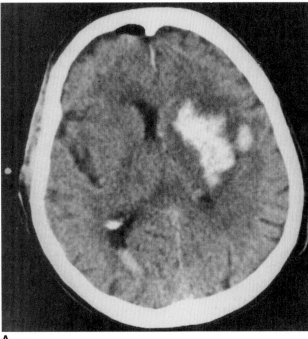

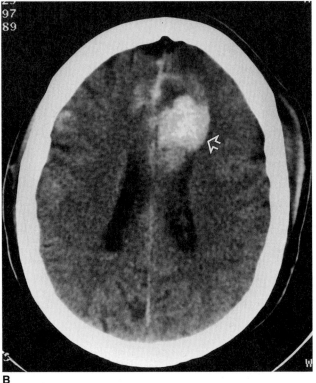

A

B

(**A** from Daffner RH, ed. Clinical Radiology: The Essentials. 2nd Ed. Philadelphia: Lippincott Williams & Wilkins, 1999:526, Figure 12.37A.)
(**B** from Daffner RH, ed. Clinical Radiology: The Essentials. 2nd Ed. Philadelphia: Lippincott Williams & Wilkins, 1999:528, Figure 12.40B.)

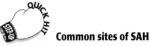

Common sites of SAH
- Junction of anterior communicating artery with anterior cerebral artery
- Junction of posterior communicating artery with the internal carotid artery
- Bifurcation of the MCA

Polycystic kidney disease is associated with berry aneurysms.

Caution: Ophthalmologic examination is mandatory to rule out **papilledema.** If papilledema is present, do not perform a lumbar puncture—you may cause a herniation. Repeat the CT scan first.

e. Use of steroids is harmful and is **not** recommended.
f. Rapid surgical evacuation of **cerebellar** hematomas can be life-saving. However, surgery is **not** helpful in most cases of **intracerebral** hemorrhage.

B. Subarachnoid hemorrhage (SAH)

1. **General characteristics**
   a. Mortality rate can be as high as 40% to 50% at 30 days.
   b. Locations—Saccular aneurysms occur at bifurcations of arteries of the circle of Willis.

2. **Causes**
   a. Ruptured berry (saccular) aneurysm is most common cause—has higher morbidity and mortality than other causes
   b. Trauma is also a common cause.
   c. AV malformation

3. **Clinical features**
   a. Sudden, severe (**often excruciating**) headache in the absence of focal neurologic symptoms; classic description is "**the worst headache of my life**" but may also be more subtle
   b. Sudden, transient loss of consciousness—in approximately 50% of patients
   c. Vomiting (common)
   d. Meningeal irritation, nuchal rigidity, and photophobia—can take several hours to develop
   e. Death—25% to 50% of patients die with the first rupture. Those who survive will recover consciousness within minutes.
   f. Retinal hemorrhages—in up to 30% of patients

4. **Diagnosis**
   a. Noncontrast CT scan—identifies the majority of SAHs. However, CT scan may be negative in up to 10% of cases.
   b. **Perform lumbar puncture if the CT scan is unrevealing or negative and clinical suspicion is high. LP is diagnostic.**
      - **Blood in the CSF** is a hallmark of SAH. (Be certain that it is not traumatic blood.)
      - **Xanthochromia** (yellow color of the CSF) is the gold standard for diagnosis of SAH. Xanthochromia results from RBC lysis. Xanthochromia implies that blood has been in CSF for several hours and that it is not due to a traumatic tap.
   c. Once SAH is diagnosed, order a cerebral angiogram. It is the definitive study for detecting the site of bleeding (for surgical clipping).
5. **Complications**
   a. Rerupture—occurs in up to 30% of patients
   b. Vasospasm—occurs in up to 50% of patients (more often with aneurysmal SAH); can cause ischemia/infarction and therefore stroke
   c. Hydrocephalus (communicating)—secondary to blood within the subarachnoid space hindering normal CSF flow
   d. Seizures may occur (blood acts as an irritant).
   e. SIADH
6. **Treatment**
   a. Surgical—consult neurosurgery. Berry aneurysms are usually treated surgically: surgically clip the aneurysm to prevent rebleeding.
   b. Medical—Therapy reduces the risks of rebleeding and cerebral vasospasm.
      - Bed rest in a quiet, dark room
      - Stool softeners to avoid straining (increases ICP and risk of repeated rerupture)
      - Analgesia for headache (acetaminophen)
      - IV fluids for hydration
      - Control of HTN—Lower the BP gradually because the elevation in BP may be a compensation for the decrease in cerebral perfusion pressure (secondary to increased ICP or cerebral arterial narrowing).
      - Calcium channel blocker (nifedipine) for vasospasm—lowers the incidence of cerebral infarction by one third

MOVEMENT DISORDERS

Parkinson's Disease

A. General characteristics
1. Results from a loss of dopamine-containing neurons—nerve cells that are located in the pigmented **substantia nigra** and the **locus ceruleus** in the midbrain
2. Onset is usually after age 50 years
3. Parkinsonism refers to symptoms and signs of Parkinson's disease and can result from many conditions (e.g., medications).
4. **Parkinson's disease is essentially a clinical diagnosis.** Laboratory studies play no role in diagnosis.

B. Clinical features
1. Pill-rolling tremor at rest (worsens with emotional stress). Tremor goes away when performing routine tasks.
2. Bradykinesia—slowness of voluntary movements
3. Rigidity is characteristic. "Cogwheel rigidity" refers to a ratchet-like jerking, which can be elicited by testing the tone in one limb while the patient clenches the opposite fist.
4. Poor postural reflexes; difficulty initiating the first step, and walking with small shuffling steps; stooped posture
5. Masked (expressionless) facies; decreased blinking

The basal ganglia/striatal region normally operates as a balanced system comprising the dopaminergic system and the cholinergic system. In Parkinson's disease, the dopaminergic pathway is compromised, and the cholinergic system operates unopposed. Therefore, the goal of treatment is either to enhance dopamine's influence or to inhibit acetylcholine's influence.

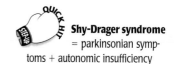
Shy-Drager syndrome = parkinsonian symptoms + autonomic insufficiency

Lewy bodies (hyalin inclusion bodies) are a key neuronal finding in the brains of patients with Parkinson's disease.

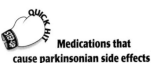

Medications that cause parkinsonian side effects

- Neuroleptic drugs (chlorpromazine, haloperidol, perphenazine)
- Metoclopramide
- Reserpine

6. Dysarthria and dysphagia, micrographia (small handwriting)
7. Impairment of cognitive function (dementia) in advanced disease
8. Autonomic dysfunction can lead to orthostatic hypotension, constipation, increased sweating, and oily skin.
9. Personality changes present in early stages. Patients become withdrawn, apathetic, and dependent on others. Depression is common and can be significant—causes worsening of parkinsonian symptoms.
10. Follows progressive course—significant disability usually presents within 5 to 10 years; indirectly leads to increased mortality

C. Treatment

1. No cure—goals are to delay disease progression and relieve symptoms.
2. Carbidopa-levodopa (Sinemet)—drug of choice for treating parkinsonian symptoms
   a. As the name implies, it is a combination of levodopa (L-Dopa) and carbidopa.
   b. It ameliorates all the symptoms of Parkinson's disease. It is the most effective of all the antiparkinsonian drugs.
   c. Side effects
      - Dyskinesias (involuntary, often choreic movements) can occur after 5 to 7 years of therapy. This is a major concern, and may warrant delay in initiating carbidopa-levodopa for as long as possible.
      - Nausea/vomiting, anorexia, HTN, hallucinations
   d. Levodopa does show an "on-off" phenomenon (over the course of the day) during treatment, which leads to fluctuations in symptoms. This is due to dose-response relationships. It often occurs in advanced disease.
3. Dopamine-receptor agonists (pergolide, bromocriptine, pramipexole)
   a. May control symptoms and delay need for levodopa for several years
   b. Initiate one of these agents when you have established the diagnosis. You may use levodopa and one of these agents at the same time.
   c. Pramipexole is the most commonly used.
   d. These can be useful for sudden episodes of hesitancy or immobility (described as "freezing").
4. Selegiline—inhibits monoamine oxidase B activity (increases dopamine activity) and reduces metabolism of levodopa. It is an adjunctive agent, and is often used in early disease.
5. Amantadine (antiviral agent)—increases the availability of endogenous dopamine with few side effects, but only transiently improves symptoms. It can be used with or without levodopa.
6. Anticholinergic drugs
   a. Trihexyphenidyl and benztropine
   b. These may be particularly helpful in patients with tremor as a major finding.
7. Amitriptyline—useful in the treatment of Parkinson's disease both as an anticholinergic agent and as an antidepressant.
8. Surgery (deep brain stimulation)—if patient does not respond to medications or in patients who develop severe disease before age 40 years

Patients with tremor as a major symptom of Parkinson's disease have a better prognosis than those who have bradykinesia as a predominant finding.

BOX 5-3 Progressive Supranuclear Palsy (PSP)

- PSP is a degenerative condition of the brainstem, basal ganglia, and cerebellum, most commonly affecting middle-aged and elderly men.
- Like Parkinson's disease, PSP causes bradykinesia, limb rigidity, cognitive decline, and follows a progressive course.
- Unlike Parkinson's disease, PSP
  - Does not cause tremor, and
  - Does cause ophthalmoplegia.

Huntington's Chorea

A. General characteristics
1. **Autosomal dominant**, so lack of family history makes this diagnosis unlikely
2. Onset is between 30 and 50 years of age. Symptoms worsen steadily, with 15 years being the typical duration from onset to death.
3. It is caused by a mutation on chromosome 4 (expanded triplet repeat sequence)—CAG leads to a loss of GABA-producing neurons in the striatum.

B. Clinical features
1. Chorea—involving the face, head and neck, tongue, trunk, and extremities
2. Altered behavior—irritability, personality changes, antisocial behavior, depression, obsessive-compulsive features, and/or psychosis
3. Impaired mentation—Progressive dementia is a key feature; 90% of patients are demented before age 50 years.
4. Gait is unsteady and irregular. Ultimately bradykinesia and rigidity prevail.
5. Incontinence

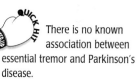

Always keep Wilson's disease in mind in a **young patient** with movement disorders (see Chapter 3).

C. Diagnosis
1. MRI shows atrophy of the head of caudate nuclei.
2. DNA testing confirms the diagnosis. Genetic counseling plays an important role.

D. Treatment: Treatment is symptomatic—there is no curative treatment. Dopamine blockers may help with the psychosis and improve chorea. Anxiolytic and antidepressant therapy may be necessary.

TREMOR

A. Physiologic tremor
1. **Causes**
   a. Fear, anxiety, fatigue
   b. Metabolic causes: hypoglycemia, hyperthyroidism, pheochromocytoma
   c. Toxic causes (e.g., alcohol withdrawal, valproic acid, lithium, methylxanthines—caffeine and theophylline)
2. **Treatment:** Treat the underlying cause, if known; otherwise, no treatment is necessary.

There is no known association between essential tremor and Parkinson's disease.

B. Essential tremor
1. Common; inherited (autosomal dominant) in up to one-third of patients
2. It is induced or exacerbated by intentional activity, such as drinking from a cup or use of utensils, and is **markedly decreased by alcohol use** (useful in diagnosis).
3. Distorted handwriting is often present. Note that bradykinesia, rigidity, shuffling gait, or postural instability are all absent.
4. Treat with propranolol.

C. Neurologic diseases (e.g., Parkinson's disease, cerebellar disease, Wilson's disease)

Ataxia

A. General characteristics
1. Gait instability
2. Loss of balance
3. Impaired limb coordination

B. Causes
1. Acquired causes: alcohol intoxication, vitamin B_{12} or thiamine deficiency, cerebellar infarction or neoplasm, demyelinating disease (multiple sclerosis [MS], AIDS), and tertiary syphilis (**tabes dorsalis**)
2. Inherited causes

TABLE 5-2	Common Tremors and Associated Features		
Feature	**Parkinsonian**	**Cerebellar**	**Essential**
Characteristic setting	Rest	With action— "intention tremor"	With certain postures (e.g., arms outstretched) or certain tasks (e.g., handwriting)
Description	Pill-rolling	Coarse	Fine
Etiology	Idiopathic or adverse effect of neuroleptic	Multiple possible etiologies	Often familial
Associated features	Rigidity, bradykinesia, shuffling gait	Ataxia, nystagmus, dysarthria	Head tremor, vocal tremulousness
Improved by	Action	Rest (no tremor at rest)	Alcohol

a. Friedreich's ataxia
- Autosomal recessive inheritance, onset by young adulthood
- Presents with ataxia, nystagmus, impaired vibratory sense and proprioception
b. Ataxia telangiectasia
- Autosomal recessive inheritance, childhood onset
- Symptoms similar to those of Friedreich's ataxia plus telangiectases
- Increased incidence of cancer

C. Treatment: Treat underlying cause if possible.

Tourette's Syndrome

A. General characteristics
1. Associated with obsessive-compulsive disorder
2. Onset before age 21 years
3. Thought to have autosomal dominant inheritance pattern
4. Not all patients with tics have Tourette's syndrome.
5. Not all patients with Tourette's syndrome experience coprolalia (involuntary swearing).

B. Clinical features (occur frequently and regularly)
1. Motor tics (multiple)
2. Phonic tics (at least one kind)

C. Treatment (if symptoms are affecting the patient's quality of life; patient education is important)
1. Clonidine
2. Pimozide
3. Haloperidol

DEMENTIA

Overview

A. General characteristics
1. Dementia is a progressive deterioration of intellectual function, typically characterized by **preservation of consciousness**.
2. The most important risk factor for dementia is increasing age.

Tics
- Motor tics (e.g., facial grimace, blinking, head jerking, shoulder shrugging)
- Phonic tics (e.g., grunting, sniffing, clearing throat, coprolalia, repetition of words)
- Conditions that must be ruled out include seizures, tardive dyskinesias, and Huntington's disease.

B. Differential diagnosis of dementia

1. Primary neurologic disorders
   a. Alzheimer's disease—accounts for 66% of all cases of dementia (see the section on Alzheimer's disease below)
   b. Vascular dementia
      - **Multi-infarct dementia** is a stepwise decline due to a series of cerebral infarctions; it may not be as prevalent as once thought.
      - Binswanger's disease—insidious onset, due to diffuse subcortical white matter degeneration, most commonly seen in patients with long-standing HTN and atherosclerosis
   c. Space-occupying lesions, such as brain tumor or chronic subdural hematoma
   d. Normal-pressure hydrocephalus—triad of dementia, gait disturbance, and incontinence; normal CSF pressure and dilated ventricles
   e. Dementia with Lewy bodies (see section below)
   f. Pick's disease—clinically identical to Alzheimer's disease
   g. Other neurologic conditions: MS, Parkinson's disease, Huntington's disease, Wilson's disease
2. Infections
   a. HIV infection (AIDS-related dementia)
   b. Neurosyphilis
   c. Cryptococcal infection of CNS
   d. Creutzfeldt-Jakob disease (spongiform encephalopathy)
   e. Progressive multifocal leukoencephalopathy
3. Metabolic disorders
   a. Thyroid disease (hypothyroidism or hyperthyroidism)
   b. Vitamin B_{12} deficiency
   c. Thiamine deficiency—common in alcoholics; if untreated can lead to Korsakoff's dementia (irreversible)
   d. Niacin deficiency — dermatitis, dementia, diarrhea, death.
4. Drugs and toxins
   a. Drug abuse; chronic alcoholism (may cause dementia independent from thiamine malnutrition)
   b. Toxic substances: aniline dyes, metals (e.g., lead)
5. Pseudodementia (depression)—Severe depression may cause a decline in cognition that is difficult to distinguish clinically from Alzheimer's disease, but is responsive to antidepressant therapy.

Forgetfulness versus dementia

- Some degree of memory loss is accepted as a normal part of aging. It may be difficult to distinguish this condition, sometimes referred to as benign forgetfulness of elderly patients, from true dementia.
- In general, benign forgetfulness does not adversely affect normal day-to-day living or baseline functioning, but it may be a risk factor for progressive dementias such as **Alzheimer's disease.**

benign forgetfulness
↓
Alzheimer's disease.

Box 5-4 Causes of Dementia

Potentially Reversible Causes of Dementia
- Hypothyroidism
- Neurosyphilis
- Vitamin B_{12}/folate deficiency/thiamine deficiency
- Medications
- Normal-pressure hydrocephalus
- Depression
- Subdural hematoma

Irreversible Causes of Dementia
- Alzheimer's disease
- Parkinson's, Huntington's
- Multi-infarct dementia
- Dementia with Lewy bodies, Pick's disease
- Unresectable brain mass
- HIV dementia
- Korsakoff's syndrome
- Progressive multifocal leukoencephalopathy ?? → BK virus.
- Creutzfeldt-Jakob disease — transmissable.

C. Clinical approach to dementia

1. Patient history—Ask patients and their family members about the nature of onset, specific deficits, physical symptoms, and comorbid conditions. Review all medications, as well as family and social history.
2. Physical examination
   a. Focus on a thorough neurologic examination and mental status examination.
   b. Gait analysis often sheds light on movement disorders, mass lesions, and non-pressure hydrocephalus.
3. Laboratory and imaging studies—Consider the following when investigating the cause of dementia: CBC with differential, chemistry panel, thyroid function tests (TSH), vitamin B_{12}, folate level, VDRL (syphilis), HIV screening, and CT scan or MRI of the head.

D. Treatment and management: general principles

1. Treat reversible causes.
2. Avoid and/or monitor doses of medications with adverse cognitive side effects (glucocorticoids, opiates, sedative hypnotics, anxiolytics, anticholinergics, lithium).
3. Treat/control comorbid medical conditions; e.g., diabetes, HTN, depression, visual and hearing impairment.
4. Pharmacologic therapy may include vitamin E, tacrine, and donepezil. The evidence supporting the efficacy of many pharmacologic treatments is inconclusive.
5. A multidisciplinary approach includes support groups for caregivers/families of patients with irreversible dementias.

Alzheimer's Disease

A. General characteristics

1. Epidemiology
   a. Alzheimer's disease is the fourth most common cause of death in the United States.
   b. Prevalence increases with age—Approximately 10% to 15% of individuals over age 65, and 15% to 30% of individuals over age 80 have Alzheimer's disease. However, many will die of other causes first.
2. Risk factors
   a. Family history (especially for early-onset Alzheimer's disease)
   b. Down's syndrome
3. Etiology is unknown, but a heritable component may be present. Chromosomes 21, 14, and 19 have been linked to Alzheimer's disease.
4. Pathology (noted at autopsy)
   a. Quantity of senile plaques (age-specific)—focal collections of dilated, tortuous neuritic processes surrounding a central amyloid core (amyloid beta-protein)
   b. Quantity of neurofibrillary tangles (age-specific)
      • Bundles of neurofilaments in cytoplasm of neurons
      • Denote neuronal degeneration

QUICK HIT

Patients with Alzheimer's disease often have **cerebral atrophy** secondary to neuronal loss. Ventricles will correspondingly be enlarged.

B. Clinical features

1. Begins insidiously but tends to progress at a steady rate
2. The average time from onset to death is 5 to 10 years (with some variability).
3. Stages
   a. Early stages—mild forgetfulness, impaired ability to learn new material, poor performance at work, poor concentration, changes in personality, impaired judgment (e.g., inappropriate humor)
   b. Intermediate stages—Memory is progressively impaired. Patients may be aware of the condition, yet denial is often present. Visuospatial disturbances are common (getting lost in a familiar place and difficulty following directions). Patients may repeat questions over and over.
   c. Later stages—Assistance is needed for activities of daily living. Patients have difficulty remembering the names of relatives/friends or major aspects of their lives. Paranoid delusions (e.g., victim of theft) and hallucinations are common.

[Handwritten margin notes:]

tacrine and donepezil – cholinesterase inhibitor.

MC causes of death
① Cardiovascular
② Cancer
③ CVA
④ Alzheimer's dx.

d. Advanced disease—Complete debilitation and dependence on others; incontinence (bowel/bladder); patient may even forget his or her own name
e. Death is usually secondary to infection or other complications of a debilitated state.

Aricept better than tacrine b/c once a day dosing and more improvement.

C. Diagnosis

1. Alzheimer's disease is essentially a **clinical diagnosis**; exclude other causes first.
2. CT scan or MRI showing diffuse cortical atrophy with enlargement of the ventricles strengthens the diagnosis.

D. Treatment

1. AChE inhibitors—Brains of patients with Alzheimer's disease have lower levels of acetylcholine. **Avoid anticholinergic medications!** Use donepezil (newer than tacrine), a cholinesterase inhibitor.   *Aricept.*
   a. Currently the first-line agent
   b. Advantages over tacrine include once-per-day dosing, more improvement in behavioral as well as cognitive domains, and fewer side effects.
2. Tacrine is currently not used as frequently because of four-times-per-day dosing and marginal improvement in cognition.
3. Certain dietary supplements (ginkgo, lecithin) have not been proven to be beneficial.
4. Vitamin E
   a. In one study, megadoses of vitamin E (2,000 IU/day) slowed disease progression and preserved function in people with moderately severe Alzheimer's disease.
   b. Full benefit remains to be defined.

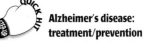

QUICK HIT

Alzheimer's disease: treatment/prevention

- No treatment has been found to have a significant effect on cognitive effects. Donepezil and tacrine are the only FDA-approved agents, but the clinical improvement with their use is marginal.
- Hormone replacement therapy is associated with a lower risk of developing Alzheimer's disease.

Dementia With Lewy Bodies

- Dementia with Lewy bodies has features of both Alzheimer's disease and Parkinson's disease, but progression may be more rapid than in Alzheimer's disease.
- Initially, visual hallucinations predominate. Other symptoms include extrapyramidal features and fluctuating mental status.
- These patients are sensitive to the adverse effects of neuroleptic agents, which often exacerbate symptoms.
- Treatment is similar to that for Alzheimer's disease, with neuroleptic agents (for hallucinations and psychotic features). Selegiline may slow the progression of disease.

ALTERED MENTAL STATUS

Acute Confusional State (Delirium)

A. General characteristics

1. Delirium is an acute period of cognitive dysfunction due to a medical disturbance or condition.
2. Elderly patients are especially prone to delirium.

B. Causes: Causes of delirium include those of coma (see Box 5-6, "SMASHED"), plus the following: "P. DIMM WIT."

1. **P** = postoperative state (compounded by pain medications)
2. **D** = dehydration and malnutrition
3. **I** = infection (sepsis, meningitis, encephalitis, urinary tract infection, and so on)
4. **M** = medications and drug intoxications—TCAs, corticosteroids, anticholinergics, hallucinogens, cocaine
5. **M** = metals (heavy metal exposure)
6. **W** = withdrawal states (from alcohol, benzodiazepines)
7. **I** = inflammation, fever
8. **T** = trauma, burns

Arousal - depends on intact
  brain stem.
Cognition - depends on intact
  cerebral cortex.

> **Box 5-5 Altered Mental Status**
>
> - Consciousness relies on arousal and cognition. Arousal is dependent on an intact brainstem (reticular activating system **in brainstem**). Cognition is dependent on an intact cerebral cortex.
> - Altered mental status, diminished level of consciousness (drowsiness, stupor, coma), and confusion are caused by many of the same conditions and **are often** variations of the same theme.
> - Depressed level of consciousness and coma can be caused by a variety of disorders. To help in classification and to organize one's thinking, it is useful to organize these causes into two categories:
>   - Diffuse injury to the brain due to any metabolic, systemic, or toxic disorder
>   - Focal intracranial structural lesions—e.g., hemorrhage, infarction, tumor

C. Clinical features

1. In contrast to both dementia and psychosis, delirium is characterized by a rapid deterioration in mental status (over hours to days), a fluctuating level of awareness, disorientation, and, frequently, abnormal vital signs.
2. Delirium may often be accompanied by acute abnormalities of perception, such as hallucinations.
3. Patients may not necessarily be agitated, but may have a slow, blunted responsiveness.

D. Diagnosis

1. Mental status examination, Mini-Mental Status Examination
2. Laboratory—e.g., chemistry panel, vitamin B_{12}, thiamine, TSH
3. LP—Perform in any febrile, delirious patient unless there are contraindications (e.g., cerebral edema).

E. Treatment

1. Treat the underlying cause.
2. Haloperidol—for agitation/psychotic-like delirious behavior
3. Supportive treatment

Coma

A. General characteristics

1. A coma is a depressed level of consciousness to the extent that the patient is completely unresponsive to any stimuli.

TABLE 5-3 Delirium Versus Dementia

Feature	Delirium	Dementia
Causes	• Infections (UTI, systemic infection) • Medications (narcotics, benzodiazepines) • Postoperative delirium (in elderly patients) • Alcoholism • Electrolyte imbalances • Medical conditions (stroke, heart disease, seizures, hepatic and renal disorders)	• Alzheimer's disease • Multi-infarct dementia • Pick's disease
Level of consciousness	Altered, fluctuating	Preserved
Hallucinations	Frequently present (visual)	Rarely present
Presence of tremor	Sometimes present (e.g., asterixis)	Usually absent unless dementia is due to Parkinson's disease
Course	• Rapid onset, **waxing and waning** • **"Sundowning"** (worsening at night) may be present	Insidious, progressive
Reversibility	Almost always reversible	Typically irreversible

---

Box 5-6   Differential Diagnosis of Coma or Stupor: SMASHED

- **S** = **s**tructural brain pathology: stroke, subdural or epidural hematoma, tumor, hydrocephalus, herniation, abscess
- **M** = **m**eningitis, mental illness (e.g., conversion disorder, catatonia—mimic coma)
- **A** = **a**lcohol, acidosis
- **S** = **s**eizures (postictal state), substrate deficiency (e.g., thiamine)
- **H** = **h**ypercapnia, hyperglycemia, hyperthermia; hyponatremia, hypoglycemia, hypoxia, hypotension/cerebral hypoperfusion, hypothermia
- **E** = **e**ndocrine causes (Addisonian crisis, thyrotoxicosis, hypothyroidism); encephalitis, encephalopathy (hypertensive, hepatic, or uremic); extreme disturbances in calcium, magnesium, phosphate
- **D** = **d**rugs (opiates, barbiturates, benzodiazepines, other sedatives); dangerous compounds (carbon monoxide, cyanide, methanol)

---

2. Causes
   a. Structural brain lesions that cause a coma are usually bilateral unless they produce enough mass effect to compress the brainstem or the opposite cerebral hemisphere (see Box 5-6).
   b. Global brain dysfunction (e.g., metabolic or systemic disorders)
   c. Psychiatric causes—Conversion disorders and malingering may be difficult to differentiate from a true coma.

B. Approach

1. Initial steps
   a. Assess vital signs. ABCs take priority.
   b. Always assume underlying trauma (stabilize cervical spine) and assess the patient for signs of underlying causes of trauma.
   c. Assess the level of consciousness using the Glasgow Coma Scale. Repeat this serially because it can change.
2. Approach to diagnosing the cause of coma
   a. Rapid motor examination—If asymmetry is noted in movements, a mass lesion is the likely cause. Metabolic or systemic causes of coma do not produce asymmetric motor abnormalities.
   b. Brainstem reflexes
      - Pupillary light reflex—If the pupils are round and symmetrically reactive (constrict to bright light), the midbrain is intact and not the cause of coma. Anisocoria (asymmetric pupils) may be a sign of uncal herniation. Keep in mind that certain eye drops or systemic medications may alter pupil size.

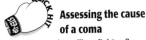
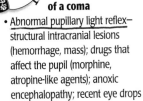

Assessing the cause of a coma
- Abnormal pupillary light reflex–structural intracranial lesions (hemorrhage, mass); drugs that affect the pupil (morphine, atropine-like agents); anoxic encephalopathy; recent eye drops
- Bilateral fixed, dilated pupils–severe anoxia
- Unilateral fixed, dilated pupil–herniation with CN III compression
- Pinpoint pupils–narcotics, ICH

TABLE 5-4   Glasgow Coma Scale

Eye opening (E)	Does not open eyes	1
	Opens to painful stimulus	2
	Opens to voice (command)	3
	Opens spontaneously	4
Motor response (M)	No movement	1
	Decerebrate posture	2
	Decorticate posture	3
	Withdraws from pain	4
	Localizes painful stimulus	5
	Obeys commands	6
Verbal response (V)	No sounds	1
	Incomprehensible sounds	2
	Inappropriate words	3
	Appropriate but confused	4
	Appropriate and oriented	5

To check whether or not brainstem is intact
1. *Pupillary light reflex*
2. *Eye movements ("dolls" maneuver)*
3. *Pts. breathing.*

• Eye movements—If the cervical spine is uninjured, perform the oculocephalic test ("doll's eyes"). When the head is turned to one side, the eyes should move conjugately to the opposite direction if the brainstem is intact.
• If the patient is breathing on her or his own, the brainstem is functioning.
c. Laboratory tests—CBC, electrolytes, calcium BUN, creatinine, glucose, plasma osmolarity, arterial blood gas, ECG
d. Toxicologic analysis of blood and urine
e. CT or MRI of the brain
f. LP—if meningitis or SAH is suspected

C. Treatment

1. Correct reversible causes and treat the underlying problem (if identified)—control airway; give supplemental oxygen, naloxone (for narcotic overdose), dextrose (for hypoglycemia). Give thiamine before a glucose load. Correct any abnormalities in BP, electrolytes, or body temperature.
2. Identify and treat herniation—lowering the ICP is critical (see Head Trauma section).

Coma pt -try - atropine, naloxone, glucose but 1st give thiamine.

Brain Herniation

A. General characteristics

1. Brain tissue moves past anatomic barriers because there is an increase in volume due to edema or mass lesion (e.g., tumor, abscess, hemorrhage).
2. Sites of herniation
   a. Uncal (transtentorial) herniation
      • Uncus compresses the midbrain
      • Compression of CN III results in ipsilateral anisocoria, sluggish pupillary light reflex (can lead to nonreactivity), and dilated pupils.
      • Contralateral hemiparesis due to compression of cerebral peduncle against bone
      • Progressive brainstem compression can lead to changes in respiration, changes in cardiovascular status, and eventually death.
   b. Tonsillar herniation
      • Medial portions of cerebellar hemispheres compress the medulla through the foramen magnum.
      • Compression of vital cardiorespiratory centers may cause rapid death.
   c. Central herniation
      • Caused by supratentorial lesions

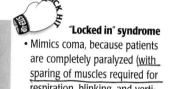

"Locked in" syndrome
• Mimics coma, because patients are completely paralyzed (with sparing of muscles required for respiration, blinking, and vertical eye movement).
• Patients are **fully aware** of their surroundings and capable of feeling pain.
• This is usually caused by infarction or hemorrhage of the ventral pons.

pontine basilar arteries

Box 5-7 Brain Death Versus Persistent Vegetative State

• Criteria for diagnosing brain death
   • **Irreversible** absence of brain and brainstem function—unresponsiveness, apnea **despite adequate oxygenation and ventilation,** no brainstem reflexes (pupils, calorics, gag, cornea, doll's eyes)
   • No drug intoxication or metabolic condition that can reversibly inhibit brain function
   • Core body temperature >32°C, 89.6°F. Brain death cannot be established in presence of hypothermia.
   • Clinical evidence or imaging study that provides a causative explanation for brain death
   • Examinations must be repeated or EEG performed. EEG shows isoelectric activity (electrical silence).
• In most states, **if a patient is proven to be brain dead,** the physician has the right to disconnect life support—the patient is legally dead. (Obviously sensitivity and consideration must be demonstrated to the family. They must be informed and given a chance to say good-bye to their loved one.)
• Patients in a "vegetative state" are completely unresponsive (comatose), but eyes are open and they appear awake. May have random head or limb movements. Patient **may** have no hope of meaningful recovery but do not meet brain death criteria. Ethical and legal issues surrounding supportive measures are much more complicated.

- Clinical findings vary—can include a change in mental status, midpoint small pupils, posturing of extremities, Cheyne-Stokes respirations, and hyperventilation.
- Causes increased muscle tone, bilateral Babinski's signs

B. Diagnosis: immediate CT scan of the head

C. Treatment
1. Intubation (using rapid-sequence technique)
2. Neurosurgical consult
3. Lower ICP (see Head Trauma section)

DEMYELINATING DISEASE

Multiple Sclerosis (MS)

A. General characteristics
1. Pathology
   a. Selective **demyelination of CNS**—Multifocal zones of demyelination (plaques) are scattered throughout the white matter. Classic location of plaques is at the angles of the lateral ventricles.
   b. Demyelination primarily involves **white matter** of the brain and spinal cord; tends to spare the gray matter/axons and the peripheral nervous system. However, improved imaging techniques are showing that cortical demyelination may be more prevalent than previously appreciated.
   c. Commonly involved tracts: pyramidal and cerebellar pathways, medial longitudinal fasciculus, optic nerve, posterior columns
2. Incidence is greater at higher latitudes. Very low incidence near the equator. Migrating from a place of high to low latitude before age 15 lowers the risk of MS.
3. Women are two to three times more likely than men to have MS.
4. Etiology is unknown, but is probably secondary to the interplay of environmental, immunologic, and genetic factors.

B. Clinical features
1. Transient sensory deficits
   a. Most common initial presentation
   b. Decreased sensation or paresthesias in upper or lower limbs
2. Fatigue—one of the most common complaints
3. Motor symptoms—mainly weakness or spasticity
   a. May appear insidiously or acutely
   b. Caused by pyramidal tract involvement (upper motor neuron involvement)

> **QUICK HIT**
> There are a variety of presenting symptoms in MS that involve many different areas of the CNS, and the inability to attribute them all to one localizing lesion is a characteristic feature of the disease.

Box 5-8   Diagnosis of Multiple Sclerosis (MS)

Clinically Definite MS
- Two episodes of symptoms
- Evidence of two white matter lesions (imaging or clinical)

Laboratory-Supported Definite MS
- Two episodes of symptoms
- Evidence of at least one white matter lesion on MRI
- Abnormal CSF (oligoclonal bands in CSF)

Probable MS
- Two episodes of symptoms and either one white matter lesion or oligoclonal bands in CSF

---

    c. Spasticity (such as leg stiffness) can impair the patient's ability to walk and maintain balance.

    d. Can lead to weakness with progression to paraparesis, hemiparesis, or quadriparesis

4. Visual disturbances

    a. **Optic neuritis**
- Monocular visual loss (in up to 20% of patients)
- Pain on movement of eyes
- Central scotoma (black spot in center of vision)
- Decreased pupillary reaction to light

    b. **Internuclear ophthalmoplegia**—strongly suggests the diagnosis
- A lesion in the medial longitudinal fasciculus results in ipsilateral medial rectus palsy on attempted lateral gaze (adduction defect) and horizontal nystagmus of abducting eye (contralateral to side of lesion).
- Diplopia can occur.

5. Cerebellar involvement—can cause ataxia, intention tremor, dysarthria

6. Loss of bladder control—consequence of upper motor neuron injury in spinal cord

7. Autonomic involvement—may present as impotence and/or constipation

8. Cerebral involvement—may occur in advanced illness and manifests as memory loss, personality change, and emotional lability; anxiety and depression are common

9. Neuropathic pain—a frustrating but common complaint that manifests as <u>hyperesthesias and trigeminal neuralgia</u>

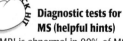

Relapses of MS produce symptoms for longer than 24 hours. They average one per year, but usually decrease in frequency over time.

C. Course

1. Most patients at initial presentation are in their 20s to 30s and present with a localizing deficit such as optic neuritis, one-sided weakness, or numbness. Patients may or may not go on to develop MS.

2. The following are the main variants of MS, showing the variability that exists in the disease progression.

    a. Clinically silent—This is also known as "stable" or "benign" MS. Some progression may occur late in the course of the disease.

    b. Relapsing/remitting (most common)—exacerbations followed by remissions

    c. Secondary progressive—Patients with relapsing/remitting disease can experience gradual worsening of symptoms that is progressive in later years.

    d. Primary progressive—This is steady progressive disease that appears later in life (after 40 years of age), and tends to have less visual and more axonal involvement.

3. Attacks average up to one per year. No one precipitant has been proven to cause attacks.

4. Prognosis is highly variable, with normal life spans in most patients.

    a. Although quality of life is diminished, many patients never develop debilitating disease.

    b. Approximately one-third of patients eventually progress to severe disability.

    c. The following increase the chances of severe disability: frequent attacks early in the disease course, onset at an older age, progressive course, and early cerebellar or pyramidal involvement.

D. Diagnosis

1. The diagnosis is essentially clinical—suspect it in young adults with relapsing and remitting neurologic signs and symptoms that are difficult to explain (due to involvement of different areas of CNS white matter). Nevertheless, on suspicion, order the MRI and consider LP (discussed below), because it is important to diagnose MS with as much certainty as possible due to the implications surrounding the management approach.

2. MRI is the test of choice (most sensitive) and is diagnostic in the majority of cases.

    a. Now considered standard of care

    b. Sensitive in identifying demyelinating lesions in CNS

Diagnostic tests for MS (helpful hints)
- MRI is abnormal in 90% of MS patients.
- CSF is abnormal in 90% of MS patients.
- Evoked potentials are abnormal in 90% of MS patients.

   c. The number of lesions on the MRI is **not** necessarily proportional to disease severity or speed of progression.

3. LP and CSF analysis—Although no laboratory tests are specific for MS, **oligoclonal bands** of immunoglobulin G are present in 90% of MS patients.

4. Evoked potentials can suggest demyelination of certain areas by measuring the speed of nerve conduction within the brain: newly remyelinated nerves will conduct sensory impulses more slowly.

E. Treatment

1. Treatment of acute attacks
   a. High-dose IV corticosteroids can shorten an acute attack. Oral steroids have not shown the same efficacy.
   b. Studies have shown that treatment of **acute** exacerbations does **not** alter the outcome or course of MS.
   c. Most acute attacks resolve within 6 weeks with or without treatment.
   d. One study showed therapeutic plasma exchange (TPE) for steroid-refractory acute demyelinating attacks had a 42% response rate.

2. Disease-modifying therapy
   a. Interferon therapy
   - Recombinant interferon β-1a, recombinant interferon β-1b, and glatiramer acetate have shown a reduction in relapse rates of 37%, 33%, and 29%, respectively.
   - The interferons can cause flulike symptoms, which can be severe and persistent.
   - Interferon therapy should be started early in the course of disease before the disability becomes irreversible.
   - Present studies have lasted less than 5 years, so long-term benefits are unknown.
   b. Nonspecific immunosuppressive therapy such as cyclophosphamide should be reserved for rapidly progressive disease, because toxic side effects are many.

3. Symptomatic therapy
   a. Baclofen for muscle spasticity
   b. Carbamazepine or gabapentin for neuropathic pain

Guillain-Barré Syndrome

A. General characteristics

1. Inflammatory demyelinating polyneuropathy that primarily affects motor nerves
2. Usually preceded by a viral or mycoplasmal infection of upper respiratory or GI tract. Common infections include *Campylobacter jejuni*, CMV, hepatitis, and HIV.
3. May also occur in Hodgkin's disease, lupus, after surgery, or after HIV seroconversion

B. Clinical features

1. Abrupt onset with rapidly **ascending weakness/paralysis** of all four extremities; frequently progresses to involve respiratory, facial, and bulbar muscles
   a. Usually symmetric (but not always)
   b. Weakness may be mild or severe.
   c. Weakness usually progresses from distal to central muscles.
   d. **If generalized paralysis is present, it can lead to respiratory arrest.**
2. Extremities may be painful, but sensory loss is not typical.
3. Sphincter control and mentation are typically spared.
4. Autonomic features (e.g., arrhythmias, tachycardia, postural hypotension) are dangerous complications.

C. Diagnosis

1. CSF analysis—elevated protein, but normal cell count
2. Electrodiagnostic studies—decreased motor nerve conduction velocity

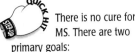 There is no cure for MS. There are two primary goals:
- Prevent relapses
- Relieve symptoms of acute exacerbations

 Prognosis for Guillain-Barré syndrome
- Signs of recovery within 1 to 3 weeks after onset favors a good prognosis. If illness continues for a longer period (e.g., beyond 6 weeks), a chronic relapsing course is more likely and prognosis is less favorable.
- It may take months before the patient recovers. A minority of patients experience recurrent attacks, and about 5% die due to respiratory failure, pneumonia, or arrhythmias.

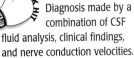 Diagnosis made by a combination of CSF fluid analysis, clinical findings, and nerve conduction velocities.

In Guillain-Barré syndrome, rapid progression to respiratory failure can occur within hours. Therefore, a timely and accurate diagnosis is critical. If you suspect Guillain-Barré syndrome, immediately admit the patient to the hospital for monitoring.

D. Treatment
1. Carefully monitor pulmonary function. Mechanical ventilation may be necessary.
2. Administer IV immunoglobulin if the patient has significant weakness. If progression continues, plasmapheresis may reduce severity of disease.
3. Do **not** give steroids. They are usually harmful and never helpful in Guillain-Barré syndrome.

CNS NEOPLASMS

Overview

A. General characteristics
1. The most common intracranial neoplasms in adults are **brain metastases** from other primary sites.
2. Among primary CNS tumors in adults, gliomas are the most common (approximately 50%), followed by meningiomas (approximately 25%).
3. Although most CNS tumors remain confined to the cranial cavity and spinal canal, all CNS tumors have malignant potential in that they may recur.

B. Clinical features
1. Nonspecific symptoms occur due to an increase in ICP (either directly by the mass effect or indirectly by obstructing the circulation of the CSF and producing hydrocephalus). Signs and symptoms depend on the severity and rate of increased ICP.
   a. Headaches—classically on awakening or with dependent head position (worrisome symptoms); usually progressive
   b. Nausea and vomiting—typically in the morning
   c. Reduction in the level of consciousness
   d. Papilledema—swollen optic disc
   e. Brain herniation may occur with extensive or rapid tumor growth.
2. Focal deficits
   a. Mass effect resulting in cranial nerve deficits
   b. Seizures—may be focal, generalized, or focal with secondary generalization; may be the only presenting sign of brain tumor
   c. Specific neurologic defects (e.g., visual disturbances, personality changes, aphasia) are dependent on location of the tumor.
   d. Sometimes the tumors themselves may cause hyperfunctioning of a given structure, such as a pituitary adenoma or a choroid plexus papilloma (overproduces CSF).

Two important indications for ordering an MRI to rule out intracranial mass
• New-onset seizure in an adult
• New and persistent or progressive headache

C. Diagnosis
1. MRI with and without gadolinium—imaging test of choice
2. Brain biopsy—only definitive way to diagnose a brain tumor and determine the specific type

D. Treatment
1. Certain types of tumors can be surgically resected and have a favorable prognosis (e.g., meningiomas, pituitary adenomas, and schwannomas).
2. However, gliomas (e.g., astrocytomas and oligodendrogliomas) usually cannot be surgically resected.
3. Radiation therapy is often given after surgery for tumors that cannot be completely resected in order to prolong survival in patients with unresectable tumors. Radiation therapy may actually cause new primary tumors, such as meningioma(s).
4. Chemotherapy is sometimes given but has limited effectiveness.
5. Controlling elevated ICP may involve steroids, mannitol, and possibly hyperventilation, depending on the severity.

Intraparenchymal Brain Tumors

A. Astrocytomas

1. Most common primary CNS neoplasms (80% of all CNS tumors) in adults
2. Arise almost exclusively in the cerebral hemispheres
3. Features
   a. These tumors infiltrate the brain and have indistinct boundaries.
   b. They tend to spread along white matter tracts and **may cross** the corpus callosum into the **opposite hemisphere**.
   c. Prognosis is poor despite advances in surgery, radiotherapy, and chemotherapy. Cure is rare. The recurrence rate is very high.
   d. Glioblastoma multiforme has the worst prognosis (90% die within 3 months), and survival beyond 2 years is rare.

B. Oligodendrogliomas

1. The peak age of occurrence is between 40 and 50 years.
2. They are malignant, but have a more indolent progression than fibrillary astrocytomas.
3. Patients survive up to 10 to 15 years after presentation.

C. Primary lymphomas

1. These are related to immunosuppression, and are encountered especially in recipients of transplanted organs and in patients with AIDS.
2. The median duration of survival is less than 2 years, and the 5-year survival is less than 5%.

D. Metastatic brain tumors

1. Almost 50% of intracranial neoplasms are metastatic.
2. The most common primary sites of neoplasms that metastasize to the brain (in order of occurrence, most frequent first) are as follows: lung, breast, skin (malignant melanoma), kidney, and GI tract.

Extraparenchymal Brain Tumors

A. Meningiomas

1. Typically occur between 40 and 50 years of age
2. Occur twice as frequently in women as in men
3. Attach to the dura—These are extracerebral, rounded masses with well-defined dural bases that compress the underlying brain.
4. Clinical presentation depends on site—Although benign, they may cause significant morbidity (and mortality), if they are large enough, due to compression of adjacent brain tissue.
5. Because of their focal and benign nature, they offer the potential for a surgical cure, but there is a high rate of recurrence.

B. Schwannomas

1. Benign tumors with no malignant potential
2. Almost always unilateral (if bilateral, this is pathognomonic for neurofibromatosis type II)

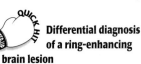

QUICK HIT

Differential diagnosis of a ring-enhancing brain lesion
- Metastatic cancer
- Brain abscess
- Glioblastoma multiforme
- Lymphoma
- Toxoplasmosis

Box 5-9 Meningeal Carcinomatosis

- Refers to cancer that metastasizes to the meninges, usually via the bloodstream
- May cause focal neurologic deficits depending on the involved locations (e.g., cranial nerve, spinal cord, or spinal root); can also cause hydrocephalus
- CSF analysis reveals malignant cells, elevated protein and lymphocytes, and decreased glucose.
- Treat with intrathecal chemotherapy.

3. Arise in the cerebellopontine angle, so they involve the 8th cranial nerve. As they grow larger, they may affect the 5th and 7th cranial nerves as well.
4. Hearing loss is usually the first symptom. Other symptoms may include tinnitus, loss of balance, nystagmus, and motor or sensory deficits involving the face. If untreated, they can cause brainstem compression.
5. Surgical excision has shown very good results. Cure is achieved if the tumor is removed completely.

HEAD TRAUMA

Overview

A. Injury assessment: With head injury, consider the implications of irreversible damage and secondary insults.
1. Irreversible damage can occur to brain tissue. There is no way to speed up recovery time for tissue that is healing.
2. Secondary insults—**Secondary insults can lead to deterioration in clinical and neurologic status. Rapid diagnosis and prevention of these secondary events are the only way to affect the ultimate prognosis.** Secondary insults can include the following:
   a. Hypotension—leads to decreased cerebral perfusion
   b. Hypoxia—can be due to a variety of mechanisms depending on injury; common causes include chest wall or pulmonary injury that impairs gas exchange, and brainstem compression leading to apnea and airway obstruction
   c. Hypercapnia—causes vasodilation and exacerbates the problem of increased intravascular volume *therefore for ↑ICP - hyperventilation works.*
   d. Increased ICP
   e. Intracranial mass effect—due to an epidural or subdural hematoma
   f. Anemia—due to blood loss in trauma

B. Key features
1. **Elevated ICP—most common cause of death after severe head injury**
   a. Normal ICP is 5 to 15 mm H_2O. ICP >20 mm H_2O is worrisome (although the precise definition of unacceptable ICP is unclear).
   b. Cerebral perfusion pressure (see Quick Hit) is important in understanding the effects of ICP and its management. If cerebral perfusion pressure is compromised due to elevated ICP, two events occur:
      • First, autoregulation is eventually lost, leading to cerebral vasodilation. Vasogenic edema occurs as fluid is lost into extravascular space, further increasing ICP.
      • Secondly, with loss of autoregulation, systemic BP becomes the sole determinant of cerebral blood flow.
   c. **Bilateral fixed and dilated pupils** suggest diffusely increased ICP.
2. Epidural or subdural hematoma (see the Epidural Hematoma section below)
3. Herniation may cause a progressive loss of consciousness, an elevation of systemic BP with widening of the pulse pressure, and the development of bradycardia, respiratory compromise, and potentially death.
4. Signs of basilar skull fracture
   a. "Raccoon eyes"—periorbital ecchymoses
   b. "Battle's sign"—postauricular ecchymoses
   c. Hemotympanum
   d. CSF rhinorrhea/otorrhea
5. Coup or contrecoup injury
   a. Coup—injury at the site of impact
   b. Contrecoup—injury at the site opposite the point of impact
6. Seizures

Mean Arterial pressure -
N°1 90

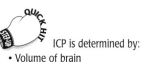
ICP is determined by:
• Volume of brain
• Volume of blood
• Volume of CSF

Two major effects of increased ICP
• Causes a decrease in cerebral perfusion pressure and thus a decrease in blood flow to the brain
• Causes transtentorial herniation; can also cause tonsillar and subfalcine herniation, but transtentorial is the most common

Cerebral perfusion pressure (mean arterial pressure minus ICP)
• Normal cerebral perfusion pressure is >50 mm Hg.
• **If ICP increases so much as to approximate mean arterial pressure, cerebral perfusion pressure is lost and brain cell death ensues.**
• In the ICU, the goal in managing a head trauma patient is to keep mean arterial pressure >80 and ICP <20. This ensures a cerebral perfusion pressure of at least 60 mm Hg.

DISEASES OF THE CENTRAL AND PERIPHERAL NERVOUS SYSTEMS

7. Diffuse axonal injury
   a. Represents global damage to the entire brain during impact
   b. The patient typically has severe neurologic dysfunction and may be in a prolonged comatose state.
   c. CT scan usually does not show an elevated ICP, but does show punctuate hemorrhages in the involved tracts.
   d. Mortality rate is 33%.

C. Treatment

1. ABCs
2. Lower ICP. General techniques:
   a. Reverse Trendelenburg position (if spine is cleared)—elevate the head of the bed.
   b. Intubation plus **hyperventilation** is effective in lowering the ICP.
      • Hyperventilation causes a decreased $PaCO_2$ and therefore prevents cerebral vasodilation. (Remember that cerebral vasodilation increases cerebral blood flow, with a subsequent increase in ICP.)
      • Maintain a $PaCO_2$ level of 30 to 35.
      • If the $PaCO_2$ level is decreased for prolonged periods, vasoconstriction can result, with subsequent ischemia.
   c. Mannitol
   d. Give narcotics (morphine or fentanyl) for sedation.
   e. Neuromuscular paralysis (vecuronium or pancuronium)
   f. Lower the body temperature slightly.
   g. If a ventricular catheter is used for ICP monitoring, drain CSF to lower the ICP.
3. Treat subdural or epidural hematoma (if present).

Epidural Hematoma

A. General characteristics

1. An epidural hematoma is a blood clot between the skull and the dura.
2. They are typically due to laceration of the middle meningeal artery when the temporal bone is fractured.

B. Clinical features

1. "Classic" presentation (actually seen in only 20% of patients) is a brief loss of consciousness followed by a lucid interval.
2. Next, the patient goes into a coma as the hematoma enlarges and compresses the midbrain (due to transtentorial herniation). The "classic" lucid interval is absent in many cases.
3. Ipsilateral blown pupil is seen in more than 50% of cases.

C. Diagnosis: CT scan for diagnosis—Epidural hematoma is seen as a lenticular-shaped, **convex** mass that overlays the brain with high attenuation (see Figure 5-5).

D. Treatment: rapid surgical decompression.

Subdural Hematoma

A. General characteristics

1. Hematoma that forms between the dura and the brain (under the dura)
2. Results from **venous bleeding** after blunt head trauma—the movement of the brain relative to the skull causes rupture of the bridging vessels.
3. Risk factors
   a. Brain atrophy (alcoholics and elderly patients)—The superficial bridging vessels have more "room" to move in response to rapid movement, thus increasing the risk of vessel rupture.
   b. Patients undergoing anticoagulation

Cushing's triad is a physiologic response to increased ICP that is due to compression of the brainstem. **If this triad is present, ICP has reached life-threatening levels.**
- Hypertension
- Bradycardia
- Respiratory irregularity

$PaCO_2$ is the most important regulator of cerebral vessel dilation/constriction. Increased $PaCO_2$ causes cerebral vasodilation.

DISEASES OF THE CENTRAL AND PERIPHERAL NERVOUS SYSTEMS

FIGURE 5-5 Epidural hematoma. Note the convex shape of the hematoma (arrows).

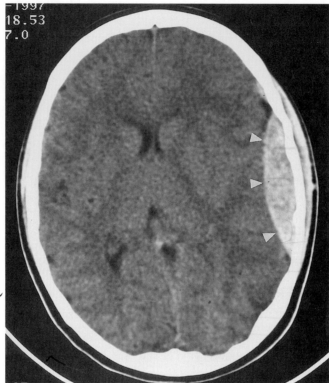

(From Daffner RH, ed. Clinical Radiology: The Essentials. 2nd Ed. Philadelphia: Lippincott Williams & Wilkins, 1999:513, Figure 12.23A.)

subdural hematoma twice more common than epidural hematoma.

4. A subdural hematoma is twice as common as an epidural hematoma.
5. The prognosis is related to the degree of associated brain injury.

B. Clinical features
1. Acute (symptoms occurring within hours or up to a few days after injury)
   a. Develop after severe head trauma
   b. Most patients are unconscious on impact. Significant brain injury is often present.
   c. Mass effect (increased ICP) causes a decline in mental status and a change in level of consciousness.
   d. Can be due to a motor vehicle accident, a fall (alcoholics and elderly patients), or a physical assault
   e. Prognosis is poor.
   f. Prompt surgical evacuation is indicated.
2. Chronic (symptoms occurring at least 1 week after injury)
   a. Sometimes due to minor injuries; patient may not remember an injury
   b. Usually seen in alcoholics or elderly patients with brain atrophy
   c. Signs and symptoms may be subtle and nonspecific. The hematoma may enlarge significantly before the patient becomes symptomatic.
   d. No loss of consciousness
   e. If small, may resolve spontaneously

C. Diagnosis: CT scan of the head—shows a crescent-shaped **(concave)** hematoma, which is usually less dense than an epidural hematoma because the blood is diluted with CSF (see Figure 5-6)

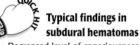

Typical findings in subdural hematomas
• Decreased level of consciousness
• Headache
• Cortical dysfunction

FIGURE 5-6 Subdural hematoma. Note the concave shape of the hematoma (arrow).

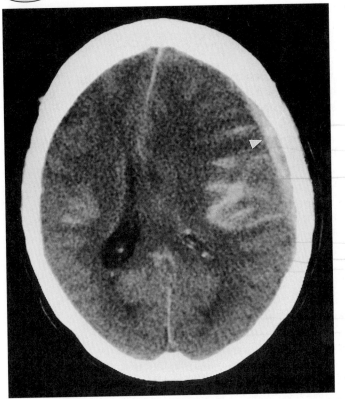

(From Daffner RH, ed. Clinical Radiology: The Essentials. 2nd Ed. Philadelphia: Lippincott Williams & Wilkins, 1999:527, Figure 12.38C.)

D. Treatment: Surgical evacuation is usually indicated for acute subdural hematomas. Chronic subdural hematomas may not require surgery, depending on the size.

Concussion

- A brain injury following blunt trauma that usually results in a brief loss of consciousness; likened to a "brain bruise"
- Patients with a history of previous concussion are four to five times more likely to have another concussion.
- Caused by electrophysiologic dysfunction of the midbrain secondary to the impact
- Usually the patient experiences confusion, dizziness, problems with concentration, and an inability to answer questions (or delay in answering) after awakening; and may also have headache, irritability, or amnesia for events before the trauma.
- Vomiting, delirium, or focal neurologic deficit suggests an elevated ICP. Rule out hematomas (epidural or subdural).
- No specific treatment exists. Recurrent elevations in ICP can lead to long-term neurologic sequelae (e.g., memory loss) or psychiatric disturbances.

NEUROMUSCULAR DISEASES

Myasthenia Gravis

A. General characteristics

1. **Autoimmune disorder**—Autoantibodies are directed against the nicotinic acetylcholine receptors of the neuromuscular junction, which leads to a reduced postsynaptic response to acetylcholine and results in significant muscle fatigue.

2. Muscles that are stimulated repeatedly (e.g., extraocular muscles) are prone to fatigue.
3. The peak incidence in women is age 20 to 30; in men, 50 to 70. It is more common in women.

> **QUICK HIT**
>
> Myasthenia gravis may be limited to extraocular muscles, especially in elderly patients.

B. Clinical features

1. **Skeletal muscle weakness**—with preservation of sensation and reflexes
   a. Weakness is exacerbated by continued use of muscle and improved by rest. Symptoms worsen toward the end of the day (due to fatigue).
   b. Involved muscles vary and may include the following:
      • Cranial muscles: extraocular muscles, eyelids (ptosis), facial muscles (facial weakness, difficulty in chewing, slurred speech)
      • Limb muscles (proximal and asymmetric)
2. Ptosis, diplopia, and blurred vision—most common initial symptoms
3. Generalized weakness, dysarthria, and dysphagia
4. The condition progresses slowly with periodic exacerbations. **Myasthenic crisis is a medical emergency that occurs in 15% of patients**. Diaphragm and intercostal fatigue result in respiratory failure, often requiring mechanical ventilation.

C. Diagnosis

1. Acetylcholine receptor antibody test is the test of choice (most specific). Nevertheless, 20% of patients with clinical manifestations of myasthenia gravis may be "antibody negative."
2. EMG shows a decremental response to repetitive stimulation of motor nerves.
3. A CT scan of the thorax can rule out **thymoma**. Thymoma is present in only 10% to 15% of patients, but the thymus is histologically abnormal in 75% of patients.
4. Edrophonium (Tensilon) test—Anticholinesterase medications cause marked improvement of symptoms, but a high false-positive rate limits utility.

D. Treatment

1. Anticholinesterase drugs (AChE inhibitors)—e.g., pyridostigmine
   a. Inhibiting AChE increases concentration of acetylcholine at the synapse by decreasing the breakdown of acetylcholine.
   b. This is a symptomatic benefit only.
2. Thymectomy
   a. This provides a symptomatic benefit and complete remission in many patients, even in the absence of a thymoma.
   b. Although usually benign, thymoma is an absolute indication for thymectomy.
3. Immunosuppressive drugs
   a. Use corticosteroids for patients with a poor response to AChE inhibitors.
   b. Azathioprine and cyclosporine are alternative third-line agents.
4. Plasmapheresis removes antibodies to acetylcholine receptors. Use it if all else fails or if the patient is in respiratory failure.
5. IV immunoglobulin therapy is now sometimes used for acute exacerbations.
6. Monitor serial forced vital capacities. A forced vital capacity of 15 mL/kg (about 1 L) is generally an indication for intubation. **Patients in myasthenic crisis have a low threshold for intubation—do not wait until the patient is hypoxic.**

> **QUICK HIT**
>
> **Medications that exacerbate symptoms of myasthenia gravis**
> • Antibiotics–aminoglycosides and tetracyclines
> • β-blockers
> • Antiarrhythmics–quinidine, procainamide, and lidocaine

Box 5-10 Lambert-Eaton Myasthenic Syndrome

• Associated with **small cell lung cancer**
• Caused by autoantibodies directed against presynaptic calcium channels
• Clinical features include proximal muscle weakness and hyporeflexia
• Distinguished from myasthenia gravis in that symptoms **improve** with repeated muscle stimulation

Duchenne's Muscular Dystrophy

A. General characteristics
1. **X-linked recessive** (almost exclusively in males) disease involving a mutation on a gene that codes for the dystrophin protein (dystrophin is absent causing muscle cells to die).
2. Characteristically, there is **no inflammation**.

B. Clinical features
1. Muscle weakness is progressive, symmetric, and starts in childhood. Proximal muscles primarily affected (pelvic girdle). Eventually involves the respiratory muscles.
2. *Gowers' maneuver*—patient uses hands to get up from floor because the weakness in the proximal lower extremity muscles makes it difficult to arise without support.
3. Enlarged calf muscles—true muscle hypertrophy at first, followed by **pseudohypertrophy** as fat replaces muscle
4. Ultimately results in wheelchair confinement, respiratory failure, and death in third decade.

C. Diagnosis
1. Serum creatine phosphokinase—levels are markedly elevated
2. DNA testing has now replaced muscle biopsy for diagnosis.

D. Treatment
1. No treatment is available at this time. Prednisone may slow the progression of disease for a limited period of time.
2. Surgery to correct progressive scoliosis is often necessary once patient becomes wheelchair dependent.

 # No treatment, Prednisone may slow it down for a limited time period.

Becker's Muscular Dystrophy

- Less common than Duchenne's muscular dystrophy
- Also X-linked recessive
- Similar to Duchenne's muscular dystrophy, but there is later onset and a less severe course. Some dystrophin is present.

NEUROCUTANEOUS SYNDROMES

Neurofibromatosis Type I (von Recklinghausen's Disease)

- Autosomal dominant disease characterized by café au lait spots, neurofibromas, and CNS tumors (gliomas, meningiomas), axillary or inguinal freckling, iris hamartomas (*Lisch's nodules*), bony lesions
- Cutaneous neurofibromas—may be disfiguring
- Complications include scoliosis, pheochromocytomas, optic nerve gliomas, renal artery stenosis, and erosive bone defects. Musculoskeletal manifestations include spinal deformity and congenital tibial dysplasia.
- Complications may require treatment. Surgically excise any symptomatic neurofibromas.

Neurofibromatosis Type II

- Autosomal dominant disease; less common than type I neurofibromatosis
- Clinical features include bilateral (sometimes unilateral) acoustic neuromas (classic finding), multiple meningiomas, café au lait spots, neurofibromas (much less common than type I), and cataracts.

Tuberous Sclerosis

- Usually autosomal dominant
- Presents with cognitive impairment, epilepsy, and skin lesions (including facial angiofibromas, adenoma sebaceum)

 Other hereditary causes of muscle weakness
- Mitochondrial disorders: associated with maternal inheritance and ragged red muscle fibers
- Glycogen storage diseases such as McArdle's disease (autosomal recessive, muscle cramping after exercise due to glycogen phosphorylase deficiency)

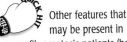 Other features that may be present in neurofibromatosis patients (both types)
- Seizures
- Mental retardation, learning disabilities
- Short height
- Macrocephalic

 In patients with neurofibromatosis, prognosis depends on the type and number of tumors and their location. Most patients can function well.

DISEASES OF THE CENTRAL AND PERIPHERAL NERVOUS SYSTEMS

- Retinal hamartomas, renal angiomyolipomas, and rhabdomyomas of the heart may also be present.
- Treat complications.

Sturge-Weber Syndrome

- Acquired disease
- Key pathologic feature is the presence of capillary angiomatoses of the pia mater
- Classic feature is facial vascular nevi (port-wine stain)
- Epilepsy and mental retardation are usually present.
- Treatment of epilepsy is often the mainstay of treatment.

Von Hippel-Lindau Disease

- Autosomal dominant
- Important features are cavernous hemangiomas of the brain or brainstem, renal angiomas, and cysts in multiple organs.
- Associated with renal cell carcinoma

SPINAL CORD DISEASES

Syringomyelia

- Central cavitation of the cervical cord due to abnormal collection of fluid within the spinal cord parenchyma (see Figure 5-7)
- Causes include cranial base malformation (patients with Arnold-Chiari malformation), intramedullary tumors, and traumatic necrosis of the cord.
- Clinical features—bilateral loss of pain and temperature sensation over the shoulders in a "capelike" distribution (lateral spinothalamic tract involvement), preservation of touch, thoracic scoliosis may occur, muscle atrophy of the hands may occur
- Diagnosed by MRI
- Treatment is surgical—syringosubarachnoid shunt

Brown-Séquard Syndrome

- Spinal cord hemisection (i.e., lesion involving either the right or the left half of the spinal cord), usually at the cervical levels (where spinal cord enlarges) (see Figure 5-7)
- Causes include trauma (e.g., stab wound) that causes hemisection of spinal cord, tumors, and abscesses (less common).
- Clinical features: **contralateral loss of pain and temperature** (spinothalamic tract), **ipsilateral hemiparesis** (corticospinal tract), and **ipsilateral loss** of position/vibration (dorsal columns)

FIGURE
5-7 Classic lesions of the spinal cord. **A.** Syringomyelia. **B.** Hemisection of the spinal cord (Brown-Séquard syndrome).

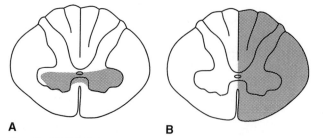

A   B

(From Fix JD. High-Yield Neuroanatomy. 2nd Ed. Philadelphia: Lippincott Williams & Wilkins, 2000:46, Figure 8-2H and E, respectively.)

Transverse Myelitis

- This is a rare condition that specifically affects the tracts across the horizontal aspect of the spinal cord at a given level. The thoracic spine is the most commonly involved.
- The cause is usually unknown, but it can occur after viral infections. Progression is usually rapid. *after flu vaccine.*
- Clinical features include lower extremity weakness or plegia, back pain, sensory deficits below the level of the lesion, and sphincter disturbance (especially urinary retention).
- MRI with contrast is the imaging study of choice.
- High-dose steroid therapy is often used, but evidence supporting its use is equivocal.
- The prognosis is highly variable and unpredictable, ranging from full recovery to death.

Horner's Syndrome

A. General characteristics

1. Results from the interruption of cervical sympathetic nerves
2. Can be preganglionic (central lesions) or postganglionic (distal to superior cervical ganglion); the former is more worrisome and requires more thorough evaluation

B. Clinical features

1. Ipsilateral ptosis—mild drooping of lid (levator palpebrae still intact)
2. Ipsilateral miosis—"pinpoint pupil"
3. Ipsilateral anhidrosis (decreased sweating on forehead)—may be difficult to detect

C. Causes

1. Idiopathic (most cases)
2. Pancoast tumor (pulmonary neoplasm of the superior sulcus at lung apex)
3. Internal carotid dissection
4. Brainstem stroke
5. Neck trauma (cervical spine injury)

Poliomyelitis

- Poliovirus affects the anterior horn cells and motor neurons of spinal cord and brainstem. Causes lower motor neuron involvement.
- Characteristic features include asymmetric muscle weakness (legs more commonly involved); absent deep tendon reflexes; flaccid, atrophic muscles; and **normal sensation**.
- Bulbar involvement (of CN IX and CN X) in 10% to 15% of cases can lead to respiratory and cardiovascular impairment.
- No treatment is available, although poliomyelitis is entirely preventable by vaccination.

MISCELLANEOUS CONDITIONS

Dizziness

A. General characteristics

1. There are three major causes of dizziness.
   a. Presyncope (lightheadedness)
   b. Vertigo (see Box 5-11 and Vertigo section below)
   c. Multisensory stimuli—This happens in times of profound shock or overwhelming sensory overload (e.g., standing over the Grand Canyon or hearing shocking news).
2. Many conditions cause a sensation of "dizziness": cerebellar disease, cerebrovascular disease, TIAs, hyperventilation, anxiety, panic attacks, and phobias.

> **Box 5-11 Vertigo**
>
> **Central Vertigo**
> - Gradual onset; other neurologic (brainstem) findings are present in most cases (e.g., weakness, hemiplegia, diplopia, dysphagia, dysarthria, facial numbness). Look for cardiovascular risk factors.
> - Accompanying nystagmus can be bidirectional or vertical (does not occur in peripheral vertigo).
>
> **Peripheral Vertigo**
> - Lesions are cochlear or retrocochlear.
> - Abrupt onset, nausea/vomiting, head position has strong effect on symptoms. Other brainstem deficits are absent, except for tinnitus/hearing loss.

B. Diagnosis
  1. Audiogram—if vestibular symptoms present
  2. CT scan/MRA—if TIA is suspected
  3. MRI of posterior fossa—if structural lesion is suspected

C. Treatment: Treat the underlying cause.

Vertigo

A. General characteristics
  1. Vertigo refers to a disturbance of the vestibular system characterized by a sensation of spinning or hallucination of movement.
  2. The initial goal is to determine whether the cause of the vertigo is peripheral (inner ear) or central (e.g., tumor, CVA).
  3. Peripheral vertigo is usually benign, but central vertigo can have serious consequences.

B. Types of peripheral vertigo
  1. Benign positional vertigo
     a. Vertigo is experienced only in specific positions or during change in position and lasts for a few moments. It has an abrupt onset as soon as the particular position is assumed.
     b. Usually presents in patients over 60 years old
     c. Often occurs after head injury
     d. Recovery is usually complete (resolves within 6 months).
  2. Ménière's disease
     a. Triad of vertigo, tinnitus, and hearing loss
     b. Attacks may last for hours to days and recur several months or years later.
     c. The hearing loss eventually becomes permanent.
  3. Acute labyrinthitis—due to viral infection of the cochlea and labyrinth; may last for several days
  4. Ototoxic drugs (aminoglycosides, some diuretics)
  5. Acoustic neuroma (schwannoma) of the 8th cranial nerve

C. Causes of central vertigo
  1. MS—demyelination of vestibular pathways of brainstem
  2. Vertebrobasilar insufficiency
  3. Migraine-associated vertigo—headache may or may not be present

Syncope

A. General characteristics
  1. Syncope refers to a transient loss of consciousness/postural tone secondary to acute decrease in cerebral blood flow.
  2. It is characterized by rapid recovery of consciousness without resuscitation.

QUICK HIT In a patient with vertigo, goal is to differentiate between peripheral (benign) and central (worrisome) vertigo (see Table 5-5). If in doubt, an MRI of the brainstem is the best imaging study to rule out an ischemic event.

DISEASES OF THE CENTRAL AND PERIPHERAL NERVOUS SYSTEMS

TABLE 5-5 Central Versus Peripheral Vertigo

Central Vertigo	Peripheral Vertigo
Gradual onset	Sudden onset
Mild intensity	Severe intensity
Mild nausea/vomiting	Intense nausea/vomiting
Associated neurologic findings typically present	No associated neurologic findings
Mild nystagmus	Relatively intense nystagmus
Position change has mild effect	Position change has intense effect
No refractoriness—can repeat the "tilt" test and patient responds every time	Rapidly refractory—cannot repeat the "tilt" test; patient will not respond again
Patient falls to same side as lesion	Patient falls to same side as lesion
Direction of nystagmus: multidirectional and even vertical	Direction of nystagmus: unilateral vertical; nystagmus is **never** peripheral.

B. Causes

1. Seizure disorder
2. Cardiac
   a. Cardiac syncope is usually sudden and without prodromal symptoms—e.g., the patient's face hits the floor.
   b. Syncope may be the first manifestation of a life-threatening cardiac condition.
   c. Causes
      - Arrhythmias (e.g., sick sinus syndrome, ventricular tachycardia, AV block, rapid supraventricular tachycardia)
      - Obstruction of blood flow (e.g., aortic stenosis, hypertrophic cardiomyopathy, pulmonary HTN, atrial myxoma, prolapsed mitral valve, severe asymmetric septal hypertrophy)
      - Massive MI
3. Vasovagal syncope ("neurocardiogenic," "vasodepressor," "simple faints")
   a. Most common cause of syncope; may account for up to 50% of all cases of syncope
   b. Most people have one episode, but for some it is a recurrent problem.
   c. Clues to diagnosis
      - Emotional stress, pain, fear, extreme fatigue, or claustrophobic situations as precipitating factors
      - Premonitory symptoms (pallor, diaphoresis, lightheadedness, nausea, dimming of vision, roaring in the ears)
      - Can occur at any age, but if the first episode is after age 40, be reluctant to make this diagnosis
      - **Tilt-table study can reproduce the symptoms in susceptible people.**
   d. Pathophysiology
      - Normally, standing up causes blood to pool in the lower extremities (leading to a decrease in cardiac output, stroke volume, and BP). These changes are compensated for by increased sympathetic tone (leading to vasoconstriction and tachycardia), and decreased parasympathetic tone.
      - In patients with vasovagal syncope, the compensatory response is interrupted in a few minutes by a paradoxical withdrawal of sympathetic stimulation and a replacement by enhanced parasympathetic (vagal) activity. This leads to an inappropriate bradycardia, vasodilation, marked decrease in BP, and cerebral perfusion.
   e. Treatment
      - Can usually be reversed by assuming the supine posture and elevating the legs
      - β-blockers and disopyramide
      - Prognosis is excellent (there is no heart disease or arrhythmias).
   f. Prevention—Avoid circumstances that precipitate attack.

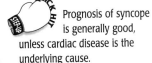 Prognosis of syncope is generally good, unless cardiac disease is the underlying cause.

 Two ways to differentiate between seizures and syncope
- In seizures, duration of unconsciousness tends to be longer. In syncope, loss of consciousness is momentary.
- In syncope, bladder control is usually retained, but in seizures it is often lost.

 Vasovagal and orthostatic syncope occur when the patient is upright (sitting up or standing). They do not occur when the patient is recumbent.

DISEASES OF THE CENTRAL AND PERIPHERAL NERVOUS SYSTEMS

4. Orthostatic hypotension (ganglionic blocking agents, diabetes, old age, prolonged bed rest)
   a. Caused by defect in vasomotor reflexes; overlaps with vasovagal syncope
   b. Common in elderly people; diabetics (autonomic neuropathy); patients taking ganglionic blocking agents, vasodilators, diuretics
   c. Posture is the main cause here. Sudden standing or prolonged standing are the precipitating causes. A positive tilt-table test result is expected.
   d. It also is associated with premonitory symptoms (lightheadedness, nausea, and so on).
   e. Treat with increased sodium intake and fluids. Consider fludrocortisone.
5. Severe cerebrovascular disease
   a. A rare cause of syncope
   b. A TIA involving the **vertebrobasilar** circulation may lead to syncope ("drop attacks").
   c. One practically never sees dizziness (or vertigo) in isolation with vertebrobasilar insufficiency—there will always be other deficits as well.
6. Other noncardiogenic causes include metabolic causes (e.g., hypoglycemia, hyperventilation), hypovolemia (e.g., hemorrhage), hypersensitivity (syncope precipitated by wearing a tight collar or turning the head), mechanical reduction of venous return (e.g., Valsalva maneuver, postmicturition), and various medications (e.g., β-blockers, nitrates, antiarrhythmic agents).

C. Diagnosis (see Figure 5-8)
1. First, attempt to rule out conditions that are life-threatening (e.g., MI, hemorrhage, and arrhythmias).
2. The main goal is to **differentiate between cardiac and noncardiac etiologies**, because the prognosis is poorest for those with underlying heart disease.
3. History
   a. Three key elements need to be determined: events before, during, and after the syncopal episode.
   b. Check the patient's medications—this is especially important in elderly patients.
   c. Seek reports from witnesses of the syncopal event.
4. Physical examination (priority given to cardiovascular system)
   a. BP and pulse measurements in supine, sitting, and standing positions
   b. Mental status (postictal state)
   c. Murmurs (aortic stenosis, hypertrophic cardiomyopathy)
   d. Carotid pulses—auscultated for bruits
   e. Apply pressure to the carotid sinus—observe for reflex bradycardia and hypotension.
5. Diagnosis
   a. **ECG** can identify life-threatening causes (ventricular tachycardia, other arrhythmias, ischemia). **Obtain for all patients.**
   b. CBC, metabolic panel, resting ECG may be appropriate
6. Additional diagnostic tests
   a. 24-hour ambulatory ECG recording (Holter monitoring) and/or event monitor—if arrhythmia is suspected and H & P and ECG are nondiagnostic
   b. Tilt-table testing—to diagnose neurocardiogenic syncope; appropriate if syncope episodes are recurrent and unexplained and there is no evidence of structural heart disease
   c. CT scan or EEG—if seizures are suspected
   d. Echocardiogram—if there is evidence of structural heart disease or abnormal ECG; evaluate LV function, hypertrophic cardiomyopathy, aortic stenosis, mitral stenosis, and so on
   e. Electrophysiologic studies in select cases

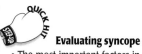

QUICK HIT

Syncope is uncommon in setting of a stroke, unless the vertebrobasilar system is involved.

QUICK HIT

Evaluating syncope
- The most important factors in decision making in syncope patients are presence/absence of structural heart disease and abnormal ECG.
- If the patient has no heart disease and syncope is unexplained, the most important test is tilt table testing for evaluation of vasovagal syncope.

FIGURE 5-8 Syncope flowchart.

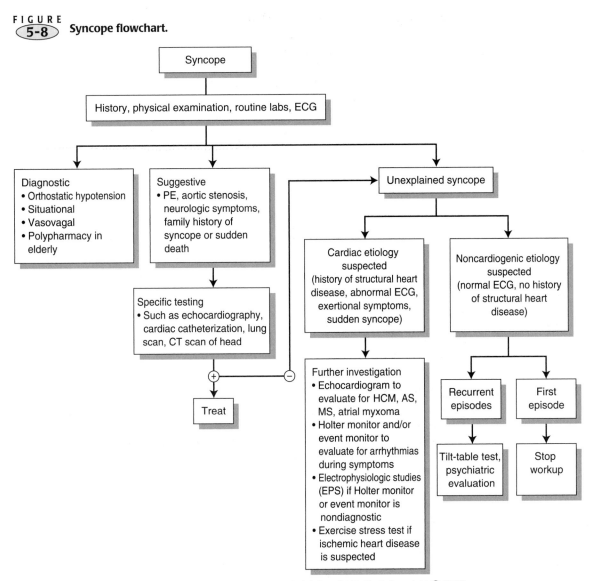

(Adapted from Heaven DJ, Sutton R. Syncope. Crit Care Med 2000;28(10 Suppl):118, Fig 1. Copyright © 2000 Lippincott Williams & Wilkins.)

Seizures

A. General characteristics

1. A seizure occurs when there is a sudden abnormal discharge of electrical activity in the brain.
2. The diagnosis of epilepsy is reserved for a syndrome of recurrent, idiopathic seizures. The ultimate cause of seizures in epilepsy is unknown.

B. Causes (four Ms, four Is)

1. Metabolic and electrolyte disturbances—hyponatremia, water intoxication, hypoglycemia or hyperglycemia, hypocalcemia, uremia, thyroid storm, hyperthermia
2. Mass lesions—brain metastases, primary brain tumors, hemorrhage
3. Missing drugs
   a. **Noncompliance with anticonvulsants** in patients with epilepsy—This is the most common reason for poor seizure control in epileptics.
   b. **Acute withdrawal from alcohol, benzodiazepines, barbiturates**
4. Miscellaneous
   a. Pseudoseizures—not true seizures but are psychiatric in origin; are often difficult to distinguish from true seizures without an EEG

> **Box 5-12   Important Aspects of H & P in a Patient Presenting With a Seizure**
>
> - Acquire a description of the seizure from bystanders (e.g., postictal state, loss of continence)
> - Determine what is the baseline state for the patient. Is the patient a known epileptic? Look into missed doses of antiepileptics, or any recent change in dosages/medications.
> - Examine the patient for any injuries—head or spine, fractures, posterior shoulder dislocation, tongue lacerations, bowel/bladder incontinence.
> - Look for signs of increased intracranial pressure.
> - Perform a complete neurologic examination.

DISEASES OF THE CENTRAL AND PERIPHERAL NERVOUS SYSTEMS

b. Eclampsia—A preeclamptic pregnant woman seizing no longer has preeclampsia! The only definitive treatment for eclampsia is delivery, but a magnesium infusion is the pharmacologic treatment of choice.

c. Hypertensive encephalopathy—Severe hypertension can cause cerebral edema.

5. Intoxications—cocaine, lithium, lidocaine, theophylline, metal poisoning (e.g., mercury, lead), carbon monoxide poisoning

6. Infections—septic shock, bacterial or viral meningitis, brain abscess

7. Ischemia—stroke, TIA (common cause of seizure in elderly patients)

8. Increased ICP – e.g., due to trauma

C. Types of epileptic seizures

1. Partial seizure—accounts for 70% of patients with epilepsy older than 18 years of age. It begins in one part of the brain (typically the temporal lobe) and initially produces symptoms that are referable to the region of the cortex involved.

   a. Simple partial seizure
      - **Consciousness remains intact.** The seizure remains localized but may evolve into a complex partial seizure
      - May involve transient unilateral clonic-tonic movement

   b. Complex partial seizure
      - **Consciousness is impaired;** postictal confusion
      - Automatisms (last 1 to 3 minutes)—purposeless, involuntary, repetitive movements (such as lip smacking or chewing); patients may become aggressive if restraint is attempted.
      - Olfactory or gustatory hallucinations

2. Generalized seizure—characterized by **loss of consciousness**. Involves disruption of electrical activity in the entire brain.

   a. Tonic-clonic (grand mal) seizure—bilaterally symmetric and without focal onset
      - Begins with sudden loss of consciousness—a fall to the ground
      - Tonic phase—The patient becomes rigid; trunk and limb extension occurs. The patient may become apneic during this phase.
      - Clonic phase—This is musculature jerking of the limbs and body for at least 30 seconds.
      - The patient then becomes flaccid and comatose before regaining consciousness.
      - Postictal confusion and drowsiness are characteristic and can last for hours, although 10 to 30 minutes is more typical.
      - Other features may include tongue biting, vomiting, apnea, and incontinence (urine and/or feces).

   b. Absence (petit mal) seizure
      - Typically involves school-age children—usually resolves as child grows older
      - Patient seems to disengage from current activity and "stare into space"—then returns to the activity several seconds later; patient looks "absent minded" during these episodes, which are often confused with "daydreaming"
      - Episodes are brief (lasting a few seconds) but may be quite frequent (up to 100 times per day).

QUICK HIT

Partial seizures may evolve into generalized seizures. When this happens, it is called **secondary generalization**.

QUICK HIT

It is important (although sometimes difficult) to differentiate between absence (petit mal) and complex partial seizures because their treatments are different. Also, absence seizures disappear in adulthood, whereas complex partial seizures do not.

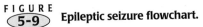

FIGURE 5-9 Epileptic seizure flowchart.

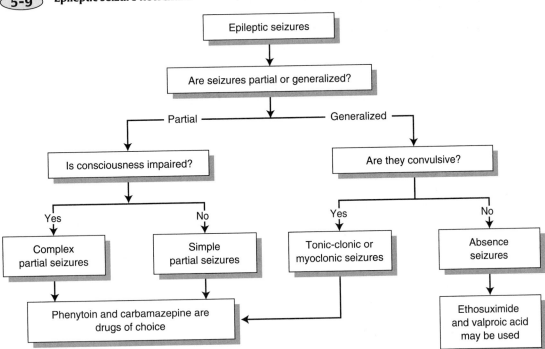

(Adapted from Humes DH, DuPont HL, Gardner LB, et al. Kelley's Textbook of Internal Medicine. 4th Ed. Philadelphia: Lippincott Williams & Wilkins, 2000:2866, Figure 426.1.)

- Impairment of consciousness but **no** loss of postural tone or continence, and no postictal confusion
- Minor clonic activity (eye blinks or head nodding) in up to 45% of cases

D. Diagnosis

1. If the patient has a known seizure disorder (epileptic), check anticonvulsant levels—this is usually the only test that is needed. Because therapeutic anticonvulsant levels are variable, **one dose may be toxic for one patient and therapeutic for another.** Therefore, take the range given in laboratory reports as a general guideline.
2. If the patient history is unclear or if this is the patient's first seizure:
   a. CBC, electrolytes, blood glucose, LFTs, renal function tests, serum calcium, urinalysis
   b. EEG
      - Although the EEG is the most helpful diagnostic test in the diagnosis of a seizure disorder, an abnormal EEG pattern alone is not adequate for the diagnosis of seizures.
      - A normal EEG in a patient with a first seizure is associated with a lower risk of recurrence.
   c. CT scan of the head—to identify a structural lesion
   d. MRI of the brain—with and without gadolinium (first without)
      - An important part of the workup of a patient with a first seizure
      - More sensitive than a CT scan in identifying structural changes, but not always practical (e.g., in an unstable patient)
   e. LP and blood cultures—if patient is febrile

E. Treatment

1. General principles
   a. For all seizures, ABCs take priority: secure airway and roll patient onto his side to prevent aspiration.

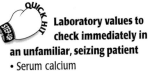

Laboratory values to check immediately in an unfamiliar, seizing patient
- Serum calcium
- Serum sodium
- Serum glucose or Accu-Chek
- BUN

DISEASES OF THE CENTRAL AND PERIPHERAL NERVOUS SYSTEMS

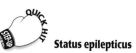

Status epilepticus

- Refers to prolonged, sustained unconsciousness with persistent convulsive activity in a seizing patient
- A medical emergency, with a mortality rate of up to 20%
- May be caused by poor compliance with medication, alcohol withdrawal, intracranial infection, neoplasm, a metabolic disorder, or a drug overdose
- Management involves establishing an airway, and giving IV diazepam, IV phenytoin, and 50 mg dextrose. Treat resistant cases with IV phenobarbital.

Remember that anticonvulsants are teratogenic (do a pregnancy test before prescribing!)

Initially ALS can involve virtually any muscle, but as the disease progresses, every region of the body becomes symmetrically involved.

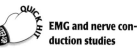

EMG and nerve conduction studies

- EMG measures the contractile properties of skeletal muscles
  - Lower motor neuron lesions: fibrillations and fasciculations at rest
  - Myopathy: no electrical activity at rest (as expected), but amplitude decreases with muscle contraction
- Nerve conduction studies
  - Demyelination decreases nerve conduction velocity (MS, Guillain-Barré syndrome)
  - Repetitive stimulation causes fatigue (myasthenia gravis)

b. Patients with a history of seizures (epilepsy)
- Seizures in these patients are usually due to **noncompliance with anticonvulsant therapy.** (Even one missed dose can result in subtherapeutic levels). Give a loading dose of the anticonvulsant medication, and continue the regular regimen as before.
- These patients should be chronically managed by a neurologist. Treatment with one of the standard antiepileptic drugs provides adequate control in 70% of adult patients. In another 15% to 20%, a combination regimen controls seizures.
- If seizures persist, increase the dosage of the first anticonvulsant until signs of toxicity appear. Add a second drug if the seizures cannot be controlled with the drug of first choice.
- If the seizures are controlled, have the patient continue the medication for at least 2 years. If the patient remains seizure-free, taper the medication(s) cautiously. Confirm this decision with a lack of seizure activity on the EEG.

c. Patient with a first seizure
- EEG and neurology consult—first steps
- Anticonvulsant therapy—weigh risks and benefits of treatment and the risk of recurrence before initiating
- With a normal EEG, the risk of recurrence is relatively low (15% in the first year), compared to the risk with an abnormal EEG (41% in the first year).

2. Anticonvulsant agents
   a. For generalized tonic-clonic seizures and partial seizures
   - Phenytoin and carbamazepine are the drugs of choice. They are equally effective, and side-effect profiles are similar.
   - Other options include phenobarbital, valproate, and primidone.
   b. For petit mal (absence) seizures—ethosuximide and valproic acid

Amyotrophic Lateral Sclerosis (ALS) or "Lou Gehrig's Disease"

A. General characteristics

1. A disorder affecting the anterior horn cells and corticospinal tracts at many levels. Corticobulbar involvement is common as well. **The presence of upper and lower motor neuron signs is a hallmark of ALS.** Note that only the motor system is involved.
2. Onset is usually between 50 and 70 years of age. (Lou Gehrig was unusually young [in his 30s] when the disease developed.) Occurrence of ALS before age 40 is uncommon.
3. Only 10% of cases are familial, with the remainder being sporadic.
4. Prognosis is dismal: 80% mortality rate at 5 years; 100% mortality rate at 10 years.

B. Clinical features

1. **Progressive muscle weakness is the hallmark feature.**
   a. Usually first noted in the legs or arms, but then spreads to other muscle groups
   b. No associated pain
   c. Muscle atrophy
2. Muscle cramps and spasticity
3. Fasciculations (unnoticed by patient)
4. Impaired speech and swallowing; dysphagia can lead to aspiration
5. Respiratory muscle weakness—dyspnea on exertion, and later, at rest; orthopnea; sleep apnea; end-stage ALS is characterized by respiratory failure
6. Weight loss and fatigue
7. The following are normal and unaffected, even in late stages.
   a. Bowel and bladder control
   b. Sensation
   c. Cognitive function
   d. Extraocular muscles

C. Diagnosis

1. EMG and nerve conduction studies can confirm degeneration of lower motor neurons and can rule out neuromuscular junction disorders.
2. Clinical or electrical evidence
   a. Involvement of two regions (probable ALS)
   b. Involvement of three to four regions (definite ALS)—affected regions include bulbar (face, larynx, tongue, jaw), cervical, thoracic, and lumbosacral

D. Treatment

1. Treatment has been very disappointing and is mainly supportive.
2. Riluzole is a glutamate-blocking agent—it may delay death by only 3 to 5 months.

Aphasia

A. General characteristics

1. Aphasia is the **loss or defect of language** (e.g., in speaking, fluency, reading, writing, comprehension of written or spoken material).
2. Most lesions that cause aphasia involve the dominant hemisphere.
   a. In 95% of right-handed people, the left cerebral hemisphere is dominant for language.
   b. In 50% of left-handed people, the left hemisphere is dominant for language (however, the right hemisphere also has language functions in most left-handed people).
3. There are four types of aphasia (described below): Wernicke's aphasia, Broca's aphasia, conduction aphasia, and global aphasia.

B. Causes

1. Stroke (most common cause)
2. Trauma to brain
3. Brain tumor
4. Alzheimer's disease

C. Types of aphasia

1. Wernicke's aphasia
   a. Receptive, fluent aphasia
   b. **Impaired comprehension of written or spoken language (key feature)**
   c. Speech is grammatically correct and is fluid but does not make much sense. Patients articulate well but often use the wrong words because they cannot understand their own words.
2. Broca's aphasia
   a. Expressive, nonfluent aphasia
   b. Speech is slow and requires effort.
   c. The patient uses short sentences (as few words as possible) without grammatical construction. The content is appropriate and meaningful.
   d. Good comprehension of language (written and spoken)
   e. Often associated with a right hemiparesis and hemisensory loss
3. Conduction aphasia
   a. Disturbance in repetition
   b. Pathology involves the connections between Wernicke's and Broca's areas.
4. Global aphasia
   a. Disturbance in all areas of language function (e.g., comprehension, speaking, reading, fluency)
   b. Often associated with a right hemiparesis

D. Treatment of aphasia

1. Most patients spontaneously recover or improve within the first month.
2. Speech therapy is helpful, but is unlikely to be of much benefit after the first few months.

QUICK HIT

The most common cause of aphasia is cerebrovascular disease. In aphasia, when speech is fluent, the lesion is posterior to the central sulcus. When speech is nonfluent, the lesion is anterior to the central sulcus.

Bell's Palsy

A. General characteristics

1. This refers to hemifacial weakness/paralysis of muscles innervated by CN VII due to swelling of the cranial nerve.
2. The prognosis is very good; 80% of patients recover fully within weeks to months.

B. Causes

1. Cause is uncertain.
2. Possible viral etiology (herpes simplex)—immunologic and ischemic factors implicated as well
3. Upper respiratory infection is a common preceding event.

C. Clinical features: There is acute onset of unilateral facial weakness/paralysis. Both upper and lower parts of the face are affected.

D. Diagnosis

1. Diagnosis is clinical, but consider Lyme disease in endemic areas as the treatment approach is different.
2. **Do not use steroids if Lyme is suspected!**
3. Consider EMG testing if paresis fails to resolve within 10 days.

E. Treatment

1. Usually none is required, as most cases resolve in 1 month
2. Short course of steroid therapy (prednisone) and acyclovir, if necessary
3. Patient should wear eye patch at night to prevent corneal abrasion (cornea is exposed due to weakness of orbicularis oculi muscle)
4. Surgical decompression of CN 7 is indicated if the paralysis progresses or if tests indicate deterioration.

Trigeminal Neuralgia (Tic Douloureux)

A. General characteristics

1. Trigeminal neuralgia is one of the most painful conditions known to mankind.
2. Usually idiopathic in origin

B. Clinical features

1. Brief (seconds to minutes) but frequent attacks of severe, lancinating facial pain
2. Involves the jaw, lips, gums, and maxillary area (ophthalmic division is less commonly affected)
3. Recurrent attacks may continue for weeks at a time.
4. No motor or sensory paralysis

C. Diagnosis

1. Clinical diagnosis
2. MRI—to rule out cerebellopontine angle tumor

D. Treatment

1. Drug of choice is carbamazepine (usually effective in relieving pain); other choices are baclofen and phenytoin, either alone or in combination with carbamazepine
2. Consider surgical decompression if medical therapy fails.
3. Patients typically experience a remitting-relapsing course. Over time, pain may become more refractory to treatment.

How to Localize a Neurologic Lesion

A. Introduction

1. Generally, neurologic deficits can be localized to one of the following 10 sites.
   a. Cerebral cortex
   b. Subcortical area

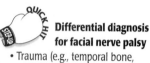

Differential diagnosis for facial nerve palsy
- Trauma (e.g., temporal bone, forceps delivery)
- Lyme disease
- Tumor (acoustic neuroma, cholesteatoma, neurofibroma)
- Guillain-Barré syndrome (palsy is usually bilateral)
- Herpes zoster

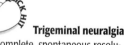

Trigeminal neuralgia
- Complete, spontaneous resolution in 85% of cases
- Mild residual disease in 10% of cases
- No resolution in 5% of cases

c. Cerebellum
d. Brainstem
e. Spinal cord
f. Plexus (plexopathy)
g. Roots (radiculopathy)
h. Peripheral nerve (peripheral neuropathy)
i. Neuromuscular junction
j. Muscle (myopathy)
2. Lesions in each of the above sites present with different neurologic findings. A good understanding of the deficits that accompany each lesion can help with localization.

FIGURE 5-10   **A. Dorsal column-medial lemniscus pathway.**

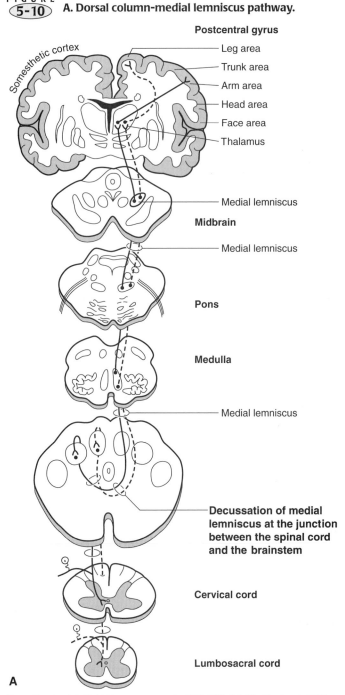

Postcentral gyrus

Somesthetic cortex

Leg area
Trunk area
Arm area
Head area
Face area
Thalamus

Medial lemniscus

Midbrain

Medial lemniscus

Pons

Medulla

Medial lemniscus

Decussation of medial lemniscus at the junction between the spinal cord and the brainstem

Cervical cord

Lumbosacral cord

A

(From Fix JD. High-Yield Neuroanatomy. 2nd Ed. Philadelphia: Lippincott Williams & Wilkins, 2000:39, Figure 7–2.)

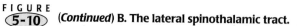

FIGURE 5-10 (*Continued*) B. The lateral spinothalamic tract.

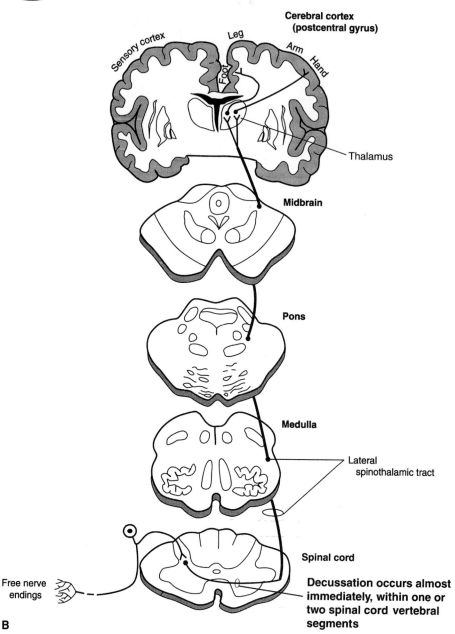

B

(From Fix JD. High-Yield Neuroanatomy. 2nd Ed. Philadelphia: Lippincott Williams & Wilkins, 2000:41, Figure 7–3.)

B. Cerebral cortex

1. Lesions in the cerebral cortex often cause two main deficits:
   a. Contralateral motor or sensory deficits (depending on which region of the cortex is involved)
   b. Aphasia
2. The hemiparesis seen with cortical lesions primarily affects the face, arms, and trunk. The legs may be affected, but typically that deficit is not as severe. This is because the neurons that control the lower extremities are in the interhemispheric fissure (see homunculus in Figure 5-10).
3. Aphasia is common when the left hemisphere is involved. Visual-spatial deficits are more common when the right hemisphere is involved.

C. Subcortical lesions

1. These involve the internal capsule, cerebral peduncles, thalamus, and pons.

FIGURE 5-10 *(Continued)* **C. The lateral and ventral corticospinal (pyramidal) tracts.**

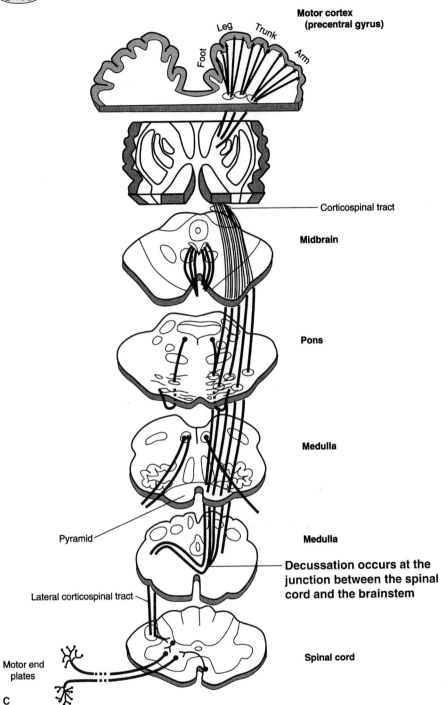

C

(From Fix JD. High-Yield Neuroanatomy. 2nd Ed. Philadelphia: Lippincott Williams & Wilkins, 2000:42, Figure 7–4.)

2. The hemiparesis is usually complete (face, arm, leg) because the neurons control-ling these structures all merge together subcortically and are very close together.

D. Cerebellum: incoordination, intention tremor, ataxia

E. Brainstem
1. Cranial nerve and spinal cord findings
2. There is a crossed hemiplegia (deficit on ipsilateral face and contralateral body) because the corticospinal tract, dorsal columns, and spinothalamic tracts cross but the cranial nerves do not.

F. Spinal cord

1. With acute injuries, spinal shock may be present and upper motor neuron signs may not be apparent initially.
2. The patient presents with upper motor neuron signs (spasticity, increased deep tendon reflexes, clonus, positive Babinski's sign), but these signs may be present with lesions in the brainstem and cortical/subcortical regions as well.
3. There is a decrease in sensation below a sharp band in the abdomen/trunk. A pin-prick is felt above this level but not below it. This is pathognomonic for spinal cord disease—the level of the lesion corresponds to the sensory level.

G. Plexus (plexopathy)

1. Deficits (motor and sensory) involve more than one nerve. Findings are variable depending on which part of the plexus is involved.
2. Trauma is the most common cause overall, especially for the brachial plexus. A post-surgical hematoma in the pelvis is a more common cause in lumbosacral plexopathy.
3. Plexuses that are commonly involved include:
   a. Brachial plexus—Erb-Duchenne type is the more common (upper trunk—C5–6 roots). Lower trunk (C8-T1) is less common.
   b. Lumbosacral plexus (L5-S3)

H. Roots (radiculopathy)

1. Pain is a key finding.
2. This affects a group of muscles supplied by a spinal root (myotome) and a sensory area supplied by a spinal root (dermatome). Therefore, the distribution of affected areas can help differentiate this from a peripheral neuropathy or a plexopathy.
3. Patients may present with weakness, atrophy, and sensory deficits in a dermatomal pattern; may include fasciculations and diminished deep tendon reflexes.

I. Peripheral nerve (peripheral neuropathy)

1. Weakness is more prominent distally at the outset (as opposed to muscle myopathy [see below])—usually asymmetric.
2. Presents with diminished deep tendon reflexes; may include sensory changes (numbness, paresthesias, tingling), muscle atrophy, and fasciculations
3. Can be due to diabetes (nerve infarction), trauma, entrapment, or vasculitis
4. Common neuropathies include radial/ulnar/median/musculocutaneous nerves, long thoracic nerve, axillary nerve, common peroneal nerve, and femoral nerve

J. Neuromuscular junction

1. Fatigability is the key finding. Muscles become weaker with use and recover with rest.
2. Normal sensation, no atrophy

K. Muscle (myopathy)

1. Myopathy refers to acquired disease (dystrophy to inherited conditions).
2. Symmetric weakness affects proximal muscles more than distal muscles (shoulders and hip muscles).
3. Presents with normal reflexes, but these may diminish late in the disease in comparison to muscle weakness
4. Normal sensation, no fasciculations
5. Muscle atrophy may occur late due to disuse (in contrast to rapid atrophy in motor neuron disease).

Connective Tissue and Joint Diseases

CONNECTIVE TISSUE DISEASES

Systemic Lupus Erythematosus (SLE)

A. General characteristics

1. An autoimmune disorder leading to inflammation and tissue damage involving multiple organ systems
2. The pathogenesis is not completely understood. SLE is an idiopathic chronic inflammatory disease with **genetic**, **environmental**, and **hormonal** factors involved in its pathogenesis.
3. The pathophysiology involves autoantibody production, deposition of immune complexes, complement activation, and accompanying tissue destruction/vasculitis.
4. Types — *Type III and Type II·*
   a. Spontaneous SLE
   b. Discoid lupus (skin lesions without systemic disease)
   c. Drug-induced lupus *(hydralazine, procainamide)*
   d. ANA-negative lupus—associated findings
      • Arthritis, Raynaud's phenomenon, subacute cutaneous lupus
      • Serology: Ro (anti-SS-A) antibody–positive, ANA-negative
      • Risk of neonatal lupus in infants of affected women

B. Clinical features

1. Constitutional symptoms: fatigue (often the sign of an impending exacerbation and a prominent finding in most patients), malaise, fever, weight loss
2. Cutaneous: butterfly rash (erythematous rash over cheeks and bridge of nose—found in one third of patients) (see Color Figure 6-1); photosensitivity; discoid lesions (erythematous raised patches with keratotic scaling); oral or nasopharyngeal ulcers; alopecia; Raynaud's phenomenon (vasospasm of small vessels when exposed to cold, usually in fingers—found in about 20% of cases)
3. Musculoskeletal: joint pain (may be the first symptom of disease—found in 90% of patients); arthritis (inflammatory and symmetric, not erosive as in RA); arthralgias; myalgia with or without myositis
4. Cardiac: pericarditis, endocarditis (Libman-Sacks endocarditis is a serious complication), myocarditis *pancarditis·*
5. Pulmonary: pleuritis (most common pulmonary finding), pleural effusion, pneumonitis (may lead to fibrosis), pulmonary HTN (rare)
6. Hematologic: hemolytic anemia with anemia or reticulocytosis of chronic disease, leukopenia, lymphopenia, thrombocytopenia } *Type II hypersensitivity·*
7. Renal: proteinuria >0.5 g/day (may have nephrotic syndrome); cellular casts; glomerulonephritis (may have hematuria); azotemia; pyuria; uremia; HTN
8. Immunologic: impaired immune response due to many factors, including autoantibodies to lymphocytes, abnormal T cell function, and immunosuppressive medications

Epidemiology of SLE
- **Women** of childbearing age account for 90% of cases.
- **African-American patients** are more frequently affected than Caucasian patients.
- Very mild in elderly patients; more severe in children
- Usually appears in late childhood or adolescence

Clinical findings associated with *neonatal lupus*
- Skin lesions
- Cardiac abnormalities (AV block, transposition of the great vessels)
- Valvular and septal defects

Clinical course of SLE
- A chronic disease characterized by exacerbations and remissions
- Malar rash, joint pain, and fatigue are the most common initial findings. With more advanced disease, renal, pulmonary, cardiovascular, and nervous systems are affected.

Box 6-1 Useful Criteria for Diagnosing SLE

A patient has SLE if four or more of these 11 criteria are present at any time.
1. Mucocutaneous signs (each counts as one)
   - Butterfly rash
   - Photosensitivity
   - Oral or nasopharyngeal ulcers
   - Discoid rash
2. Arthritis
3. Pericarditis, pleuritis
4. Hematologic disease—hemolytic anemia with reticulocytosis, leukopenia, lymphopenia, thrombocytopenia
5. Renal disease: proteinuria >0.5 g/day, cellular casts
6. CNS—seizures, psychosis
7. Immunologic manifestations—positive LE preparation, false-positive test result for syphilis, anti-ds DNA, anti-Sm Ab
8. ANAs

QUICK HIT

Conditions in which ANAs are elevated
- SLE
- RA
- Scleroderma
- Sjögren's syndrome
- Mixed connective tissue disease
- Polymyositis and dermato-myositis
- Drug-induced lupus

9. GI: nausea/vomiting, dyspepsia, dysphagia, peptic ulcer disease
10. CNS: seizures, psychosis (may be subtle), depression, headaches, TIA, cerebrovascular accident
11. Other findings include conjunctivitis and an increased incidence of Raynaud's phenomenon and Sjögren's syndrome.

C. Diagnosis (see Box 6-1 and Figure 6-1)
1. **Positive ANA screening test**—sensitive but not specific; almost all patients with SLE have elevated serum ANA levels.
2. **Anti-ds DNA** (in 40%) and **anti-Sm Ab** (in 30%)—The presence of either of these is diagnostic of SLE—very specific (but obviously not sensitive).
3. Anti-ss DNA (in 70%)
4. **Antihistone Abs** (in 70%) are present in 100% of cases of drug-induced lupus. If negative, drug-induced lupus can be excluded.
5. Ro (SS-A) and La (SS-B) are found in 15% to 35%. Associated with:
   a. Sjögren's syndrome.
   b. Subacute cutaneous SLE
   c. Neonatal lupus (with congenital heart block)
   d. Complement deficiency (C2 and C4)
   e. ANA-negative lupus (see Table 6-2)
6. Positive LE preparation: ANAs bind to nuclei of damaged cells, producing LE bodies.
7. False-positive test result for syphilis
8. Complement levels are usually decreased.
9. CBC, renal function tests (BUN, creatinine), urinalysis, serum electrolytes
10. Anticardiolipin and lupus anticoagulant

D. Treatment
1. Avoid sun exposure because it can exacerbate cutaneous rashes.
2. NSAIDs—for less severe symptoms

Box 6-2 Drug-Induced Lupus

- Certain drugs may produce a lupus-like syndrome that is similar to SLE except that it does not affect the CNS or kidneys.
- If renal or CNS involvement is present, it is **not** drug-induced lupus. In addition, the classic butterfly rash, alopecia, and ulcers are typically not seen in drug-induced lupus.
- Most patients improve after withdrawal of the offending drug. Therefore, the prognosis is obviously more favorable.
- Commonly implicated agents include hydralazine, procainamide, isoniazid, chlorpromazine, methyldopa, and quinidine.
- Laboratory findings in drug-induced lupus: antihistone antibodies are always present; there is an absence of anti-ds DNA and anti-Sm Ab.

Box 6-3 **Antiphospholipid Antibody Syndrome**

- A hypercoagulable state that can be idiopathic or associated with SLE (or other collagen vascular diseases such as scleroderma)
- Typical findings
  - Recurrent venous thrombosis—pulmonary embolism is a risk
  - Recurrent arterial thrombosis
  - Recurrent fetal loss (abortions)
  - Thrombocytopenia
  - Livedo reticularis (rash).
- Laboratory findings: presence of lupus anticoagulant, anticardiolipin antibody, or both. Prolonged PTT or PT is not corrected by adding normal plasma.
- Treatment is long-term anticoagulation (INR of 2.5 to 3.5).

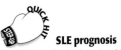

SLE
MCC of Death → Renal
function and opportunistic
infections.

3. Either local or systemic corticosteroids—for acute exacerbations
4. Systemic steroids for severe manifestations
5. Antimalarial agents such as hydroxychloroquine—for constitutional, cutaneous, and articular manifestations
6. Cytotoxic agents such as cyclophosphamide—for active glomerulonephritis
7. Monitor the following and treat appropriately:
   a. Renal disease, which produces the most significant morbidity
   b. HTN

Scleroderma (Systemic Sclerosis)

A. General characteristics
1st sign- could be edematous (inflammation) in the extremities →
bilateral fibrosis
1. A chronic connective tissue disorder that can lead to widespread fibrosis.
2. Pathophysiology: Cytokines stimulate fibroblasts, causing an abnormal amount of collagen deposition. **It is the high quantity of collagen that causes the problems associated with this disease (composition of the collagen is normal).**
3. Scleroderma is more common in women. Average age of onset is 35 to 50 years.
4. There are two types of scleroderma: diffuse and limited (see Table 6-4).
   (classification on the basis of skin involvement).

B. Clinical features
1. Raynaud's phenomenon
   a. Present in almost all patients; usually appears before other findings
   b. Caused by vasospasm and thickening of vessel walls in the digits
   c. Can lead to digital ischemia, with ulceration and infarction/gangrene
   d. Cold temperature and stress bring about color changes of fingers—blanching first, then cyanotic, and then red. *White → Blue → Red.*
2. Cutaneous fibrosis
   a. Tightening of skin of the face and extremities (**sclerodactyly** refers to a claw-like appearance of the hand)
   b. Can lead to contractures, disability, and disfigurement
3. GI involvement
   a. Occurs in most patients (both diffuse and limited)
   b. Findings include dysphagia/reflux from esophageal immobility (up to 90% of patients), delayed gastric emptying, constipation/diarrhea, abdominal distention, and pseudo-obstruction. Prolonged acid reflux may eventually lead to esophageal strictures.

QUICK HIT

SLE prognosis
- Most patients do not achieve normal life expectancy. With proper treatment, severe organ damage can be prevented and symptoms controlled in many cases.
- The most common causes of death are opportunistic infections and renal failure.

QUICK HIT

Differential diagnosis of Raynaud's phenomenon
- Primary–no other disorder exists
- Scleroderma
- SLE
- Mixed connective tissue disease
- Vasculitis (e.g., Buerger's disease)
- Certain medications (e.g., β-blockers, nicotine, bleomycin)
- Disorders that disrupt blood flow or vessels, such as thromboangiitis obliterans

---

Box 6-4 **Lupus Glomerulonephritis (GN)**

Lupus GN is the most common finding (usually present at diagnosis). There are five types of renal involvement.
- Type I (5%): minimal lesions—renal failure is very rare
- Type II (20%): mesangial lupus GN—renal failure is rare
- Type III (25%): focal proliferative GN—renal failure is uncommon
- Type IV (40%): diffuse proliferative GN—renal failure is common
- Type V (10%): membranous lupus GN—renal failure is uncommon

TABLE 6-1 **Common Laboratory Markers in Rheumatologic Diseases**

Laboratory Marker	Conditions	Comments
ANAs	• SLE (almost all patients) • Scleroderma • Sjögren's syndrome • Polymyositis	Highly sensitive for SLE but not for the others
RF	• RA (70% of patients) • Healthy population (up to 3%)	Neither sensitive nor specific for RA
C-ANCA	Wegener's granulomatosis	Sensitive and specific Can vary with disease activity
P-ANCA	Polyarteritis nodosa	70% to 80% sensitive for microscopic PAN Not specific
Lupus anticoagulant	Antiphospholipid antibody syndrome	
ESR	• Infection (acute or chronic) • Malignancy • Rheumatologic diseases • Miscellaneous (tissue necrosis, pregnancy)	• Low sensitivity and specificity • Major uses: diagnose/rule out inflammatory process and monitor course of inflammatory conditions
C-reactive protein	• Inflammatory states and infection • Miscellaneous conditions (e.g., MI, vasculitis, trauma, malignancy, pancreatitis)	• Primarily used for infection—much more sensitive and specific than ESR • If levels are markedly elevated (>15), bacterial infection is likely present.

TABLE 6-2 **Antinuclear Antibodies in Rheumatologic Diseases**

Antibody	Normal (%)	SLE (%)	Drug LE (%)	MCTD* (%)	Sjögren's Syndrome (%)	Scleroderma (%)	CREST (%)	Dermatomyositis/ Polymyositis (%)	RA (%)
ANA	1–10	95	100	95	70	80	80	80	50
Anti-ds DNA	—	60	—	—	30	—	—	—	—
Antihistones	—	60	90	—	—	—	—	—	—
Anti-uroporphyrin isomerase ribonucleoprotein	—	40	—	(90)	—	15	10	15	
Anti-Sm	—	40	—	—	—	—	—	—	—
Anti-Ro	—	40	—	—	50	—	—	—	5
Anti-leucine aminopeptidase	—	15	—	—	60	—	—	—	—
Antiscleroderma-70	—	—	—	—	—	20	10	—	—
Anticentromere	—	—	—	—	—	30	(80)	—	—

*MCTD, mixed connective tissue disease.

Adapted from Humes DH, DuPont HL, Gardner LB, et al. Kelley's Textbook of Internal Medicine. 4th Ed. Philadelphia: Lippincott Williams & Wilkins, 2000:1454, Table 188.1.

FIGURE
6-1   **Diagnosis of SLE.**

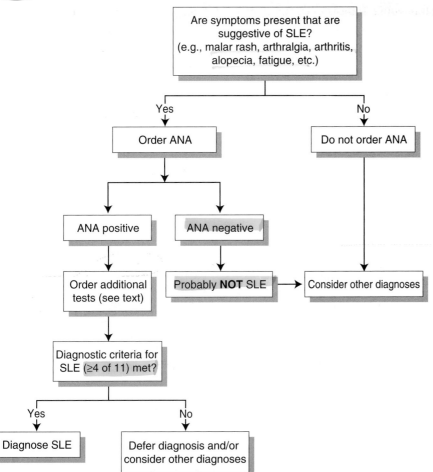

(Adapted from Humes DH, DuPont HL, Gardner LB, et al. Kelley's Textbook of Internal Medicine. 4th Ed. Philadelphia: Lippincott Williams & Wilkins, 2000:1387, Figure 178-3.)

TABLE 6-3   HLA Associations With Rheumatic Diseases

Disease	Associated HLA
SLE	HLA-DR2 and HLA-DR3
Sjögren's syndrome	HLA-DR3
RA	HLA-DR4
Ankylosing spondylitis, Reiter's syndrome, psoriatic arthritis	HLA-B27

The degree of skin involvement predicts prognosis: diffuse scleroderma has a worse prognosis than limited scleroderma.

- Twenty percent of patients with scleroderma have Sjögren's syndrome.
- In patients with Sjögren's syndrome, search for an occult lymphoma (look for lymphadenopathy and hepatosplenomegaly).

40% → B cell lymphoma.

4. Pulmonary involvement
   a. Most common cause of death from scleroderma
   b. Interstitial fibrosis and/or pulmonary HTN may be present also.
5. Cardiac involvement: pericardial effusions, myocardial involvement that can lead to CHF, arrhythmias
6. Renal involvement (renal crisis—rapid malignant hypertension) occurs in patients with diffuse disease (rare today).

C. Diagnosis
1. Diagnostic tests are of limited utility. Almost all patients have elevated ANAs (high sensitivity, low specificity).
2. **Anticentromere antibody** is very specific for the limited form.
3. **Anti-topoisomerase I** (antiscleroderma-70) Ab is very specific for the diffuse form.
4. Barium swallow (esophageal dysmotility) and pulmonary function test are used to detect complications.

D. Treatment
1. No effective cure
2. Treat symptoms—NSAIDs for musculoskeletal pains, H_2 blockers or proton pump inhibitors for esophageal reflux
3. Raynaud's phenomenon—Avoid cold and smoking, keep hands warm; if severe, use calcium channel blockers.
4. Treat pulmonary and renal complications if present.

Sjögren's Syndrome

A. General characteristics
1. Sjögren's syndrome is an autoimmune disease most commonly seen in women. Lymphocytes infiltrate and destroy the lacrimal and salivary glands.
2. A multiorgan disease (can also involve the skin, lungs, thyroid, vessels, and liver)
3. Primary versus secondary Sjögren's syndrome

TABLE 6-4 Diffuse Versus Limited Scleroderma	
Diffuse *(Systemic sclerosis)*	**Limited** *(CREST)*
Widespread skin involvement	Skin involvement limited to distal extremities (and face, neck)—sparing of the trunk
Rapid onset of symptoms (skin and other complications occur rapidly after onset of Raynaud's phenomenon)	Delayed onset: Skin involvement occurs slowly after the onset of Raynaud's phenomenon. Therefore, the patient has a long history of Raynaud's phenomenon before other symptoms begin.
Significant visceral involvement (i.e., fibrosis of internal organs)—lungs, heart, GI tract, kidneys	Visceral involvement occurs late—pulmonary HTN and ischemic vascular disease; minimal constitutional symptoms
Associated with ANAs but absence of anticentromere antibody	Anticentromere antibody is found in most patients.
Poorer prognosis—10-year survival is 40% to 65%	Better prognosis than diffuse form Normal life span is expected in most cases, unless severe pulmonary HTN develops.
• Peripheral edema (of hands and legs), polyarthritis, fatigue and weakness (muscle involvement), carpal tunnel syndrome • Renal failure can occur, but now rare • Interstitial lung disease more common	CREST syndrome is a variant. **C**alcinosis of the digits **R**aynaud's phenomenon **E**sophageal motility dysfunction **S**clerodactyly of the fingers **T**elangiectases (over the digits and under the nails)

pulmonary HTN.

a. Primary Sjögren's syndrome: dry eyes and dry mouth, along with lymphocytic infiltration of the minor salivary glands (on histology); patients do not have another rheumatologic disease

b. Secondary Sjögren's syndrome: dry eyes and dry mouth along with a connective tissue disease (RA, systemic sclerosis, SLE, polymyositis)

4. Patients have increased risk of non-Hodgkin's lymphoma. Malignancy is the most common cause of death.

B. Clinical features

1. Dry eyes—burning, redness, blurred vision
2. Dry mouth
3. Arthralgias, arthritis, fatigue
4. Many extraglandular manifestations (more common in primary disease), such as chronic arthritis, interstitial nephritis, and vasculitis

C. Diagnosis

1. ANAs are present in 95% of patients. RF is present in 50% to 75% of patients with secondary disease.
2. Ro (SS-A) present in 55% of patients, and La (SS-B) Abs present in 40% of patients.
3. Nonspecific findings: increased erythrocyte sedimentation rate (ESR), normocytic, normochromic anemia, leukopenia

D. Treatment

1. Pilocarpine (enhances secretions)
2. Artificial tears for dry eyes ✓
3. Good oral hygiene ✓
4. NSAIDs, steroids for arthralgias, arthritis
5. Patients with secondary Sjögren's syndrome—therapy for connective tissue disease

> **QUICK HIT**
> Patients with antibodies to Ro (SS-A) are at increased risk of having a child with neonatal SLE (with congenital heart block). ,

Mixed Connective Tissue Disease

- Mixed connective tissue disease is an "overlap" syndrome with clinical features similar to those of SLE, RA, systemic sclerosis, and polymyositis. Findings consistent with each of these diseases do not necessarily occur simultaneously. It usually takes some time for a pattern to be identified and a diagnosis of mixed connective tissue disease to be made.
- Clinical findings include pulmonary involvement, esophageal dysfunction, polyarthritis, sclerodactyly, cutaneous manifestations, myopathy, and Raynaud's phenomenon.
- The presence of anti-U1-RNP Abs is a key laboratory finding. High ANA and RF may be present.
- Treatment varies according to which specific disease predominates.

RHEUMATOID ARTHRITIS (RA)

A. General characteristics

1. RA is a chronic **inflammatory** autoimmune disease involving the **synovium of joints**. The inflamed synovium can cause damage to cartilage and bone.
2. It is a systemic disease that has many extra-articular manifestations (see below).
3. The usual age of onset is 20 to 40 years; it is more common in women than in men (3:1).
4. Disease severity is variable—some patients have moderate restrictions and are capable of performing activities of daily living, whereas others are confined to a wheelchair or bed.
5. Etiology is uncertain. It may be caused by an infection or a series of infections (most likely viral), but genetic predisposition is necessary.

B. Clinical features

1. **Symmetrical** inflammatory polyarthritis (symmetrical joint swelling is the most common sign)—can involve every joint in the body **except the DIP joints**.

[handwritten margin notes: MCC of death. SLE - opportunistic infections / Renal. Systemic sclerosis - Pulmonary. Sjogren — non-hodgkin lymphoma.]

> **Box** 6-5 **Diagnosis of Rheumatoid Arthritis**
>
> A patient has RA if four or more of these seven criteria are present at any time.
> 1. Morning stiffness for at least 6 weeks
> 2. Arthritis of three or more joints lasting at least 6 weeks—MCP, PIP, wrist, elbow, knee, ankle, MIP joints
> 3. Symmetric arthritis for at least 6 weeks
> 4. Arthritis of hand joints for at least 6 weeks—PIP, MCP, or wrist joint
> 5. Rheumatoid nodules
> 6. Serum RF
> 7. Radiographic changes consistent with RA (erosions and periarticular decalcification)

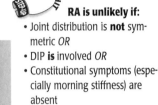

RA is unlikely if:
- Joint distribution is **not** symmetric *OR*
- DIP **is** involved *OR*
- Constitutional symptoms (especially morning stiffness) are absent

  a. Pain on motion of joints/tenderness in joints
  b. Joints commonly involved include **joints of the hands (PIP, MCP) and wrists,** knees, ankles, elbows, hips, and shoulders.
  c. Characteristic hand deformities
  - Ulnar deviation of the MCP joints (see Figure 6-3A)
  - *Boutonnière deformities* of the PIP joints (PIP flexed, DIP hyperextended) (see Figure 6-3C)
  - *Swan-neck contractures* of the fingers (MCP flexed, PIP hyperextended, DIP flexed) (see Figure 6-3B)

FIGURE
6-2 The clinical course of rheumatoid arthritis can be grouped into four classes of patients.

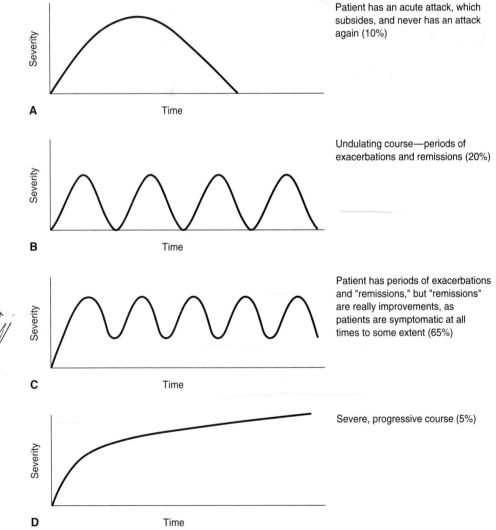

Patient has an acute attack, which subsides, and never has an attack again (10%)

Undulating course—periods of exacerbations and remissions (20%)

Patient has periods of exacerbations and "remissions," but "remissions" are really improvements, as patients are symptomatic at all times to some extent (65%)

Severe, progressive course (5%)

FIGURE
6-3 Rheumatoid arthritis. **A.** Ulnar deviation at metacarpophalangeal joints.
B. Swan-neck deformity. **C.** Boutonnière deformity.

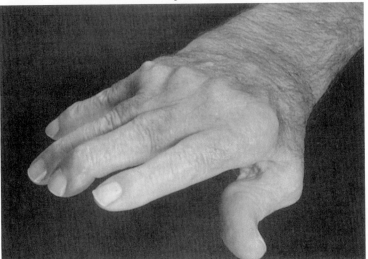

A

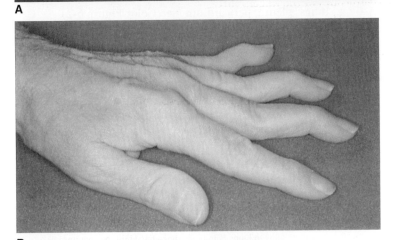

B

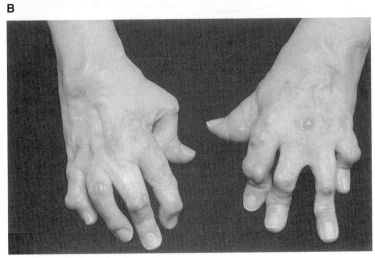

C

(From Hunder GG. Atlas of Rheumatology. 3rd Ed. Philadelphia: Lippincott Williams & Wilkins, 2000:11, Figures 1-27, 1-28, and 1-29A, respectively; and Curr Med 2002:11.)

2. Constitutional symptoms can be prominent
  a. **Morning stiffness** (present in all patients)—improves as the day progresses
  b. Low-grade fever, weight loss
  c. Fatigue can be prominent because this is a systemic disease.
3. Cervical spine involvement is common at C1-C2 (subluxation and instability), but it is less common in the lower cervical spine.
  a. Instability of the cervical spine is a potentially life-threatening complication of RA. Most patients do not have neurologic involvement, but if they do, it can be progressive and fatal if not treated surgically.
  b. This is seen in 30% to 40% of patients. All patients with RA should have cervical spine radiographs before undergoing any surgery (due to risk of neurologic injury during intubation).
4. Cardiac involvement may include pericarditis, pericardial effusions, conduction abnormalities, and valvular incompetence.
5. Pulmonary involvement—usually pleural effusions; interstitial fibrosis may occur
6. Ocular involvement—episcleritis or scleritis
7. Soft tissue swelling (rather than bony enlargement)
8. Drying of mucous membranes: Sjögren's xerostomia
9. Subcutaneous **rheumatoid nodules** over extensor surfaces, may also occur in visceral structures—e.g., lungs, pleura, pericardium (see Color Figure 6-2)

TABLE 6-5 **Extra-articular Manifestations in Rheumatoid Arthritis**

Constitutional symptoms	Malaise, anorexia, some weight loss, fever
Cutaneous	• Skin becomes thin and atrophic and bruises easily • Vasculitic changes/ulcerations involving fingers, nail folds • Subcutaneous **rheumatoid nodules** (elbows, sacrum, occiput)—**pathognomonic for RA**
Pulmonary	• Pleural effusions (very common)—**Pleural fluid characteristically has very low glucose** and low complement. • Pulmonary fibrosis—with a restrictive pattern on pulmonary function tests and a honeycomb pattern on CXR • Pulmonary infiltrates • Rheumatic nodules in lungs (similar to those on skin)—can cavitate or become infected
Cardiac	• Rheumatic nodules in heart—can lead to conduction disturbances (heart block and bundle branch block) • Pericarditis—in 40% of patients with RA • Pericardial effusion
Eyes	• Scleritis • Scleromalacia—softening of the sclera; if not treated may perforate, leading to blindness • Dry eyes (and dry mucous membranes in general); may develop Sjögren's syndrome
Nervous system	Mononeuritic multiplex—infarction of nerve trunk Patient cannot move the arm or leg; implies systemic vasculitis, which is a bad sign.
Felty's syndrome	• Triad of RA, neutropenia, and splenomegaly • Also anemia, thrombocytopenia, and lymphadenopathy • Associated with high titers of RF and extra-articular disease • Increased susceptibility to infection • Usually occurs fairly late in the disease process
Blood	• Anemia of chronic disease: mild, normocytic, normochromic anemia • Thrombocytosis
Vasculitis	A microvascular vasculitis—can progress to mesenteric vasculitis, PAN, or other vascular syndromes

TABLE 6-6 Synovial Fluid Analysis

Condition	Appearance of Fluid	WBC/mm³	PMNs	Other Findings
Normal	Clear	<200	<25%	
Noninflammatory arthritis (OA/trauma)	Clear, yellow; possibly red if traumatic	<2,000	<25%	RBCs for trauma
Inflammatory arthritis (RA, gout, pseudogout, Reiter's syndrome)	Cloudy yellow	>5,000	50% to 70%	Positively birefringent crystals with pseudogout; negatively birefringent crystals with gout
Septic arthritis (bacterial, tuberculosis)	Turbid, purulent	Usually >50,000	>70%	Synovial fluid culture positive for most cases of bacterial arthritis except gonococcal (only 25% are positive)

    a. Pathognomonic for RA

    b. Nearly always occurs in seropositive patients (i.e., those with RF)

C. Diagnosis

1. Laboratory findings

    a. High titers of RF are associated with more severe disease and are generally nonspecific. RF is eventually present in 80% of patients with RA (may be absent early in the disease), but is also present in up to 3% of the healthy population.

    b. Elevated ESR, C-reactive protein (Non-specific)

    c. Normocytic normochromic anemia (anemia of chronic disease)

2. Radiographs

    a. Loss of juxtaarticular bone mass (periarticular osteoporosis) near the finger joints

    b. **Narrowing of the joint space** (due to thinning of the articular cartilage) is usually seen late in the disease.

    c. **Bony erosions** at the margins of the joint

3. Synovial fluid analysis (see Table 6-6) is nonspecific.

D. Treatment

1. Principles of treatment

    a. The goals of treatment are to prevent or halt joint destruction and to come as close to clinical remission as possible while avoiding the toxicity of anti-RA medication.

    b. Treatment must be individualized to the patient. A treatment regimen that works for one patient may not work for another.

2. Exercise helps to maintain range of motion and muscle strength.

3. Symptomatic treatment

    a. NSAIDs are the drugs of choice for control of pain. They play an important role in controlling inflammation and should be part of most treatment regimens.

    b. Corticosteroids (low-dose)—Use these if NSAIDs do not provide adequate relief.

      • Short-term treatment may be appropriate.

      • Avoid long-term, high-dose steroids.

      • Long term, **low-dose** corticosteroids may actually alter the course of the disease (have been shown to diminish radiographic progression)—more studies are needed before this can be considered a disease-modifying drug.

QUICK HIT

Poor prognostic indicators in RA
• High RF titers
• Subcutaneous nodules
• Erosive arthritis
• Autoantibodies to RF

QUICK HIT

In RA, changes in joints are usually more extensive than in OA because the entire synovium is involved in RA. Note that osteophytes (characteristic of OA) are **not** present in RA.

QUICK HIT

Variants of RA
• **Felty's syndrome:** anemia, neutropenia, splenomegaly, and RA
• **Juvenile RA:** begins before 18 years of age. Extra-articular manifestations may predominate (**Still's disease**), or arthritis may predominate.

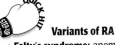

CONNECTIVE TISSUE AND JOINT DISEASES

4. Disease-modifying drugs
   a. General principles
      • Can reduce morbidity and mortality (by nearly 30%)—by limiting complications, slowing progression of disease, and preserving joint function
      • Should be initiated early (at the time of diagnosis)
      • They have a slow onset of action (6 weeks or longer for effect to be seen), so begin treating RA while waiting for the disease-modifying therapy to take effect. Once the effect is evident, gradually taper and discontinue NSAIDs and corticosteroids and continue the disease-modifying program.
   b. First-line agents
      • Methotrexate
         • Most popular treatment right now—first-line therapy.
         • Initial improvement is seen in 4 to 6 weeks. Nearly 80% of treated patients will experience moderate to excellent symptomatic benefit from treatment; remission is rare.
         • Side effects include GI upset, oral ulcers (stomatitis), mild alopecia, bone marrow suppression, hepatocellular injury, and idiosyncratic interstitial pneumonitis, which may lead to pulmonary fibrosis.
         • Closely monitor liver and renal function
         • Supplement with folate.
      • Hydroxychloroquine
         • This is an alternative first-line agent, but usually not as effective as methotrexate.
         • It requires eye examinations every 6 months because of risk of visual loss due to retinopathy (although quite rare).
      • Sulfasalazine—alternate first-line agent, but less effective than methotrexate
   c. Second-line agents include gold compounds, penicillamine, azathioprine, and cyclosporine.
5. Surgery (in severe cases)
   a. Synovectomy (arthroscopic) decreases joint pain and swelling but does not prevent x-ray progression and does not improve joint range of motion.
   b. Joint replacement surgery for severe pain unresponsive to conservative measures

New - biologicals → humera

CRYSTAL-INDUCED ARTHRITIDES

Gout

A. General characteristics
1. Gout is inflammatory monoarticular arthritis caused by crystallization of monosodium urate in joints. Hyperuricemia is a hallmark of the disease, but it does not by itself indicate gout.
2. Ninety percent of patients are men over 30 years of age. Women are not affected until after menopause.
3. Pathogenesis
   a. Increased production of uric acid
      • Hypoxanthine-guanine phosphoribosyltransferase deficiency—e.g., in Lesch-Nyhan syndrome
      • Phosphoribosyl pyrophosphate synthetase overactivity
      • Increased cell turnover associated with a number of conditions, including cancer chemotherapy, chronic hemolysis, and hematologic malignancies
   b. Decreased excretion of uric acid (accounts for 90% of cases)
      • Renal disease
      • NSAIDs, diuretics
      • Acidosis

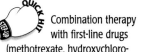

QUICK HIT

Combination therapy with first-line drugs (methotrexate, hydroxychloroquine, and sulfasalazine) produces higher remission rates.

First line therapy for RA is actually DMARDS.

CONNECTIVE TISSUE AND JOINT DISEASES

4. Pathophysiology of inflammation
   a. PMNs play a key role in the acute inflammation of gout.
   b. It develops when uric acid crystals collect in the synovial fluid as the extracellular fluid becomes saturated with uric acid.
   c. IgGs coat monosodium urate crystals, which are phagocytized by PMNs, leading to the release of inflammatory mediators and proteolytic enzymes from the PMNs, which then result in inflammation.

B. Clinical features (four stages)

1. Asymptomatic hyperuricemia
   a. Increased serum uric acid level in absence of clinical findings of gout, may be present without symptoms for 10 to 20 years or longer
   b. Should not be treated because over 95% of patients remain asymptomatic
2. Acute gouty arthritis
   a. Peak age of onset is 40 to 60 years of age for men
   b. Initial attack usually involves one joint of the lower extremity
      • Sudden onset of exquisite pain—The patient may be unable to tolerate a bed sheet on affected joint. Pain often wakes the patient from sleep.
      • Most often affects the big toe—the first metatarsophalangeal joint (podagra). Other common joints affected are ankles and knees.
   c. Pain and cellulitic changes—erythema, swelling, tenderness, and warmth
   d. Fever may or may not be present.
   e. As it resolves, the patient may have desquamation of overlying skin.
3. Intercritical gout
   a. An asymptomatic period after the initial attack. The patient may not have another attack for years.
   b. Sixty percent of patients have a recurrence within 1 year. Some patients (fewer than 10%) never have another attack of gout.
   c. There is a 75% likelihood of a second attack within the first 2 years.
   d. Attacks tend to become polyarticular with increased severity over time.
4. Chronic tophaceous gout
   a. Occurs in people who have had poorly controlled gout for more than 10 to 20 years.
   b. Tophi
      • Aggregations of urate crystals surrounded by giant cells in an inflammatory reaction
      • Seen only after several attacks of acute gout; noted after an average of 10 years following the initial attack
      • Tophi cause deformity and destruction of hard and soft tissues. In joints, they lead to destruction of cartilage and bone, triggering secondary degeneration and development of arthritis. They may be extra-articular.
   c. Common locations of tophi: extensor surface of forearms, elbows, knees, Achilles tendons, and pinna of external ear

C. Diagnosis

1. Joint aspiration and synovial fluid analysis (under a polarizing microscope) is the only way to make a definitive diagnosis—**needle-shaped and negatively birefringent urate crystals** appear in synovial fluid.
2. Serum uric acid is **not** helpful in diagnosis because it can be normal even during an acute gouty attack.
3. Radiographs reveal punched-out erosions with an overhanging rim of cortical bone.

D. Treatment

1. In all stages, avoid secondary causes of hyperuricemia.
   a. Medications that increase uric acid levels (thiazide and loop diuretics)
   b. Obesity
   c. Reduce alcohol intake.
   d. Reduce dietary purine intake.

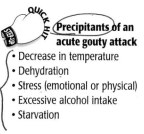

Precipitants of an acute gouty attack
• Decrease in temperature
• Dehydration
• Stress (emotional or physical)
• Excessive alcohol intake
• Starvation

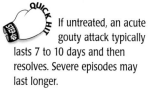

If untreated, an acute gouty attack typically lasts 7 to 10 days and then resolves. Severe episodes may last longer.

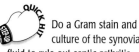

Do a Gram stain and culture of the synovial fluid to rule out septic arthritis, which is the most worrisome diagnosis on the differential list.

Complications of gout
• Nephrolithiasis—risk is small (less than 1% per year)
• Degenerative arthritis occurs in less than 15% of patients. Incidence is decreasing due to effective treatment of hyperuricemia and consequent prevention of tophaceous gout.

FIGURE
6-4 Posteroanterior radiographs of the hand showing the typical pattern of involvement for **(A)** osteoarthritis (osteophytes, subchondral sclerosis, joint space narrowing) (arrows) and **(B)** rheumatoid arthritis (periarticular erosions, osteopenia) (arrows). Anteroposterior radiographs of the hip in patients with **(C)** osteoarthritis, showing typical superolateral migration of the femoral head (arrow), and **(D)** rheumatoid arthritis, showing axial migration of the femoral head (arrow).

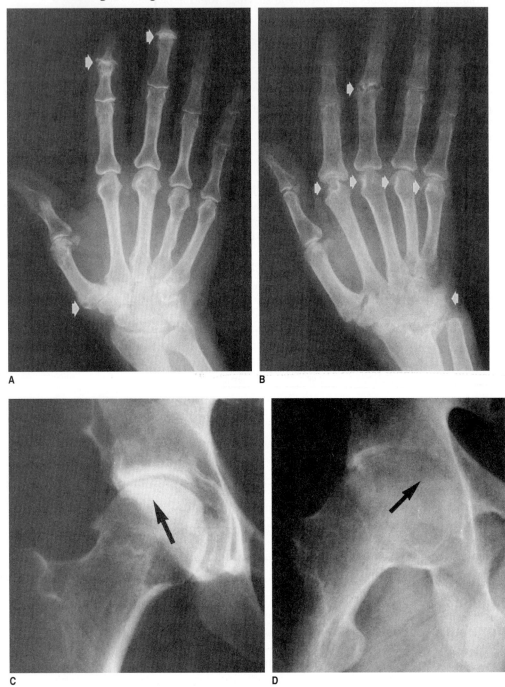

(**A** and **B** from Humes DH, DuPont HL, Gardner LB, et al. Kelley's Textbook of Internal Medicine. 4th Ed. Philadelphia: Lippincott Williams & Wilkins, 2000:1463, Figures 190.4A and B.)
(**C** and **D** from Humes DH, DuPont HL, Gardner LB, et al. Kelley's Textbook of Internal Medicine. 4th Ed. Philadelphia: Lippincott Williams & Wilkins, 2000:1466, Figures 190.9A and B.)

FIGURE
6-5 Gout: common sites of involvement

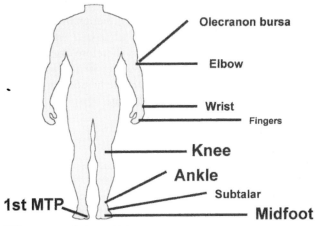

- Olecranon bursa
- Elbow
- Wrist
- Fingers
- **Knee**
- **Ankle**
- Subtalar
- **1st MTP**
- **Midfoot**

MTP, metatarsophalangeal joint.
(From Stoller JK, Ahmad M, Longworth DL: The Cleveland Clinic Intensive Review of Internal Medicine. 3rd Ed. Philadelphia: Lippincott Williams & Wilkins, 2002:374, Figure 30.6.)

2. Acute gout
   a. Bed rest is important. Early ambulation may precipitate a recurrence.
   b. NSAIDs
      • Treatment of choice in acute gout (indomethacin is traditionally used, but other NSAIDs are effective)
      • Very effective in relieving pain promptly; best if initiated early—a delay in initiating therapy can impair response.
   c. Colchicine
      • An alternative for patients who cannot take NSAIDs or did not respond to NSAIDs
      • Effective but less favored because 80% of treated patients develop significant nausea/vomiting, abdominal cramps, and severe diarrhea. Compliance tends to be low due to these side effects.
      • It is contraindicated in renal insufficiency and cytopenia.
   d. Corticosteroids
      • Oral prednisone (7- to 10-day course) if patient does not respond to or cannot tolerate NSAIDs and colchicine
      • Intra-articular corticosteroid injections (if only one joint is involved)— dramatic relief of symptoms
3. Prophylactic therapy
   a. Wait until patient has had at least two acute gouty attacks (or perhaps three) before initiating prophylactic therapy. Two attacks per year is sometimes used as a rough guideline. This is because the second attack may take years to occur (if at all), and so the risk-to-benefit ratio for prophylactic medication (allopurinol or uricosuric agents) is not favorable after one gouty attack.
   b. When giving prophylaxis, add either colchicine or an NSAID for 3 to 6 months to prevent an acute attack. The colchicine or NSAID can then be discontinued, and the patient can remain on the uricosuric agent or allopurinol indefinitely.
   c. The choice of whether to use uricosuric drugs or allopurinol depends on how much uric acid is excreted in the urine in a 24-hour period.
      • Uricosuric drugs (probenecid, sulfinpyrazone)—If the 24-hour urine uric acid is <800 mg/day, this indicates undersecretion of urate. These drugs increase renal excretion of uric acid; use them only in patients with normal renal function. They are contraindicated if the patient has a history of renal stones.
      • Allopurinol (a xanthine oxidase inhibitor, decreases uric acid synthesis)—If the 24-hour urine uric acid is >800 mg/day, this indicates overproduction. Never give this for acute gout; it makes it worse. Use once-daily dosing. It is well tolerated.

Uric acid levels in pt. w/ tophaceous gout should be reduced to 6 mg/dL to dissolve tophi and other urate deposits in the tissue.

 QUICK HIT In acute gout, avoid aspirin (can aggravate the problem) and acetaminophen (has no anti-inflammatory properties).

CONNECTIVE TISSUE AND JOINT DISEASES

Pseudogout (Calcium Pyrophosphate Deposition Disease)

A. General characteristics

1. Calcium pyrophosphate crystals deposit in joints, leading to inflammation.
2. Risk factors
   a. Deposition increases with age and with OA of the joints. Therefore, pseudogout is common in elderly patients with degenerative joint disease.
   b. Other conditions that may increase crystal deposition include hemochromatosis, hyperparathyroidism, hypothyroidism, and Bartter's syndrome.

B. Clinical features

1. The most common joints affected are knees and wrists.
2. It is classically monoarticular, but can be polyarticular as well.

C. Diagnosis

1. Joint aspirate is required for definitive diagnosis—**weakly positively birefringent, rod-shaped and rhomboidal crystals** in synovial fluid (calcium pyrophosphate crystals)
2. Radiographs—chondrocalcinosis (cartilage calcification)

FIGURE 6-6 Evaluation of joint pain.

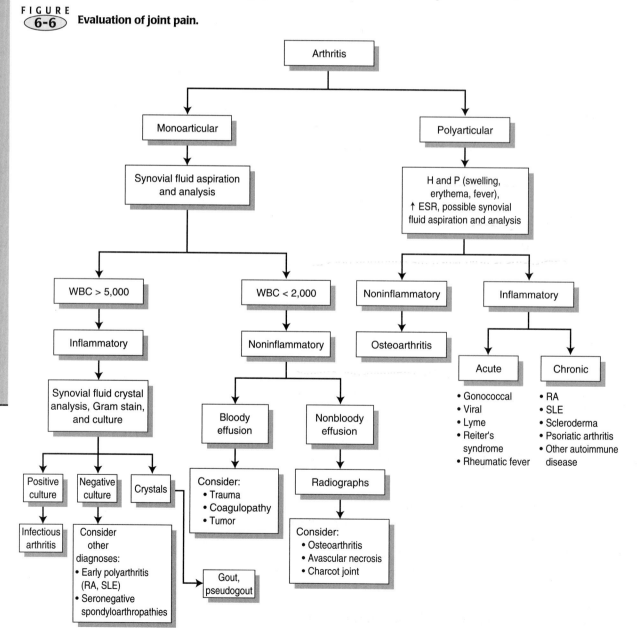

TABLE 6-7 Major Arthritides	Osteoarthritis	Rheumatoid Arthritis	Gouty Arthritis
Onset	Insidious	Insidious	Sudden
Common locations	Weight-bearing joints (knees, hips, lumbar/cervical spine), hands	Hands (PIP, MCP), wrists, ankles, knees	Great toe, ankles, knees, elbows
Presence of inflammation	No	Yes	Yes
Radiographic changes	Narrowed joint space, osteophytes, subchondral sclerosis, subchondral cysts	Narrowed joint space, bony erosions	Punched-out erosions with overhanging rim of cortical bone
Laboratory findings	None	Elevated ESR, RF, anemia	Crystals
Other features	• No systemic findings • Bouchard's nodes and Heberden's nodes in hands	• Systemic findings—extra-articular manifestations common • Ulnar deviation, swan-neck, and boutonnière deformity	• Tophi • Nephrolithiasis

D. Treatment
1. Treat the underlying disorder (if identified).
2. Symptomatic management is similar to that for gout (NSAIDs, colchicine, intra-articular steroid injections).
3. Total joint replacement is appropriate if symptoms are debilitating.

MYOPATHIES AND PAIN SYNDROMES

Idiopathic Inflammatory Myopathies

A. General characteristics
1. The term polymyositis is used when the condition does not involve the skin (usually occurs in adults). The term dermatomyositis is used when polymyositis is associated with a characteristic skin rash.
2. More common in female patients.
3. Classification
   a. **Polymyositis**
   b. **Dermatomyositis**
   c. Childhood onset dermatomyositis—subcutaneous calcifications
   d. Myositis associated with collagen vascular disease
   e. Myositis associated with malignancy
   f. **Inclusion body myositis**—"oddball" for the following reasons: affects male more than female patients, absence of autoantibodies, distal muscle involvement, and relatively low creatine kinase (CK); prognosis is poor

B. Causes
1. Hypothesis: A genetically susceptible individual plus an environmental trigger leads to immune activation, which results in chronic inflammation.
2. Pathologic changes in muscle
   a. Dermatomyositis—humoral immune mechanisms
   b. Polymyositis and inclusion body myositis—cell-mediated process

C. Clinical features
1. Features common to both polymyositis and dermatomyositis

> **Box** 6-6 **Diagnostic Criteria for Polymyositis**
>
> If two of first four → possible polymyositis
> If three of first four → probable polymyositis
> If all four → definite polymyositis
> - Symmetric proximal muscle weakness
> - Elevation in serum creatine phosphokinase
> - EMG findings of a myopathy
> - Biopsy evidence of myositis
> - Characteristic rash of dermatomyositis

     a. **Symmetrical proximal muscle weakness** that develops subacutely over weeks or several months
- The earliest and most severely affected muscle groups are the neck flexors, shoulder girdle, and pelvic girdle muscles.
- Distal extremity weakness is less frequent and typically less severe.

     b. Myalgia in 33% of patients

     c. Dysphagia in up to 30% of patients (involvement of esophageal muscles)

2. Features unique to dermatomyositis
   a. *Heliotrope rash* (butterfly)—around eyes, bridge of nose, cheeks
   b. *Gottron's papules*—papular, erythematous, scaly lesions over the knuckles (MCP, PIP, DIP)
   c. *V sign*—rash on the face, neck, and anterior chest
   d. *Shawl sign*—rash on shoulders and upper back, elbows, and knees
   e. Periungual erythema with telangiectases
   f. Subcutaneous calcifications in children—can be extremely painful

3. Associated findings
   a. In both polymyositis and dermatomyositis
      - Arthralgias (common)
      - CHF and conduction defects (rare)
      - Interstitial lung disease (in minority of patients)
   b. In dermatomyositis only
      - Vasculitis of the GI tract, kidneys, lungs, and eyes (more common in children)
      - There is an increased incidence of malignancy in older adults (lung, breast, ovary, GI tract, and myeloproliferative disorders). Once dermatomyositis is diagnosed, make an effort to uncover an occult malignancy. Dermatomyositis associated with malignancy often remits once the tumor is removed.

D. Diagnosis

1. Laboratory
   a. CK level is significantly elevated. CK levels correspond to the degree of muscle necrosis, so one can monitor the disease severity.
   b. LDH, aldolase, AST, ALT elevated
   c. ANA in over 50%
   d. Anti-synthetase antibodies (anti-Jo-1 antibodies)—abrupt onset of fever, cracked hands, Raynaud's phenomenon, interstitial lung disease, arthritis; does not respond well to therapy
   e. Anti-signal recognition particle
      - Cardiac manifestations (common)
      - Worst prognosis of all subsets
   f. Anti-Mi-2 antibodies—better prognosis
2. EMG—abnormal in 90% of patients
3. Muscle biopsy
   a. Shows inflammation and muscle fiber fibrosis in *all three*
   b. Dermatomyositis—perivascular and perimysial
   c. Polymyositis and inclusion body myositis—endomysial

E. Treatment

1. Corticosteroids are the initial treatment. Continue until symptoms improve, and then taper very slowly (up to 2 years may be necessary).
2. Immunosuppressive agents (for patients who do not respond to steroids)—methotrexate, cyclophosphamide, chlorambucil
3. Physical therapy

Inclusion Body Myositis

- More common in men (elderly)
- Insidious onset of slowly progressive proximal **and** distal weakness, often leads to delay in diagnosis
- There is early weakness and atrophy of quadriceps, forearm flexors, and tibialis anterior muscles. Involvement is asymmetrical. Facial weakness occurs in one-third of patients, and dysphagia in one-half of patients.
- Patients can also have loss of deep tendon reflexes (nerves are not involved in polymyositis and dermatomyositis).
- Extramuscular manifestations are rare.
- Diagnosis—slight elevation of CK levels (relatively low)
- Poor response to therapy

Polymyalgia Rheumatica

A. General characteristics

1. Usually occurs in elderly patients (rare before age 50). The mean age of onset is 70, and it is more common in women.
2. The cause is unknown, but an autoimmune process may be responsible. There is a possible genetic link (association with HLA-DR4 allele).
3. Self-limited disease (duration of 1 to 2 years)

B. Clinical features

1. Hip and shoulder muscle pain (bilateral)
   a. Often begins abruptly (but may be gradual)
   b. Stiffness in shoulder and hip regions after a period of inactivity is the most prominent symptom.
   c. Pain occurs on movement; muscle strength is normal.
   d. Profound morning stiffness is common.
2. Constitutional symptoms are usually present: malaise, fever, depression, weight loss, and fatigue.
3. Joint swelling
   a. Up to 20% of patients have synovitis in knees, wrists, or hand joints (can be confused with RA).
   b. Synovitis and tenosynovitis around the shoulder may lead to rotator cuff tendonitis or adhesive capsulitis.
4. Signs and symptoms of temporal arteritis (if present)

C. Diagnosis

1. Essentially a clinical diagnosis
2. ESR is usually elevated and aids in diagnosis.
   a. Almost always >50, frequently >100
   b. Correlates with disease activity

D. Treatment: Corticosteroids

1. Response usually occurs within 1 to 7 days. Corticosteroids are not curative, but are effective in suppressing inflammation until the disease resolves itself.
2. After 4 to 6 weeks, begin to taper slowly.
3. Most patients (60% to 70%) can stop corticosteroids within 2 years. A few patients have symptoms for up to 10 years.

QUICK HIT

About 10% of people with polymyalgia rheumatica develop temporal arteritis; whereas up to 40% to 50% of people with temporal arteritis have coexisting polymyalgia rheumatica.

CONNECTIVE TISSUE AND JOINT DISEASES

Fibromyalgia

A. General characteristics

1. Adult women account for 80% to 90% of cases.
2. Chronic nonprogressive course with waxing and waning in severity; many patients improve with time
3. **Key to diagnosis: multiple trigger points** (points that are tender to palpation)
   a. Symmetrical
   b. Eighteen characteristic locations have been identified, including occiput, neck, shoulder, ribs, elbows, buttocks, and knees.
4. Etiology is unknown—somatization is not a proven cause.

B. Clinical features

1. **Stiffness**, body aches (musculoskeletal), fatigue
   a. Pain is constant and aching, and is aggravated by weather changes, stress, sleep deprivation, and cold temperature. It is worse in the morning.
   b. Rest, warmth, and mild exercise improve the pain.
2. Sleep patterns are disrupted, and sleep is unrefreshing.
3. Anxiety and depression are common.

C. Diagnosis

1. Diagnostic criteria
   a. Widespread pain including axial pain for at least 3 months
   b. Pain in at least 11 of 18 possible tender point sites
2. Before confirming the diagnosis, rule out/consider the following conditions: myofascial syndromes, rheumatoid disease, polymyalgia rheumatica, ankylosing spondylitis, spondyloarthropathy, chronic fatigue syndrome, Lyme disease, hypothyroidism, polymyositis, depression and somatization disorder, and hypertrophic osteoarthropathy.

D. Treatment and management

1. Advise the patient to stay active and productive.
2. Medications are generally not effective. SSRIs and TCAs have shown some effect and may be beneficial. Avoid narcotics.
3. Cognitive-behavioral therapy, exercise, consider psychiatric evaluation

SERONEGATIVE SPONDYLOARTHROPATHIES

Ankylosing Spondylitis

A. General characteristics

1. Strong association with HLA-B27 (90% of patients) (see Table 6-3). Three times more common in male than in female patients.
2. Look for positive family history of ankylosing spondylitis, inflammatory bowel disease, or psoriasis.
3. Bilateral sacroiliitis is a prerequisite for making the diagnosis.
4. Onset is in adolescence or young adulthood.
5. It is characterized by "fusion" of the spine in an ascending manner (from lumbar to cervical spine).
6. Course
   a. There is a slow progression, but the course is highly variable; acute exacerbations are common.
   b. Life expectancy is usually normal.
   c. The first 10 years of the disease can give an indication of long-term severity.

B. Clinical features

1. Low back pain and stiffness (secondary to sacroiliitis)—limited motion in lumbar spine
2. Neck pain and limited motion in cervical spine—occurs later in course of disease

> **Box 6-7 Seronegative Spondyloarthropathies**
>
> Diseases that belong to the seronegative spondyloarthropathies include the following:
> - Ankylosing spondylitis
> - Reactive arthritis (and Reiter's syndrome)
> - Psoriatic arthritis
> - Arthropathy of inflammatory bowel disease (IBD)
> - Undifferentiated spondyloarthropathies
>
> The seronegative spondyloarthropathies have the following **in common:**
> - Negative RF
> - Strong association with HLA-B27 antigen
> - Oligoarthritis (asymmetrical)
> - Enthesitis (inflammation at sites of insertion of fascia, ligament, or tendon to bone)
> - Inflammatory arthritis (axial and sacroiliac joints)
> - Extra-articular features (eyes, skin, genitourinary tract)
> - Familial predisposition

3. Enthesitis—inflammation at tendinous insertions into bone (Achilles tendon and supraspinatus tendon)
4. With extensive spinal involvement, the spine becomes brittle and is prone to fractures with minimal trauma. Severe spinal cord injury can occur with such trauma.
5. Chest pain and diminished chest expansion—due to thoracic spine involvement
6. Shoulder and hip pain—Most commonly, the peripheral joints are affected.
7. Constitutional symptoms—fatigue, low-grade fever, weight loss
8. Extra-articular manifestations
   a. Eye involvement (most common)—acute anterior uveitis or iridocyclitis
   b. Other extra-articular features are rare, but may involve the following systems: cardiac, renal, pulmonary, and nervous systems.
9. Loss of normal posture as disease advances

C. Diagnosis
1. Imaging studies of lumbar spine and pelvis (plain film, MRI, or CT) reveal sacroiliitis—sclerotic changes in the sacroiliac area. Eventually, the vertebral columns fuse, producing "**bamboo spine.**"
2. Elevated ESR in up to 75% of patients (due to inflammation)—nonspecific
3. HLA-B27 is not necessary for diagnosis.

D. Treatment
1. NSAIDs (indomethacin) for symptomatic relief
2. Physical therapy (maintaining good posture, extension exercises)
3. Surgery may be necessary in some patients with severe spinal deformity.
4. Patients with ankylosing spondylitis who sustain even minor trauma and who complain of neck or back pain should be strictly immobilized to prevent spinal cord injury until thorough imaging studies are obtained.

Reactive Arthritis

A. General characteristics
1. Reactive arthritis is asymmetric inflammatory oligoarthritis of lower extremities (upper extremities less common). The arthritis is preceded by an infectious process that is remote from the site of arthritis (1 to 4 weeks prior), usually after enteric or urogenital infections.
2. It occurs mostly in HLA-B27–positive individuals.
3. **Reiter's syndrome** is an example of reactive arthritis, but most patients do not have the classic findings of Reiter's syndrome (see Box 6-8), so the term reactive arthritis is now used.
4. The organisms usually associated with reactive arthritis include *Salmonella, Shigella, Campylobacter, Chlamydia, Yersinia.*

In ankylosing spondylitis, the low back pain and stiffness are characteristically worse in the morning and better as the day progresses. They improve with exercise and a hot shower and worsen with rest or inactivity.

Complications of ankylosing spondylitis
- Restrictive lung disease
- Cauda equina syndrome
- Spine fracture with spinal cord injury
- Osteoporosis
- Spondylodiscitis

Reactive arthritis is a clinical diagnosis. If any patient has an acute asymmetric arthritis that progresses sequentially from one joint to another, reactive arthritis should be in the differential diagnosis.

> **Box 6-8 Reiter's Syndrome**
>
> - Classic triad of arthritis, urethritis, and ocular inflammation (conjunctivitis or anterior uveitis): "Can't see" (uveitis), "can't pee" (urethritis), "can't climb a tree" (arthritis).
> - Classic symptoms of Reiter's syndrome may not always occur together.
> - Patient can develop reactive arthritis after nongonococcal urethritis or after enteric infections with any one of the following: *Salmonella*, *Shigella flexneri*, *Campylobacter jejuni*, *Yersinia enterocolitica*.

B. Clinical features
1. Look for evidence of infection (GI or genitourinary) 1 to 4 weeks before the onset of symptoms.
2. Asymmetric arthritis—New joints may be involved sequentially over days. Joints are painful, with effusions and lack of mobility.
3. Fatigue, malaise, weight loss, and fever are common.
4. Joint pain may persist or recur over a long-term period.

C. Diagnosis: Send synovial fluid for analysis (to rule out infection or crystals).

D. Treatment
1. NSAIDs are first-line therapy.
2. If there is no response, then try sulfasalazine and immunosuppressive agents such as azathioprine.
3. Antibiotic use is controversial—usually not given.

Psoriatic Arthritis

- Develops in fewer than 10% of patients with psoriasis
- It is typically gradual in onset. Patients usually have skin disease for months to years before the arthritis develops.
- Usually asymmetric and polyarticular
- Upper extremities most often involved; smaller joints more common than large joints
- Initial treatment is NSAIDs, but persistent arthritis may require drugs used to treat RA.

VASCULITIS

Temporal Arteritis

A. General characteristics
1. Also known as "giant cell arteritis"

QUICK HIT

The term **undifferentiated spondyloarthropathy** is used when a patient has features of reactive arthritis but there is no evidence of previous infection (in the GI or genitourinary tract) and the classic findings of Reiter's syndrome are absent.

TABLE 6-8 Causes of Joint Pain	
Polyarticular Joint Pain	**Monoarticular Joint Pain**
RA	Osteoarthritis
SLE	Gout
Viral arthritis	Pseudogout
Reiter's syndrome	Trauma
Rheumatic fever	Septic arthritis
Lyme disease	Hemarthrosis
Gonococcal arthritis	
Drug-induced arthritis	

Box 6-9 Vasculitis

- In all of the vasculitic syndromes, blood vessels are inflamed and vascular necrosis can result. Findings depend on the size of the vessel involved and the location of involvement (target organ ischemia).
- If any patient has a systemic illness that has not been explained by another process (or has ischemia involving one or more systems), entertain the diagnosis of vasculitis.
- Classified according to size of vessel
  - Large vessel: Takayasu's arteritis, temporal arteritis
  - Medium vessel: polyarteritis nodosa, Kawasaki's disease (a pediatric disease), Wegener's granulomatosis, Churg-Strauss syndrome, microscopic polyangiitis
  - Small vessel: Henoch-Schönlein purpura, hypersensitivity vasculitis, Behçet's syndrome

---

2. Vasculitis of unknown cause; typical patient is >50 years of age; twice as common in women as men
3. The temporal arteries are most frequently affected, but it may involve other arteries, such as the aorta or carotids.
4. Associated with increased risk of aortic aneurysm and aortic dissection

B. Clinical features
1. Constitutional symptoms of malaise, fatigue, weight loss, and low-grade fever
2. Headaches—may be severe
3. Visual impairment (**in only 25% to 50%**)
   a. Caused by involvement of ophthalmic artery
   b. Optic neuritis; amaurosis fugax; may lead to **blindness** in up to 50% if not treated early and aggressively
4. Jaw pain with chewing—intermittent claudication of jaw/tongue when chewing
5. Tenderness over temporal artery; absent temporal pulse
6. Palpable nodules
7. **40% of patients also have polymyalgia rheumatica.**

C. Diagnosis
1. ESR elevated (but normal ESR does not exclude the diagnosis).
2. Biopsy of the temporal artery has a sensitivity of 90%. A single negative biopsy does not exclude the diagnosis.

D. Treatment
1. Use high-dose steroids (prednisone) early to prevent blindness.
   a. Start treatment **immediately**, even if temporal arteritis is only suspected. **Do not wait for biopsy results.** If visual loss is present, admit the patient to the hospital for IV steroids; otherwise, start oral prednisone.
   b. If the diagnosis is confirmed, continue treatment for at least 4 weeks, then taper gradually, but maintain steroid therapy for up to 2 to 3 years. Relapse is likely to occur if steroids are stopped prematurely.
2. Follow up on ESR levels to monitor effectiveness of treatment.
3. Visual loss in one eye may be temporary or permanent. Prompt and aggressive steroid treatment is primarily given to prevent involvement of the other eye, but it may improve the visual outcome in the affected eye as well.
4. Even if untreated, the disease is usually eventually self-limiting in most patients, although vision loss may be permanent.

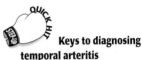

Keys to diagnosing temporal arteritis
- Age >50 years
- New headache
- Tender/palpable temporal artery
- High ESR
- Jaw claudication

If temporal arteritis is suspected, begin prednisone and order a temporal artery biopsy.

• Discrepancies of BP (arm versus leg)
• Arterial bruits

Takayasu's Arteritis

A. General characteristics
1. Most common in young Asian women
2. Vasculitis of aortic arch and its major branches—potentially leading to stenosis or narrowing of vessels
3. Diagnosed via arteriogram

B. Clinical features
1. Constitutional symptoms—fever, night sweats, malaise, arthralgias, fatigue
2. Pain and tenderness over involved vessels
3. Absent pulses in carotid, radial, or ulnar arteries; aortic regurgitation may be present
4. Signs and symptoms of ischemia eventually develop in areas supplied by involved vessels.
5. Severe complications include limb ischemia, aortic aneurysms, aortic regurgitation, stroke, and secondary HTN due to renal artery stenosis. The main prognostic predictor is presence or absence of these complications.

C. Treatment
1. Steroids may relieve the symptoms.
2. Treat HTN.
3. Surgery or angioplasty may be required to recannulate stenosed vessels. Bypass grafting is sometimes necessary.

Churg-Strauss Syndrome

• Vasculitis involving many organ systems (respiratory, cardiac, GI, skin, renal, neurologic)
• Clinical features include constitutional findings (fever, fatigue, weight loss); prominent respiratory tract findings (asthma, dyspnea); and skin lesions (subcutaneous nodules, palpable purpura).
• Diagnosis is made by biopsy of lung or skin tissue (prominence of eosinophils). **It is associated with p-ANCA.**
• The prognosis is poor, with a 5-year survival of 25% (death is usually due to cardiac or pulmonary complications). With treatment (steroids), the 5-year prognosis improves to 50%.

Wegener's Granulomatosis

A. General characteristics: Vasculitis predominantly involving the kidneys and upper and lower respiratory tract (sometimes other organs as well)

B. Clinical features
1. Upper respiratory symptoms (e.g., sinusitis); purulent or bloody nasal discharge
2. Oral ulcers (may be painful)
3. Pulmonary symptoms (cough, hemoptysis, dyspnea)
4. Renal involvement (glomerulonephritis—may have rapidly progressive renal failure)
5. Eye disease (conjunctivitis, scleritis)
6. Musculoskeletal (arthralgias, myalgias)
7. Tracheal stenosis
8. Constitutional findings (e.g., fever, weight loss)

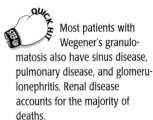

QUICK HIT
Most patients with Wegener's granulomatosis also have sinus disease, pulmonary disease, and glomerulonephritis. Renal disease accounts for the majority of deaths.

C. Diagnosis

1. Chest radiograph is abnormal (nodules or infiltrates).
2. Laboratory findings: markedly elevated ESR; anemia (normochromic normocytic); hematuria; **positive c-ANCA in 90% of patients**—sensitive and specific; thrombocytopenia may be present
3. Open lung biopsy confirms diagnosis.

D. Prognosis and treatment

1. Prognosis is poor—most patients die within 1 year after the diagnosis.
2. A combination of cyclophosphamide and corticosteroids can induce remissions in many patients, but a relapse may occur at any time.
3. Consider renal transplantation if the patient has end-stage renal disease (ESRD).

> **QUICK HIT**
> There is no pulmonary involvement in polyarteritis nodosa (which distinguishes it from Wegener's granulomatosis).

Polyarteritis Nodosa (PAN)

A. General characteristics

1. Vasculitis of medium-sized vessels involving the nervous system and GI tract
2. Can be associated with hepatitis B, HIV, and drug reactions
3. Pathophysiology: PMN invasion of all layers and fibrinoid necrosis plus resulting intimal proliferation lead to reduced luminal area, which results in ischemia, infarction, and aneurysms.

B. Clinical findings

1. Early symptoms are fever, weakness, weight loss, myalgias and arthralgias, and abdominal pain (bowel angina).
2. Other findings are HTN, mononeuritic multiplex, and livedo reticularis.

C. Diagnosis

1. Diagnosis is made by biopsy of involved tissue or mesenteric angiography.
2. ESR is usually elevated, and p-ANCA may be present.
3. Test for fecal occult blood.

D. Prognosis and treatment: The prognosis is poor, but is improved to a limited extent with treatment. Start with corticosteroids. If PAN is severe, add cyclophosphamide.

Behçet's Syndrome

- An autoimmune, multisystem vasculitic disease; cause is unknown
- Clinical features: recurrent oral and genital ulcerations (usually painful), arthritis (knees and ankles most common), eye involvement (uveitis, optic neuritis, iritis, conjunctivitis), CNS involvement (meningoencephalitis, intracranial HTN), fever, and weight loss.
- Diagnosis is made by biopsy of involved tissue (laboratory tests are not helpful).
- Treatment is steroids, which are helpful.

Buerger's Disease (Thromboangiitis Obliterans)

- Occurs mostly in young men who **smoke cigarettes**
- Acute inflammation of small- and medium-sized arteries and veins, affecting arms and legs
- May lead to gangrene
- Clinical features include ischemic claudication; cold, cyanotic, painful distal extremities; paresthesias of distal extremities; and ulceration of digits.
- Smoking cessation is mandatory to reduce progression.

Hypersensitivity Vasculitis

- Small-vessel vasculitis that is a hypersensitivity reaction in response to a drug (penicillin, sulfa drugs), infection, or other stimulus
- Skin is predominantly involved—palpable purpura, macules, or vesicles (common on lower extremities) can occur. Lesions can be painful.
- Constitutional symptoms (fever, weight loss, fatigue) may be present.
- Diagnosis is made by biopsy of tissue.
- Prognosis is very good—spontaneous remissions are common.
- Withdrawal of the offending agent and steroids are the treatments of choice.

* Acute treatment for knee sprains
- RICE - Rest, Ice, Compression, elevation (symptomatic treatment).
- Obtain a knee radiograph for → >55 yrs, tenderness at the head of fibula/patella, inability to flex 90° or bear weight both immediately and during evaluation.

Diseases of the Renal and Genitourinary System

RENAL FAILURE

Acute Renal Failure (ARF)

A. General characteristics

1. Definition: A rapid decline in renal function, with an increase in serum creatinine level (a relative increase of 50% or an absolute increase of 0.5 to 1.0 mg/dL).
2. ARF may be oliguric, anuric, or nonoliguric. Severe ARF may occur without a reduction in urine output (nonoliguric ARF).
3. Weight gain and edema are the most common clinical findings in patients with ARF. This is due to a positive water and sodium (Na^+) balance.
4. Characterized by **azotemia** (elevated BUN and Cr)
   a. Elevated BUN is also seen with catabolic drugs (e.g., steroids), GI/soft tissue bleeding, and dietary protein intake. *ex. patient not eating but then put on a PEG tube.*
   b. Elevated Cr is also seen with increased muscle breakdown and various drugs. *statins* The baseline Cr level varies proportionately with muscle mass.

   Normal BUN - 7-18
   N'l Creatnine - 0.6-1.2

5. Prognosis
   a. More than 80% of patients in whom ARF develops recover completely. However, the prognosis varies widely depending on the severity of renal failure and the presence of comorbid conditions.
   b. The older the patient and the more severe the insult, the lower is the likelihood of complete recovery.
   c. The most common cause of death is infection (75% of all deaths), followed by cardiorespiratory complications.

B. Categories

1. Prerenal failure
   a. Most common cause of ARF
   b. **Potentially reversible**
   c. Etiology (decrease in systemic arterial blood volume or renal perfusion)—can complicate any disease that causes hypovolemia, *(CHF)* low cardiac output, or systemic vasodilation *(sepsis)*
      - Hypovolemia—dehydration, excessive diuretic use, poor fluid intake, vomiting, diarrhea, burns, hemorrhage
      - CHF
      - Peripheral vasodilation—sepsis, excessive antihypertensive medications
      - Renal arterial obstruction
      - Cirrhosis, hepatorenal syndrome
      - In patients with decreased renal perfusion, NSAIDs, ACE inhibitors, and cyclosporin can precipitate prerenal failure.

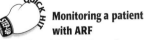

Types of ARF (see Figure 7-1)
- **Prerenal ARF**—decrease in renal blood flow (60% to 70% of cases)
- **Intrinsic ARF**—damage to renal parenchyma (25% to 40% of cases)
- **Postrenal ARF**—urinary tract obstruction (5% to 10% of cases)

Monitoring a patient with ARF
- Daily weights, intake and output
- BP
- Serum electrolytes
- Watch Hb and Hct for anemia.
- Watch for infection.

Box 7-1   Diagnostic Approach in ARF

- History and physical examination
- The first thing to do is to determine the duration of renal failure. A baseline Cr level provides this information.
- The second task is to determine whether ARF is due to prerenal, intrarenal, or postrenal causes. This is done via a combination of history, physical examination, and laboratory findings.
  —Signs of volume depletion and CHF suggest a **prerenal** etiology.
  —Signs of an allergic reaction (rash) suggest acute interstitial nephritis (an intrinsic renal etiology).
  —A suprapubic mass, BPH, or bladder dysfunction suggests a **postrenal** etiology.
- Medication review
- Urinalysis
- Urine chemistry (FENa, osmolality, urine Na^+, urine Cr)
- Renal ultrasound (to rule out obstruction)

QUICK HIT

Prerenal failure versus ATN

	Prerenal Failure	ATN
Urine osmolarity	>500	>350
Urine Na^+	<20	>40
FENa	<1%	>1%
Urine sediment	Scant	Full brownish pigment, granular casts with epithelial casts

QUICK HIT

Note that prerenal azotemia and ischemic ARF are part of a spectrum of manifestations of renal hypoperfusion. The latter differs in that injury to renal tubular cells occurs.

d. Pathophysiology
- Renal blood flow decreases enough to lower the GFR, which leads to decreased clearance of metabolites (BUN, Cr, uremic toxins).
- Because the renal parenchyma is undamaged, tubular function (and therefore the concentrating ability) is preserved. Therefore the kidney responds appropriately, conserving as much sodium and water as possible.
- This form of ARF is reversible on restoration of blood flow, but if hypoperfusion persists, ischemia results and can lead to acute tubular necrosis (ATN) (see below).

e. Clinical features—signs of volume depletion (dry mucous membranes, hypotension, tachycardia, decreased tissue turgor, oliguria/anuria)

f. Laboratory findings
- **Oliguria—always** found in prerenal failure (this is to preserve volume)
- Increased BUN to serum Cr ratio (**>20:1** is the classic ratio)—because kidney can reabsorb urea
- Increased urine osmolality (>500 mOsm/kg H_2O)—because the kidney is able to reabsorb water
- Decreased urine Na^+ (<20 mEq/L with fractional excretion of sodium [FENa] <1%) because Na^+ is avidly reabsorbed
- Increased urine/plasma Cr ratio (>40:1)—because much of the filtrate is reabsorbed (but not the creatinine)
- Bland urine sediment

2. Intrinsic renal failure
a. Kidney tissue is damaged such that glomerular filtration and tubular function are significantly impaired. The kidneys are unable to concentrate urine effectively.
b. Causes
- Tubular disease (ATN)—can be caused by ischemia (most common cause), nephrotoxins (see Box 7-2)
- Glomerular disease (acute glomerulonephritis [GN])—e.g., Goodpasture's syndrome, Wegener's granulomatosis, poststreptococcal GN, lupus

Box 7-2   Causes of Acute Tubular Necrosis (ATN)

- **Ischemic ARF**
  - Secondary to **severe decline in renal blood flow,** as in shock, hemorrhage, sepsis, disseminated intravascular coagulation, heart failure
  - Ischemia results in the death of tubular cells.
- **Nephrotoxic ARF**
  - Injury secondary to substances that directly injure renal parenchyma and result in cell death
  - Causes include antibiotics (aminoglycosides), radiocontrast agents, NSAIDs (especially in the setting of CHF), poisons, myoglobinuria (from muscle damage, rhabdomyolysis, strenuous exercise), hemoglobinuria (from hemolysis), chemotherapeutic drugs (cisplatin), and kappa and gamma light chains produced in multiple myeloma.

Box 7-3 Course of ATN

- Onset (insult)
- **Oliguric phase**
  - Azotemia and uremia—average length 10 to 14 days
  - Urine output <400 to 500 mL/day
- **Diuretic phase**
  - Begins when urine output is >500 mL/day
  - High urine output due to the following: fluid overload (excretion of retained salt, water, other solutes that were retained during oliguric phase); osmotic diuresis due to retained solutes during oliguric phase; tubular cell damage (delayed recovery of epithelial cell function relative to GFR)
- **Recovery phase**—recovery of tubular function

- Vascular disease—e.g., renal artery occlusion, TTP, HUS
- Interstitial disease—e.g., allergic interstitial nephritis, often due to a hypersensitivity reaction to medication (see Tubulointerstitial Diseases section)

c. Clinical features depend on the cause. Edema is usually present. Recovery may be possible but takes longer than in prerenal failure.

d. Laboratory findings
  - Decreased BUN-to-serum Cr ratio (<20:1) in comparison with prerenal failure. Both BUN and Cr levels are still elevated, but less urea is reabsorbed than in prerenal failure.
  - Increased urine Na^+ (>40 mEq/L with FENa >2% to 3%)—because Na^+ is poorly reabsorbed
  - Decreased urine osmolality (<350 mOsm/kg H_2O)—because renal water reabsorption is impaired
  - Decreased urine–plasma Cr ratio (<20:1)—because filtrate cannot be reabsorbed

3. Postrenal failure
  a. Least common cause of ARF
  b. Obstruction of urinary tract (with intact kidney) causes increased tubular pressure (urine produced cannot be excreted), which leads to decreased GFR. Blood supply and renal parenchyma are intact.
  c. Renal function is restored if obstruction is relieved before the kidneys are damaged.
  d. Postrenal obstruction, if untreated, can lead to ATN.
  e. Causes
    - Urethral obstruction secondary to enlarged prostate (BPH) is the most common cause.
    - Obstruction of solitary kidney
    - Nephrolithiasis
    - Obstructing neoplasm (bladder, cervix, prostate, and so on)
    - Retroperitoneal fibrosis
    - Ureteral obstruction is an uncommon cause because obstruction must be bilateral to cause renal failure.

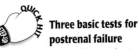

Three basic tests for postrenal failure
- Physical examination–palpate the bladder
- Ultrasound–look for obstruction, hydronephrosis
- Catheter–look for urine

Diagnosis of ARF is usually made by finding elevated BUN and Cr levels. The patient is usually asymptomatic.

TABLE 7-1 Studies to Differentiate Prerenal From Intrinsic ARF

	Prerenal	Intrinsic Renal
Urinalysis	Hyaline casts	Abnormal
BUN/Cr ratio	>20:1	<20:1
FENa	<1%	>2%–3%
Urine osmolality	>500 mOsm	250–300 mOsm
Urine sodium	<20	>40

FIGURE
7-1   Causes of ARF.

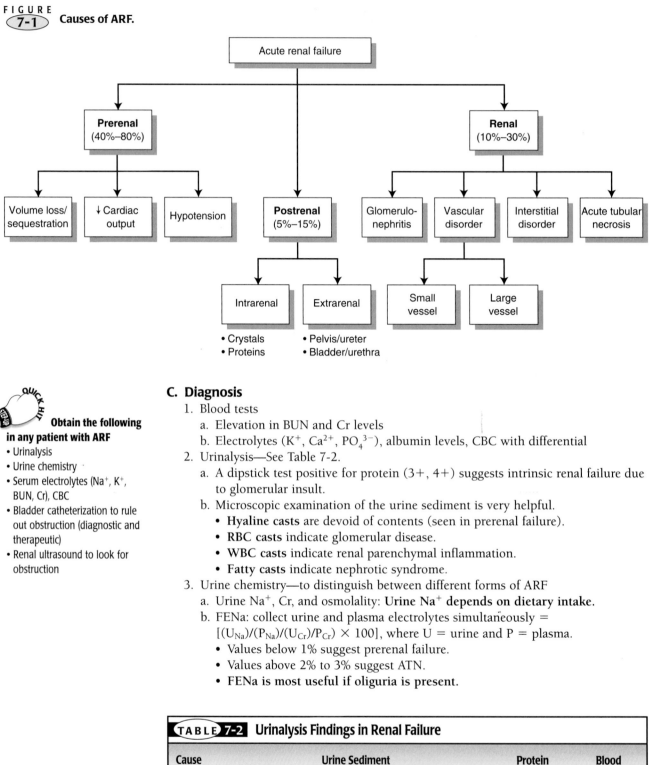

C. Diagnosis

1. Blood tests
   a. Elevation in BUN and Cr levels
   b. Electrolytes (K^+, Ca^{2+}, PO_4^{3-}), albumin levels, CBC with differential
2. Urinalysis—See Table 7-2.
   a. A dipstick test positive for protein (3+, 4+) suggests intrinsic renal failure due to glomerular insult.
   b. Microscopic examination of the urine sediment is very helpful.
      • **Hyaline casts** are devoid of contents (seen in prerenal failure).
      • **RBC casts** indicate glomerular disease.
      • **WBC casts** indicate renal parenchymal inflammation.
      • **Fatty casts** indicate nephrotic syndrome.
3. Urine chemistry—to distinguish between different forms of ARF
   a. Urine Na^+, Cr, and osmolality: **Urine Na^+ depends on dietary intake.**
   b. FENa: collect urine and plasma electrolytes simultaneously = $[(U_{Na})/(P_{Na})/(U_{Cr})/P_{Cr}) \times 100]$, where U = urine and P = plasma.
      • Values below 1% suggest prerenal failure.
      • Values above 2% to 3% suggest ATN.
      • **FENa is most useful if oliguria is present.**

Obtain the following in any patient with ARF
- Urinalysis
- Urine chemistry
- Serum electrolytes (Na^+, K^+, BUN, Cr), CBC
- Bladder catheterization to rule out obstruction (diagnostic and therapeutic)
- Renal ultrasound to look for obstruction

TABLE 7-2 Urinalysis Findings in Renal Failure

Cause	Urine Sediment	Protein	Blood
Prerenal	Benign sediment—few hyaline casts	Negative	Negative
Intrarenal			
Acute tubular necrosis	"Muddy brown" casts, renal tubular cells/casts, granular casts	Trace	Negative
Acute glomerulonephritis	Dysmorphic RBCs, RBCs with casts, WBCs with casts, fatty casts	4+	3+
Acute interstitial nephritis	RBCs, WBCs, WBCs with casts, eosinophils	1+	2+
Postrenal	Benign; may or may not see RBCs, WBCs	Negative	Negative

c. Renal failure index = $(u_{Na}/[u_{Cr}/p_{Cr}]) \times 100)$
- Values below 1% suggest prerenal failure.
- Values above 1% suggest ATN.

4. Urine culture and sensitivities—if infection is suspected
5. Renal ultrasound
   a. Useful for evaluating kidney size and **for excluding urinary tract obstruction (i.e., postrenal failure)**—presence of bilateral hydronephrosis or hydroureter
   b. **Order for most patients with ARF**—unless the cause of the ARF is obvious and is not postrenal
6. CT scan (abdomen and pelvis)—may be helpful in some cases; usually done if renal ultrasound shows an abnormality such as hydronephrosis
7. Renal biopsy—useful occasionally if there is suspicion of acute GN or acute allergic interstitial nephritis
8. Renal arteriography—to evaluate for possible renal artery occlusion; should be performed only if specific therapy will make a difference

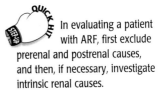

In evaluating a patient with ARF, first exclude prerenal and postrenal causes, and then, if necessary, investigate intrinsic renal causes.

D. Complications

1. ECF volume expansion and resulting pulmonary edema—Treat with a diuretic (furosemide). If there is no response within 2 hours, consider dialysis.
2. Metabolic
   a. **Hyperkalemia**—due to decreased excretion of K^+ and the movement of potassium from ICF to ECF due to tissue destruction and acidosis
   b. **Metabolic acidosis** (with increased anion gap)—due to decreased excretion of hydrogen ions; if severe (below 16 mEq/L), correct with sodium bicarbonate
   c. Hypocalcemia—loss of ability to form active vitamin D and rapid development of PTH resistance
   d. Hyponatremia may occur if water intake is greater than body losses, or if a volume-depleted patient consumes excessive hypotonic solutions. (Hypernatremia may also be seen in hypovolemic states.)
   e. Hyperphosphatemia
   f. Hyperuricemia
3. Uremia—Toxic end products of metabolism accumulate (especially from protein metabolism).
4. Infection
   a. A common and serious complication of ARF (occurs in 50% to 60% of cases). The cause is probably multifactorial, but uremia itself is thought to impair immune functions.
   b. Examples include pneumonia, UTI, wound infection, and sepsis.

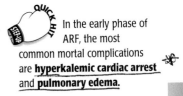

In the early phase of ARF, the most common mortal complications are **hyperkalemic cardiac arrest** and **pulmonary edema.**

E. Treatment

1. General measures
   a. Avoid medications that decrease renal blood flow (NSAIDs) and/or that are nephrotoxic (e.g., aminoglycosides, radiocontrast agents).
   b. Adjust medication dosages for level of renal function.
   c. Correct fluid imbalance.
      - If the patient is volume depleted, give IV fluids. However, many patients with ARF are volume overloaded (especially if they are oliguric or anuric), so diuresis may be necessary.
      - The goal is to strike a balance between correcting volume deficits and avoiding volume overload (while maintaining adequate urine output).
      - Monitor fluid balance by daily weight measurements (most accurate estimate) and intake–output records.
   d. Correct electrolyte disturbances if present.
   e. Optimize cardiac output. BP should be approximately 120 to 140/80 to 90.
   f. Order dialysis if symptomatic uremia, intractable acidemia, hyperkalemia, or volume overload develop.
2. Prerenal
   a. Treat the underlying disorder.

F I G U R E
7-2   Evaluation of ARF.

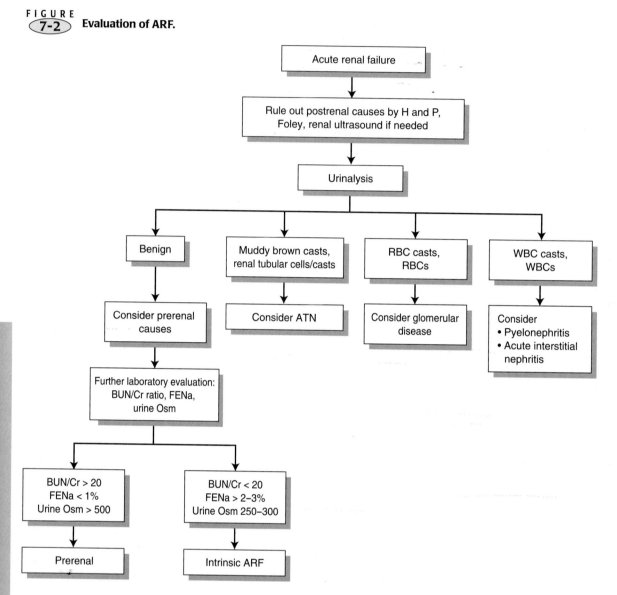

TABLE 7-3	Prognostic Factors in ARF	
Severity of renal failure	Magnitude of increase in Cr Presence of oliguria Fractional excretion of sodium Requirement for dialysis Duration of severe renal failure Marked abnormalities on urinalysis
Underlying health of patient	Age Presence, severity, and reversibility of underlying disease
Clinical circumstances	Cause of renal failure Severity and reversibility of acute process(es) Number and type of other failed organ systems Development of sepsis and other complications

Adapted from Schrier RW, ed. Diseases of the Kidney and Urinary Tract. Vol II. 7th Ed. Philadelphia: Lippincott Williams & Wilkins, 2001:1128, Table 41–14.

b. Give NS to maintain euvolemia and restore blood pressure—do not give to patients with edema or ascites. Stopping antihypertensive medications may be necessary.

c. Eliminate any offending agents (ACE inhibitors, NSAIDs).

d. If the patient is unstable, Swan-Ganz monitoring is indicated for accurate assessment of intravascular volume.

3. Intrinsic

a. Once ATN develops, therapy is supportive. Eliminate the cause/offending agent.

b. If the patient is oliguric, a trial of furosemide may help to increase urine flow. This improves fluid balance.

4. Postrenal—A bladder catheter may be inserted to decompress the urinary tract. Consider urology consultation.

Chronic Renal Failure (CRF)

A. General characteristics

1. **Irreversible**, progressive reduction in GFR and other renal functions that occurs over a period of months to years

2. Causes

   a. **Diabetes is the most common cause** (30% of cases).

   b. **HTN is responsible for 25% of cases.**

   c. Chronic GN accounts for 15% of cases.

   d. Interstitial nephritis, polycystic kidney disease, obstructive uropathy

   e. Any of the causes of ARF may lead to CRF if prolonged and/or if treatment is delayed.

3. Severity

   a. Mild CRF—GFR between 70 and 120 mL/min

   b. Moderate CRF—GFR between 30 and 70 mL/min

   c. Severe CRF—GFR <30 mL/min

   d. ESRD—GFR <10 mL/min

4. Pathophysiology

   a. Plasma Cr varies inversely with GFR.

   b. Cr clearance is the most common clinical measure of GFR.

   c. An increase in plasma Cr indicates disease progression, whereas a decrease suggests recovery of renal function (assuming muscle mass has not changed).

5. More common in African-American than in Caucasian patients.

B. Clinical features—any of the following may be present:

1. Cardiovascular

   a. HTN

   • Secondary to salt and water retention—Decreased GFR stimulates renin–angiotensin system and aldosterone secretion to increase, which leads to an increase in BP.

   • Renal failure is the most common cause of secondary HTN.

   b. CHF—due to volume overload, HTN, and anemia

   c. Pericarditis (uremic)

2. GI (usually due to uremia)

   a. Nausea, vomiting

   b. Loss of appetite (anorexia)

3. Neurologic

   a. Symptoms include lethargy, somnolence, confusion, peripheral neuropathy, and uremic seizures. Physical findings include weakness, asterixis, and hyper-reflexia. Patients may show "restless legs"—neuropathic pain in the legs that is only relieved with movement.

   b. Hypocalcemia can cause lethargy, confusion, and tetany.

4. Hematologic

   a. Normocytic normochromic anemia (secondary to deficiency of erythropoietin)—may be severe

   b. Bleeding secondary to platelet dysfunction (due to uremia); avoid antiplatelet agents

 Whenever a patient has elevated Cr levels, the first thing to do is determine the patient's **baseline** Cr level, if possible. This helps determine whether the patient has ARF, CRF, or chronic renal insufficiency/failure with superimposed ARF. (This condition is known as "acute on chronic" renal failure.)

• **Azotemia** refers to the elevation of BUN.
• **Uremia** refers to the signs and symptoms associated with accumulation of nitrogenous wastes due to impaired renal function. It is difficult to predict when uremic symptoms will appear, but it rarely occurs unless the BUN is >60 mg/dL.

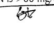 When a patient's renal function is irreversibly compromised but **not** failed, the term **chronic renal insufficiency** is used. It is generally applied to those with a chronic elevation of serum creatinine to 1.5 to 3.0 mg/dL.

TABLE 7-4 Differentiation of ARF Versus CRF	
Favors Chronic	**Favors Acute**
History of kidney disease, HTN, abnormal urinalysis, edema	—
Small kidney size on renal ultrasound	—
—	Return of renal function to normal with time
Hyperkalemia, acidemia, hyperphosphatemia, anemia	Hyperkalemia, acidemia, hyperphosphatemia, anemia
—	Urine output <500 mL/day without uremic symptoms
Urinalysis with broad casts (i.e., more than two to three WBCs in diameter)	—

Adapted from Schrier RW, ed. Diseases of the Kidney and Urinary Tract. Vol II. 7th Ed. Philadelphia: Lippincott Williams & Wilkins, 2001:1098, Figure 41–5.

5. Endocrine/metabolic
   a. Calcium-phosphorus disturbances
      • Decreased renal clearance of phosphate leads to **hyperphosphatemia**, which results in decreased renal production of 1,25-dihydroxy vitamin D. This leads to **hypocalcemia**, which causes secondary hyperparathyroidism.
      • So, **hypo**calcemia and **hyper**phosphatemia are usually seen, but long-standing secondary hyperparathyroidism and calcium-based phosphate binders may sometimes cause **hypercalcemia**.
      • Secondary hyperparathyroidism causes **renal osteodystrophy**, which causes bone pain and fractures.
      • Hyperphosphatemia may cause calcium and phosphate to precipitate, which causes vascular calcifications that may result in necrotic skin lesions. This is called **calciphylaxis**.
   b. Sexual/reproductive symptoms due to hypothalamic-pituitary disturbances and gonadal response to sex hormones: in men, decreased testosterone; in women, amenorrhea, infertility, and hyperprolactinemia
   c. Pruritus (multifactorial etiology)—common and difficult to treat
6. Fluid and electrolyte problems (see Chapter 8)
   a. Volume overload—watch for pulmonary edema
   b. Hyperkalemia—due to decreased urinary secretion
   c. Hypermagnesemia—occurs secondary to reduced urinary loss
   d. Hyperphosphatemia—see above
   e. Metabolic acidosis—due to loss of renal mass (and thus decreased ammonia production) and the kidney's inability to excrete H^+
7. Immunologic—Uremia inhibits cellular and humoral immunity.

C. Diagnosis
1. Urinalysis—examine sediment (see ARF)
2. Measure Cr clearance to estimate GFR
3. CBC (anemia, thrombocytopenia)
4. Serum electrolytes (e.g., K^+, Ca^{2+}, PO_4^{3-}, serum protein)
5. Renal ultrasound—evaluate size of kidneys/rule out obstruction
   a. Small kidneys are suggestive of chronic renal insufficiency with little chance of recovery.
   b. Presence of normal-sized or large kidneys does not exclude CRF.
   c. Renal biopsy—in select cases to determine specific etiology

D. Treatment

1. Diet
   a. Low protein—to 0.7 to 0.8 g/kg body weight per day
   b. Use a low-salt diet if HTN, CHF, or oliguria are present.
   c. Restrict potassium, phosphate, and magnesium intake.
2. ACE inhibitors—dilate efferent arteriole of glomerulus
   a. If used early on, they reduce the risk of progression to ESRD because they slow the progression of proteinuria.
   b. Use with great caution because they can cause hyperkalemia.
3. BP control
   a. Strict control decreases the rate of disease progression.
   b. ACE inhibitors are the preferred agents. Multiple drugs, including diuretics, may be required.
4. Glycemic control (if the patient is diabetic) prevents worsening of proteinuria.
5. Correction of electrolyte abnormalities
   a. Correct hyperphosphatemia with calcium citrate (a phosphate binder).
   b. Patients with chronic renal disease are generally treated with long-term oral calcium and vitamin D in an effort to prevent secondary hyperparathyroidism and uremic osteodystrophy.
   c. Acidosis—Treat the underlying cause (renal failure). Patients may require oral bicarbonate replacement.
6. Anemia—Treat with erythropoietin.
7. Pulmonary edema—Arrange for dialysis if the condition is unresponsive to diuresis.
8. Pruritus—Try capsaicin cream or cholestyramine and UV light.
9. Dialysis (See indications in the Dialysis section.)
10. Transplantation is the only cure.

QUICK HIT

In a patient with CRF, symptomatic volume overload and severe hyperkalemia are the most common complications that require urgent intervention.

Dialysis

A. General characteristics

1. Overview
   a. Dialysis is the artificial mechanism by which fluid and toxic solutes are removed from the circulation when the kidneys cannot do so sufficiently.
   b. In all forms of dialysis, the blood interfaces with an artificial solution resembling human plasma (called the dialysate), and diffusion of fluid and solutes occurs across a semipermeable membrane.
   c. **The two major methods of dialyzing a patient are hemodialysis and peritoneal dialysis** (discussed below).
   d. The majority of dialysis patients in the United States receive hemodialysis at hospitals or dialysis centers, but more and more patients are opting for CAPD (chronic ambulatory peritoneal dialysis).
2. Settings in which dialysis is considered
   a. CRF—Dialysis serves as a bridge to renal transplantation or as a permanent treatment when the patient is not a transplantation candidate.
   b. ARF—Dialysis is often required as a temporary measure until the patient's renal function improves.
   c. Overdose of medications or ingestions of substances cleared by the kidneys—Some, but not all medications and toxins can be dialyzed (see Quick Hit).

QUICK HIT

Life-threatening complications in CRF
- Hyperkalemia—Obtain an ECG (be aware that potassium levels can be high without ECG changes).
- Pulmonary edema secondary to volume overload—Look for recent weight gain.
- Infection (e.g., pneumonia, UTI, sepsis)

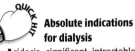

QUICK HIT

Absolute indications for dialysis
- **A**cidosis—significant, intractable metabolic acidosis
- **E**lectrolytes—severe, persistent hyperkalemia
- **I**ntoxications—methanol, ethylene glycol, lithium, aspirin
- **O**verload—hypervolemia not managed by other means
- **U**remia (severe)—based on clinical presentation, not laboratory values (e.g., uremic pericarditis is an absolute indication for dialysis)

B. Specific indications for dialysis

1. Nonemergent indications
   a. Cr and BUN levels are not absolute indications for dialysis.
   b. Symptoms of uremia
      - Nausea and vomiting
      - Lethargy/deterioration in mental status, encephalopathy, seizures
      - Pericarditis
2. Emergent indications (usually in the setting of renal failure)

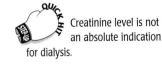

QUICK HIT

Creatinine level is not an absolute indication for dialysis.

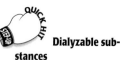

Dialyzable substances
• Salicylic acid
• Lithium
• Ethylene glycol
• Magnesium-containing laxatives

a. Life-threatening manifestations of volume overload
  • Pulmonary edema
  • Hypertensive emergency refractory to antihypertensive agents
b. Severe, refractory electrolyte disturbances, e.g., hyperkalemia, hypermagnesemia
c. Severe metabolic acidosis
d. Drug toxicity/ingestions (particularly in patients with renal failure): methanol, ethylene glycol, lithium, aspirin

C. Hemodialysis

1. Process
   a. The patient's blood is pumped by an artificial pump outside of the body through the dialyzer, which typically consists of fine capillary networks of semipermeable membranes. The dialysate flows on the outside of these networks, and fluid and solutes diffuse across the membrane.
   b. The patient's blood must be heparinized to prevent clotting in the dialyzer.
2. Frequency: Most hemodialysis patients require 3 to 5 hours of dialysis 3 days per week.
3. Access
   a. Use the central catheter placed in the subclavian vein for temporary access.
   b. Arteriovenous fistula
      • This is the best form of permanent dialysis access.
      • It requires vascular surgery to connect the radial artery to veins in the forearm.
      • Allow time for the fistula to mature.
      • An audible bruit over the fistula indicates that it is patent.
   c. An alternative to an arteriovenous fistula is an implantable graft.
4. Alternatives to traditional hemodialysis
   a. Continuous arteriovenous hemodialysis (CAVHD) and continuous venovenous hemodialysis (CVVHD) are often used in hemodynamically unstable patients, such as ICU patients with ARF.
   b. Lower flow rates of blood and dialysate enable dialysis to occur while minimizing rapid shifts in volume and osmolality.
   c. They require highly efficient dialyzers to be effective.
5. Advantages of hemodialysis
   a. It is considered more efficient than peritoneal dialysis. High flow rates and efficient dialyzers shorten the period of time required for dialysis.
   b. It can be initiated more quickly than peritoneal dialysis, using temporary vascular access in the emergent setting.
6. Disadvantages of hemodialysis
   a. It is less similar to the physiology of natural kidney function than is peritoneal dialysis, predisposing the patient to the following:
      • Hypotension due to rapid removal of extravascular volume
      • Hypo-osmolality due to solute removal
   b. Requires vascular access

D. Peritoneal dialysis

1. Process
   a. The peritoneum serves as the dialysis membrane. Dialysate fluid is infused into the peritoneal cavity, then fluids and solutes from the peritoneal capillaries diffuse into the dialysate fluid, which is drained from the abdomen.
   b. A **hyperosmolar** (high-glucose) solution is used, and water is removed from the blood via osmosis.
2. Frequency: Dialysate fluid is drained and replaced every hour in acute peritoneal dialysis, but only once every 4 to 8 hours in CAPD.
3. Access
   a. With CAPD, dialysate is infused into the peritoneal fluid via an implanted catheter.
   b. A temporary catheter is used for acute peritoneal dialysis.

4. Advantages
   a. The patient can learn to perform dialysis on his or her own.
   b. It mimics the physiology of normal kidney function more closely than hemodialysis in that it is more continuous.
5. Disadvantages
   a. High glucose load may lead to hyperglycemia and hypertriglyceridemia.
   b. Peritonitis is a significant potential complication.
   c. The patients must be highly motivated to self-administer it.
   d. Cosmetic—There is increased abdominal girth due to dialysate fluid.

E. Limitations and complications of dialysis
1. Limitations—Dialysis does not replicate the kidney's synthetic functions. Therefore, dialysis patients are still prone to erythropoietin and vitamin D deficiency, with their associated complications.
2. Complications associated with hemodialysis
   a. Hypotension—may result in myocardial ischemia, fatigue, and so on
   b. The relative hypo-osmolality of the ECF compared with the brain may result in nausea, vomiting, headache, and rarely, seizures or coma.
   c. "First-use syndrome"—Chest pain, back pain, and rarely, anaphylaxis may occur immediately after a patient uses a new dialysis machine.
   d. Complications associated with anticoagulation—hemorrhage, hematoma, etc.
   e. Infection of vascular access site—may lead to sepsis
   f. Hemodialysis-associated amyloidosis of β_2 microglobulin in bones and joints
3. Complications associated with peritoneal dialysis
   a. Peritonitis, often accompanied by fever and abdominal pain—usually can be treated with intraperitoneal antibiotics; cloudy peritoneal fluid is key sign
   b. Abdominal/inguinal hernia—increased risk due to elevated intra-abdominal pressures
   c. Hyperglycemia—especially with diabetic patients
   d. Protein malnutrition

PROTEINURIA AND HEMATURIA

Proteinuria

A. General characteristics
1. Defined as the urinary excretion of >150 mg protein/24 hr
2. Classification
   a. Glomerular
      • Due to increased glomerular permeability to proteins
      • Can lead to nephrotic syndrome
      • May be seen in all types of GN
      • Protein loss tends to be more severe than in nonglomerular causes.
   b. Tubular
      • Small proteins normally filtered at the glomerulus then reabsorbed by the tubules appear in the urine because of abnormal tubules (i.e., due to decreased tubular reabsorption).
      • Proteinuria tends to be less severe.
      • Causes include sickle cell disease, urinary tract obstruction, and interstitial nephritis.
   c. Overflow proteinuria—Increased production of small proteins overwhelms the tubules' ability to reabsorb them (e.g., Bence Jones protein in multiple myeloma).
   d. Other causes of proteinuria (all of the following can affect renal blood flow):
      • UTI
      • Fever, heavy exertion/stress, CHF
      • Pregnancy
      • Orthostatic proteinuria—occurs when patient is standing but not when recumbent; self-limited and benign

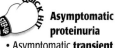

Asymptomatic proteinuria
• Asymptomatic **transient** proteinuria has an excellent prognosis (no further evaluation necessary).
• Asymptomatic **persistent** proteinuria and symptomatic proteinuria require further workup (high chance of renal disease in these patients).

> **Box 7-4** **Urinalysis**
>
> Collection—a clean-catch, midstream urine sample (after cleaning urethral meatus) is usually adequate for urinalysis and urine culture in adults.
>
> Urinalysis consists of the following three steps.
> - Visual inspection of urine—examine color, clarity
> - Dipstick reactions
>   - pH—This depends on acid-base status. The average is about 6, but can range from 4.5 to 8.0.
>   - Specific gravity—This is directly proportional to urine osmolality (and therefore solute concentration in urine). Normal is 1.002 to 1.035. It increases with volume depletion and decreases with volume overload. Appropriate changes in specific gravity with volume status of the patient indicate adequate tubular function (i.e., renal concentrating ability).
>   - Protein—Proteinuria is defined as >150 mg/day; nephrotic syndrome, >3.5 g/day. The following are rough guidelines: Trace = 50 to 150 mg/day; 1+ = 150 to 500 mg/day; 2+ = 0.5 to 1.5 g/day; 3+ = 2 to 5 g/day; 4+ = >5 g/day.
>   - Glucose—Excessive glucose indicates diabetes. Absence of glucosuria does **not** rule out diabetes, however.
>   - Blood—hematuria—see text
>   - Ketones—DKA, starvation
>   - Nitrite—suggests presence of bacteria in urine
>   - Leukocyte esterase—suggests presence of WBC in urine; if negative, infection is unlikely
> - Microscopic examination of urine sediment
>   - Look for casts, cells, bacteria, WBCs, RBCs (number, shape), crystals

Nephrotic syndrome (handwritten annotation)

QUICK HIT

Three key features of nephrotic syndrome
- Proteinuria
- Hypoalbuminemia
- Hyperlipidemia

3. Nephrotic syndrome
   a. Key features
      - **Urine protein** excretion rate >3.5 g/24 hr
      - **Hypoalbuminemia**—Hepatic albumin synthesis cannot keep up with these urinary protein losses. The result is decreased plasma oncotic pressure, which leads to edema.
      - **Edema**—This is often the initial complaint (from pedal edema to periorbital to anasarca, ascites, pleural effusion). It results from hypoalbuminemia. Increased aldosterone secretion exacerbates the problem (increases sodium reabsorption).
      - **Hyperlipidemia** and lipiduria—increased hepatic synthesis of LDL and VLDL because liver is revving up albumin synthesis.
      - Hypercoagulable state (due to loss of certain anticoagulants in the urine)—increased risk of thromboembolic events (deep venous thrombosis, pulmonary embolism, renal vein thrombosis)
      - Increased incidence of infection—results from loss of immunoglobulins in the urine
   b. Nephrotic syndrome usually indicates significant glomerular disease (either primary or secondary to systemic illness); the underlying cause is abnormal glomerular permeability.
   c. Causes
      - Primary glomerular disease (50% to 75% of cases of nephrotic syndrome)—Membranous nephropathy is most common in adults (50% of cases), followed by FSGS (25%) and membranoproliferative GN (15%). Minimal change disease is the most common cause in children (75% of cases).

        ① Membranous ② FSGS ③ MPGN (handwritten annotation)

      - Systemic disease—diabetes, collagen vascular disease, SLE, RA, Henoch-Schönlein purpura, polyarteritis nodosa (PAN), Wegener's granulomatosis
      - Amyloidosis, cryoglobulinemia
      - Drugs/toxins—captopril, heroin, heavy metals, NSAIDs, penicillamine
      - Infection—bacterial, viral, protozoal
      - Multiple myeloma, malignant HTN, transplant rejection

B. Diagnosis
   1. Urine dipstick test (read color changes)
      a. Specific for albumin—detects concentrations of 30 mg/dL or higher

b. Graded 0, trace, 1+ (15 to 30 mg/dL) through 4+ (>500 mg/dL)
c. More sensitive to albumin than to immunoglobulins, thus can lead to false-negative results when predominant urinary protein is globulin (e.g., light chains in myeloma)

2. Urinalysis
  a. Initial test once proteinuria is detected by dipstick test.
  b. Examination of urine sediment is important
    • RBC casts suggest GN.
    • WBC casts suggest pyelonephritis and interstitial nephritis.
    • Fatty casts suggest nephrotic syndrome (lipiduria).
  c. If urinalysis confirms the presence of protein, a 24-hour urine collection (for albumin and Cr) is appropriate to establish the presence of significant proteinuria.

3. Test for microalbuminuria
  a. Corresponds to albumin excretion of 30 to 300 mg/day. *microalbuminuria*
  b. This is below the range of sensitivity of standard dipsticks. Special dipsticks can detect microgram amounts of albumin. If the test result is positive, perform a radioimmunoassay (the most sensitive and specific test for microalbuminuria).
  c. **Microalbuminuria can be an early sign of diabetic nephropathy.**

4. Other tests to determine etiology (may or may not be necessary depending on case)
  a. Cr clearance—best test of renal function
  b. Serum BUN and Cr
  c. CBC—to detect anemia due to renal failure
  d. Serum albumin level—varies inversely with degree of proteinuria
  e. Renal ultrasound—to detect obstruction, masses, cystic disease
  f. Intravenous pyelogram (IVP)—to detect chronic pyelonephritis
  g. ANA levels (lupus), anti–glomerular basement membrane, hepatitis serology, antistreptococcal antibody titers, complement levels, cryoglobulin studies
  h. Serum and urine electrophoresis (myeloma)
  i. Renal biopsy—if no cause is identified by less invasive means

C. Treatment

1. Asymptomatic proteinuria
  a. If it is transient, no further workup or treatment is necessary.
  b. If it is persistent, further testing is indicated. Start by checking BP and examining urine sediment. Treat the underlying condition and associated problems (e.g., hyperlipidemia).

2. Symptomatic proteinuria—Further testing is always required.
  a. Treat the underlying disease (diabetes, multiple myeloma, SLE, minimal change disease).
  b. ACE inhibitors—These decrease urinary albumin loss. They are an essential part of treatment for diabetics with HTN and should be started before fixed albuminuria is present.
  c. Diuretics—if edema is present
  d. Limit dietary protein.
  e. Treat hypercholesterolemia (using diet or a lipid-lowering agent).
  f. Vaccinate against influenza and pneumococcus—there is an increased risk of infection in these patients.

Hematuria

A. General characteristics

1. Hematuria is defined as >3 erythrocytes/HPF on urinalysis.
2. Microscopic hematuria is more commonly glomerular in origin; gross hematuria is more commonly nonglomerular or urologic in origin.
3. **Consider gross painless hematuria to be a sign of bladder or kidney cancer until proven otherwise.**
4. This may lead to obstruction if large clots form in the lower GI tract. Excessive blood loss can lead to iron deficiency anemia.

QUICK HIT

Gross hematuria is a common presenting sign in patients with bladder cancer (up to 85% of cases) and patients with renal cell carcinoma (up to 40% of cases).

QUICK HIT

Infection (cystitis, urethritis, prostatitis) accounts for 25% and stones for 20% of all cases of atraumatic hematuria.

QUICK HIT

Menstrual blood can contaminate a urine sample and lead to a false-positive dipstick reading for hematuria.

QUICK HIT

If hematuria is microscopic, think of glomerular disease. If gross, think of postrenal causes (trauma, stones, malignancy). Infection can cause either gross or microscopic hematuria.

QUICK HIT

If the patient has no other symptoms associated with the hematuria, and thorough workup fails to reveal a cause, the prognosis is excellent. (There is usually mild glomerular/interstitial disease.)

QUICK HIT

Rapid progressive glomerulonephritis is a clinical syndrome that includes any type of GN in which rapid deterioration of renal function occurs over weeks to months, leading to renal failure and ESRD.

B. Causes

1. Kidney stones
2. Infection (UTI, urethritis, pyelonephritis)
3. Bladder or kidney cancer
4. Glomerular disease, immunoglobulin (Ig) A nephropathy
5. Trauma (Foley catheter placement, blunt trauma, invasive procedures)
6. Strenuous exercise (marathon running), fever—Hematuria is generally harmless.
7. Systemic diseases (SLE, rheumatic fever, Henoch-Schönlein purpura, Wegener's granulomatosis, HUS, Goodpasture's syndrome, PAN)
8. Bleeding disorders (e.g., hemophilia, thrombocytopenia)
9. Sickle cell disease
10. Medications (cyclophosphamide, anticoagulants, salicylates, sulfonamides)
11. Analgesic nephropathy
12. Polycystic kidney disease, simple cysts
13. BPH—rarely causes isolated hematuria

C. Diagnosis

1. Urine dipstick—sensitivity in identifying hematuria is >90%
2. Urinalysis—crucial in evaluation of hematuria
   a. Examine urine sediment—This is very important in identifying possible renal disease.
   b. If RBC casts and proteinuria are also present, a glomerular cause is almost always present (usually GN).
   c. If pyuria is present, send for urine culture.
   d. If dipstick is positive for blood, but urinalysis does not reveal microscopic hematuria (no RBCs), hemoglobinuria or myoglobinuria is likely present.
3. Urine specimen—for cytology
   a. To detect cancers (bladder cancer is the main concern)
   b. **If suspicion for malignancy is high, perform a cystoscopy to evaluate the bladder regardless of cytology results.**
4. 24-hour urine—Test for Cr and protein to assess renal function. Collect if proteinuria is present. (If it is heavy, glomerular disease is likely.)
5. Blood tests—coagulation studies, CBC, BUN/Cr
6. IVP, CT scan, ultrasound—if no cause is identified by the above tests; look for stones, tumors, cysts, ureteral strictures, or vascular malformations
7. Renal biopsy—if there is suspicion of glomerular disease

D. Treatment: Treat the underlying cause; maintain urine volume.

GLOMERULAR DISEASE (GLOMERULONEPHROPATHIES)

Overview

A. General characteristics

1. Glomerular disease can be primary (intrinsic renal pathology) or secondary (to a systemic disease). Two important categories of glomerular pathology are diseases that present with nephrotic syndrome and those that present with nephritic syndrome. Many conditions have features of both. See Table 7-5.
2. There is a wide range in the rate of disease progression, varying from days to weeks in the acute glomerular diseases, to years in the chronic disorders.

B. Causes

1. GN is usually caused by immune-mediated mechanisms.
2. Other mechanisms include metabolic and hemodynamic disturbances.

C. Clinical features

1. Glomerular disorders are characterized by impairment in selective filtration of blood, resulting in excretion of larger substances such as plasma proteins and blood cells. As disease advances, GFR decreases proportionately, leading to renal failure and the possible need for dialysis and/or transplantation.

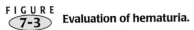

FIGURE 7-3 Evaluation of hematuria.

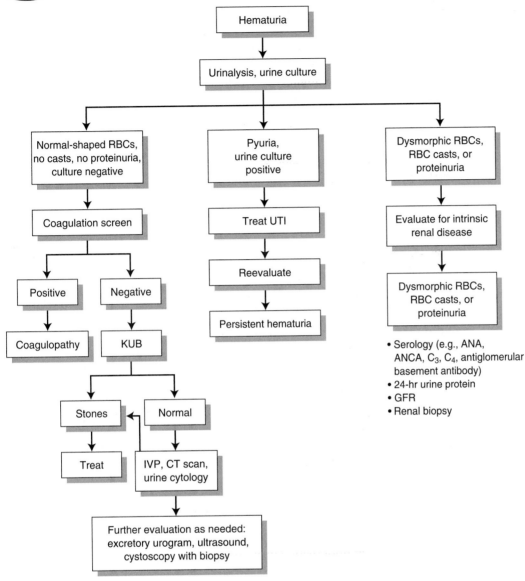

2. The classic features of glomerular disease are proteinuria, hematuria, or both. Nephrotic range proteinuria is pathognomonic for glomerular disease.

D. Diagnosis
1. Urinalysis (hematuria, proteinuria, RBC casts)
2. Blood tests (renal function tests)
3. Needle biopsy of the kidney

E. Treatment depends on the disease, but often involves use of steroids and cytotoxic agents.

Primary Glomerular Disorders

A. Minimal change disease
1. Nephrotic syndrome—most common presentation
2. Most common in children—Hodgkin's disease and non-Hodgkin's lymphoma have been associated with minimal change disease.
3. No histologic abnormalities on light microscopy; fusion of foot processes on electron microscopy

 Possible presentations of glomerular disease
- Isolated proteinuria
- Isolated hematuria
- Nephritic syndrome—hematuria, HTN, azotemia
- Nephrotic syndrome—proteinuria, edema, hypoalbuminemia, hyperlipidemia

	Nephritic Syndrome	Nephrotic Syndrome
TABLE 7-5	**Nephritic Versus Nephrotic Syndrome**	
Pathogenesis	Inflammation of glomeruli due to any of the causes of glomerulonephritis	Abnormal glomerular permeability due to a number of conditions
Causes	Poststreptococcal glomerulonephritis is the most common cause, but may be due to any of the causes of glomerulonephritis	Many conditions. Membranous glomerulonephritis is the most common cause in adults. Other causes include diabetes, SLE, drugs, infection, glomerulonephritis (focal segmental and others). Minimal change disease is the most common cause in children.
Laboratory findings	Hematuria ARF—azotemia, oliguria Proteinuria, if present, is mild and not in nephrotic range	Urine protein excretion rate <3.5 g/24 hr Hypoalbuminemia Hyperlipidemia, fatty casts in urine
Clinical findings	HTN Edema	Edema Hypercoagulable state Increased risk of infection

4. Excellent prognosis; responsive to steroid therapy (4 to 8 weeks), although relapses may occur

B. Focal segmental glomerulosclerosis (FSGS)

1. This accounts for 25% of cases of nephrotic syndrome in adults. Hematuria and HTN are often present.
2. It has a fair to poor prognosis. It is generally resistant to steroid therapy— patients develop renal insufficiency within 5 to 10 years of diagnosis. The course is progressive.
3. The treatment regimen is controversial, but remission has been achieved in 50% of patients with the use of cytotoxic agents, steroids, and immunosuppressive agents.

C. Membranous glomerulonephritis

1. Usually presents with nephrotic syndrome; glomerular capillary walls are thickened.
2. Primary disease is idiopathic. The secondary form is due to infection (hepatitis C virus, hepatitis B virus, syphilis, malaria), drugs (gold, captopril, penicillamine), neoplasm, or lupus.
3. The prognosis is fair to good. The course is variable; remission is common (in 40% of cases), but renal failure develops in 33% of patients. Steroid therapy does not change the survival rate.

D. IgA nephropathy (Berger's disease)

1. Asymptomatic recurrent hematuria/mild proteinuria is common. **This is the most common cause of glomerular hematuria.** Gross hematuria after an upper respiratory infection (or exercise) is common.
2. Renal function is usually normal.
3. Mesangial deposition of IgA and C3 are seen on electron microscopy.
4. The prognosis in most patients is good with preservation of renal function (renal insufficiency may develop in 25%).
5. Some advocate steroids for unstable disease, but no therapy has been proven to be effective.

E. Hereditary nephritis (Alport's syndrome)

1. X-linked or autosomal-dominant inheritance with variable penetrance

COLOR PLATES

3-1 Kayser-Fleisher ring.

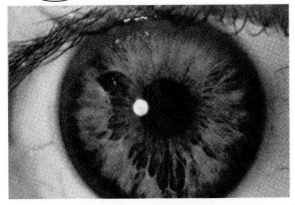

(Used with permission from Humes DH, DuPont HL, Gardner LB, et al. Kelley's Textbook of Internal Medicine, 4th Ed. Philadelphia: Lippincott Williams & Wilkins, 2000, Figure 105.4 in color plate section.)

4-1 Exophthalmos (thyrotoxicosis).

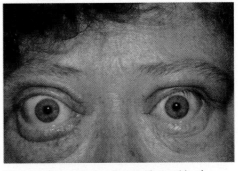

(From Goodheart HP. Goodheart's Photoguide of Common Skin Disorders, 2nd Ed. Philadelphia: Lippincott Williams & Wilkins, 2003, Photo 25.9.)

6-1 SLE butterfly rash.

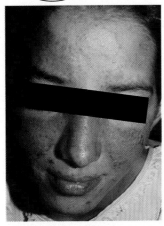

(From Goodheart HP. Goodheart's Photoguide of Common Skin Disorders, 2nd Ed. Philadelphia: Lippincott Williams & Wilkins, 2003, Figure 25.24.)

6-2 Rheumatoid nodules of the hand.

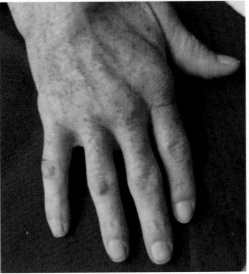

(Image provided by Stedman's.)

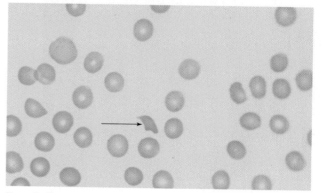
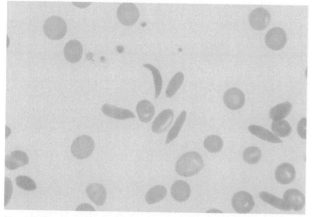
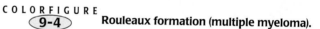
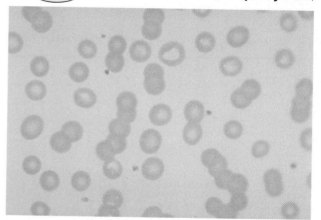

Herpes simplex virus.

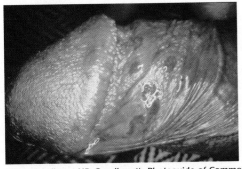

(From Goodheart HP. Goodheart's Photoguide of Common Skin Disorders, 2nd Ed. Philadelphia: Lippincott Williams & Wilkins, Figure 19.13, 2003.)

Chancre of primary syphilis.

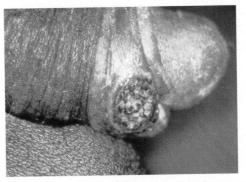

(From Goodheart HP. Goodheart's Photoguide of Common Skin Disorders, 2nd Ed. Philadelphia: Lippincott Williams & Wilkins, Figure 19.15, 2003.)

Chancroid.

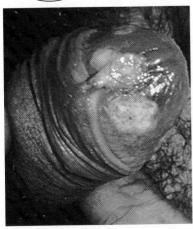

(From Goodheart HP. Goodheart's Photoguide of Common Skin Disorders, 2nd Ed. Philadelphia: Lippincott Williams & Wilkins, Figure 19.14, 2003.)

Erythema migrans (Lyme disease).

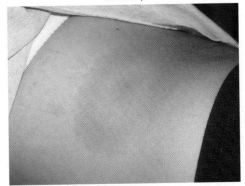

(From Goodheart HP. Goodheart's Photoguide of Common Skin Disorders, 2nd Ed. Philadelphia: Lippincott Williams & Wilkins, Figure 7.19, 2003.)

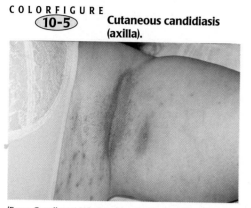

(From Goodheart HP. Goodheart's Photoguide of Common Skin Disorders, 2nd Ed. Philadelphia: Lippincott Williams & Wilkins, Figure 3.25, 2003.)

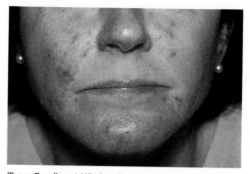

(From Goodheart HP. Goodheart's Photoguide of Common Skin Disorders, 2nd Ed. Philadelphia: Lippincott Williams & Wilkins, Figure 1.14, 2003.)

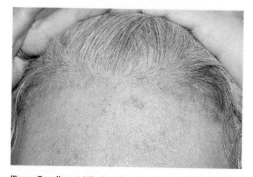

(From Goodheart HP. Goodheart's Photoguide of Common Skin Disorders, 2nd Ed. Philadelphia: Lippincott Williams & Wilkins, Figure 2.58, 2003.)

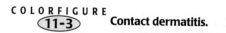
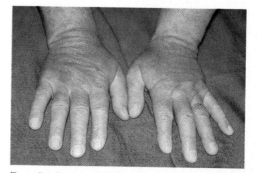

(From Goodheart HP. Goodheart's Photoguide of Common Skin Disorders, 2nd Ed. Philadelphia: Lippincott Williams & Wilkins, Figure 2.41, 2003.)

Pityriasis rosea.

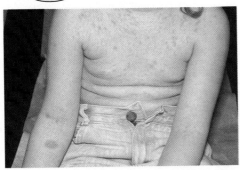

(From Goodheart HP. Goodheart's Photoguide of Common Skin Disorders, 2nd Ed. Philadelphia: Lippincott Williams & Wilkins, Figure 4.3, 2003.)

spontaneous resolution

Erythema nodosum.

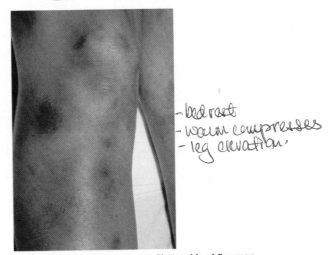

*- bad rash
- warm compresses
- leg elevation.*

(From Goodheart HP. Goodheart's Photoguide of Common Skin Disorders, 2nd Ed. Philadelphia: Lippincott Williams & Wilkins, Figure 25.17, 2003.)

**Erythema multiforme.
(A) Bulla. (B) Target (or iris) lesion.**

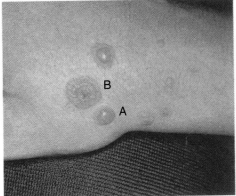

(From Bickley LS, Szilagyi P. Bates' Guide to Physical Examination and History Taking, 8th Ed. Philadelphia: Lippincott Williams & Wilkins, Table 4.8, 2003.)

**Human papilloma virus
(genital wart).**

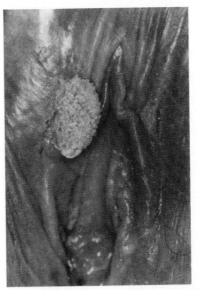

(From Wilkinson EJ, Stone IK. Atlas of Vulvar Disease. Baltimore: Williams & Wilkins, Figure 17.9a, 1994.)

Molluscum contagiosum.

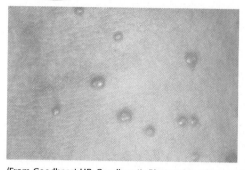

(From Goodheart HP. Goodheart's Photoguide of Common Skin Disorders, 2nd Ed. Philadelphia: Lippincott Williams & Wilkins, Figure 6.13, 2003.)

Herpes zoster.

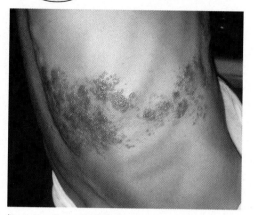

(From Goodheart HP. Goodheart's Photoguide of Common Skin Disorders, 2nd Ed. Philadelphia: Lippincott Williams & Wilkins, Figure 6.33, 2003.)

Scabies.

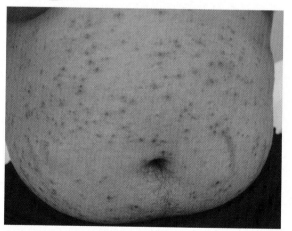

(Image provided by Stedman's.)

Actinic keratosis.

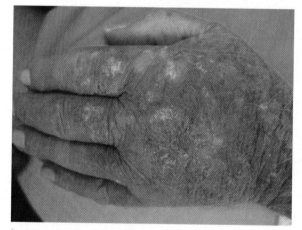

(Image provided by Stedman's.)

11-12 **Basal cell carcinoma.**

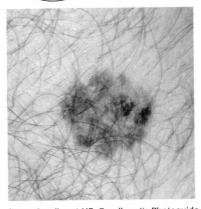

(Image provided by Stedman's.)

11-13 **Squamous cell carcinoma.**

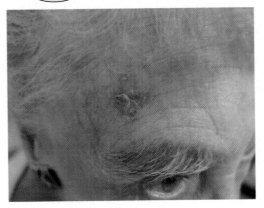

(Image provided by Stedman's.)

11-14 **Malignant melanoma.**

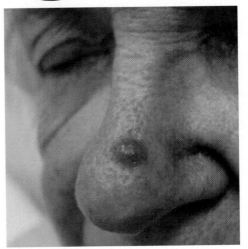

(From Goodheart HP. Goodheart's Photoguide of Common Skin Disorders, 2nd Ed. Philadelphia: Lippincott Williams & Wilkins, Figure 21.20, 2003.)

11-15 **Psoriasis.**

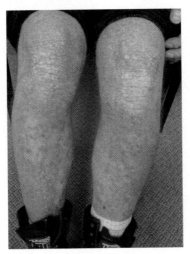

(Image provided by Stedman's.)

11-16 **Seborrheic keratosis.**

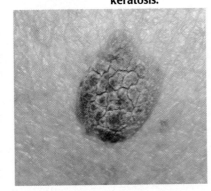

(From Goodheart HP. Goodheart's Photoguide of Common Skin Disorders, 2nd Ed. Philadelphia: Lippincott Williams & Wilkins, Figure 21.13, 2003.)

11-17 Urticaria.

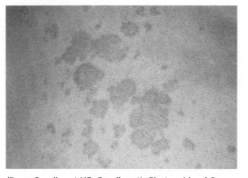

(From Goodheart HP. Goodheart's Photoguide of Common Skin Disorders, 2nd Ed. Philadelphia: Lippincott Williams & Wilkins, Figure G.11, 2003.)

11-18 Angioedema.

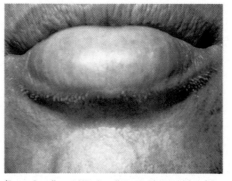

(From Goodheart HP. Goodheart's Photoguide of Common Skin Disorders, 2nd Ed. Philadelphia: Lippincott Williams & Wilkins, Figure 20.1, 2003.)

12-1 Cotton wool spots (hypertension).

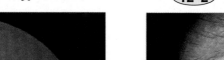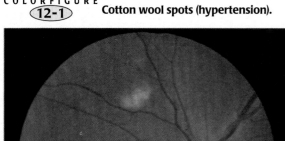

(From Stoller JK, Ahmad M, Longworth DL. The Cleveland Clinic Intensive Review of Internal Medicine, 3rd Ed. Philadelphia: Lippincott Williams & Wilkins, Figure 6.1, 2002.)

12-2 Cataract.

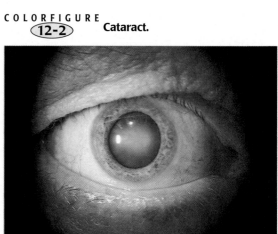

(From Tasman W, Jaeger E. The Wills Eye Hospital Atlas of Clinical Ophthalmology, 2nd Ed. Philadelphia: Lippincott Williams & Wilkins, Figure 12.2, 2001.)

2. Features include hematuria, pyuria, proteinuria, high-frequency hearing loss without deafness, progressive renal failure
3. No effective treatment

Secondary Glomerular Disorders

A. Diabetic nephropathy—most common cause of ESRD (see Chapter 4)

B. Hypertensive nephropathy—(see Renal Vasculature Disease section)

C. Lupus—(see Chapter 6)

D. Membranoproliferative glomerulonephritis
1. Usually due to hepatitis C infection; other causes include hepatitis B, syphilis, and lupus
2. Common association with cryoglobulinemia
3. The prognosis is poor. Renal failure develops in 50% of patients. Treatment is rarely effective.

E. Poststreptococcal GN—most common cause of nephritic syndrome
1. This occurs after infection with group A β-hemolytic streptococcal infection of the upper respiratory tract (or skin—impetigo). The GN develops about 10 to 14 days after infection.
2. It primarily affects children (ages 2 to 6 years).
3. Features include **hematuria**, edema, HTN, low complement levels, and proteinuria.
4. Antistreptolysin-O may be elevated.
5. It is self-limited (usually resolves in weeks to months) with an excellent prognosis. Some cases develop into rapidly progressive GN (more commonly in adults).
6. Therapy is primarily supportive: antihypertensives, loop diuretics for edema; the use of antibiotics is controversial.

F. Goodpasture's syndrome
1. Classic triad of proliferative GN (usually crescentic), pulmonary hemorrhage, and IgG anti–glomerular basement membrane antibody
2. Clinical features include fever, myalgia, rapidly progressive renal failure, hemoptysis, cough, and dyspnea.
3. Lung disease precedes kidney disease by days to weeks. It is associated with a variable course.

G. Dysproteinemias—amyloidosis, light chain/heavy chain diseases

H. Sickle cell nephropathy—(see Renal Vascular Disease section)

I. HIV nephropathy
1. Characteristics include proteinuria, edema, and hematuria.
2. Histopathology resembles FSGS.
3. Improvement is seen with prednisone, ACE inhibitors, and antiretroviral therapy.

J. Glomerulonephritis in endocarditis
1. This results from an immune-complex mechanism. However, a nonimmune mechanism (septic emboli, ischemia, antibiotic related) should be considered as well.
2. Therapy involves treating the underlying infection.

K. Wegener's granulomatosis—(see Chapter 6)

L. Polyarteritis nodosa—(see Chapter 6)

TUBULOINTERSTITIAL DISEASES

Acute Interstitial Nephritis (AIN)

A. General characteristics
1. Inflammation involving interstitium (tissue that surrounds glomeruli and tubules)
2. Accounts for 10% to 15% of cases of ARF
3. Causes
   a. **Acute allergic reaction to a medication is the most common cause**—e.g., penicillins, NSAIDs, diuretics (furosemide, thiazide), anticoagulants, phenytoin, sulfonamides
   b. Infection (especially in children)—due to a variety of agents, including streptococcus spp. and *Legionella pneumophila*
   c. Collagen vascular diseases—e.g., sarcoidosis

B. Clinical features
1. AIN causes ARF and its associated symptoms.
2. Rash, fever, and eosinophilia are classic findings.
3. Pyuria and hematuria may be present.

C. Diagnosis
1. Renal function tests (increased BUN and Cr levels)
2. Urinalysis
   a. **Eosinophils in the urine suggest the diagnosis, given the proper history and findings.**
   b. Mild proteinuria or microscopic hematuria may be present.
3. Note that it is often impossible to distinguish AIN from ATN based on clinical grounds alone. Renal biopsy is the only way to distinguish between the two, but is usually not performed given its invasiveness.

D. Treatment
1. Removing the offending agent is usually enough to reverse the clinical findings.
2. Treat infection if present.

Chronic Interstitial Nephritis

- A slowly progressive form of interstitial nephritis that can lead to progressive scarring of the interstitium, renal failure, and ESRD over time (years)
- Renal papillary necrosis may be present.
- Unlike with AIN, there are no signs or symptoms of hypersensitivity in chronic interstitial nephritis.
- Causes include prolonged urinary tract obstruction, reflux nephropathy, heavy use of analgesics, heavy metal exposure (lead, cadmium), and arteriolar nephrosclerosis with associated HTN.

Renal Papillary Necrosis

- Most commonly associated with analgesic nephropathy, diabetic nephropathy, sickle cell disease, urinary tract obstruction, UTI, chronic alcoholism, and renal transplant rejection
- Diagnosis is typically made by excretory urogram—note change in papilla or medulla.
- The course is variable. Some patients have rapid progression, whereas others have a more indolent, chronic course.
- Sloughed, necrotic papillae can cause ureteral obstruction.
- Treat the underlying cause, and stop the offending agents.

Renal Tubular Acidosis (RTA)

A. General characteristics
1. RTA is a disorder of the renal tubules that leads to a non–anion gap hyperchloremic metabolic acidosis. Glomerular function is normal.

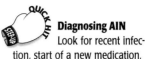

Diagnosing AIN
Look for recent infection, start of a new medication, rash, fever, general aches/pains, and signs/symptoms of ARF.

The diagnosis of AIN can be made if the patient is known to have been exposed to one of the offending agents, and has the following: rash, fever, acute renal insufficiency, and eosinophilia.

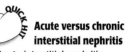

Acute versus chronic interstitial nephritis
- **Acute** interstitial nephritis causes a rapid deterioration in renal function and is associated with interstitial eosinophils or lymphocytes.
- **Chronic** interstitial nephritis has a more indolent course and is associated with tubulointerstitial fibrosis and atrophy.

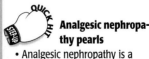

Analgesic nephropathy pearls
- Analgesic nephropathy is a form of toxic injury to the kidney due to excessive use of over-the-counter analgesics (those that contain phenacetin, acetaminophen, NSAIDs, or aspirin).
- It can manifest as interstitial nephritis or renal papillary necrosis.
- It may lead to acute or chronic renal failure.

2. It is characterized by a decrease in the H^+ excreted in the urine, leading to acidemia and urine alkalosis.
3. There are three types of RTA (types 1, 2, and 4). (Type 3 RTA is a term that is no longer used.)

B. Type 1 (distal)

1. The defect is an inability to secrete H^+ at the distal tubule (therefore new bicarbonate cannot be generated). This inability to acidify the urine results in metabolic acidosis. Although normally the urine pH can be as low as 4.7, in distal RTA the urine pH cannot be lowered below 6, regardless of the severity of metabolic acidosis.
2. It leads to increased excretion of ions (sodium, calcium, potassium, sulfate, phosphate), with the following effects:
   a. Decrease in ECF volume
   b. **Hypokalemia**
   c. **Renal stones/nephrocalcinosis** (due to increased calcium and phosphate excretion into alkaline urine)
   d. Rickets/osteomalacia in children
3. Leads to hypokalemic, hyperchloremic, non–anion gap metabolic acidosis
4. Symptoms are secondary to nephrolithiasis and nephrocalcinosis. Up to 70% of patients have kidney stones.
5. Causes: congenital, multiple myeloma, nephrocalcinosis, nephrotoxicity (e.g., amphotericin B toxicity), autoimmune diseases (lupus, Sjögren's syndrome), medullary sponge kidney, and analgesic nephropathy
6. Treatment
   a. Correct acidosis with sodium bicarbonate. This can also help prevent kidney stones, which is a major goal of therapy.
   b. Administer phosphate salts (promotes excretion of titratable acid).

C. Type 2 (proximal)

1. The defect is an inability to reabsorb HCO_3^- at the proximal tubule, resulting in **increased excretion of bicarbonate in the urine** and metabolic acidosis. The patient also loses K^+ and Na^+ in the urine.
2. Characterized by hypokalemic, hyperchloremic non–anion gap metabolic acidosis (as in type 1 RTA).
3. Causes
   a. Fanconi's syndrome (in children)
   b. Cystinosis, Wilson's disease, lead toxicity, multiple myeloma, nephrotic syndrome, amyloidosis
4. Nephrolithiasis and nephrocalcinosis do not occur (as they do in type 1 RTA).
5. Treatment: Treat the underlying cause.
   a. Do not give bicarbonate to correct the acidosis because it will be excreted in the urine.
   b. Sodium restriction increases sodium reabsorption (and thus bicarbonate reabsorption) in the proximal tubule.

D. Type 4

1. This can result from any condition that is associated with hypoaldosteronism, or increased renal resistance to aldosterone.
2. It is common in patients with interstitial renal disease and diabetic nephropathy.
3. It is characterized by decreased Na^+ absorption and decreased H^+ and K^+ secretion in the distal tubule.
4. Unlike other types of RTA, **type 4 results in hyperkalemia** and acidic urine (although a non–anion gap metabolic acidosis still occurs).
5. Nephrolithiasis and nephrocalcinosis are rare.

Hartnup Syndrome

• Autosomal recessive inheritance of defective amino acid transporter

- Results in decreased intestinal and renal reabsorption of neutral amino acids, such as tryptophan, causing nicotinamide deficiency
- Clinical features are similar to those of pellagra: dermatitis, diarrhea, ataxia, and psychiatric disturbances.
- Give supplemental nicotinamide if the patient is symptomatic.

Fanconi's Syndrome

- Fanconi's syndrome is a hereditary or acquired proximal tubule dysfunction that leads to defective transport of some of the following: glucose, amino acids, sodium, potassium, phosphate, uric acid, and bicarbonate.
- It is associated with glucosuria, phosphaturia (leads to skeletal problems: rickets/impaired growth in children; osteomalacia, osteoporosis, and pathologic fractures in adults), proteinuria, polyuria, dehydration, type 2 RTA, hypercalciuria, and hypokalemia.
- Treat with phosphate, potassium, alkali and salt supplementation, as well as adequate hydration.

RENAL CYSTIC DISEASES

Adult Polycystic Kidney Disease

A. General characteristics
1. An autosomal dominant condition
2. The course is variable, but ESRD commonly develops in 50% of patients (by late 50s or 60s); remainder have a normal lifespan.

B. Clinical features
1. Hematuria
2. Abdominal pain
3. HTN (in >50% of cases)
4. Palpable kidneys on abdominal examination
5. Complications/associated findings
   a. **Intracerebral berry aneurysm (in 5% to 20% of cases)**
   b. Infection of renal cysts; bleeding into cysts
   c. Renal failure (late in the disease)
   d. Kidney stones
   e. Heart valve abnormalities (especially mitral valve prolapse)
   f. Cysts in other organs (liver, spleen, pancreas, brain)
   g. Diverticula (colon)
   h. Hernias (abdominal/inguinal)

C. Diagnosis
1. Ultrasound is confirmatory—multiple cysts appear on the kidney.
2. CT scan and MRI are alternatives.

D. Treatment
1. No curative therapy is available.
2. Drain cysts if symptomatic.
3. Treat infection with antibiotics.
4. Control HTN.

Medullary Sponge Kidney

- Characterized by cystic dilation of the collecting ducts
- May present with hematuria, UTIs, or nephrolithiasis
- Thought to be associated with hyperparathyroidism and parathyroid adenoma
- Diagnosed by IVP
- No treatment is necessary other than the prevention of stone formation and the treatment of recurrent UTIs.

Simple Renal Cysts

- Very common (50% of people over age 50); incidence increases with age
- May be single or multiple; usually asymptomatic and discovered incidentally on abdominal ultrasound or other imaging study
- No treatment is necessary in most cases.

RENAL VASCULAR DISEASE

Renal Artery Stenosis (Renovascular Hypertension)

A. General characteristics
1. Renal artery stenosis causes a decrease in blood flow to the juxtaglomerular apparatus. As a result, the renin-angiotensin-aldosterone system becomes activated, leading to HTN.
2. **This is the most common cause of secondary HTN.**

B. Causes
1. Atherosclerosis
   a. Accounts for two-thirds of cases (most often in elderly men)
   b. Bilateral in up to one-third of cases
   c. Smoking and high cholesterol levels are predisposing factors.
2. Fibromuscular dysplasia
   a. Usually seen in young females
   b. Bilateral in 50% of patients

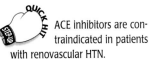

ACE inhibitors are contraindicated in patients with renovascular HTN.

C. Clinical features
1. HTN—Look for a sudden onset of HTN in a patient without a family history. HTN is often severe (may cause malignant HTN) and refractory to medical therapy.
2. Decreased renal function
3. Abdominal bruit (RUQ, LUQ, or epigastrium) is present in 50% to 80% of patients; it is especially common in patients with fibromuscular hyperplasia.

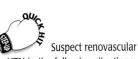

Suspect renovascular HTN in the following situations:
- Malignant HTN
- Sudden onset of HTN
- HTN that suddenly worsens
- HTN that does not respond to standard medical therapy

D. Diagnosis
1. Renal arteriogram is the gold standard, but **contrast dye can be nephrotoxic—do not use it in patients with renal failure.**
2. MRA is a new test that has high sensitivity and specificity. The magnetic dye is not nephrotoxic so it **can** be used in patients with renal failure.
3. The captopril renal scintigram (scan) is a good noninvasive study if renal function is normal.

E. Treatment
1. Revascularization with percutaneous transluminal renal angioplasty (PRTA) is the initial treatment in most patients; it has a higher success rate and a lower restenosis rate with fibromuscular dysplasia than with the atherosclerotic type.
2. Surgery if PRTA is not successful (bypass)
3. Conservative medical therapy (ACE inhibitors, calcium channel blockers) alone only if PRTA or surgery are contraindicated

Renal Vein Thrombosis

- May be seen in the following clinical settings: nephrotic syndrome, invasion of renal vein by renal cell carcinoma, trauma, pregnancy/oral contraceptives, extrinsic compression (retroperitoneal fibrosis, aortic aneurysm, lymphadenopathy), or severe dehydration (in infants)
- Clinical features depend on the acuity and severity of the process and include decreased renal perfusion (can lead to renal failure), flank pain, HTN, hematuria, and proteinuria.
- Diagnostic tests include selective renal venography visualizing the occluding thrombus (definitive study) or IVP.
- Anticoagulate to prevent pulmonary embolism.

Atheroembolic Disease of the Renal Arteries

- Refers to showers of cholesterol crystals that dislodge from plaques in large arteries and embolize to the renal vasculature
- Can occur in other organs as well, such as the retina, brain, or skin
- Refer to cholesterol embolization syndrome in Chapter 1.

Hypertensive Nephrosclerosis

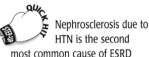

Nephrosclerosis due to HTN is the second most common cause of ESRD (diabetes is the most common cause).

A. Definition: Systemic HTN increases capillary hydrostatic pressure in the glomeruli, leading to benign or malignant sclerosis.

1. Benign nephrosclerosis—Thickening of the glomerular afferent arterioles develops in patients with long-standing HTN.
   a. Results in mild to moderate increase in Cr levels, microscopic hematuria, and mild proteinuria
   b. Advanced disease can lead to ESRD.
2. Malignant nephrosclerosis—This can develop in a patient with long-standing benign HTN or in a previously undiagnosed patient.
   a. Characterized by a rapid decrease in renal function and accelerated HTN due to diffuse intrarenal vascular injury
   b. African-American men are the most susceptible.
   c. Clinical manifestations include:
      - Markedly elevated BP (papilledema, cardiac decompensation, CNS findings)
      - Renal manifestations: a rapid increase in Cr, proteinuria, hematuria, RBC and WBC casts in urine sediment, and sometimes nephrotic syndrome
      - Microangiopathic hemolytic anemia may also be present.

B. Treatment

1. The most important treatment for both benign and malignant forms is controlling the BP (see Chapter 1). It is not clear which blood pressure agents should be used in the chronic setting, or how effective they are once frank albuminuria is present.
2. In advanced disease, treat as for CRF.

Scleroderma

In rare cases, this may cause malignant HTN. See Chapter 6.

Sickle Cell Nephropathy

- This refers to a sickling of RBCs in the microvasculature, which leads to infarction, mostly in the renal papillae. Recurrent papillary infarction can lead to papillary necrosis, renal failure, and a high frequency of UTIs.
- Nephrotic syndrome can develop (which can lead to renal failure).
- It progresses to ESRD in approximately 5% of patients.
- Ischemic injury to the renal tubules can occur, which increases the risk of dehydration (impaired urine concentration), precipitating sickling crises.
- ACE inhibitors may be helpful.

STONES AND OBSTRUCTIONS

Nephrolithiasis

A. General characteristics

1. Nephrolithiasis is the development of stones within the urinary tract.
2. Sites of obstruction
   a. Ureterovesicular junction—most common site of impaction
   b. Calyx of the kidney
   c. Ureteropelvic junction
   d. Intersection of the ureter and the iliac vessels (near the pelvic brim)

3. Risk factors
    a. Low fluid intake—most common and preventable risk factor
    b. Family history
    c. Conditions known to precipitate stone formation (e.g., gout, Crohn's disease, hyperparathyroidism, type 1 RTA)
    d. Medications (e.g., loop diuretics, acetazolamide, antacids, chemotherapeutic drugs that cause cell breakdown [uric acid stones])
    e. Male gender (three times more likely to have urolithiasis)
    f. UTIs (especially with urease-producing bacteria)
4. Types of stones
    a. Calcium stones (most common form)
        • **Account for 80% to 85% of urinary stones**; composed of calcium oxalate or calcium phosphate or both
        • Bipyramidal or biconcave ovals
        • **Radiodense (i.e., visible on an abdominal radiograph)**
        • Secondary to hypercalciuria and hyperoxaluria, which can be due to a variety of causes
    b. Uric acid stones (second most common)
        • Account for 10% of stones
        • These are associated with hyperuricemia, secondary to gout or to chemotherapeutic treatment of leukemias and lymphomas with high cell destruction. The release of purines from dying cells leads to hyperuricemia.
        • Flat square plates
        • **Stones are radiolucent (cannot be seen on an abdominal radiograph)**—require CT, ultrasound, or IVP for detection
    c. Struvite stones (staghorn stones)
        • Account for 5% to 10% of stones
        • Radiodense (visible on an abdominal radiograph); rectangular prisms
        • Occur in patients with recurrent UTIs due to urease-producing organisms (Proteus, Klebsiella, Serratia, Enterobacter spp)
        • They are facilitated by alkaline urine: urea-splitting bacteria convert urea to ammonia, thus producing the alkaline urine.
        • The resultant ammonia combines with magnesium and phosphate to form struvite calculi.
    d. Cystine stones
        • Account for 1% of urinary stones
        • Genetic predisposition—cystinuria
        • Hexagon-shaped crystals are poorly visualized.
5. Clinical course
    a. If a stone is >1 cm, it is unlikely to pass spontaneously. **Stones <0.5 cm usually do pass spontaneously.**
    b. Recurrence is common. Up to 50% of patients have recurrences within 10 years of having the first stone.

B. Clinical features

1. Renal colic—refers to the pain associated with passing a kidney stone into the ureter, with ureteral obstruction and spasm
    a. Description of pain—begins suddenly and soon becomes severe (patient cannot sit still—usually writhes in excruciating pain)
    b. Location of pain—begins in the flank and radiates anteriorly toward the groin (i.e., follows path of the stone)
2. Nausea and vomiting are common
3. Hematuria (in over 90% of cases)
4. UTI

C. Diagnosis

1. Laboratory testing
    a. Urinalysis

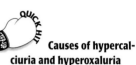

Causes of hypercalciuria and hyperoxaluria
Causes of hypercalciuria
• ↑ intestinal absorption of calcium
• ↓ renal reabsorption of calcium, leading to ↑ renal excretion of calcium
• ↑ bone resorption of calcium
• Primary hyperparathyroidism
• Sarcoidosis
• Malignancy
• Vitamin D excess
Causes of hyperoxaluria
• Severe steatorrhea of any cause can lead to calcium oxalate stones (due to ↑ absorption of oxalate)
• Small bowel disease, Crohn's disease
• Pyridoxine deficiency

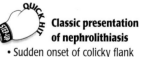

Classic presentation of nephrolithiasis
• Sudden onset of colicky flank pain that radiates into groin
• Urinalysis showing hematuria

- Reveals either microscopic or gross hematuria
- Reveals an associated UTI if pyuria or bacteruria are present
- Examine the urinary sediment for crystals (calcium, cystine, uric acid, or struvite crystals).
- Determine the urinary pH—alkaline urine might indicate the presence of urease-producing bacteria that cause an infection stone. Acidic urine is suggestive of uric acid stones.

Hematuria plus pyuria indicates a stone with concomitant infection.

  b. Urine culture—Obtain if infection is suspected.
  c. 24-hour urine—Collect to assess Cr, calcium, uric acid, oxalate, and citrate levels.
  d. Serum chemistry—Obtain BUN and Cr levels (for evaluation of renal function) and also calcium, uric acid, and phosphate levels.
2. Imaging
  a. Plain radiograph of the kidneys, ureter, and bladder (KUB) (see Figure 7-4)
    - Initial imaging test for detecting stones
    - Cystine and uric acid stones are not usually visible on plain films.
  b. CT scan (spiral CT) without contrast
    - Most sensitive test for detecting stones
    - All stones, even radiolucent ones such as uric acid stones and cystine stones, are visible on the CT scan.
  c. IVP
    - Most useful test for defining degree and extent of urinary tract obstruction
    - This is usually not necessary for the diagnosis of renal calculi. IVP may be appropriate for deciding whether a patient needs procedural therapy.
  d. Renal ultrasonography
    - Helps in detecting hydronephrosis or hydroureter
    - False-negative results are common in early obstruction. Also, there is a low yield in visualizing the stone.

Having the stone for analysis is very helpful both in treatment and in preventing recurrence. Likewise, reporting a history of stones and their composition (if determined) is very helpful. The patient should attempt to recover the stone that is passed (strain urine).

D. Treatment

1. General measures (for all types of stones)
  a. Analgesia: IV morphine, parenteral NSAIDs (ketorolac)
  b. Vigorous fluid hydration—beneficial in all forms of nephrolithiasis
  c. Antibiotics—if UTI is present
  d. Outpatient management is appropriate for most patients. Indications for hospital admission include:
    - Pain not controlled with oral medications
    - Anuria (usually in patients with one kidney)
    - Renal colic plus UTI and/or fever
    - Large stone (>1 cm) that is unlikely to pass spontaneously
2. Specific measures (based on severity of pain)
  a. Mild to moderate pain: high fluid intake, oral analgesia while waiting for stone to pass spontaneously (give the patient a urine strainer)
  b. Severe pain (especially with vomiting)
    - Prescribe IV fluids and pain control.
    - Obtain a KUB and an IVP to find the site of obstruction.
    - If a stone does not pass spontaneously after 3 days, consider urologic surgery.
  c. Ongoing obstruction and persistent pain not controlled by narcotics—Surgery is necessary.
    - Extracorporeal shock wave lithotripsy
      - Most common method
      - It breaks the stone apart; once the calculus is fragmented, the stone can pass spontaneously.
      - Best for stones that are >5 mm but <2 cm in diameter
    - Percutaneous nephrolithotomy
      - If lithotripsy fails
      - Best for stones >2 cm in diameter
3. Prevention of recurrences
  a. Dietary measures

> **Box 7-5 Prostate-Specific Antigen (PSA), Digital Rectal Examination (DRE), and Transrectal Ultrasonography (TRUS)**
>
> - If PSA level >10 ng/mL, TRUS with biopsy is indicated, regardless of DRE findings.
> - If DRE is abnormal, TRUS with biopsy is indicated, regardless of PSA level.
> - If PSA is <4.0 ng/mL and DRE is negative, annual follow-up is indicated.
> - If PSA is 4.1 to 10.0 and DRE is negative, there is controversy over what to do next.

2. Risk factors
   a. Age (most important risk factor)
   b. African-American race
   c. High-fat diet
   d. Positive family history
   e. Exposure to herbicides and pesticides—Certain occupations, such as farming and work in industrial chemical industry, present a higher risk.

B. Clinical features

1. Early—It is most commonly asymptomatic. Cancer begins in the periphery of the gland and moves centrally. Thus, obstructive symptoms occur late. In fact, by the time prostate cancer causes urinary obstruction, it often has metastasized to bone or lymph nodes.
2. Later—Symptoms due to obstruction of the urethra occur: difficulty in voiding, dysuria, and increased urinary frequency.
3. Late—bone pain from metastases (most commonly vertebral bodies, pelvis, and long bones in legs), weight loss

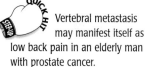 Vertebral metastasis may manifest itself as low back pain in an elderly man with prostate cancer.

C. Diagnosis

1. Digital rectal examination (DRE)
   a. Carcinoma is characteristically hard, nodular, and irregular.
   b. Normal prostate feels like a thenar eminence. Cancer feels like a knuckle.
   c. When palpable, 60% to 70% have spread beyond the prostate.
   d. If DRE is abnormal, transrectal ultrasonography (TRUS) is indicated, regardless of the prostate-specific antigen (PSA) level.
2. PSA—Use as a screening test is controversial.
   a. PSA is not cancer-specific. PSA levels also increase as a result of the following:
      - Prostatic massage (but DRE does not change PSA levels)
      - Needle biopsy
      - Cystoscopy
      - BPH
      - Prostatitis
      - Advanced age
   b. Refinements of the PSA assay
      - Age-adjusted PSA (because PSA normally increases with age)
      - PSA velocity—analysis of the rate of increase in the level with time
      - Quantifying free and protein-bound forms of serum PSA—PSA produced by prostate cancer tends to be bound by plasma proteins, whereas PSA produced by normal cells is more likely to be free in plasma.
      - PSA density—correlation of PSA levels with prostate volume
3. TRUS with biopsy
   a. May need to repeat biopsies for definitive diagnosis
   b. Indications
      - PSA >10 ng/dL (or possibly lower)
      - PSA velocity >0.75 per year
      - Abnormal DRE
4. Other tests in the evaluation include a bone scan, plain radiographs of the pelvis and spine, and a CT scan of the pelvis to evaluate for metastatic disease.

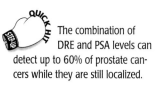 The combination of DRE and PSA levels can detect up to 60% of prostate cancers while they are still localized.

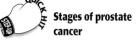 **Stages of prostate cancer**
- Stage A—nonpalpable; confined to prostate
- Stage B—palpable nodule, but confined to prostate
- Stage C—extends beyond capsule without metastasis
- Stage D—metastatic disease

D. Treatment

1. Localized disease (to prostate)—The definitive therapy is radical prostatectomy. However, watchful waiting is warranted in older men (i.e., those whose remaining natural life expectancy is <10 years) who are asymptomatic.
2. Locally invasive disease—**Give radiation therapy plus androgen deprivation** (not curative, but decreases the local spread).
3. Metastatic disease—Reduce the amount of testosterone with any of the following:
   a. Orchiectomy (removes testes)
   b. Antiandrogens
   c. Luteinizing hormone-releasing hormone agonists (Leuprolide)

Renal Cell Carcinoma

A. General characteristics

1. It is twice as common in men as in women.
2. Most cases are sporadic; less than 2% occur as part of autosomal dominant von Hippel-Lindau syndrome.
3. The cause is unknown.
4. Areas of metastasis include the lung, liver, brain, and bone. Tumor thrombus can invade the renal vein or inferior vena cava, resulting in hematogenous dissemination.

B. Risk factors

1. Cigarette smoking
2. Phenacetin analgesics (high use)
3. Adult polycystic kidney disease
4. Chronic dialysis (multicystic disease develops)
5. Exposure to heavy metals (mercury, cadmium)

C. Clinical features

1. Hematuria is most common symptom (gross or microscopic)—occurs in 70% of patients
2. Abdominal or flank pain—occurs in 50% of patients
3. Abdominal (flank) mass—occurs in 40% of patients
4. Weight loss, fever
5. Paraneoplastic syndromes (uncommon)—These tumors can ectopically secrete erythropoietin (causing polycythemia), PTH-like hormone (causing hypercalcemia), renin (causing HTN), cortisol (causing Cushing's syndrome), or gonadotropins (causing feminization or masculinization).

D. Diagnosis

1. Renal ultrasound—for detection of renal mass
2. Abdominal CT (with and without contrast)—optimal test for diagnosis and staging; perform if ultrasound shows a mass or cysts

E. Treatment—Radical nephrectomy (excision of kidney and adrenal gland, including Gerota's fascia with excision of nodal tissue along the renal hilum) for stages I to IV

Bladder Cancer

A. General characteristics

1. Bladder carcinoma is the most common type of tumor of the genitourinary tract; 90% of bladder cancers are transitional cell carcinomas. Transitional cell carcinomas can occur anywhere from the kidney to the bladder (e.g., renal pelvis, ureter), but 90% of these carcinomas are in the bladder.
2. The most common route of spread is local extension to surrounding tissues.
3. **It is likely to recur after removal.**
4. Risk factors
   a. Cigarette smoking (major risk factor)
   b. Industrial carcinogens (aniline dye, azo dyes)

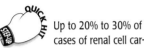

Up to 20% to 30% of cases of renal cell carcinoma are discovered incidentally on a CT scan or ultrasound performed for other reasons.

The classic triad of hematuria, flank pain, and abdominal mass occurs in less than 10% of patients with renal cell carcinoma.

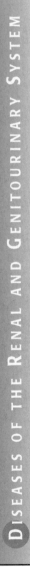

DISEASES OF THE RENAL AND GENITOURINARY SYSTEM

    c. Radiation, biologic agents (coffee, artificial sweeteners)

    d. Long-term treatment with cyclophosphamide (may cause hemorrhagic cystitis and increase risk of transitional cell carcinoma)

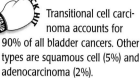

Transitional cell carcinoma accounts for 90% of all bladder cancers. Other types are squamous cell (5%) and adenocarcinoma (2%).

B. Clinical features

1. Initial presenting sign is **hematuria** in most cases (painless hematuria is the classic presentation).
2. Irritable bladder symptoms, such as dysuria frequency

C. Diagnosis

1. Urinalysis and urine culture—to rule out infection
2. Urine cytology—to detect malignant cells
3. IVP
4. Cystoscopy and biopsy (definitive test)
5. Chest radiograph and CT scan—for staging

D. Treatment (depends on the stage of disease)

1. Stage 0 (superficial, limited to mucosa; also known as carcinoma in situ)—intravesical chemotherapy
2. Stage A (involves lamina propria)
    a. Transurethral resection of the bladder tumor
    b. Tends to recur, so frequent cystoscopy and removal of recurrent tumors are indicated
3. Stage B (muscle invasion)—radical cystectomy, lymph node dissection, removal of prostate/uterus/ovaries/anterior vaginal wall, and urinary diversion (e.g., ileal conduit)
4. Stage C (extends to perivesicular fat)—Treatment is the same as for stage B.
5. Stage D (metastasis to lymph nodes, abdominal organs, or distant sites)—Consider cystectomy and systemic chemotherapy.

Testicular Cancer

A. General characteristics

1. Most common in men 20 to 35 years of age, but can occur in men of any age
2. Has a relatively high cure rate compared with other cancers
3. Types
    a. Germ cell tumors (account for 95% of all testicular cancers)—most common in men 20 to 40 years of age; curable in >95% of cases
      • Seminomas (35%)—most common; slow growth and late invasion; most radiosensitive
      • Nonseminomatous (65%)—usually contain cells from at least two of the following four types (mixed cell type): embryonal carcinoma (high malignant potential, hemorrhage and necrosis are common; metastases to the abdominal lymphatics and the lungs may occur as an early event); choriocarcinoma (most aggressive type; rare; metastases usually occur by time of diagnosis); teratoma (rarely metastasize); yolk sac carcinoma (rare in men, usually occurs in young boys)
    b. Non–germ cell tumors (account for 5% of all testicular cancers)—are usually benign
      • Leydig cell tumors are hormonally active—most are benign and are treated with surgery. Prognosis is poor if metastasis occurs. They may secrete a variety of steroid hormones, including estrogen and androgens, and are associated with precocious puberty in children and gynecomastia in adults.
      • Sertoli cell tumors are usually benign.

In a patient with a scrotal mass, perform a careful physical examination to determine its site of origin because testicular cancers are almost always malignant, whereas extratesticular tumors within the scrotum are almost always benign.

B. Risk factors

1. Cryptorchidism—surgical correction does not eliminate risk
2. Klinefelter's syndrome

C. Clinical features

1. Painless mass/lump/firmness of the testicle—because of lack of pain, may go unnoticed by patient until advanced

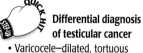

Differential diagnosis of testicular cancer
- Varicocele–dilated, tortuous veins in testicle
- Testicular torsion
- Spermatocele (testicular cyst)
- Hydrocele (fluid in testicle)
- Epididymitis
- Lymphoma

DISEASES OF THE RENAL AND GENITOURINARY SYSTEM

2. Gynecomastia may be present because some of the nonseminomatous germ cell tumors produce gonadotropins.

D. Diagnosis
1. Physical examination (testicular mass)
2. Testicular ultrasound—initial test for localizing the tumor
3. Tumor markers—helpful in diagnosis, staging, and monitoring response to therapy
   a. β-hCG
      - Always elevated in choriocarcinoma
      - May be elevated in other types of nonseminomatous germ cell tumors as well
   b. AFP
      - Increased in embryonal tumors (in 80% of cases)
      - Choriocarcinoma and seminoma never have an elevated AFP.
4. CT scan and chest radiograph for staging

E. Treatment
1. If testicular cancer is suspected based on physical examination or ultrasound, the testicle should be removed surgically (to confirm diagnosis). An inguinal approach is used because a scrotal incision may lead to tumor seeding of the scrotum.
2. After orchiectomy, perform a CT scan of the chest, abdomen, and pelvis for staging.
3. Perform β-hCG and AFP measurement after orchiectomy for comparison with the preoperative values.
4. Further treatment depends on the histology of the tumor.
   a. Seminoma—inguinal orchiectomy and radiation (very radiosensitive)
   b. Nonseminomatous disease—orchiectomy and retroperitoneal lymph node dissection with or without chemotherapy

Penile Cancer

- The peak incidence of this tumor is in men in their seventh decade.
- Circumcision may have a protective effect because penile cancer is very rare in those who have been circumcised.
- It is associated with herpes simplex virus and HPV 18 infection.
- It presents as an exophytic mass on the penis.
- Treatment of the primary disease is local excision.

MISCELLANEOUS CONDITIONS

Testicular Torsion

- Twisting of the spermatic cord leading to arterial occlusion and venous outflow obstruction; ischemia can lead to testicular infarction
- Usually seen in adolescent male patients
- Clinical features include acute severe testicular pain, swollen and tender scrotum, and an elevated testicle (as twisting occurs, the testicle moves to a higher position in scrotum).
- **This is a surgical emergency.** The treatment is immediate surgical detorsion and orchiopexy to the scrotum (perform bilaterally to prevent torsion in the contralateral testicle). **If surgery is delayed beyond 6 hours, infarction may occur, and the testicle may not be salvageable.**
- Orchiectomy is appropriate if a nonviable testicle is found.

Epididymitis

- Epididymitis is infection of the epididymis. The common offending organism in children and elderly patients is *Escherichia coli*; in young men, sexually transmitted diseases are more common (gonorrhea, *Chlamydia*).
- Clinical features include a swollen, tender testicle; dysuria; fever/chills; scrotal pain; and a scrotal mass.
- Rule out testicular torsion, and administer antibiotics.

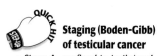

Staging (Boden-Gibb) of testicular cancer
- Stage A—confined to testis/cord
- Stage B—retroperitoneal lymph node spread (below diaphragm)
- Stage C—distant metastasis

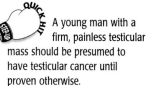

A young man with a firm, painless testicular mass should be presumed to have testicular cancer until proven otherwise.

Do not confuse testicular cancer with testicular torsion or epididymitis.

Epididymitis may be difficult to differentiate from testicular torsion.
- Torsion has a more acute onset.
- Torsion is not associated with fever.

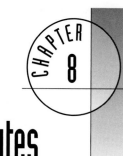

Fluids, Electrolytes, and Acid-Base Disorders

VOLUME DISORDERS

Approach to Volume Disorders

A. Normal body fluid compartments

1. Men: Total body water (TBW) = 60% of body weight.
2. Women: TBW = 50% of body weight.
3. Percentage of TBW decreases with age and increasing obesity (TBW decreases because fat contains very little water).
4. Distribution of water
   a. Intracellular fluid (ICF) is two-thirds of TBW (or 40% of body weight)—the largest proportion of TBW is in skeletal muscle mass.
   b. Extracellular fluid (ECF) is one third of TBW (or 20% of body weight).
      - Plasma is one-third of ECF, 1/12 of TBW, and 5% of body weight.
      - Interstitial fluid is two-thirds of ECF, one-fourth of TBW, and 15% of body weight.
5. Water exchange
   a. Normal intake: 1,500 mL in fluids taken PO per day; 500 mL in solids or product of oxidation
   b. Normal output
      - From 800 to 1,500 mL in urine per day is the normal range. Minimum urine output to excrete products of catabolism is about 500 to 600 mL/day, assuming normal renal concentrating ability.
      - Output of 250 mL/day occurs in stool.
      - From 600 to 900 mL/day in insensible losses occurs. This is highly variable but increases with fever, sweating, hyperventilation, and tracheostomies (unhumidified air)—see below.
   c. Remember the Starling equation and forces: fluid shift depends on hydrostatic and oncotic pressures.

B. Assessing volume status

1. This is not a simple task. For example, a patient with lower extremity edema may be euvolemic, or may be total-body overloaded but intravascularly depleted. Skin turgor and mucous membranes are very difficult to assess and are not always reliable indicators of volume status.
2. Tracking input and output is not an exact science either because there is no accurate way of calculating insensible losses. Monitoring urine output is very important in the assessment of volume status: **normal urine output in adults is more than 1.0 mL/kg per hour.** Low urine output could be a sign of volume depletion.
3. Daily weights may give a more accurate assessment of volume trends.

 For body fluid compartments, remember the 60-40-20 rule.
- TBW is 60% of body weight (50% for women).
- ICF is 40% of body weight.
- ECF is 20% of body weight (interstitial fluid 15% and plasma 5%).

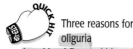 Three reasons for oliguria
- Low blood flow to kidney (assess heart)
- Kidney problem
- Postrenal obstruction (place a Foley catheter)

FIGURE
8-1 **Body fluid compartments.**

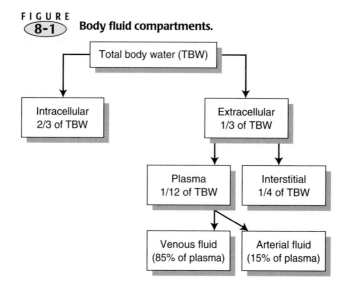

4. Keep in mind the larger picture of the patient's condition.
   a. In general, patients with sepsis, fever, burns, or open wounds have high insensible losses (and higher metabolic demands).
   b. For each degree of atmospheric temperature over 37°C, the body's water loss increases by approximately 100 mL/day.
   c. Patients with liver failure, nephrotic syndrome, or any condition causing hypoalbuminemia tend to third-space fluid out of the vasculature and may be total-body hypervolemic but intravascularly depleted.
   d. Patients with CHF may have either pulmonary edema or anasarca, depending on which ventricle is involved.
   e. Patients with ESRD are very prone to hypervolemia for obvious reasons.

C. Fluid replacement therapy
1. Normal saline (NS)—often used to increase intravascular volume if the patient is dehydrated or has lost blood; usually not the best option in patients with CHF unless the patient needs urgent resuscitation
2. D51/2NS (hypertonic)
   a. Often the standard maintenance fluid (often given with 20 mEq of KCl/L of fluid)
   b. Has some glucose, which can spare muscle breakdown, and has water for insensible losses
3. D5W (hypotonic)
   a. Used to dilute powdered medicines
   b. May sometimes be indicated in correcting hypernatremia
   c. Only 1/12 remains intravascular because it diffuses into the TBW compartment, so not effective in maintaining intravascular volume
4. Lactated Ringer's solution—This is excellent for replacement of intravascular volume; it is not a maintenance fluid. It is the most common trauma resuscitation fluid. Do not use if hyperkalemia is a concern (contains potassium).

Hypovolemia

A. Causes
1. GI losses due to vomiting, nasogastric suction, diarrhea, fistula drainage, etc.
2. Third-spacing due to ascites, effusions, bowel obstruction, crush injuries, burns
3. Inadequate intake
4. Polyuria—e.g., diabetic ketoacidosis (DKA)
5. Sepsis, intra-abdominal and retroperitoneal inflammatory processes
6. Trauma, open wounds, sequestration of fluid into soft tissue injuries
7. Insensible losses—evaporatory losses through skin (75%) and the respiratory tract (25%)

> **QUICK HIT**
> If a patient is receiving hypotonic solutions (1/2 NS, 1/4 NS), water is initially transferred from the ECF to intracellular space to equilibrate osmotic pressures in both compartments.

> **Box** **8-1** **Calculation of Maintenance Fluids**
>
> - 100/50/20 rule:
>   - 100 mL/kg for first 10 kg, 50 mL/kg for next 10 kg, 20 mL/kg for every 1 kg over 20
>   - Divide total by 24 for hourly rate
>   - For example, for a 70-kg man: $100 \times 10 = 1,000$; $50 \times 10 = 500$, 20×50 kg = 1,000. Total = 2,500. Divide by 24 hours: **104 mL/hr**
> - 4/2/1 rule:
>   - 4 mL/kg for first 10 kg, 2 mL/kg for next 10 kg, 1 mL/kg for every 1 kg over 20
>   - For example, for a 70-kg man: $4 \times 10 = 40$; $2 \times 10 = 20$; $1 \times 50 = 50$. Total = **110 mL/hr**

B. Clinical features

1. CNS findings: mental status changes, sleepiness, apathy, coma
2. Cardiovascular findings (due to decrease in plasma volume): orthostatic hypotension, tachycardia, decreased pulse pressure, decreased central venous pressure (CVP) and pulmonary capillary wedge pressure (PCWP)
3. Skin: poor skin turgor, hypothermia, pale extremities, dry tongue
4. Oliguria
5. Ileus, weakness
6. Acute renal failure due to prerenal azotemia (fractional excretion of sodium <1%)

C. Diagnosis

1. Monitor urine output and daily weights. If the patient is critically ill and has cardiac or renal dysfunction, consider placing a Swan-Ganz catheter (to measure CVP and PCWP).
2. Elevated serum sodium, low urine sodium, and a BUN/Cr ratio of >20:1 suggest hypoperfusion to the kidneys, which usually (not always) represents hypovolemia.
3. Increased hematocrit: 3% increase for each liter of deficit
4. The concentration of formed elements in the blood (RBCs, WBCs, platelets, plasma proteins) increases with an ECF deficit and decreases with an ECF excess.

D. Treatment

1. Correct volume deficit
   a. Use bolus to achieve euvolemia. Begin with isotonic solution (lactated Ringer's or NS).
   b. Again, frequent monitoring of HR, BP, urine output, and weight is essential.
   c. **Maintain urine output at 0.5 to 1 mL/kg per hour.**
   d. Blood loss—Replace blood loss with crystalloid at a 3:1 ratio.
2. Maintenance fluid
   a. D51/2NS solution with 20 mEq KCl/L is the most common adult maintenance fluid. (Dextrose is added to inhibit muscle breakdown.)
   b. There are two methods of calculating the amount of maintenance fluid (see Box 8-1).

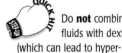 Do **not** combine bolus fluids with dextrose (which can lead to hyperglycemia) or potassium (which can lead to hyperkalemia).

Hypervolemia

A. Causes

1. Iatrogenic (parenteral overhydration)
2. Fluid-retaining states: CHF, nephrotic syndrome, cirrhosis, ESRD

B. Clinical features

1. Weight gain
2. Peripheral edema (pedal or sacral), ascites, or pulmonary edema
3. Jugular venous distention

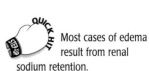 Most cases of edema result from renal sodium retention.

4. Elevated CVP and PCWP
5. Pulmonary rales
6. Low hematocrit and albumin concentration

C. Treatment
1. Fluid restriction
2. Judicious use of diuretics
3. Monitor urine output and daily weights, and consider Swan-Ganz catheter placement depending on the patient's condition.

SODIUM

Overview of Sodium Homeostasis

A. Salt and water regulation
1. Na^+ regulation is intimately associated with water homeostasis, yet it is regulated by independent mechanisms.
2. Changes in Na^+ **concentration** are a reflection of water homeostasis, whereas changes in Na^+ **content** are a reflection of Na^+ homeostasis.
3. Disturbance of Na^+ balance may lead to hypovolemia or hypervolemia, and disturbance of water balance may lead to hyponatremia or hypernatremia.

B. Sodium homeostasis
1. Sodium is actively pumped out of cells and is therefore restricted to the extracellular space. It is the main osmotically active cation of the ECF.
2. An increase in sodium intake results in an increase in ECF volume, which results in an increase in GFR and sodium excretion. A decline in the extracellular circulating volume results in a decreased GFR and a reduction in sodium excretion.
3. Diuretics inhibit Na^+ reabsorption through various mechanisms in the renal tubular system. Furosemide and other loop diuretics inhibit the Na^+-K^+-Cl^- transporter in the thick ascending limb of the loop of Henle, whereas thiazide diuretics inhibit the Na^+-Cl^+ cotransporter at the early distal tubule. However, the majority of Na^+ reabsorption occurs in the proximal tubule.
4. A decrease in renal perfusion pressure results in activation of the renin-angiotensin-aldosterone system. Aldosterone increases sodium reabsorption and potassium secretion from the late distal tubules.

C. Water homeostasis
1. Osmoreceptors in the hypothalamus are stimulated by plasma hypertonicity (usually >295 mOsm/kg); activation of these stimulators produces thirst.
2. Hypertonic plasma also stimulates the secretion of antidiuretic hormone (ADH) from the posterior pituitary gland. When ADH binds to V_2 receptors in the renal collecting ducts, water channels are synthesized and more water is reabsorbed.
3. ADH is suppressed as plasma tonicity decreases.
4. Ultimately, the amount of water intake and output (including renal, GI, and insensible losses from the skin and respiratory tract) must be equivalent over time to preserve a steady state.
5. When a steady state is not achieved, hyponatremia or hypernatremia usually occurs.

Hyponatremia

A. General characteristics
1. This refers to too much water in relation to sodium in the serum.
2. It is typically defined as a plasma Na^+ concentration <135 mmol/L.
3. Symptoms usually begin when the Na^+ level falls to >120 mEq/L. An important exception is increased intracranial pressure (ICP) (e.g., after head injury). As ECF osmolality decreases, water shifts into brain cells, further increasing ICP. (Therefore, it is critical to keep serum sodium normal or slightly high in such patients.)

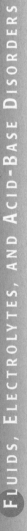

FLUIDS, ELECTROLYTES, AND ACID-BASE DISORDERS

QUICK HIT
• Aldosterone increases sodium reabsorption.
• ADH increases water reabsorption.

QUICK HIT
• Hyponatremia and hypernatremia are caused by too much or too little **water.**
• Hypovolemia and hypervolemia are caused by too much or too little **sodium.**

B. Causes and classification (based on serum osmolality)

1. **Hypotonic hyponatremia**—"true hyponatremia"—serum osmolality <280 mOsm/kg
   a. Hypovolemic
      - Low urine sodium (<10 mEq/L)—implies increased sodium retention by the kidneys to compensate for **extrarenal losses** (e.g., diarrhea, vomiting, nasogastric suction, diaphoresis, third-spacing, burns, pancreatitis) of **sodium-containing fluid**
      - High urine sodium (>20 mEq/L)—renal salt loss is likely—e.g., diuretic excess, decreased aldosterone (ACE inhibitors), ATN
   b. Euvolemic—no evidence of ECF expansion or contraction on clinical grounds
      - SIADH
      - Psychogenic polydipsia
      - Postoperative hyponatremia
      - Hypothyroidism
      - Administration/intake of a relative excess of free water—if a patient is given D5W (or other hypotonic solution) to replace fluids, or if water alone is consumed after intensive exertion (with profuse sweating)
      - Drugs—haloperidol (Haldol), cyclophosphamide, certain antineoplastic agents
   c. Hypervolemic (low urine sodium)—This is due to water-retaining states. The relative excess of water in relation to sodium results in hyponatremia.
      - CHF
      - Nephrotic syndrome (renal failure)
      - Liver disease
2. Isotonic hyponatremia (pseudohyponatremia)
   a. An increase in plasma solids lowers the plasma sodium **concentration**. But the **amount** of sodium in plasma is normal (hence, **pseudo**hyponatremia).
   b. This can be caused by any condition that leads to elevated protein or lipid levels.
3. Hypertonic hyponatremia
   a. Caused by the presence of osmotic substances that cause an **osmotic shift of water out of cells.** These substances cannot cross the cell membrane and therefore create osmotic gradients.
   b. These substances include:
      - Glucose—**Hyperglycemia** increases osmotic pressure and water shifts from cells into ECF, leading to a dilutional hyponatremia. For every 100 mg/dL increase in blood glucose level above normal, the serum sodium level decreases about 3 mEq/L. Note that the actual sodium content in the ECF is unchanged.
      - Mannitol, sorbitol, glycerol, maltose
      - Radiocontrast agents

[handwritten margin note: hypomagnasemia / hypocalcemia / hyponatremia } hyperirritability= ↑ deep tendon reflexes.]

C. Clinical features

1. **Neurologic symptoms predominate**—caused by "water intoxication"—osmotic water shifts, which leads to increased ICF volume, specifically brain cell swelling or cerebral edema
   a. Headache, delirium, irritability
   b. Muscle twitching, weakness
   c. Hyperactive deep tendon reflexes
2. Increased ICP, seizures, coma
3. GI—nausea, vomiting, ileus, watery diarrhea
4. Cardiovascular—hypertension due to increased ICP
5. Increased salivation and lacrimation
6. Oliguria progressing to anuria—**may not be reversible if therapy is delayed**

D. Diagnosis (see Figure 8-2)

1. Plasma osmolality—low in a patient with true hyponatremia
2. Urine osmolality
   a. Low if the kidneys are responding appropriately by diluting the urine—e.g., primary polydipsia
   b. Elevated if there are increased levels of ADH—e.g., SIADH, CHF, and hypothyroidism

Excessive water intake alone rarely leads to hyponatremia because the kidneys have a great capacity to excrete water.

As opposed to acute water intoxication, when hyponatremia develops gradually (over a few days), the clinical features do not appear until a relatively lower sodium level is reached.

FLUIDS, ELECTROLYTES, AND ACID-BASE DISORDERS

FIGURE
8-2 Evaluation of hyponatremia.

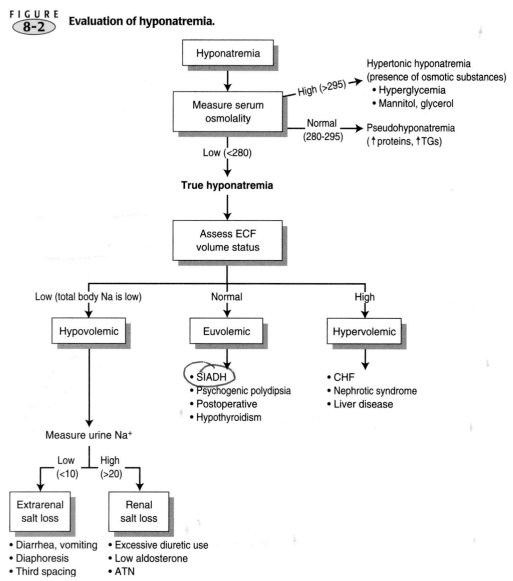

(Adapted from Harwood-Nuss A, Wolfson AB. The Clinical Practice of Emergency Medicine. 3rd Ed. Philadelphia: Lippincott Williams & Wilkins, 2001:849, Figure 173.1.)

3. Urine sodium concentration
   a. Urine Na^+ should be low in the setting of hyponatremia.
   b. Urine Na^+ concentration >20 mmol/L is consistent with a salt-wasting nephropathy or hypoaldosteronism. Diuretics may produce this as well.
   c. Urine Na^+ concentration >40 mmol/L is consistent with (but does not define) SIADH.

E. Treatment
1. Isotonic and hypertonic hyponatremias—Diagnose and treat the underlying disorder.
2. Hypotonic hyponatremia
   a. Mild (Na^+ 12-0-130 mmol/L)—Withhold free water, and allow the patient to reequilibrate spontaneously.
   b. Moderate (Na^+ 110 to 120 mmol/L)—loop diuretics (given with saline to prevent renal concentration of urine due to high ADH)
   c. Severe (Na^+ <110 mmol/L or if symptomatic)—Give hypertonic saline to increase serum sodium by 1 to 2 mEq/L per hour until symptoms improve.
      • Hypertonic saline rapidly increases the tonicity of ECF.
      • Do not increase sodium more than 8 mmol/L during the first 24 hours. An overly rapid increase in serum sodium concentration may produce **central pontine demyelination**.

Hypernatremia

A. General characteristics

1. Defined as a plasma Na^+ concentration >145 mmol/L
2. Refers to excess sodium in relation to water; can result from water loss or sodium infusion
3. Assess ECF volume clinically, as follows:
   a. Hypovolemic hypernatremia (sodium stores are depleted, but more water loss than sodium loss)
      - Renal loss—from diuretics, **osmotic diuresis** (most commonly due to glycosuria in diabetics), renal failure
      - Extrarenal loss—from **diarrhea**, diaphoresis, respiratory losses
   b. Isovolemic hypernatremia (sodium stores normal, water lost)
      - **Diabetes insipidus**
      - Insensible respiratory (tachypnea)
   c. Hypervolemic hypernatremia (sodium excess)—occurs infrequently
      - Iatrogenic—most common cause of hypervolemic hypernatremia (e.g., large amounts of parenteral $NaHCO_3$, TPN)
      - Exogenous glucocorticoids
      - Cushing's syndrome
      - Saltwater drowning
      - Primary hyperaldosteronism

B. Clinical features

1. Neurologic symptoms predominate
   a. Altered mental status, restlessness, weakness, focal neurologic deficits
   b. Can lead to confusion, seizures, coma
2. Tissues and mucous membranes are dry; salivation decreases.

 Most cases of hypernatremia are due to the following types of water loss.
- Nonrenal loss: insensible loss, GI tract (diarrhea)
- Renal loss: osmotic diuresis, diabetes insipidus

 Excessively rapid correction of hypernatremia can lead to **cerebral edema** as water shifts into brain cells. Therefore, the rate of correction should not exceed 12 mEq/L per day (should be <8 mEq/L in the first 24 hours).

 Clinical features of hypernatremia are secondary to osmotic effects on the brain (water shifts out of brain cells, leaving them dehydrated). Symptoms are more prominent and severe when sodium levels increase rapidly.

FIGURE 8-3 Evaluation of hypernatremia.

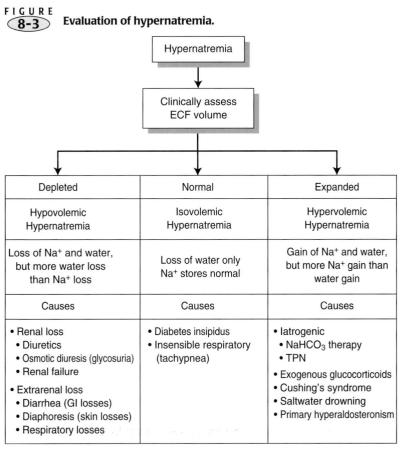

Depleted	Normal	Expanded
Hypovolemic Hypernatremia	Isovolemic Hypernatremia	Hypervolemic Hypernatremia
Loss of Na^+ and water, but more water loss than Na^+ loss	Loss of water only Na^+ stores normal	Gain of Na^+ and water, but more Na^+ gain than water gain
Causes	Causes	Causes

• Renal loss
• Diuretics
• Osmotic diuresis (glycosuria)
• Renal failure
 	
• Extrarenal loss
• Diarrhea (GI losses)
• Diaphoresis (skin losses)
• Respiratory losses
	• Diabetes insipidus
	• Insensible respiratory (tachypnea)
		• Iatrogenic
		  • $NaHCO_3$ therapy
		  • TPN
		• Exogenous glucocorticoids
		• Cushing's syndrome
		• Saltwater drowning
		• Primary hyperaldosteronism

(Adapted from Glasscock RJ, Massry SG. Massry and Glassock's Textbook of Nephrology. 4th Ed. Philadelphia: Lippincott Williams & Wilkins, 2000.)

C. Diagnosis
1. Urine volume should be low if the kidneys are responding appropriately.
2. Urine osmolality should be >800 mOsm/kg.
3. Desmopressin should be given to differentiate nephrogenic from central diabetes insipidus if diabetes insipidus is suspected (see Chapter 4).

D. Treatment
1. Hypovolemic hypernatremia—Give isotonic NaCl to restore hemodynamics. Correction of hypernatremia can wait until the patient is hemodynamically stable, then replace the free water deficit (see Box 8-1).
2. Isovolemic hypernatremia—Patients with diabetes insipidus require vasopressin. Prescribe oral fluids, or if the patient cannot drink, give D5W.
3. Hypervolemic hypernatremia—Give diuretics (furosemide) and D5W to remove the excess sodium. Dialyze patients with renal failure.

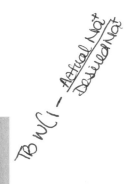

QUICK HIT

Calculating free water deficit

Water deficit = TBW (1 − actual Na^+ ÷ desired Na^+)

(handwritten margin note) $TB \, nCl - \frac{Actual \, Na^+}{Desired \, Na^+}$

CALCIUM

Calcium Metabolism

A. Normal serum calcium: The normal serum calcium (Ca^{2+}) range is 8.5 to 10.5 mg/dL. Calcium balance is regulated by hormonal control, but levels are also affected by albumin and pH.
1. Albumin
   a. Calcium in plasma exists in two forms.
      - Protein-bound form: Most calcium ions are bound to albumin, so the total calcium concentration fluctuates with the protein (albumin) concentration.
      - Free ionized form: **physiologically active** fraction; under tight hormonal control (PTH), **independent of albumin levels**
   b. In hypoalbuminemia the total calcium is low, but ionized calcium is normal, and can be estimated by the following formula: total calcium − (serum albumin × 0.8).
2. Changes in pH alter the ratio of calcium binding. An increase in pH increases the binding of calcium to albumin. Therefore, in alkalemic states (especially acute respiratory alkalosis), total calcium is normal, but ionized calcium is low and the patient frequently manifests signs and symptoms of hypocalcemia.

QUICK HIT

Maintenance of calcium balance is a function of PTH, calcitonin, and vitamin D, and their target organs: bone, kidney, and gut.

B. Hormonal control
1. PTH— ↑ plasma Ca^{2+} and ↓ plasma PO_4^{3-} by acting on:
   a. Bone: ↑ bone resorption
   b. Kidney: ↑Ca^{2+} reabsorption, ↓ PO_4^{3-} reabsorption
   c. Gut: activation of vitamin D
2. Calcitonin— ↓ plasma Ca^{2+} and ↓ plasma PO_4^{3-} by acting on:
   a. Bone: ↓ bone resorption
   b. Kidney: ↓ Ca^{2+} reabsorption, ↑ PO_4^{3-} reabsorption
   c. Gut: ↓ postprandial Ca^{2+} absorption
3. Vitamin D— ↑ plasma Ca^{2+} and ↑ plasma PO_4^{3-} by acting on:
   a. Bone: ↑ bone resorption
   b. Kidney: ↑ Ca^{2+} reabsorption, ↓ PO_4^{3-} reabsorption
   c. Gut: ↑ Ca^{2+} absorption, ↑ PO_4^{3-} reabsorption

Hypocalcemia

QUICK HIT

Ionized calcium may be low with normal serum calcium levels in acute alkalotic states.

A. Causes
1. Hypoparathyroidism (most common cause)—usually due to surgery on the thyroid gland (with damage to nearby parathyroids)
2. Acute pancreatitis—Deposition of calcium deposits lowers serum Ca^{2+} levels.
3. Renal insufficiency—mainly due to decreased production of 1,25-dihydroxy vitamin D
4. Hyperphosphatemia—PO_4^{3-} precipitates with Ca^{2+}, resulting in calcium phosphate deposition.

5. Pseudohypoparathyroidism—autosomal recessive disease causing congenital end-organ resistance to PTH (so PTH levels are actually high); also characterized by mental retardation and short metacarpal bones
6. Hypomagnesemia—results in decreased PTH secretion
7. Vitamin D deficiency
8. Malabsorption—short bowel syndrome
9. Blood transfusion (with citrated blood)—Calcium binds to citrate.
10. Osteoblastic metastases
11. Hypoalbuminemia—but ionized fraction is normal so hypoalbuminemia is clinically irrelevant

B. Clinical features

1. Asymptomatic
2. Rickets and osteomalacia
3. Increased neuromuscular irritability
   a. Numbness/tingling—circumoral, in fingers, in toes
   b. Tetany
      - Hyperactive deep tendon reflexes
      - *Chvostek's sign*—Tapping a facial nerve leads to a contraction (twitching) of facial muscles.
      - *Trousseau's sign*—Inflate BP cuff to a pressure higher than the patient's systolic BP for 3 minutes (occludes blood flow in forearm). This elicits carpal spasms.
   c. Grand mal seizures
4. Basal ganglia calcifications
5. Cardiac manifestations
   a. Arrhythmias
   b. Prolonged QT interval on ECG—Hypocalcemia should always be in the differential diagnosis for a prolonged QT interval.

> **QUICK HIT**
> Hospitalized patients frequently have low serum albumin concentrations. Therefore, if you see a low calcium level, look at the albumin level (it is usually low as well). A low serum **ionized calcium** level is much less common.

C. Diagnosis

1. To evaluate for the above-listed etiologies, obtain the following: BUN, Cr, magnesium, albumin, and ionized calcium. Amylase, lipase, and liver function tests may also be warranted.
2. Serum PO_4^{3-}: high in renal insufficiency and in hypoparathyroidism, low in primary vitamin D deficiency
3. PTH
   a. Low in hypoparathyroidism
   b. Elevated in vitamin D deficiency
   c. Very high in pseudohypoparathyroidism

D. Treatment

1. If symptomatic, provide emergency treatment with IV calcium gluconate. Make sure that magnesium is replaced.
2. For long-term management, use oral calcium supplements (calcium carbonate) and vitamin D.
3. For PTH deficiency
   a. Replacement therapy with vitamin D (or calcitriol) plus a high oral calcium intake.
   b. Thiazide diuretics—Lower urinary calcium, and prevent urolithiasis

Hypercalcemia

A. Causes

1. Endocrinopathies
   a. Hyperparathyroidism—increased Ca^{2+}, low PO_4^{3-}
   b. Renal failure—usually results in **hypo**calcemia, but sometimes secondary hyperparathyroidism elevates PTH levels high enough to cause **hyper**calcemia
   c. Paget's disease of the bone—due to osteoclastic bone resorption
   d. Hyperparathyroidism, acromegaly, Addison's disease

2. Malignancies
   a. Metastatic cancer—Bony metastases result in bone destruction due to osteoclastic activity. Most tumors that metastasize to bone cause both osteolytic and osteoblastic activity (prostate cancer, mainly osteoblastic; kidney carcinoma, usually osteolytic).
   b. Multiple myeloma—secondary to two causes
      • Lysis of bone by tumor cells
      • Release of osteoclast-activating factor by myeloma cells
   c. Tumors that release PTH-like hormone (e.g., lung cancer)
3. Pharmacologic
   a. Vitamin D intoxication—increased GI absorption of calcium
   b. Milk-alkali syndrome—hypercalcemia, alkalosis, and renal impairment due to excessive intake of calcium and certain absorbable antacids (calcium carbonate, milk)
   c. Drugs—thiazide diuretics (inhibit renal excretion), lithium (increases PTH levels in some patients, e.g., squamous cell carcinoma)
4. Other
   a. Sarcoidosis—increased GI absorption of calcium
   b. Familial hypercalciuric hypercalcemia

B. Clinical features
1. "Stones"
   a. Nephrolithiasis
   b. Nephrocalcinosis
2. "Bones"
   a. Bone aches and pains
   b. Osteitis fibrosa cystica ("brown tumors") predisposes to pathologic fractures.
3. "Grunts and groans"
   a. Muscle pain and weakness
   b. Pancreatitis
   c. Peptic ulcer disease
   d. Gout
   e. Constipation
4. "Psychiatric overtones"—depression, fatigue, anorexia, sleep disturbances, anxiety, lethargy
5. Other findings
   a. Polydipsia, polyuria
   b. Hypertension
   c. Weight loss
   d. ECG—shortened QT interval
   e. Patients may be asymptomatic.

C. Diagnosis
1. Same laboratory tests as in hypocalcemia
2. Radioimmunoassay of PTH: elevated in primary hyperparathyroidism, low in occult malignancy
3. Radioimmunoassay of PTH-related protein: elevated in malignancy
4. Bone scan or bone survey to identify lytic lesions
5. Urinary cAMP: markedly elevated in primary hyperparathyroidism

D. Treatment
1. Increase urinary excretion.
   a. IV fluids (normal saline)—first step in management
   b. Diuretics (furosemide)—further inhibit calcium reabsorption
2. Inhibit bone resorption in patients with osteoclastic disease (e.g., malignancy).
   a. Bisphosphonates (pamidronate)
   b. Calcitonin
3. Give glucocorticoids if vitamin D-related mechanisms (intoxication, granulomatous disorders) and multiple myeloma are the cause of the hypercalcemia. However, glucocorticoids are ineffective in most other forms of hypercalcemia.

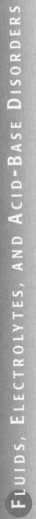

• In **hyper**calcemia, ECG shows shortening of the QT interval.
• In **hypo**calcemia, ECG shows a prolongation of the QT interval.

4. Use hemodialysis for renal failure patients.
5. Phosphate is effective but incurs the risk of metastatic calcification.

POTASSIUM

Potassium Metabolism

- **Normal K$^+$ levels:** 3.5 to 5.0 mEq/L
- **Location in the body**—Most of the body's potassium (98%) is intracellular.
- **Hypokalemia**—Alkalosis and insulin administration may cause hypokalemia because they cause a shift of potassium into the cells.
- **Hyperkalemia**—Acidosis and anything resulting in cell lysis increases serum K$^+$ (both force K$^+$ out of cells into the ECF).
- **Potassium secretion**—Most of the excretion of potassium occurs through the kidneys (80%); the remainder occurs via the GI tract. Aldosterone plays an important role in renal potassium secretion.

Serum potassium is affected by pH: alkalosis can lead to hypokalemia, whereas acidosis can lead to hyperkalemia.

Hypokalemia

A. Causes
1. GI losses
   a. Vomiting and nasogastric drainage (volume depletion and metabolic alkalosis also result)
   b. Diarrhea
   c. Laxatives and enemas
   d. Intestinal fistulae
   e. Decreased potassium absorption in intestinal disorders

Interpretation of urine potassium in hypokalemia
- Low with GI losses (<20 mEq/L)
- High with renal losses (>20 mEq/L)

2. Renal losses
   a. Diuretics
   b. Renal tubular or parenchymal disease
   c. Primary and secondary hyperaldosteronism
   d. Excessive glucocorticoids
   e. Magnesium deficiency
   f. Bartter's syndrome—chronic volume depletion secondary to an autosomal-recessive defect in salt reabsorption in the thick ascending limb of the loop of Henle leads to hyperplasia of juxtaglomerular apparatus, which leads to increased renin levels and secondary aldosterone elevations.

Diarrhea is a common cause of both hypokalemia and non-anion gap metabolic acidosis.

3. Other causes
   a. Insufficient dietary intake
   b. Insulin administration
   c. Certain antibiotics
   d. Profuse sweating
   e. Epinephrine (β_2 agonists)—Hypokalemia occurs in 50% to 60% of trauma patients, perhaps due to increased epinephrine levels.

The presence or absence of HTN is useful in differentiating causes of hypokalemia. If the patient is hypertensive, excessive aldosterone activity is likely. If the patient is normotensive, either GI or renal loss of K$^+$ is likely.

B. Clinical features
1. Arrhythmias—prolongs normal cardiac conduction
2. Muscular weakness, fatigue, paralysis, and muscle cramps
3. Decreased deep tendon reflexes
4. Paralytic ileus
5. Polyuria and polydipsia
6. Nausea/vomiting
7. Exacerbates digitalis toxicity

 Arrhythmias are the most dangerous complications of hypokalemia. ECG changes in hypokalemia appear as follows:
- T wave flattens out; if severe, T wave inverts
- U wave appears

C. Treatment
1. Identify and treat the underlying cause.
2. Discontinue any medications that can aggravate hypokalemia.

F I G U R E
8-4 Diagnostic evaluation of hypokalemia.

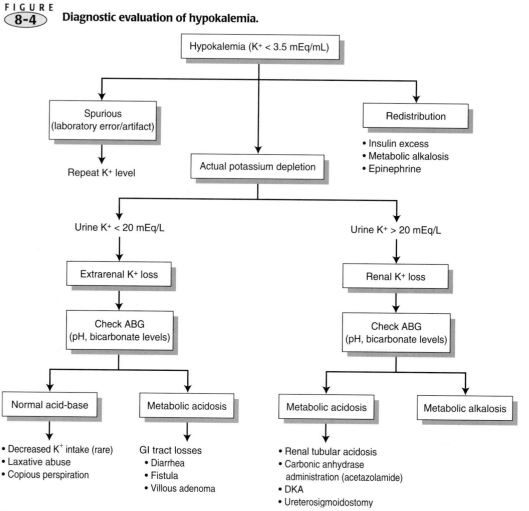

(Adapted from Humes DH, DuPont HL, Gardner LB, et al. Kelley's Textbook of Internal Medicine. 4th Ed. Philadelphia: Lippincott Williams & Wilkins, 2000:1165, Figure 146.2.)

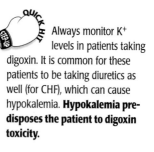

QUICK HIT

Always monitor K^+ levels in patients taking digoxin. It is common for these patients to be taking diuretics as well (for CHF), which can cause hypokalemia. **Hypokalemia predisposes the patient to digoxin toxicity.**

QUICK HIT

Hyperkalemia inhibits renal ammonia synthesis and reabsorption. Thus, net acid excretion is impaired and results in metabolic acidosis. This further exacerbates hyperkalemia due to K^+ movement out of cells.

3. Oral KCl is the preferred (safest) method of replacement and is appropriate in most instances. Always retest the K^+ levels after administration.
   a. Using 10 mEq of KCl increases K^+ levels by 0.1 mEq/L.
   b. It comes in slow-acting and fast-acting forms.
4. IV KCl can be given if the hypokalemia is severe (<2.5), or if the patient has arrhythmias secondary to the hypokalemia.
   a. Give slowly to avoid hyperkalemia.
   b. Monitor K^+ concentration and monitor cardiac rhythm when giving IV potassium.
   c. Infusion pearls
      • Maximum infusion rate of 10 mEq/hr in peripheral IV line
      • Maximum infusion rate of 20 mEq/hr in central line
      • May add 1% lidocaine to bag to decrease pain (potassium burns!)

Hyperkalemia

A. Causes

1. Increased total body potassium
   a. Renal failure (acute or chronic)
   b. Addison's disease
   c. Potassium-sparing diuretics (spironolactone)
   d. Hyporeninemic hypoaldosteronism
   e. ACE inhibitors

    f. Iatrogenic overdose—Exercise particular caution when administering potassium to patients with renal failure.

    g. Blood transfusion

2. Redistribution—translocation of potassium from intracellular to extracellular space

    a. Acidosis (not organic acidosis)

    b. Tissue/cell breakdown—rhabdomyolysis (muscle breakdown), hemolysis, burns

    c. GI bleeding

    d. Insulin deficiency—Insulin stimulates the Na^+-K^+-ATPase and causes K^+ to shift into cells. Therefore, insulin deficiency and hypertonicity (high glucose) promote K^+ shifts from ICF to ECF.

    e. Rapid administration of β-blocker

3. Pseudohyperkalemia (spurious)

    a. This refers to an artificially elevated plasma K^+ concentration due to K^+ movement out of cells immediately before or after venipuncture. Contributing factors include **prolonged use of a tourniquet with or without repeated fist clenching.** This can cause acidosis and subsequent K^+ loss from cells. Nevertheless, plasma (not serum) K^+ should be normal. (Repeat the test to confirm this.)

    b. Other contributing factors include leukocytosis, hemolysis, and thrombocytosis.

B. Clinical features

1. **Arrhythmias**—The most important effect of hyperkalemia is on the heart. Check an ECG immediately in a hyperkalemic patient.

2. Muscle weakness and (rarely) flaccid paralysis

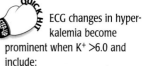 ECG changes in hyperkalemia become prominent when K^+ >6.0 and include:
- Peaked T waves (by 10 mm)
- A prolonged PR interval
- Widening of QRS and merging of QRS with T wave
- Ventricular fibrillation and cardiac arrest (with increasing levels of K^+)

FIGURE 8-5 Diagnostic evaluation of hyperkalemia.

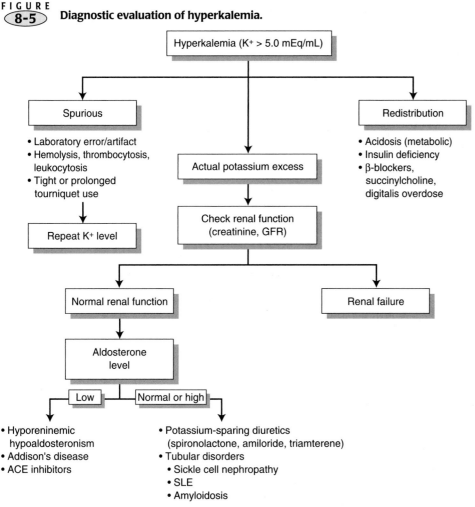

(Adapted from Humes DH, DuPont HL, Gardner LB, et al. Kelley's Textbook of Internal Medicine. 4th Ed. Philadelphia: Lippincott Williams & Wilkins, 2000:1168, Figure 147.1.)

3. Decreased deep tendon reflexes
4. Respiratory failure
5. Nausea/vomiting, intestinal colic, diarrhea

C. Treatment

1. If the hyperkalemia is severe, or if ECG changes are present, first give **IV calcium.**
   a. Calcium stabilizes the resting membrane potential of the myocardial membrane—i.e., it decreases membrane excitability.
   b. Use caution in giving calcium to patients on digoxin. (Hypercalcemia predisposes the patient to digoxin toxicity.)
2. Shift potassium into the intracellular compartment.
   a. **Glucose and insulin**—Glucose alone will stimulate insulin from β-cells, but exogenous insulin is more rapid. Give both to prevent hypoglycemia.
   b. Sodium bicarbonate
      • Increases pH level, which shifts K^+ into cells
      • An emergency measure in severe hyperkalemia
3. Remove potassium from the body.
   a. **Kayexalate**—GI potassium exchange resin (Na^+/K^+ exchange in GI tract), absorbs K^+ in the colon, preventing reabsorption (passed in stool)
   b. **Hemodialysis**
      • Most rapid and effective way of lowering plasma K^+
      • Reserved for intractable hyperkalemia and for those with renal failure
   c. Diuretics (furosemide)

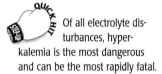

Of all electrolyte disturbances, hyperkalemia is the most dangerous and can be the most rapidly fatal.

MAGNESIUM

Overview

• Normal Mg^{2+} levels: 1.8 to 2.5 mg/dL
• **Location in the body**—Most of the magnesium in the body (two-thirds) is in bones. The remainder (one-third) is intracellular. Only 1% of magnesium is extracellular.
• **Influences on magnesium excretion**—Many hormones can alter urinary magnesium excretion (e.g., insulin/glucagons, PTH, calcitonin, ADH, and steroids).
• **Magnesium absorption and balance**
   • About 30% to 40% of dietary magnesium is absorbed in the GI tract, but this percentage increases when magnesium levels are low.
   • The kidney has a great capacity to reabsorb magnesium and is the major regulator of magnesium balance.

Hypomagnesemia

A. Causes

1. GI causes
   a. Malabsorption, steatorrheic states (most common cause)
   b. Prolonged fasting
   c. Fistulas
   d. Patients receiving TPN without Mg^{2+} supplementation
2. Alcoholism (common cause)
3. Renal causes
   a. SIADH
   b. Diuretics
   c. Bartter's syndrome
   d. Drugs: gentamicin, amphotericin B, cisplatin
   e. Renal transplantation
4. Other causes: postparathyroidectomy, DKA, thyrotoxicosis, lactation, burns, pancreatitis

Hypomagnesemia makes hypokalemia and hypocalcemia more difficult to treat.

FLUIDS, ELECTROLYTES, AND ACID-BASE DISORDERS

B. Clinical features

1. Marked neuromuscular and CNS hyperirritability
   a. Muscle twitching, weakness, tremors
   b. Hyperreflexia, seizures
   c. Mental status changes
2. Effect on calcium levels: **Coexisting hypocalcemia is common** because of decreased release of PTH and bone resistance to PTH when Mg^{2+} is low.
3. Effect on potassium levels
   a. **Coexisting hypokalemia**—in up to 50% of cases
   b. In muscle and myocardium, when either intracellular Mg^{2+} or K^+ decreases, a corresponding decrease in the other cation takes place.
4. ECG changes—prolonged QT interval, T wave flattening, and ultimately, torsade de pointes

C. Treatment

1. For mild hypomagnesemia—oral Mg^{2+} (e.g., magnesium oxide)
2. For severe hypomagnesemia—parenteral Mg^{2+} (e.g., magnesium sulfate)

Hypermagnesemia

A. Causes

1. Renal failure (most common cause)
2. Early-stage burns, massive trauma or surgical stress, severe ECF volume deficit, severe acidosis
3. Excessive intake of magnesium-containing laxatives or antacids combined with renal insufficiency
4. Adrenal insufficiency
5. Rhabdomyolysis
6. Iatrogenic—in the obstetric setting in women with preeclampsia or eclampsia

B. Clinical features

1. Nausea, weakness
2. Facial paresthesias
3. Progressive loss of deep tendon reflexes
4. ECG changes resemble those seen with hyperkalemia (increased P-R interval, widened QRS complex, and elevated T waves).
5. Somnolence leading to coma and muscular paralysis occur late.
6. Death is usually caused by respiratory failure or cardiac arrest.

C. Treatment

1. Withhold exogenously administered magnesium.
2. Prescribe IV calcium gluconate for emergent symptoms (cardioprotection).
3. Administer saline and furosemide.
4. Order dialysis in renal failure patients.

PHOSPHATE

Overview

- **Normal phosphate levels:** 3.0 to 4.5 mg/dL
- **Location in the body**—Most of the phosphorus is in the bones (85%); the remainder is intracellular in soft tissues (15%) and a very small amount (0.1%) in ECF.
- **Influence on phosphate absorption**—Vitamin D controls phosphorus absorption in the GI tract.
- **Phosphate excretion and balance**—PTH controls phosphorus excretion in the kidney— PTH increases renal phosphorus excretion by inhibiting reabsorption. The function of the kidney in maintaining phosphate balance is very important.

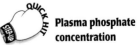

Plasma phosphate concentration
- Normal: 3.0 to 4.5 mg/dL
- **Hypo**phosphatemia: <2.5 mg/dL
- **Hyper**phosphatemia: >5 mg/dL

FLUIDS, ELECTROLYTES, AND ACID-BASE DISORDERS

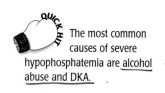

The most common causes of severe hypophosphatemia are <u>alcohol abuse</u> and <u>DKA.</u>

Hypophosphatemia

A. Causes

1. Decreased intestinal absorption due to alcohol abuse, vitamin D deficiency, malabsorption of phosphate, excessive use of phosphate-binding antacids, hyperalimentation (TPN), and/or starvation
2. <u>Increased renal excretion</u>
   a. Excess PTH states (vitamin D deficiency, hyperparathyroidism)
   b. Hyperglycemia (glycosuria), oncogenic osteomalacia, ATN, <u>renal tubular acidosis</u>, and so on
   c. Hypokalemia or hypomagnesemia
3. Other causes: respiratory alkalosis, anabolic steroids, severe hyperthermia DKA, hungry bones syndrome (deposition of bone material after parathyroidectomy)

B. Clinical features

1. None, if the hypophosphatemia is mild
2. Any of the following, if the hypophosphatemia is severe
   a. Neurologic: encephalopathy, confusion, seizures, numbness, paresthesias
   b. Musculoskeletal: muscular weakness, myalgias, bone pain, <u>rickets/osteomalacia</u>
   c. Hematologic: hemolysis, RBC dysfunction, WBC dysfunction, platelet dysfunction
   d. Cardiac: cardiomyopathy and myocardial depression secondary to low ATP levels, <u>may lead to cardiac arrest</u>
   e. Rhabdomyolysis
   f. Anorexia
   g. <u>Difficulty in ventilator weaning</u>

C. Treatment

1. If mild (>1 mg/dL), oral supplementation: <u>Neutra-Phos capsules, K-Phos tablets,</u> milk (excellent source of phosphate)
2. If severe/symptomatic or if patient is NPO: parenteral supplementation

Hyperphosphatemia

A. Causes

1. Decreased renal excretion of PO_4^{3-} due to renal insufficiency (most common cause), bisphosphonates, hypoparathyroidism, vitamin D intoxication, and/or tumor calcinosis
2. Increased phosphate administration (e.g., PO_4^{3-} repletion or PO_4^{3-} enemas)
3. Rhabdomyolysis, cell lysis, or acidosis (releases PO_4^{3-} into the ECF)

B. Clinical features

1. This results in metastatic calcification and soft-tissue calcifications; a calcium-phosphorus product (<u>serum calcium × serum phosphorus</u>) >70 indicates that calcification is likely to occur.
2. The associated hypocalcemia can lead to neurologic changes (tetany, neuromuscular irritability).

C. Treatment

1. Phosphate-binding antacids containing aluminum hydroxide or carbonate (bind phosphate in bowel and prevent its absorption)
2. Hemodialysis (if patient has renal failure)

ACID-BASE DISORDERS

Metabolic Acidosis

A. General characteristics

1. Metabolic acidosis is characterized by decreased blood pH and a decreased plasma bicarbonate concentration. The goal is to identify the underlying condition that is causing the metabolic acidosis.

[Handwritten margin notes:]
Renal insufficiency → MCC for hypermg²⁺ & hyperphosphatemia

could be caused by cocaine, vasoconstriction

↑PO₄²⁺ → ↓Ca²⁺ ↓ tetany Neuromuscular irritability

Box 8-2   Effects of Acidosis and Alkalosis

- **Acidosis**
  - Right shift in oxygen–hemoglobin dissociation curve diminishes affinity of hemoglobin for oxygen (so increases oxygen delivery to tissues)
  - Depresses CNS
  - Decreases pulmonary blood flow
  - Arrhythmias
  - Impairs myocardial function
  - Hyperkalemia —
- **Alkalosis** ($\uparrow HCO_3^-$)
  - Decreases cerebral blood flow
  - Left shift in oxygen–hemoglobin dissociation curve increases affinity of hemoglobin for oxygen (so decreases oxygen delivery to tissues)
  - Arrhythmias
  - Tetany, seizures   *b/c HCO₃ binds to Ca²⁺ → hypocalcemia → tetany.*

Lactic Acidosis   mild 2-5   severe >5
(1) Type A - tissue hypoperfusion mito don't have enough O₂ for aerobic glycosis → therefore anaerobic glycolysis.
(2) Type B - No clinical evidence of inadequate tissue O₂ delivery ex. Metformin.

---

2. Anion gap (AG)
   a. AG (mEq/L) = $[Na^+] - ([Cl^-] + [HCO^{3-}])$
   b. Reflects ions present in serum but unmeasured (i.e., proteins, phosphates, organic acids, sulfates)
   c. Normal values are 8 to 15 mEq/L, but this varies to some extent.
3. Pathophysiology
   a. When fixed acid (lactate) is added, the H^+ from fixed acid is buffered by the bicarbonate system. CO_2 is formed and removed by lungs. $H^+ + HCO_3^- \Leftrightarrow H_2CO_3 \Leftrightarrow H_2O + CO_2$. HCO_3^- levels decrease in ECF; therefore, kidneys reabsorb more HCO_3^- (new) to maintain pH.
   b. Three situations can arise.
      - The change in AG equals the change in HCO_3^- (see Figure 8-7A): simple metabolic acidosis—The addition of acid causes the AG to increase proportionally.
      - The change in AG is less than the change in HCO_3^- (see Figure 8-7B): **normal AG acidosis PLUS high AG acidosis**—If after the addition of acid, the HCO_3^- is lower than the calculated prediction, then you started with a lower HCO_3^-.
      - The change in AG is greater than the change in HCO_3^- (see Figure 8-7C): **metabolic alkalosis PLUS high AG acidosis**—When you have a high AG, the acid has to be buffered by HCO_3^-, so HCO_3^- decreases. If HCO_3^- does not decrease, it means you started at a higher HCO_3^-.

ΔAG/ΔHCO₃ → simple metabolic acidosis
ΔAG/ΔHCO₃ <1 → N'l AG acidosis + high AG acidosis
ΔAG/ΔHCO₃ >1 → Met. alkalosis + high AG acidosis

B. Causes
1. Increased AG acidosis
   a. Ketoacidosis
      - Diabetes mellitus
      - Prolonged starvation
      - Prolonged alcohol abuse
   b. Lactic acidosis—can occur in many different conditions
      - Low tissue perfusion (decreased oxygen delivery to tissues)   *b/c it goes to anaerobic glycolysis.*
      - Shock states (septic, cardiogenic, hypovolemic)
      - Excessive expenditure of energy (e.g., seizures)
   c. Renal failure—decreased NH_4^+ excretion (thus decreasing net acid)—Decreased excretion of organic anions, sulfate, and phosphate increases AG.
   d. Intoxication
      - Salicylate (aspirin)
      - Methanol
      - Ethylene glycol
2. Normal AG acidosis (hyperchloremic metabolic acidosis)—The low HCO_3^- is associated with high Cl^-, so that the AG remains normal
   a. Renal loss of bicarbonate

QUICK HIT The bicarbonate level obtained in a serum chemistry panel (venous CO_2) is a measured value (more reliable), whereas the level obtained in an arterial blood gas is a calculated value (less reliable).

QUICK HIT Salicylate overdose causes both primary respiratory alkalosis **and** primary metabolic acidosis.

FLUIDS, ELECTROLYTES, AND ACID-BASE DISORDERS

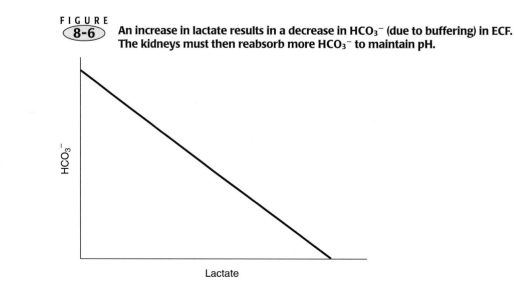

Box 8-3 Arterial Blood Gas Interpretation

- **CO₂ level**
  - If elevated, think of either respiratory acidosis or compensation for metabolic alkalosis.
  - If low, think of either respiratory alkalosis or compensation for metabolic acidosis.
- **HCO₃⁻ level**
  - If elevated, think of either metabolic alkalosis or compensation for respiratory acidosis.
  - If low, think of either metabolic acidosis or compensation for respiratory alkalosis.
  - The **base excess/base deficit** values in arterial blood gas indicate the amount of acid or base that is needed to titrate the plasma pH to 7.40 (with a Paco₂ of 40).

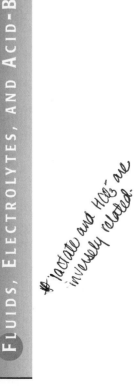

Na⁺
K⁺
K⁺ absorbed
HCO₃
Cl⁻

resulting in acidosis and hypokalemia.

- Proximal tubular acidosis—This is characterized by decreased HCO_3^- reabsorption. Causes include multiple myeloma, cystinosis, and Wilson's disease.
- Distal tubular acidosis—This is characterized by the inability to make HCO_3^-. Causes include SLE, Sjögren's syndrome, and taking amphotericin B.
- Carbonic anhydrase inhibition (e.g., acetazolamide—a diuretic)

b. GI loss of HCO_3^-
  - Diarrhea—HCO_3^- loss in diarrhea (**most common cause of non-AG acidosis**)
  - Pancreatic fistulas—pancreatic secretions contain high HCO_3^- levels
  - Small bowel fistulas
  - Ureterosigmoidostomy—colon secretes HCO_3^- in urine in exchange for Cl^-

done as a Rx. for bladder Ca s/p bladder removal, or for bladder exstrophy. but now more commonly performed ileal conduit.

C. Clinical features

1. Hyperventilation (deep rhythmic breathing), also known as Kussmaul's respiration
   a. This is a typical compensation (i.e., response) for a metabolic acidosis and is a cardinal feature of metabolic acidosis; it is usually seen in severe metabolic acidosis (pH < 7.20).
   b. It is less prominent when the acidosis is chronic.
2. Decreased cardiac output and decreased tissue perfusion
   a. Occurs with severe metabolic acidosis (blood pH <7.2)
   b. Acidosis diminishes tissue responsiveness to catecholamines. This can lead to an undesirable chain of events: poor tissue perfusion → lactic acidosis → decreased cardiac output → hypotension → further decrease in tissue perfusion.

lactate and HCO₃⁻ are inversely related.

FIGURE 8-6 An increase in lactate results in a decrease in HCO_3^- (due to buffering) in ECF. The kidneys must then reabsorb more HCO_3^- to maintain pH.

D. Diagnosis

1. History is important.
2. Calculate the AG.
3. Winter's formula: **expected $Paco_2$ = 1.5 (measured HCO_3^-) + 8 ± 2.**
   a. Predicts the expected respiratory compensation ($Paco_2$ level) to metabolic acidosis: If the $Paco_2$ does not fall within an acceptable range, then the patient has another primary acid-base disorder.

FIGURE 8-7

A. Simple metabolic acidosis. The change in AG is equal to the change in HCO_3^-. As you add acid, HCO_3^- decreases, and AG increases proportionately. **B.** Normal anion gap acidosis PLUS high anion gap acidosis. The change in AG is less than the change in HCO_3^-. If after the addition of acid, HCO_3^- is lower than predicted, then you started at a lower HCO_3^- level (*). **C.** Metabolic alkalosis plus high anion gap acidosis. The change in AG is less than the change in HCO_3^- If after the addition of acid, the *decrease* in HCO_3^- is less than expected, then you started at a higher HCO_3^- level (*).

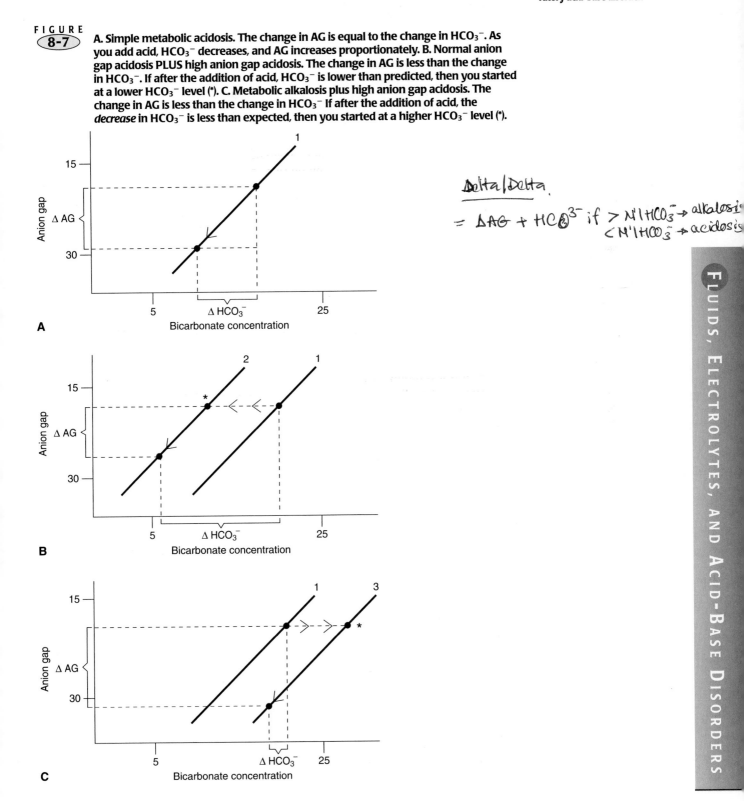

FLUIDS, ELECTROLYTES, AND ACID-BASE DISORDERS

Metabolic acidosis w/ respiratory acidosis → bad sign b/c failure of compensation → impending respiratory failure.

b. If the Pa_{CO_2} falls within the predicted range, then the patient has a simple metabolic acidosis with an appropriate secondary hypocapnia.

c. If the actual Pa_{CO_2} is higher than the calculated Pa_{CO_2}, then the patient has metabolic acidosis with respiratory acidosis. **This is a serious finding because this failure of compensation can be a sign of impending respiratory failure.**

d. If the actual Pa_{CO_2} is lower than the calculated Pa_{CO_2}, then the patient has metabolic acidosis with respiratory alkalosis.

E. Treatment

1. Treatment varies depending on the cause.
2. Sodium bicarbonate is sometimes needed (especially for normal AG acidosis). In correcting metabolic acidosis (correct severe acidosis to a pH of 7.20) realize that this HCO_3^- takes 24 hours to get to the brain. During this time, hyperventilation continues. Therefore, Pa_{CO_2} remains low while HCO_3^- is increasing—a dangerous combination ($[H^+] = 24\ [Pa_{CO_2} \div HCO_3^-]$).
3. Mechanical ventilation may be required if the patient is fatigued from prolonged hyperventilation, especially in DKA.

Metabolic Alkalosis

A. General characteristics

1. Metabolic alkalosis is characterized by an increased blood pH and plasma HCO_3^-.
2. Uncomplicated metabolic alkalosis is typically transient, because kidneys can normally excrete the excess HCO_3^-.
3. Consider two events in metabolic alkalosis:
   a. Event that initiates the metabolic alkalosis (loss of H^+ via gastric drainage, vomiting, and so on), or increased HCO_3^- concentration due to ECF volume contraction
   b. Mechanism that **maintains** the metabolic alkalosis due to the kidney's inability to excrete the excess HCO_3^-

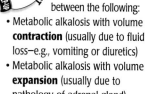

QUICK HIT In evaluating a patient with metabolic alkalosis, the first step is to determine whether the ECF volume has contracted or expanded, and why.

QUICK HIT Exogenous bicarbonate loading (administering bicarbonate) can cause metabolic alkalosis, but this usually occurs in ESRD.

B. Causes

1. Saline-sensitive metabolic alkalosis (urine chloride <10 mEq/L)—characterized by ECF contraction and hypokalemia
   a. Vomiting or nasogastric suction—When the patient loses HCl, gastric HCO_3^- generation occurs, which causes alkalosis.
   b. Diuretics—These decrease the ECF volume. Body HCO_3^- content remains normal, but plasma HCO_3^- increases because of ECF contraction.
   c. Villous adenoma of colon, diarrhea with high chloride content
2. Saline-resistant metabolic alkalosis (urine chloride >20 mEq/L)—characterized by ECF expansion and hypertension (due to increased mineralocorticoids)
   a. Most are secondary to adrenal disorders (primary hyperaldosteronism). Increased levels of mineralocorticoid secretion lead to increased tubular reabsorption of Na^+ and HCO_3^-, and an excessive loss of Cl^- in the urine. The result is metabolic alkalosis and expansion of the ECF compartment (because of increased Na^+ reabsorption).
   b. Other causes include Cushing's syndrome, severe K^+ deficiency, Bartter's syndrome, and diuretic abuse.

QUICK HIT It is useful to distinguish between the following:
- Metabolic alkalosis with volume **contraction** (usually due to fluid loss—e.g., vomiting or diuretics)
- Metabolic alkalosis with volume **expansion** (usually due to pathology of adrenal gland)
An easy way to make this distinction is via the chloride concentration in the urine.

C. Clinical features

1. There are no characteristic signs or symptoms.
2. The patient's medical history is most helpful (look for vomiting, gastric drainage, diuretic therapy, and so on).

D. Diagnosis

1. Elevated HCO_3^- level, elevated blood pH
2. Hypokalemia is common (due to renal loss of K^+).
3. Pa_{CO_2} is elevated as a compensatory mechanism (due to hypoventilation). It is rare for a compensatory increase in Pa_{CO_2} to exceed 50 to 55 mm Hg (the respiratory rate

to achieve this is so low that PaO_2 would be decreased). A higher value implies a superimposed respiratory acidosis.

4. The urine chloride level is very important in distinguishing between saline-sensitive and saline-resistant types.

Always order urine Cl^- when have a pt. w/ metabolic alkalosis. b/c treatment differs b/n saline sensitive and saline resistant.

E. Treatment

1. Treat the underlying disorder that caused the metabolic alkalosis.
2. Normal saline plus potassium will restore the ECF volume if the patient is volume contracted.
3. Address the underlying cause (or prescribe spironolactone) if the patient is volume expanded.

Respiratory Acidosis

A. General characteristics

1. Defined as a reduced blood pH and $PaCO_2$ >40 mm Hg
2. Renal compensation (increased reabsorption of HCO_3^-) begins within 12 to 24 hours and takes 5 days or so to complete.
   a. Acute respiratory acidosis
      - There is an immediate compensatory elevation of HCO_3^-.
      - There is an increase of 1 mmol/L for every 10 mm Hg increase in $PaCO_2$.
   b. Chronic respiratory acidosis
      - Renal adaptation occurs, and HCO_3^- increases by 4 mmol/L for every 10 mm Hg increase in $PaCO_2$.
      - This is generally seen in patients with underlying lung disease, such as chronic obstructive pulmonary disease (COPD).

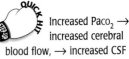 **QUICK HIT** Any disorder that reduces CO_2 clearance (i.e., inhibits adequate ventilation) can lead to respiratory acidosis.

COPD → mainly ventilatory defect. Pneumonias → Lung involvement → problem w/ hypoxemia → ↑ A-a gradient.

B. Causes—alveolar hypoventilation

1. Primary pulmonary diseases—e.g., COPD, airway obstruction
2. Neuromuscular diseases—e.g., myasthenia gravis
3. CNS malfunction—injury to brainstem
4. Drug-induced hypoventilation (e.g., from morphine, anesthetics, or sedatives)—Narcotic overdose in postoperative patients is a possibility (look for pinpoint pupils).
5. Respiratory muscle fatigue

C. Clinical features

1. Somnolence, confusion, and myoclonus with asterixis
2. Headaches, confusion, and papilledema are signs of acute CO_2 retention.

↑ CO_2 → CNS BV vasodilation.

QUICK HIT Increased $PaCO_2$ → increased cerebral blood flow, → increased CSF pressure, which results in generalized CNS depression.

D. Treatment

1. Verify patency of the airway.
2. If PaO_2 is low (<60 mm Hg), initiate supplemental oxygen. **Caution:** In patients who are "CO_2 retainers" (e.g., COPD patients), oxygen can exacerbate the respiratory acidosis, so administer oxygen judiciously. (See the discussion under Acute Respiratory Failure in Chapter 2.)
3. Correct reversible causes.
4. Any measure to improve alveolar ventilation
   a. Aggressive pulmonary toilet
   b. Correct reversible pulmonary disease (e.g., treat pneumonia).
   c. Remove obstruction.
   d. If there is drug-induced hypoventilation, clear the agent from the body (**naloxone!**).
   e. Administer bronchodilators.
5. Intubation and mechanical ventilation may be necessary to relieve the acidemia and hypoxia that result from hypoventilation. The following situations require intubation:
   a. Severe acidosis
   b. $PaCO_2$ >60 or inability to increase PaO_2 with supplemental oxygen
   c. If patient is obtunded or shows deterioration in mental status
   d. Impending respiratory fatigue (ensues with prolonged labored breathing)

Respiratory Alkalosis

A. General characteristics

1. Characterized by an increased blood pH and decreased Pa_{CO_2}
2. In order to maintain blood pH within the normal range, HCO_3 must decrease, so renal compensation occurs (i.e., HCO_3^- excretion increases). However, this does not occur acutely, but rather over the course of several hours.
   a. Acutely, for each 10 mm Hg decrease in Pa_{CO_2}, plasma HCO_3^- decreases by 2 mEq/L and blood pH increases by 0.08 mEq/L.
   b. Chronically, for each 10 mm Hg decrease in Pa_{CO_2}, plasma HCO_3^- decreases by 5 to 6 mEq/L and blood pH decreases by 0.02 mEq/L.

B. Causes—alveolar hyperventilation

1. Anxiety
2. Pulmonary embolism, pneumonia, asthma
3. Sepsis
4. Hypoxia—leads to increased respiratory rate
5. Mechanical ventilation
6. Pregnancy—Increased serum progesterone levels cause hyperventilation.
7. Liver disease (cirrhosis)
8. Medication (salicylate toxicity)
9. Hyperventilation syndrome

C. Clinical features

1. Symptoms are mostly related to decreased cerebral blood flow (vasoconstriction): lightheadedness, dizziness, anxiety, paresthesias, and perioral numbness.
2. Tetany (indistinguishable from hypocalcemia)
3. Arrhythmias (in severe cases)

D. Treatment

1. Correct the underlying cause.
2. Sometimes this does not need to be treated (e.g., in the case of pregnancy).
3. An inhaled mixture containing CO_2 or breathing into a paper bag may be useful.

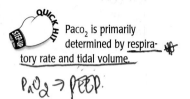

QUICK HIT

Pa_{CO_2} is primarily determined by respiratory rate and tidal volume.

$Pa_{O_2} \rightarrow PEEP$.

QUICK HIT

Any disorder that increases the respiratory rate inappropriately can lead to respiratory alkalosis.

CHAPTER 9

Hematologic Diseases and Neoplasms

ANEMIAS

Basics of Anemia

A. General characteristics

1. Anemia is defined as a reduction in Hct or Hb concentration.
2. When red cell mass (as measured by Hb or less precisely by Hct) decreases, several compensatory mechanisms maintain oxygen delivery to the tissues. These mechanisms include:
   a. Increased cardiac output (heart rate and stroke volume)
   b. Increased extraction ratio
   c. Rightward shift of the oxyhemoglobin curve (increased 2,3-diphosphoglycerate [2,3-DPG])
   d. Expansion of plasma volume
3. As a general rule, blood transfusion is not recommended unless either of the following is true.
   a. The Hb concentration is <7 g/dL, *OR*
   b. The patient requires increased oxygen-carrying capacity (e.g., patients with coronary artery disease or some other cardiopulmonary disease).
4. If anemia develops rapidly, symptoms are more likely to be present, because there is little time for compensatory mechanisms. When onset is gradual, compensatory mechanisms are able to maintain oxygen delivery, and symptoms may be minimal or absent.

B. Clinical features

1. A variety of nonspecific complaints—headache, fatigue, poor concentration, diarrhea, nausea, vague abdominal discomfort
2. Pallor—best noted in the conjunctiva
3. Hypotension and tachycardia
4. Signs of the underlying cause—jaundice if hemolytic anemia, blood in stool if GI bleeding

C. Diagnosis

1. Hb and Hct
   a. Formula for converting Hb to Hct: Hb × 3 = Hct (1 unit of packed RBCs (PRBCs) increases Hb level by 1 point, and Hct by 3 points)
   b. If the patient has good cardiac function and intravascular volume is adequate, low Hb and Hct levels are tolerated—even an Hb of 7 or 8 provides sufficient oxygen-carrying capacity for most patients. However, anemia is not tolerated as well in patients with impaired cardiac function.

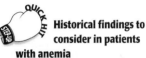

Historical findings to consider in patients with anemia
- Family history of hemophilia, G6PD deficiency, thalassemia
- Bleeding (melena, recent trauma/surgery, hematemesis)
- Chronic illnesses (e.g., renal failure)
- Alcoholism (folate, vitamin B$_{12}$, iron deficiency)

 # most likely to see bx if acute anemia.

Pseudoanemia refers to a decrease in hemoglobin and hematocrit secondary to dilution (i.e., secondary to acute volume infusion or overload).

Box 9-1 Transfusion Pearls

- PRBCs (contains no platelets or clotting factors)
  - Mix with normal saline to infuse faster (not with lactated Ringer's solution because calcium causes coagulation within the IV line).
  - Each unit raises the hematocrit by 3 to 4 points.
  - Typically administered in 2 units—each unit may be given to an adult over 90 to 120 minutes.
  - Always check CBC after the transfusion is completed.
- Fresh frozen plasma (FFP)   *only clotting factors*
  - Contains all of the clotting factors
  - Contains **no** RBCs/WBCs/platelets
  - Given for high PT/PTT, coagulopathy, and deficiency of clotting factors – FFP can be given if you cannot wait for Vitamin K to take effect, or if patient has liver failure (in which case Vitamin K will not work).
  - Follow up PT and PTT to assess response
- Cryoprecipitate
  - Contains factor VIII and fibrinogen
  - For hemophilia A, decreased fibrinogen (DIC), and vWD
- Platelet transfusions—1 unit raises platelet count by 10,000
- Whole blood only for massive blood loss (rarely used)

---

2. Reticulocyte index
   a. The reticulocyte count is an important initial test in evaluating anemia because it indicates whether effective erythropoiesis is occurring in the bone marrow. Effective erythropoiesis is dependent on adequate raw materials (iron, vitamin B_{12}, folate) in the bone marrow, absence of intrinsic bone marrow disease (e.g., aplastic anemia), adequate erythropoietin from the kidney, and survival of reticulocytes (no premature destruction before leaving the bone marrow).
   b. A reticulocyte index >2% implies excessive RBC destruction or loss. The bone marrow is responding to increased RBC requirements.
   c. A reticulocyte index <2% implies inadequate RBC production by the bone marrow.
3. Blood smear and RBC indices (especially mean corpuscular volume [MCV])—see below

QUICK HIT

Note that all causes of anemia are initially normocytic because it takes some time for the abnormal-sized RBCs to outnumber the normal-sized ones.

Box 9-2 Hemolytic Transfusion Reactions Are Divided Into Intravascular and Extravascular Hemolysis

- **Intravascular hemolysis** (also called acute hemolytic reactions)   *Acute*
  - Very serious and life threatening—This is caused by ABO-mismatched blood transfused into patient. (Usually due to clerical error.) For example, if B blood is given to a type A patient, anti-B IgM antibodies attach to all of the infused B RBCs, they activate a complement pathway, and produce a massive intravascular hemolysis as C9 punches holes through RBC membranes.
  - Symptoms include fever/chills, nausea/vomiting, pain in the flanks/back, chest pain, and dyspnea.
  - Complications include hypovolemic shock (hypotension, tachycardia), DIC, and renal failure with hemoglobinuria.
  - Management involves stopping the transfusion immediately and aggressively replacing the fluid to avoid shock and renal failure.
- **Extravascular hemolysis** (also called delayed hemolytic transfusion reaction)   *Delayed*
  - Extravascular hemolysis is less severe and in most cases is self-limited; it may occur within 3 to 4 weeks after a transfusion.
  - It is caused by one of the minor RBC antigens. For example, if a patient is Kell antigen-negative and has anti-Kell IgG antibodies from a previous exposure to the antigen, reexposure of her memory B cells to Kell antigen on RBCs will result in synthesis of IgG anti-Kell antibodies. These antibodies coat all of the Kell antigen-positive donor RBCs, which will be removed extravascularly by macrophages in the spleen, liver, and bone marrow.
  - Symptoms are subtle and include fever, jaundice, and anemia.
  - Management: None. The prognosis is good.

D. Diagnosing the cause of anemia (general approach) (see Figure 9-1)

1. If the reticulocyte index <2, examine the smear and RBC indices.

   a. If microcytic anemia (MCV < 80), the differential diagnosis includes the following:
   - **Iron deficiency anemia—most common cause**
   - Anemia of chronic disease—Iron is present in the body but is not available for hemoglobin synthesis (iron trapping in macrophages).
   - Thalassemias—defective synthesis of globin chains
   - Ring sideroblastic anemias (includes lead poisoning, pyridoxine deficiency, toxic effects of alcohol)—This is a defective synthesis of protoporphyrins. Iron accumulates in mitochondria.

   b. If macrocytic anemia (MCV >100), the differential diagnosis includes the following:
   - Nuclear defect (MCV increases significantly)—vitamin B_{12} deficiency and folate deficiency
   - Liver disease (MCV increases up to 115)—due to altered metabolism of plasma lipoproteins into their membranes, altering RBC shape (and increasing volume)
   - Stimulated erythropoiesis (MCV increases up to 110)—Reticulocytes are larger than mature RBCs, resulting in an increase in polychromatophilic RBCs.

liver dx— also causes macrocytic anemia.

FIGURE 9-1 Evaluation of anemia.

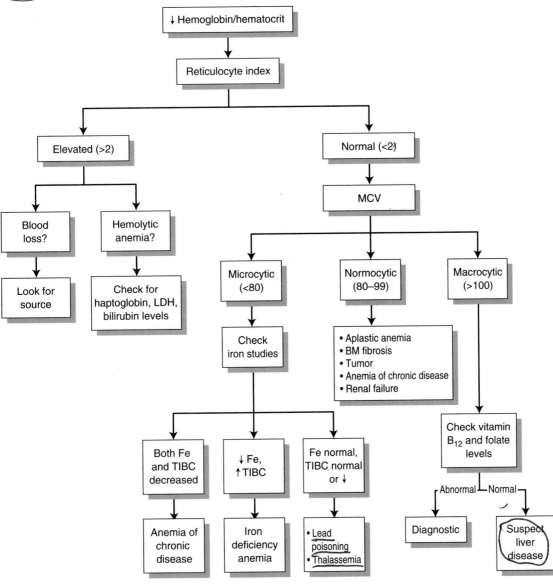

In an anemic patient, the first step is to assess volume status and hemodynamic stability. If unstable, transfuse PRBCs before attempting to find the cause of the anemia.

first ⇒ stabilize the patient.

In elderly patients with iron deficiency anemia, you must rule out colon cancer.

c. If normocytic anemia, the differential diagnosis includes the following:
- Aplastic anemia
- Bone marrow fibrosis
- Tumor
- Anemia of chronic disease (chronic inflammation, malignancy)
- Renal failure (decreased erythropoietin production)

2. If the reticulocyte index >2, do the following.
   a. Suspect acute blood loss—look for the source of the bleeding.
   b. Suspect hemolysis (see below).

Microcytic Anemias

Iron Deficiency Anemia

A. Causes
1. Most common cause of anemia worldwide
2. Causes
   a. Chronic blood loss
      - Most common cause of iron deficiency anemia in adults
      - Menstrual blood loss is the most common source. **In the absence of menstrual bleeding, GI blood loss is most likely.**
   b. Dietary deficiency/increased iron requirements—primarily seen in these three age groups:
      - **Infants and toddlers**—Occurs especially if the diet is predominantly human milk (low in iron). Children in this age group also have an increased requirement for iron because of accelerated growth. It is most common between 6 months and 3 years of age.
      - **Adolescents**—Rapid growth increases iron requirements. Adolescent women are particularly at risk due to loss of menstrual blood.
      - **Pregnant women**—Pregnancy increases iron requirements.

B. Clinical features
1. Pallor
2. Fatigue, generalized weakness
3. Dyspnea on exertion
4. Orthostatic lightheadedness
5. Hypotension, if acute
6. Tachycardia

C. Diagnosis
1. Laboratory tests (see Table 9-1)
   a. Decreased serum ferritin—most reliable test available
   b. Increased TIBC
   c. Elevated transferrin levels
   d. Decreased serum iron
   e. Microcytic, hypochromic RBCs on peripheral smear (see Color Figure 9-1)

TABLE 9-1	Iron Studies in Microcytic Anemias			
	Serum Ferritin	Serum Iron	TIBC	RDW
Iron deficiency anemia	Low	Low	High	High
Anemia of chronic disease	Normal/high	Low	Normal/low	Normal
Thalassemia	Normal/high	Normal/high	Normal	Normal/high

2. Bone marrow biopsy—the gold standard, but rarely performed. Indicated if laboratory evidence of iron deficiency anemia is present and no source of blood loss is found.

3. Guaiac stool test—if GI bleeding is suspected.

D. Treatment

1. Oral iron replacement (ferrous sulfate)
   a. A trial should be given to a menstruating woman. However, in men and post-menopausal women with iron deficiency anemia, attempt to determine the source of blood loss.
   b. Side effects include constipation, nausea, and dyspepsia.

2. Parenteral iron replacement
   a. Iron dextran can be administered IV or IM.
   b. This is rarely necessary because most patients respond to oral iron therapy. It may be useful in patients with poor absorption, patients who require more iron than oral therapy can provide, or patients who cannot tolerate oral ferrous sulfate.

3. Blood transfusion is **not** recommended unless anemia is severe or the patient has cardiopulmonary disease.

Thalassemias

A. General characteristics

1. Inherited disorders characterized by inadequate production of either the α- or β-globin chain of hemoglobin

2. They are classified according to the chain that is deficient.

3. β-thalassemias
   a. β-chain production is deficient, but the synthesis of α-chains is unaffected.
   b. Excess α-chains bind to and damage the RBC membrane.
   c. It is most often found in people of Mediterranean, Middle Eastern, and Indian ancestry.
   d. Severity varies with different mutations.

4. α-thalassemias
   a. There is a decrease in α-chains, which are a component of all types of hemoglobins.
   b. The β-globin chains form tetramers, which are abnormal hemoglobins.
   c. The severity depends on the number of gene loci that are deleted/mutated—it ranges from an asymptomatic carrier state to prenatal death.

B. β-Thalassemias

1. Thalassemia major (Cooley's anemia; homozygous β-chain thalassemia)—occurs predominantly in Mediterranean populations
   a. Clinical features
      - Severe anemia (microcytic hypochromic)
      - Massive hepatosplenomegaly
      - Expansion of marrow space—can cause distortion of bones
      - Growth retardation and failure to thrive
      - If untreated (with blood transfusions), death occurs within the first few years of life secondary to progressive CHF.
   b. Diagnosis
      - Hemoglobin electrophoresis—**Hb F is elevated.**
      - Peripheral blood smear—**microcytic hypochromic anemia**
   c. Treatment—Frequent PRBC transfusions are required to sustain life.

2. Thalassemia minor (heterozygous β-chain thalassemia)
   a. Clinical features: Patients are usually asymptomatic. A mild microcytic, hypochromic anemia is the only symptom.
   b. Diagnosis: hemoglobin electrophoresis
   c. Treatment: usually not necessary (Patients are not transfusion-dependent.)

The MCH and MCHC are of little value clinically. They are neither sensitive nor specific for any diagnosis. However, mean corpuscular volume (MCV) is very valuable in diagnosing the cause of anemia.

The RDW measures the variation in RBC size. The RDW is usually abnormal in iron deficiency, but is generally normal in all of the other microcytic anemias.

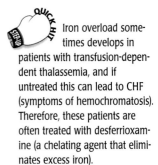

Iron overload sometimes develops in patients with transfusion-dependent thalassemia, and if untreated this can lead to CHF (symptoms of hemochromatosis). Therefore, these patients are often treated with desferrioxamine (a chelating agent that eliminates excess iron).

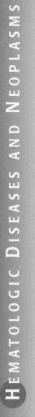

QUICK HIT

If iron deficiency anemia is suspected, but the anemia does not respond to iron therapy, obtain a hemoglobin electrophoresis to rule out α- and β-thalassemia.

QUICK HIT

The most common type of thalassemia is thalassemia minor (β-thalassemia minor is more common than α-thalassemia minor). Both of these conditions can be mistaken for iron deficiency.

3. Thalassemia intermedia
   a. Usually involves both β-globin genes
   b. Severity of anemia is intermediate.
   c. Patients usually are not transfusion-dependent.

C. α-thalassemias
   1. Silent carriers—mutation/deletion of only one α locus
      a. Asymptomatic
      b. Normal hemoglobin and hematocrit level
      c. No treatment necessary
   2. α-thalassemia trait (or minor)—mutation/deletion of two α loci
      a. Characterized by mild microcytic hypochromic anemia
      b. Common in African-American patients
      c. No treatment necessary
   3. Hb H disease—mutation/deletion of three α loci
      a. Hemolytic anemia, splenomegaly
      b. Significant microcytic, hypochromic anemia
      c. Hemoglobin electrophoresis shows Hb H.
      d. Treatment is often the same as for patients with β-thalassemia major. Splenectomy is sometimes helpful.
   4. Mutation/deletion of all four α loci—This is either fatal at birth (hydrops fetalis) or shortly after birth.

Sideroblastic Anemia

- Caused by abnormality in RBC iron metabolism
- Hereditary or acquired—Acquired causes include drugs (chloramphenicol, INH, alcohol), exposure to lead, collagen vascular disease, and neoplastic disease (myelodysplastic syndromes).
- Clinical findings: increased serum iron and ferritin, normal TIBC; ringed sideroblasts in bone marrow
- Treatment: Remove offending agents. Consider pyridoxine.

Normocytic Anemias

Anemia of Chronic Disease

- Occurs in the setting of chronic infection (e.g., tuberculosis, lung abscess), cancer (e.g., lung, breast, Hodgkin's disease), inflammation (rheumatoid arthritis, systemic lupus erythematosus [SLE]), or trauma. The release of inflammatory cytokines has a suppressive effect on erythropoiesis.
- It may be difficult to differentiate from iron deficiency anemia.
- Laboratory findings: Low serum iron, low TIBC, and low serum transferrin levels occur. Serum ferritin levels are increased.
- The anemia is usually normocytic and normochromic, but may be microcytic and hypochromic as well.
  - No specific treatment is necessary other than treatment of the underlying process. Do not give iron. The anemia is usually mild and well-tolerated.

Aplastic Anemia

A. General characteristics
   1. Bone marrow failure leading to **pancytopenia** (anemia, neutropenia, thrombocytopenia)
   2. Causes
      a. Idiopathic—majority of cases
      b. Radiation exposure
      c. Medications—e.g., chloramphenicol, sulfonamides, gold, carbamazepine
      d. Viral infection—e.g., human parvovirus, hepatitis C, hepatitis B, Epstein-Barr virus (EBV), cytomegalovirus, herpes zoster varicella, HIV
      e. Chemicals—e.g., benzene, insecticides

B. Clinical features
1. Symptoms of anemia—fatigue, dyspnea
2. Signs and symptoms of thrombocytopenia—e.g., petechiae, easy bruising
3. Increased incidence of infections (due to neutropenia)
4. Can transform into acute leukemia

C. Diagnosis
1. Normocytic, normochromic anemia
2. Perform a bone marrow biopsy for definitive diagnosis—this reveals hypocellular marrow and the absence of progenitors of all three hematopoietic cell lines.

D. Treatment
1. Bone marrow transplantation
2. Transfusion of PRBCs and platelets, if necessary (use judiciously)
3. Immunosuppression

Macrocytic Anemias

Vitamin B₁₂ Deficiency

A. General characteristics
1. Vitamin B_{12} is involved in two important reactions.
   a. As a cofactor in conversion of homocysteine to methionine
   b. As a cofactor in conversion of methylmalonyl CoA to succinyl CoA
2. Vitamin B_{12} stores in the liver are plentiful, and can sustain an individual for 3 or more years.
3. The main dietary sources of vitamin B_{12} are meat and fish.
4. Vitamin B_{12} is bound to intrinsic factor (produced by gastric parietal cells), so it can be absorbed by the terminal ileum.

B. Causes (almost all cases are due to impaired absorption)
1. Pernicious anemia (lack of intrinsic factor)—most common cause in the Western hemisphere
2. Gastrectomy
3. Poor diet (e.g., strict vegetarianism); alcoholism
4. Crohn's disease, ileal resection (terminal ileum)
5. Other organisms competing for vitamin B_{12}
   a. *Diphyllobothrium latum* infestation (fish tapeworm)
   b. Blind-loop syndrome (bacterial overgrowth)

Pernicious anemia is a special case of vitamin B_{12} deficiency. It is an autoimmune disorder resulting in inadequate production of intrinsic factor, which leads to impaired absorption of vitamin B_{12} in the terminal ileum.

C. Clinical features
1. Anemia
2. Sore tongue (stomatitis and glossitis)
3. Neuropathy—can distinguish between vitamin B_{12} deficiency and folate deficiency
   a. Demyelination in posterior columns, in lateral corticospinal tracts and spinocerebellar tracts—leads to a loss of position/vibratory sensation in lower extremities, ataxia, and upper motor neuron signs (increased deep tendon reflexes, spasticity, weakness, Babinski sign)
   b. Can lead to urinary and fecal incontinence, impotence
   c. Can lead to dementia—Investigate in the workup for dementia.

In a patient with megaloblastic anemia, always try to determine whether folate or vitamin B_{12} deficiency is the cause, because folate supplements can improve the anemia of vitamin B_{12} deficiency, but not the neurologic impairment. Therefore, **if the vitamin B_{12} deficiency remains untreated, irreversible neurologic disease can result.**

D. Diagnosis
1. Peripheral blood smear
   a. Megaloblastic anemia—macrocytic RBCs (MCV >100)
   b. Hypersegmented neutrophils (see Color Figure 9-1)
2. Serum vitamin B_{12} level is low (<100 pg/mL)
3. Serum methylmalonic acid and homocysteine levels—These are elevated in vitamin B_{12} deficiency and are useful if the vitamin B_{12} level is borderline.

Note that patients with vitamin B_{12} deficiency can have moderate to severe neurologic symptoms with little to no anemia (i.e., blood counts may be normal). Delay in diagnosis and treatment may lead to irreversible neurologic disease.

The serum homocysteine level is increased in both folate deficiency and vitamin B_{12} deficiency. However, serum methylmalonic acid levels are only increased with vitamin B_{12} deficiency.

4. Perform a Schilling test—provides information regarding the cause of the vitamin B_{12} deficiency
   a. Give an IM dose of unlabeled vitamin B_{12} to saturate binding sites.
   b. Give an oral dose of radioactive vitamin B_{12}; measure the amount of vitamin B_{12} in urine and plasma to determine how much vitamin B_{12} was absorbed.
   c. Repeat the test (oral radioactive vitamin B_{12}) with the addition of intrinsic factor. If malabsorption is the problem, adding intrinsic factor will not do anything. However, if pernicious anemia is present, adding intrinsic factor will improve serum vitamin B_{12} levels.

E. Treatment: Parenteral therapy is preferred—cyanocobalamin (vitamin B12) IM once per month

Folate Deficiency

A. General characteristics
1. Folic acid stores are limited. Inadequate intake of folate over a 3-month period can lead to deficiency.
2. Green vegetables are the main source of folate. Overcooking of vegetables can remove folate.

B. Causes
1. Inadequate dietary intake such as "tea and toast" (most common cause)
2. Alcoholism
3. Long-term use of oral antibiotics
4. Increased demand
5. Pregnancy
6. Hemolysis
7. Use of folate antagonists such as methotrexate
8. Anticonvulsant medications (phenytoin)
9. Hemodialysis

C. Clinical features: similar to those in vitamin B_{12} deficiency without the neurologic symptoms

D. Treatment: daily oral folic acid replacement

Hemolytic Anemias

Overview

A. General characteristics
1. Premature destruction of RBCs that may be due to a variety of causes
2. Bone marrow is normal and responds appropriately by increasing erythropoiesis, leading to an elevated reticulocyte count. However, if erythropoiesis cannot keep up with the destruction of RBCs, anemia results.
3. Hemolytic anemia can be acute or chronic with a corresponding variation in clinical features.
4. Hemolytic anemias can be classified based on mechanism, as follows:
   a. Hemolysis due to factors external to RBC defects—**most cases are acquired**
      • Immune hemolysis
      • Mechanical hemolysis (e.g., prosthetic heart valves, microangiopathic hemolytic anemia)
      • Medications, burns, toxins (e.g., from a snake bite or brown recluse spider); infection (malaria, clostridium), and so on
   b. Hemolysis due to intrinsic RBC defects—**most cases are inherited**
      • Hemoglobin abnormality: sickle cell anemia, hemoglobin C disease, thalassemias

- Membrane defects: hereditary spherocytosis, paroxysmal nocturnal hemoglobinuria
- Enzyme defects: glucose-6-phosphate dehydrogenase (G6PD) deficiency, pyruvate kinase deficiency

5. Hemolytic anemias can be classified based on the predominant site of hemolysis, as follows:
   a. Intravascular hemolysis—within the circulation
   b. Extravascular hemolysis—within the reticuloendothelial system, primarily the spleen

B. Clinical features

1. Signs and symptoms of anemia
2. Signs and symptoms of underlying disease (e.g., bone crises in sickle cell disease)
3. Jaundice
4. Dark urine color (due to hemoglobinuria, not bilirubin) may be present. This indicates an intravascular process.
5. Hepatosplenomegaly, cholelithiasis, lymphadenopathy (in chronic cases)

C. Diagnosis

1. Hb/Hct—level depends on degree of hemolysis and reticulocytosis
2. Elevated reticulocyte count due to increased RBC production
3. Peripheral smear
   a. Schistocytes suggest intravascular hemolysis ("trauma" or mechanical hemolysis) (see Color Figure 9-2).
   b. Spherocytes or helmet cells suggest extravascular hemolysis (depending on the cause).
   c. Sickled RBCs—sickle cell anemia
   d. Heinz bodies in G6PD deficiency
4. Haptoglobin levels—**low** in hemolytic anemias (especially intravascular hemolysis). Haptoglobin binds to hemoglobin, so its absence means that hemoglobin was destroyed.
5. LDH level is elevated—LDH is released when RBCs are destroyed.
6. Elevated indirect (unconjugated) bilirubin levels due to degradation of heme because RBCs are destroyed
7. Direct Coombs test (detects antibody or complement on RBC membrane)—positive in autoimmune hemolytic anemia
8. Osmotic fragility—see below

D. Treatment

1. Treat underlying cause.
2. Transfusion of PRBCs if severe anemia is present or patient is hemodynamically compromised.
3. Folate supplements (folate is depleted in hemolysis)

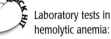
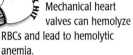
The following are relevant in the history of a patient with hemolytic anemia: ethnic background, family history of jaundice/anemia, medications.

Mechanical heart valves can hemolyze RBCs and lead to hemolytic anemia.

Laboratory tests in hemolytic anemia:
- Elevated reticulocyte count, LDH
- Decreased haptoglobin and hemoglobin/hematocrit

Physical injury to RBCs leads to the presence of fragmented RBCs called **schistocytes** and **helmet cells** on the blood smear. This can occur in TTP, DIC, and patients with prosthetic heart valves.

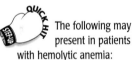
The following may present in patients with hemolytic anemia:
- Jaundice, increased bilirubin
- Decreased haptoglobin
- Increased LDH

Box 9-3 Almost Every Organ Can Be Involved in Sickle Cell Disease

- Blood—chronic hemolytic anemia, aplastic crises
- Heart—high-output CHF due to anemia
- CNS—stroke
- GI tract—gallbladder disease (stones), splenic infarctions, abdominal crises
- Bones—painful crises, osteomyelitis, avascular necrosis
- Lungs—infections, acute chest syndrome
- Kidneys—hematuria, papillary necrosis, renal failure
- Eyes—proliferative retinopathy, retinal infarcts
- Genitalia—priapism

Sickle Cell Anemia

A. General characteristics

1. Causes
   a. **Autosomal recessive** disorder that results when the normal Hb A is replaced by the mutant Hb S. Sickle cell disease is caused by inheritance of two Hb S genes (homozygous).
   b. Hb S may be distinguished from Hb A by electrophoresis because of the substitution of an uncharged valine for a negatively charged glutamic acid at the 6th position of the β-chain.
   c. Under reduced oxygen conditions (e.g., acidosis, hypoxia, changes in temperature, dehydration, and infection) the Hb molecules polymerize, causing the RBCs to sickle. Sickled RBCs obstruct small vessels, leading to ischemia.
2. Sickle cell trait
   a. About 1 in 12 people of African descent carry the sickle cell trait; they are heterozygous. The sickle cell trait also appears in Italians, Greeks, and Saudi Arabians.
   b. Patients with sickle cell trait are not anemic and have a normal life expectancy.
3. Screening can identify asymptomatic carriers (sickle cell trait), for whom genetic counseling may be provided.
4. Prognosis
   a. Survival correlates with the frequency of vaso-occlusive crises—more frequent crises are associated with a shorter lifespan.
   b. If there are more than three crises per year, the median age of death is 35 years. Patients with fewer crises per year may live into their 50s.
   c. In general, sickle cell disease reduces life expectancy by 25 to 30 years.

B. Clinical features

1. Severe, lifelong **hemolytic anemia**
   a. Jaundice, pallor
   b. Gallstone disease (very common)—pigmented gallstones
   c. The anemia itself is well compensated and is rarely transfusion dependent.
   d. High-output heart failure may occur over time (secondary to anemia)—many adults eventually die of CHF.
   e. Aplastic crises
      • These are usually provoked by a viral infection such as **human parvovirus B19**, which reduces the ability of the bone marrow to compensate.
      • Treatment is blood transfusion—the patient usually recovers in 7 to 10 days.
2. Findings secondary to vaso-occlusion
   a. **Painful crises** involving **bone**—Bone infarction causes severe pain. This is the most common clinical manifestation.
      • Bone pain usually involves multiple sites (e.g., tibia, humerus, femur). It may or may not be bilateral.
      • The pain is self-limiting and usually lasts 2 to 7 days.
   b. **Hand–foot syndrome** (dactylitis)
      • Painful swelling of dorsa of hands and feet seen in infancy and early childhood (usually 4 to 6 months)
      • Often the first manifestation of sickle cell disease
      • Caused by avascular necrosis of the metacarpal and metatarsal bones
   c. **Acute chest syndrome**
      • Due to repeated episodes of pulmonary infarctions
      • Clinical presentation is similar to pneumonia
      • Associated with chest pain, respiratory distress, pulmonary infiltrates, and hypoxia
   d. Repeated episodes of splenic infarctions—These lead to autosplenectomy as the spleen is reduced to a small, calcified remnant. The spleen is large in childhood but is no longer palpable by 4 years of age.
   e. Avascular necrosis of joints—most common in hip (decreased blood supply to femoral head) and shoulder (decreased blood supply to humeral head)

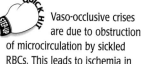

Sickle cell crises vary in severity and frequency among patients. They are typically followed by periods of remission. Some patients have many painful events requiring multiple hospitalizations per year; others have very few crises.

Vaso-occlusive crises are due to obstruction of microcirculation by sickled RBCs. This leads to ischemia in various organs, producing the characteristic "painful crises."

f. Priapism
  - Erection due to vaso-occlusion, usually lasting between 30 minutes and 3 hours
  - Usually subsides spontaneously, after urine is passed, after light exercise, or after a cold shower
  - A trial of hydralazine or nifedipine or use of an antiandrogen (e.g., stilbestrol) may prevent further episodes.
  - Sustained priapism (lasting more than 3 hours) is rare (less than 2%), but is a medical emergency. 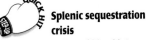 → blood transfusion

g. CVAs (stroke)—the result of cerebral thrombosis; primarily affects children
h. Ophthalmologic complications—e.g., retinal infarcts, vitreous hemorrhage, proliferative retinopathy, retinal detachment
i. Renal papillary necrosis with hematuria (usually painless)
  - A common complication—up to 20% of patients
  - Seldom requires hospitalization and may cease spontaneously
j. Chronic leg ulcers due to vaso-occlusion (decreased blood flow to superficial vessels)—typically over lateral malleoli
k. Abdominal crisis may occur in adulthood—mimics acute abdomen

3. Infectious complications
  a. Functional asplenia results in increased susceptibility to infections (particularly encapsulated bacteria such as *Haemophilus influenzae*, *Streptococcus pneumoniae*).
  b. Predisposition to *Salmonella* osteomyelitis—also due to splenic malfunction

4. Delayed growth and sexual maturation, especially in boys

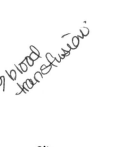

QUICK HIT

Splenic sequestration crisis
- Sudden pooling of blood into the spleen results in rapid development of splenomegaly and hypovolemic shock
- A potentially fatal complication of sickle cell disease (and β-thalassemia) occurring more commonly in children (because they have intact spleens)

C. Diagnosis: Laboratory tests
1. Anemia is the most common finding.
2. Peripheral smear—sickle-shaped RBCs (see Color Figure 9-3)
3. Hemoglobin electrophoresis is required for diagnosis. In most cases, diagnosis is made from newborn screening tests.

D. Treatment
1. Advise the patient as follows.
   a. Avoid high altitudes (low oxygen tension can precipitate crisis).
   b. Maintain fluid intake (dehydration can precipitate crisis).
   c. Treat infections promptly (infection/fever can precipitate crisis).
2. Early vaccination for *S. pneumoniae*, *H. influenzae*, and *Neisseria meningitidis*
3. Prophylactic penicillin for children until 6 years of age—start at 4 months
4. Folic acid supplements (due to chronic hemolysis)
5. Management of painful crises
   a. Hydration—oral hydration if mild episode, otherwise give IV fluids (normal saline)
   b. Morphine for pain control—do not underestimate patient's pain.
   c. Keep the patient warm.
   d. Supplemental oxygen if hypoxia is present
6. Hydroxyurea
   a. Enhances Hb F levels, which interferes with the sickling process
   b. Results in reduced incidence of painful crises
   c. Accelerates healing of leg ulcers and may reduce recurrence
7. Blood transfusion
   a. Not used unless absolutely necessary
   b. Base the need for transfusion on the patient's clinical condition and not on the Hb levels. Transfusion should be considered in acute chest syndrome, stroke, priapism that does not respond to fluids/analgesia, and cardiac decompensation.
8. Bone marrow transplantation—This has been performed successfully to treat sickle cell anemia, but is not routinely performed due to matched donor availability and risk of complications. It may be more cost-effective in the long run than conservative therapy.
9. Gene therapy offers hope for the future.

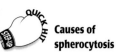

Causes of spherocytosis
- Hereditary spherocytosis
- G6PD deficiency
- ABO incompatibility (but not Rh incompatibility)
- Hyperthermia
- Autoimmune hemolytic anemia

Hereditary Spherocytosis

A. General characteristics

1. Hereditary spherocytosis is an autosomal dominant inheritance of a defect in the gene coding for spectrin and other RBC proteins. Spectrin content is decreased but is not totally absent.
2. There is a loss of RBC membrane surface area without a reduction in RBC volume, necessitating a spherical shape. The spherical RBCs become trapped and destroyed in the spleen (by macrophages)—hence the term extravascular hemolysis.

B. Clinical features

1. Hemolytic anemia (can be severe)
2. Jaundice
3. Splenomegaly
4. Gallstones
5. Occasional hemolytic crises

C. Diagnosis

1. RBC **osmotic fragility** to hypotonic saline
   a. Tests the ability of RBCs to swell in a graded series of hypotonic solutions
   b. Because of their shape, spherocytes tolerate less swelling before they rupture; thus, they are osmotically fragile. The RBCs undergo lysis at a higher (thus earlier) oncotic pressure.
2. Elevated reticulocyte count, elevated MCHC
3. Peripheral blood smear would reveal spherocytes (sphere-shaped RBCs).
4. Direct Coombs test result is negative. This is helpful in distinguishing this disease from autoimmune hemolytic anemia, in which spherocytes are also seen.

D. Treatment: Splenectomy is the treatment of choice.

Glucose-6-Phosphate Dehydrogenase (G6PD) Deficiency

A. General characteristics

1. An X-linked recessive disorder that primarily affects men
2. Known precipitants include sulfonamides, nitrofurantoin, primaquine, dimercaprol, fava beans, and infection.
3. Types of G6PD deficiency
   a. A mild form is present in 10% of African-American men (A-variant)
      - In this form, hemolytic episodes are usually self-limited because they mainly involve only the older RBCs and spare the younger RBCs. (The younger RBCs have sufficient G6PD to prevent RBC destruction.)
      - Hemolytic episodes are usually triggered by infection or by drugs such as antimalarials (primaquine) and sulfur-containing antibiotics (sulfonamide or trimethoprim sulfamethoxazole).
   b. A more severe form is present in people of Mediterranean descent.
      - In this form, young as well as old RBCs are G6PD-deficient.
      - Causes severe hemolytic anemia when exposed to fava beans
      - May require transfusions until the drug is eliminated from the body

B. Clinical features

1. Episodic hemolytic anemia that is usually drug-induced
2. Dark urine and jaundice on physical examination

C. Diagnosis

1. Peripheral blood smear
   a. Shows **"bite cells"**—RBCs after the removal of the Heinz bodies look as if they have "bites" taken out of them. The "bitten" areas are secondary to phagocytosis of Heinz bodies by splenic macrophages.

- Deficiency of G6PD results in an accumulation of unneutralized H_2O_2, which denatures Hb, precipitating Heinz body formation within RBCs.
- Heinz bodies attach to RBC membranes, reducing their flexibility and making them prone to sequestration by the spleen.

b. **Heinz bodies** (abnormal hemoglobin precipitates within RBCs) are visible with special stains.
2. Deficient NADPH formation on G6PD assay
3. Measurement of G6PD levels is diagnostic; however, G6PD levels may be normal during the hemolytic episode because the RBCs that are most deficient in G6PD have already been destroyed. Repeating the test at a later date facilitates diagnosis.

D. Treatment
1. Avoid drugs that precipitate hemolysis.
2. Maintain hydration.
3. Perform RBC transfusion when necessary.

Autoimmune Hemolytic Anemia (AIHA)

A. General characteristics
1. Production of autoantibodies toward RBC membrane antigen(s) which leads to destruction of these RBCs
2. The type of antibody produced (immunoglobulin [Ig] G or IgM) determines the prognosis, site of RBC destruction, and response to treatment.
3. The course is variable, but tends to be more fulminant in children than in adults.
4. Warm AIHA (more common than cold AIHA)
   a. Autoantibody is IgG, which binds optimally to RBC membranes at 37°C (hence "warm")
   b. Results in **extravascular hemolysis**—The primary site of RBC sequestration is the spleen. Splenomegaly is a common feature.
   c. Causes
      • Primary (idiopathic)
      • Secondary to lymphomas, leukemias (chronic lymphocytic leukemia [CLL]), other malignancies, collagen vascular diseases (especially SLE), drugs such as α-methyldopa
5. Cold AIHA
   a. Autoantibody is IgM, which binds optimally to RBC membrane at cold temperatures (usually 0°C to 5°C)
   b. Produces complement activation and **intravascular hemolysis**—primary site of RBC sequestration is the liver
   c. Causes—can be idiopathic (elderly) or due to infection (such as *Mycoplasma pneumoniae* infection or infectious mononucleosis)

B. Clinical features
1. Signs and symptoms of anemia (e.g., fatigue, pallor)
2. Jaundice if significant hemolysis is present
3. Features of the underlying disease

C. Diagnosis
1. Direct Coombs test
   a. If RBCs are coated with IgG (positive direct Coombs test), then the diagnosis is warm AIHA.
   b. If RBCs are coated with complement alone, then the diagnosis is cold AIHA.
2. If there is a positive cold agglutinin titer, then the diagnosis is cold AIHA.
3. Spherocytes may be present in warm AIHA.

D. Treatment
1. Often, no treatment is necessary in either type of AIHA, because the hemolysis is mild. If it is more severe, the therapeutic approach depends on the type of autoantibody causing the hemolysis.
2. Warm AIHA
   a. Glucocorticoids are the mainstay of therapy.
   b. Splenectomy—Use for patients whose condition does not respond to glucocorticoids.

   c. Immunosuppression (azathioprine or cyclophosphamide) may be beneficial.
   d. RBC transfusions—if absolutely necessary
   e. Folic acid supplements
3. Cold AIHA
   a. Avoiding exposure to cold—prevents bouts of hemolysis and anemia
   b. RBC transfusions—if absolutely necessary
   c. Various chemotherapeutic agents
   d. Steroids are not beneficial.

Paroxysmal Nocturnal Hemoglobinuria (PNH)

A. General characteristics
1. An acquired disorder that affects hematopoietic stem cells and cells of all blood lineages
2. This is caused by a deficiency of anchor proteins that link complement-inactivating proteins to blood cell membranes. The deficiency of this anchoring mechanism results in an unusual susceptibility to complement-mediated lysis of RBCs, WBCs, and platelets.

B. Clinical features
1. Chronic intravascular hemolysis—results in chronic paroxysmal hemoglobinuria, elevated LDH
2. Normochromic normocytic anemia (unless iron deficiency anemia is present)
3. Pancytopenia
4. Thrombosis of venous systems can occur—e.g., of the hepatic veins (Budd-Chiari syndrome)
5. May evolve into aplastic anemia, myelodysplasia, myelofibrosis, and acute leukemia
6. Abdominal, back, and musculoskeletal pain

C. Diagnosis
1. Ham's test: The patient's cells are incubated in acidified serum, triggering the alternative complement pathway, resulting in lysis of PNH cells but not normal cells.
2. Sugar water test: The patient's serum is mixed in sucrose. In PNH, hemolysis ensues.
3. Flow cytometry of anchored cell surface proteins (CD55, CD59)—much more sensitive and specific for PNH

D. Treatment
1. Glucocorticoids (prednisone) are the usual initial therapy, but many patients do not respond.
2. Bone marrow transplantation

PLATELET DISORDERS

Thrombocytopenia

A. General characteristics
1. Platelet counts <150,000. Normal is 150,000 to 400,000/μL
2. Causes
   a. Decreased production
      • Bone marrow failure: acquired (aplastic anemia), congenital (Fanconi's syndrome), congenital intrauterine rubella
      • Bone marrow invasion: tumors, leukemia, fibrosis
      • Bone marrow injury: drugs (ethanol, gold, cancer chemotherapy agents, chloramphenicol), chemicals (benzene), radiation, infection
   b. Increased destruction
      • Immune: infection, drug-induced, immune thrombocytopenic purpura (ITP), SLE, heparin-induced thrombocytopenia (HIT) type 2, HIV-associated thrombocytopenia

- Nonimmune: disseminated intravascular coagulation (DIC), thrombotic thrombocytopenic purpura (TTP), HIT type 1
  c. Sequestration from splenomegaly
  d. Dilutional—after transfusions or hemorrhage
  e. Pregnancy—usually an incidental finding (especially third trimester) but can also occur in setting of preeclampsia or eclampsia (remember HELLP syndrome)

HIT
- HIT type 1: Heparin directly causes platelet aggregation; seen <48 hours after initiating heparin; no treatment is needed.
- HIT type 2: Heparin induces antibody-mediated injury to platelet; seen 3 to 12 days after initiating heparin; heparin should be discontinued immediately.

B. Diagnosis
1. CBC—platelet count
2. Bleeding time, prothrombin time (PT), partial thromboplastin time (PTT)
3. To determine the cause of thrombocytopenia, the following may be helpful: examination of peripheral blood smear, bone marrow biopsy.

C. Clinical features
1. Cutaneous bleeding: petechiae (most common in dependent areas), ecchymoses at sites of minor trauma
2. Mucosal bleeding: epistaxis, menorrhagia, hemoptysis, bleeding in GI and genitourinary tracts
3. Excessive bleeding after procedures or surgery
4. Intracranial hemorrhage and heavy GI bleeding can be life-threatening and occur when platelet levels are severely low.
5. Unlike coagulation disorders (e.g., hemophilia), heavy bleeding into tissues and joints (hemarthroses, hematomas) is not seen in thrombocytopenia.

D. Treatment
1. Treat the underlying cause.
2. Platelet transfusion—Use depending on the cause and severity of thrombocytopenia.
3. Discontinue NSAIDs, other antiplatelet agents, and anticoagulants.

Immune Thrombocytopenic Purpura (ITP)

A. General characteristics
1. This results from autoimmune antibody formation against host platelets. These antiplatelet antibodies (IgG) coat and damage platelets, which are then removed by splenic macrophages (reticuloendothelial system binds self-immunoglobulins attached to the platelet).
2. Occurs in two forms
   a. Acute form
      - Seen in children
      - Preceded by a viral infection (in most cases)
      - Usually self-limited—80% resolve spontaneously within 6 months
   b. Chronic form
      - Usually seen in adults, most commonly in women between 20 and 40 years of age
      - Spontaneous remissions are rare.

TABLE 9-2 Severity of Thrombocytopenia and Associated Risk

Platelet Count	Risk
>100,000	Abnormal bleeding (even after trauma or surgery) is unusual
20,000 to 70,000	Increased bleeding hemorrhage during surgery or trauma
<20,000	Minor spontaneous bleeding: easy bruising, petechiae, epistaxis, menorrhagia, bleeding gums
<5,000	Major spontaneous bleeding: intracranial bleeding, heavy GI bleeding

B. Clinical features

1. Petechiae and ecchymoses on the skin
2. Bleeding of the mucous membranes
3. No splenomegaly

C. Diagnosis

1. The platelet count is frequently less than 20,000. The remainder of the blood count is normal (unless significant bleeding has occurred, in which case the Hb/Hct is decreased and the reticulocyte count is increased).
2. Peripheral smear shows decreased platelets.
3. Bone marrow aspiration shows increased megakaryocytes.
4. There is an increased amount of platelet-associated IgG.

D. Treatment

1. Adrenal corticosteroids
2. IV immune globulin—saturates the reticuloendothelial system binding sites for platelet-bound self-immunoglobulin, so there is less platelet uptake and destruction by the spleen
3. Splenectomy—induces remission in 70% to 80% of the cases of chronic ITP
4. Platelet transfusions—for life-threatening and serious hemorrhagic episodes

Thrombotic Thrombocytopenic Purpura (TTP)

A. General characteristics

1. TTP is a rare disorder of platelet consumption. The cause is unknown.
2. Hyaline microthrombi (mostly platelet thrombi) occlude small vessels—any organ may be involved. They cause mechanical damage to RBCs (schistocytes on peripheral smear).
3. This is a life-threatening emergency that is responsive to therapy (see below). If untreated, death occurs within a few months.

B. Clinical features

1. Hemolytic anemia (microangiopathic)
2. Thrombocytopenia
3. Acute renal failure (mild)
4. Fever
5. Fluctuating, transient neurologic signs—can range from mental status change to hemiplegia

C. Treatment

1. Plasmapheresis (large volume)
   a. Begin as soon as diagnosis is established (delay in treatment is life-threatening)
   b. Response is usually good (monitor platelet count, which should increase)
2. Corticosteroids and splenectomy—may be of benefit in some cases
3. Platelet transfusions are contraindicated.

Bernard-Soulier Syndrome

- Autosomal recessive disease
- Disorder of platelet adhesion (to subendothelium) due to deficiency of platelet glycoprotein GPIb-IX
- On peripheral blood smear, platelets are abnormally large.
- Platelet count is mildly low.

Glanzmann's Thrombasthenia

- Autosomal recessive disease
- Disorder of platelet aggregation due to deficiency in platelet glycoprotein GPIIb-IIIa
- Bleeding time is prolonged.
- Platelet count is normal.

TTP

- There is no consumption of clotting factors in TTP, so PT and PTT are normal.
- TTP = HUS + fever + altered mental status
- HUS = microangiopathic hemolytic anemia + thrombocytopenia + renal failure

FIGURE
9-2 Classification of platelet disorders.

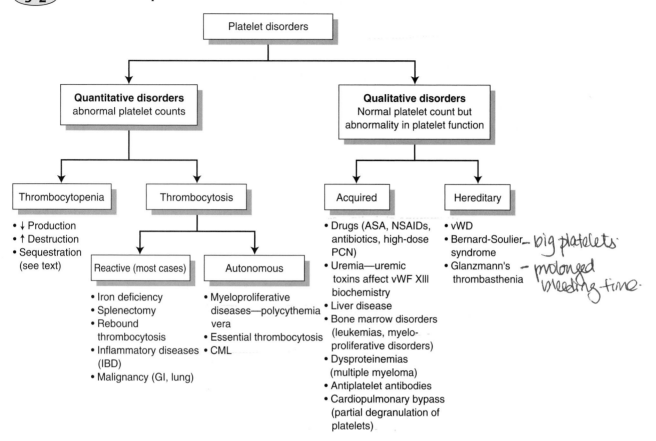

Handwritten annotations: "big platelets" (pointing to Bernard-Soulier), "prolonged bleeding time" (pointing to Glanzmann's)

Figure contents:

- **Platelet disorders**
  - **Quantitative disorders** — abnormal platelet counts
    - **Thrombocytopenia**
      - ↓ Production
      - ↑ Destruction
      - Sequestration (see text)
    - **Thrombocytosis**
      - **Reactive (most cases)**
        - Iron deficiency
        - Splenectomy
        - Rebound thrombocytosis
        - Inflammatory diseases (IBD)
        - Malignancy (GI, lung)
      - **Autonomous**
        - Myeloproliferative diseases—polycythemia vera
        - Essential thrombocytosis
        - CML
  - **Qualitative disorders** — Normal platelet count but abnormality in platelet function
    - **Acquired**
      - Drugs (ASA, NSAIDs, antibiotics, high-dose PCN)
      - Uremia—uremic toxins affect vWF XIII biochemistry
      - Liver disease
      - Bone marrow disorders (leukemias, myeloproliferative disorders)
      - Dysproteinemias (multiple myeloma)
      - Antiplatelet antibodies
      - Cardiopulmonary bypass (partial degranulation of platelets)
    - **Hereditary**
      - vWD
      - Bernard-Soulier syndrome
      - Glanzmann's thrombasthenia

DISORDERS OF COAGULATION

von Willebrand's Disease (vWD)

A. General characteristics

1. Autosomal dominant disorder characterized by deficiency or defect of factor VIII–related antigen (von Willebrand's factor [vWF])
2. vWF enhances platelet aggregation and adhesion (the first steps in clot formation). It also acts as a carrier of factor VIII in blood.
3. The most common inherited bleeding disorder (affects 1% to 3% of population)

TABLE 9-3 vWF Versus Factor VIII Coagulant Protein

	vWF (Also Known as Factor VIII–Related Antigenic Protein)	Factor VIII Coagulant Protein
Site of synthesis	Endothelial cells and megakaryocytes	Liver
Functions	• Platelet adhesion—mediates the adhesion of platelets to the injured vessel walls (i.e., it reacts with platelet GPIb/IX and subendothelium) • Binds the factor VIII coagulant protein and protects it from degradation	Fibrin clot formation
Inheritance pattern	Autosomal dominant	X-linked recessive
vWD	Low	Reduced
Hemophilia	Normal	Very low

Factor VIII has two portions: the coagulant portion (factor VIII coagulant protein) and an antigenic portion (factor VIII antigenic protein). The latter is synonymous with vWF.

Other causes of impaired platelet function include uremia as well as the use of NSAIDs and aspirin.

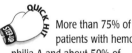

- In many patients, vWD is mild, and is not diagnosed until surgery or trauma.
- In general, bleeding in vWD is much milder than in hemophilia. Spontaneous hemarthroses do not occur.

Suspect hemophilia if unsuspected hemorrhage occurs in a male patient with a positive family history.

More than 75% of patients with hemophilia A and about 50% of patients with hemophilia B are HIV-positive. However, these statistics should be decreasing with time, thanks to modern screening of donor blood.

Detection of factor VIII inhibitor

- If normal plasma is mixed with plasma from a hemophiliac patient, PTT becomes normal.
- If PTT fails to normalize, this is diagnostic of the presence of a factor VIII inhibitor.

4. There are three major subtypes with varying severity.
   a. Type 1 (most common form)—decreased levels of vWF
   b. Type 2 (less common)—exhibits qualitative abnormalities of vWF
   c. Type 3 (least common form)—absent vWF (very severe disease)

B. Clinical features
1. Cutaneous and mucosal bleeding—epistaxis, easy bruising, excessive bleeding from scratches and cuts, gingival bleeding
2. Menorrhagia (affects more than 50% of women with vWD)
3. GI bleeding is possible.

C. Diagnosis
1. Diagnosis is derived from clinical findings and laboratory information, which can be variable.
2. **Prolonged bleeding time** (but normal platelet count)—PTT may be prolonged (a normal PTT does not exclude this diagnosis).
3. Decreased plasma vWF, decreased factor VIII activity
4. Reduced ristocetin-induced platelet aggregation

D. Treatment
1. DDAVP (desmopressin)—induces endothelial cells to secrete vWF.
   a. Treatment of choice for type 1 vWD (the most common type)
   b. Some patients with type 2 vWD may respond to DDAVP, but it is not effective in type 3 vWD.
2. Factor VIII concentrates (containing high-molecular-weight vWF)
   a. Give to all patients with vWD (any type) after major trauma or during surgery
   b. Recommended for type 3 vWD (and type 2 patients not responsive to DDAVP)
3. Cryoprecipitate is not recommended as treatment for vWD because it carries the risk of viral transmission.
4. Avoid aspirin/NSAIDs (exacerbate bleeding tendency).

Hemophilia A

A. General characteristics
1. X-linked recessive disorder—affects male patients primarily (approximately 1 in 10,00 male patients)
2. Caused by deficiency or defect of factor VIII coagulant protein
3. Bleeding tendency is related to factor VIII activity (see Table 9-4).

B. Clinical features
1. Hemarthrosis
   a. Knees are the most common site, but any joint can be involved.
   b. Progressive joint destruction can occur secondary to recurrent hemarthroses.
      - Maintaining normal factor VIII levels (by prophylactic administration of factor VIII concentrate) can minimize joint destruction.
      - Synovectomy (arthroscopic) or radiosynovectomy may be needed if severe recurrent hemarthrosis occur despite optimal medical management.
2. Intracranial bleeding
   a. Second most common cause of death (AIDS due to past history of transfusion [before screening was initiated] is most common)
   b. Any head trauma is potentially life-threatening and requires urgent evaluation.
3. Intramuscular hematomas
4. Retroperitoneal hematomas
5. Hematuria or hemospermia

C. Diagnosis
1. Prolonged PTT
2. Low factor VIII coagulant level and normal levels of vWF

TABLE 9-4	Classification of Severity of Hemophilia	
Classification	Amount (or Activity) of Factor VIII	Clinical Feature
Subclinical	10% of normal factor VIII	Usually asymptomatic
Mild factor VIII deficiency	5% to 10% of normal factor VIII	Bleeding after injuries/surgery
Moderate factor VIII deficiency	1% to 5% of normal factor VIII	Rare spontaneous bleeding; severe bleeding after trauma or surgery
Severe factor VIII deficiency—accounts for about 60% of all cases—diagnosed in infancy or early childhood	<1% of normal factor VIII	Spontaneous bleeding in joints (hemarthrosis) and soft tissues; severe hemorrhage after surgery and trauma

D. Treatment

1. Acute hemarthrosis
   a. Analgesia (codeine with or without acetaminophen)—Avoid aspirin and NSAIDs.
   b. Immobilization of the joint, ice packs, non–weight-bearing
2. Clotting factor replacement
   a. Factor VIII concentrate is the mainstay of therapy (both plasma-derived and recombinant factor VIII are available)—for acute bleeding episodes and before surgery or dental work
   b. Cryoprecipitate and fresh frozen plasma (FFP) are not recommended because of the risk of viral transmission.
3. Desmopressin (DDAVP) —This may be helpful in patients with mild disease. It can increase the levels of factor VIII up to fourfold.
4. Gene therapy offers hope for the future.

Hemophilia B

- Caused by deficiency of factor IX
- X-linked recessive disorder
- Much less common than hemophilia A
- Clinical features are identical to those of hemophilia A.
- Treatment involves administration of factor IX concentrates. DDAVP does not play a role in treatment.

Disseminated Intravascular Coagulation (DIC)

A. General characteristics

1. DIC is characterized by abnormal activation of the coagulation sequence, leading to formation of microthrombi throughout the microcirculation. This causes consumption of platelets, fibrin, and coagulation factors. Fibrinolytic mechanisms are activated, leading to hemorrhage. Therefore, bleeding and thrombosis occur simultaneously.
2. Most common in critically ill patients (in ICU), but can occur in healthy patients as well
3. Can be acute (and fatal), or more gradual
4. Causes
   a. Infection—most common cause, especially gram-negative sepsis, but any infection can cause DIC
   b. Obstetric complications (placenta and uterus have increased tissue factor)—amniotic fluid emboli (often acute and fatal); retained dead fetus (often chronic); abruptio placentae

- PT: reflects extrinsic pathway (prolonged by warfarin)
- PTT: reflects intrinsic pathway (prolonged by heparin)
- Thrombin time: measure of fibrinogen concentration
- Bleeding time: reflects platelet function

- Normal PT = 11–15 sec
- Normal PTT = 25–40 sec
- Normal bleeding time = 2–7 min

Whenever a coagulopathy is present, consider vitamin K deficiency and liver disease in the differential diagnosis (in addition to DIC).
• Liver disease: PT and PTT are elevated, but TT, fibrinogen, and platelets are usually normal.
• Vitamin K deficiency: PT is prolonged, but PTT, TT, platelet count, and fibrinogen level S are normal.

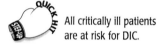

Complications of DIC
• Hemorrhage—Intracranial bleeding is a common cause of death.
• Thromboembolism—stroke, pulmonary embolism, bowel infarction, acute renal failure, arterial occlusion

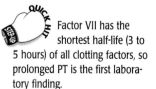

All critically ill patients are at risk for DIC.

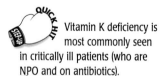

Vitamin K deficiency is most commonly seen in critically ill patients (who are NPO and on antibiotics).

Factor VII has the shortest half-life (3 to 5 hours) of all clotting factors, so prolonged PT is the first laboratory finding.

c. Major tissue injury—trauma, major surgery, burns, fractures
d. Malignancy—lungs, pancreas, prostate, GI tract, acute promyelocytic leukemia
e. Shock, circulatory collapse
f. Snake venom (rattlesnakes)

B. Clinical features
1. Bleeding tendency (more common in acute cases)
   a. Superficial hemorrhage (ecchymoses, petechiae, purpura)
   b. Bleeding from GI tract, urinary tract, gingival or oral mucosa
   c. Oozing from sites of procedures, incisions, and so on
2. Thrombosis—occurs most often in chronic cases. End-organ infarction may develop; all tissues are at risk, especially the CNS and kidney.

C. Diagnosis
1. The following are all increased: (see Table 9-5)
   a. PT, PTT, bleeding time, TT
   b. Fibrin split products (due to activation of fibrinolytic system)
   c. D-dimer
2. The following are decreased:
   a. Fibrinogen level
   b. Platelet count (thrombocytopenia)
3. Peripheral smear reveals schistocytes from damage of RBCs as they go through the microcirculation (with microthrombi).

D. Treatment
1. Management of the condition that precipitated DIC
2. Supportive measures may be indicated if severe hemorrhage is present (these are only temporizing measures).
   a. FFP replaces all the clotting factors.
   b. Platelet transfusions
   c. Cryoprecipitate replaces clotting factors and fibrinogen.
   d. Low doses of heparin (IV or SC) inhibit clotting and can prevent consumption of clotting factors. The use of heparin is controversial; give only in rare cases in which thrombosis dominates the clinical picture.
   e. Other supportive measures include oxygen and IV fluids. Maintain BP and renal perfusion.

Vitamin K Deficiency

A. General characteristics
1. Several clotting factors depend on vitamin K as a cofactor in their synthesis by the liver (factors II, VII, IX, and X; protein C and S). The process is posttranslational modification (gamma-carboxylation).
2. Sources of vitamin K include diet (e.g., leafy green vegetables) and synthesis by intestinal bacterial flora.
3. Causes
   a. Broad-spectrum antibiotics (suppression of gut flora) in patients who are NPO (inadequate dietary intake)
   b. Patients on TPN (unless vitamin K is added)
   c. Malabsorption of fat-soluble vitamins (small bowel disease, inflammatory bowel disease, obstructive jaundice)
   d. Warfarin—a vitamin K antagonist (causes production of inactive clotting factors)

B. Clinical features
1. Hemorrhage—Serious bleeding can develop.
2. PT is initially prolonged (factor VII has the shortest half-life). PTT prolongation follows (as other factors diminish).

C. Treatment

1. Vitamin K replacement (oral or subcutaneous)—It may take a few days for PT to return to normal.
2. If bleeding is severe and emergency treatment is necessary, FFP should be transfused.

Coagulopathy of Liver Disease

A. General characteristics

1. All clotting factors are produced by the liver (except vWF).
2. Liver disease must be severe for coagulopathy to develop. Therefore, if the coagulopathy is due to liver failure, the overall prognosis for the patient is very poor.
3. The following are the reasons coagulopathy develops in liver failure:
   a. There is a decreased synthesis of clotting factors.
   b. Cholestasis leads to decreased vitamin K absorption, which leads to vitamin K deficiency.
   c. Hypersplenism (splenomegaly due to portal hypertension) causes thrombocytopenia.

B. Clinical features

1. Abnormal bleeding—GI bleeding is the most common, primarily due to varices secondary to portal hypertension, but exacerbated by the coagulopathy.
2. Prolonged PT and PTT (especially PT)

C. Treatment

1. FFP (contains all clotting factors)—if PT or PTT is prolonged or if bleeding is present
2. Vitamin K in certain cases (cholestasis)
3. Platelet transfusion—if thrombocytopenia is present
4. Cryoprecipitate—if there is a deficiency of fibrinogen

 QUICK HIT Prolonged PT is a poor prognostic indicator in cirrhosis because synthesis of clotting factors is not **significantly** impaired until liver disease is advanced.

QUICK HIT Patients with antithrombin III deficiency do not respond to heparin. (Heparin requires the presence of AT III.)

Inherited Hypercoagulable States

A. Causes

1. Antithrombin (AT) III deficiency
   a. Autosomal dominant inheritance
   b. AT III is an inhibitor of thrombin, so a deficiency leads to increased thrombosis.
2. Antiphospholipid antibody syndrome
   a. Acquired hypercoagulability state
   b. Can present with arterial or venous thrombosis
3. Protein C deficiency
   a. Autosomal dominant inheritance

TABLE 9-5 Laboratory Findings for Bleeding Disorders

Condition	Platelet Count	Bleeding Time	PT	PTT
Hemophilia	NL*	NL	NL	Increased
vWD	NL	Increased	NL	Increased
ITP	Decreased	Increased	NL	NL
TTP	Decreased	Increased	NL	NL
DIC	Decreased	Increased	Increased	Increased
Heparin	NL or decreased	NL	NL	Increased
Warfarin	NL	NL	Increased	NL
Liver disease	NL	NL	Increased	Increased

*NL = normal

> **Box 9-4** **Secondary Hypercoagulable States or Risk Factors**
>
> - Malignancy (especially pancreas, GI, lung, and ovaries)
> - Antiphospholipid antibody syndrome—the lupus anticoagulant
> - Pregnancy—up to 2 months postpartum
> - Immobilization, causing stasis of blood
> - Myeloproliferative disorders
> - Oral contraceptives
> - Postoperative state (especially after orthopedic procedures)
> - Trauma
> - Nephrotic syndrome
> - Heparin-induced thrombocytopenia or DIC
> - Paroxysmal nocturnal hemoglobinuria
> - Heart failure—causes stasis of blood

QUICK HIT

In many cases, inherited hypercoagulable diseases cause thrombotic events when other risk factors (e.g., immobilization, pregnancy) are also present.

QUICK HIT

- Check for any secondary hypercoagulable states or risk factors (see Box 9-4) in any patient with a DVT, PE, or any thrombotic event, especially if recurrent. Once these are ruled out, search for an inherited hypercoagulable state.
- It is very important to identify the patient with an inherited hypercoagulable state because prophylactic anticoagulation should be started and genetic counseling may be appropriate.

   b. Protein C is an inhibitor of factors V and VIII, so a deficiency leads to unregulated fibrin synthesis.
4. Protein S deficiency—Protein S is a cofactor of protein C, so a deficiency leads to decreased protein C activity.
5. Factor V Leiden (activated protein C resistance)
   a. A mutation in factor V gene
   b. Protein C can no longer inactivate factor V, leading to unregulated prothrombin activation, and thus an increase in thrombotic events.
6. Prothrombin gene mutation
7. Hyperhomocystinemia

B. Clinical features
1. Venous thromboembolism (deep venous thrombosis [DVT] and pulmonary embolism [PE]) are the most common sequelae. Such hypercoagulable disorders are usually not diagnosed until the patient has had several episodes of DVT or PE.
2. Suspect an inherited hypercoagulable state if one or more of the following are present.
   a. The patient has a family history of DVT, PE, or thrombotic events.
   b. The patient has recurrent episodes of DVT, PE, or thrombotic events.
   c. The patient's first thrombotic event was before age 40.
   d. The patient experiences thrombosis in unusual sites, e.g., in mesenteric veins, inferior vena cava, renal veins, or cerebral veins.

C. Diagnosis: Functional assays are available for antithrombin, antiphospholipid antibodies, protein C, protein S, factor V Leiden, prothrombin gene mutation, and hyperhomocystinemia.

D. Treatment
1. Standard treatment for DVT or PE as in patients without primary hypercoagulable states
2. Patients with any of these disorders who have had two or more thromboembolic events should be permanently anticoagulated with warfarin.

ANTICOAGULATION

Heparin

A. Mechanism of action
1. Potentiates the action of antithrombin to primarily inhibit clotting factors IIa and Xa
2. Prolongs PTT
3. Half-life of standard heparin is 1 hour. It is longer for low-molecular-weight heparins (LMWHs) (longer than 3 hours and up to 24 hours, depending on the product).

B. Indications for use

1. Venous thromboembolism: DVT, PE
2. Acute coronary syndromes: unstable angina, myocardial infarction
3. Low-dose standard heparin or LMWH for DVT prophylaxis
4. Atrial fibrillation in acute setting
5. After vascular bypass grafting

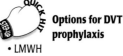

Options for DVT prophylaxis
- LMWH
- Low-dose unfractionated heparin
- Pneumatic compression boots

C. Administration

1. Standard heparin
   a. A therapeutic dose is usually given intravenously, initiated with a bolus of 70 to 80 U/kg and followed by continuous IV infusion (15 to 18 U/kg/hr infusion). Therapeutic PTT is usually 60 to 90 seconds, but this varies depending on the clinical situation.
   b. A prophylactic dose is given subcutaneously—low-dose heparin (5,000 U SC subcutaneously every 12 hours). PTT monitoring is not necessary with SC dosing.
2. LMWH
   a. Therapeutic dose—given as a weight-adjusted dose
   b. Prophylactic dose—varies depending on type of product

D. Adverse effects

1. Bleeding
2. Heparin-induced thrombocytopenia (HIT)—lower incidence with LMWHs
3. Possible osteoporosis—lower incidence with LMWHs
4. Transient alopecia
5. Rebound hypercoagulability after removal due to depression of AT III

E. Contraindications to heparin

1. Previous HIT
2. Active bleeding, GI bleeding, intracranial bleeding
3. Hemophilia, thrombocytopenia
4. Severe HTN
5. Recent surgery on eyes, spine, brain

F. Reversing the effects of heparin and LMWHs

1. The half-life of standard heparin is short, so it will cease to have an effect within 4 hours of its cessation.
2. One can give protamine sulfate to reverse the effects of heparin if necessary (effectiveness is not proven, but it is the only potential antidote that exists in the case of severe bleeding).
3. LMWH has a longer half-life than standard heparin, so it takes longer for the effects to fade.

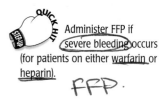

Administer FFP if severe bleeding occurs (for patients on either warfarin or heparin).

FFP.

Low-Molecular-Weight Heparin (LMWH)

A. Mechanism of action

1. LMWHs mostly inhibit factor Xa (equivalent inhibition of factor Xa as standard heparin), but have less inhibition of factor IIa (thrombin) and platelet aggregation.
2. They cannot be monitored by PT or PTT because they do not affect either.

B. Indications for use

1. LMWHs are being used more now because of their greater convenience compared with standard heparin, as well as a decreased risk of side effects (HIT, osteoporosis).
   a. They are given subcutaneously (no IV administration).
   b. PTT monitoring is not necessary.
   c. They are easier to use as an outpatient—the patient may be discharged if stable, and the patient can continue LMWH until the level of long-term anticoagulation (warfarin) is therapeutic.

2. Excreted via kidneys
3. It is much more expensive than standard heparin, but often more cost-effective in the long run due to reduced testing, nursing time, and hospital length of stay.

Warfarin

A. Mechanism of action
1. A vitamin K antagonist—leads to a decrease in vitamin K–dependent clotting factors (II, VII, IX, X) and proteins C and S
2. Causes prolongation of PT (and increase in INR)
3. It takes 4 to 5 days for the anticoagulant effect to begin. Therefore, start heparin as well if the goal is acute anticoagulation because heparin has an immediate effect. Once warfarin is therapeutic (checking by INR), then stop the heparin and continue warfarin for as long as necessary.

B. Indications for use: same as heparin but used for long-term anticoagulation

C. Administration
1. Given orally
2. Heparin is initiated first—as soon as PTT is therapeutic, initiate warfarin. Continue heparin for at least 4 days after starting warfarin. Once INR is therapeutic on warfarin, stop the heparin.
3. The level of anticoagulation is monitored by the INR. In most cases, an INR of 2 to 3 is therapeutic.

D. Adverse effects
1. Hemorrhage
2. Skin necrosis is a rare but serious complication. It is caused by rapid decrease in protein C (a vitamin K–dependent inhibitor of factors Va and VIIIa).
3. **Teratogenic—avoid during pregnancy!**
4. Should not be given to alcoholics or to any patient who is prone to frequent falls because an intracranial bleed in a patient on warfarin can be catastrophic

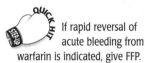

If rapid reversal of acute bleeding from warfarin is indicated, give FFP.

E. Reversing the effects of warfarin
1. Discontinue warfarin and administer vitamin K.
2. The half-life of warfarin is much longer than that of heparin—it takes 5 days to correct the effects of warfarin on stopping the medication. Vitamin K infusion corrects an abnormal PT within 4 to 10 hours if the patient has normal liver function.
3. Giving vitamin K makes it difficult to return the patient to therapeutic INR levels if anticoagulation is to be continued.

PLASMA CELL DISORDERS

Multiple Myeloma

A. General characteristics
1. Multiple myeloma is neoplastic proliferation of a single plasma cell line that produces monoclonal immunoglobulin. This leads to enormous copies of one specific immunoglobulin (usually of the IgG or IgA type).
2. Incidence is increased after age 50; it is twice as common in African-American patients as in Caucasian patients.
3. The etiology is unclear.
4. As the disease process advances, bone marrow elements are replaced by malignant plasma cells. Therefore, anemia, leucopenia, and thrombocytopenia may be present in advanced disease.

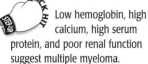

Low hemoglobin, high calcium, high serum protein, and poor renal function suggest multiple myeloma.

B. Clinical features

1. Skeletal manifestations
   a. Bone pain due to osteolytic lesions, fractures, and vertebral collapse—occurs especially in the low back or chest (ribs) and jaw (mandible)
   b. Pathologic fractures
   c. Loss of height secondary to collapse of vertebrae
2. Anemia (normocytic normochromic)—present in most patients due to bone marrow infiltration and renal failure
3. Renal failure—mainly due to the following conditions:
   a. Myeloma nephrosis—Immunoglobulin precipitation in renal tubules leads to tubular casts of Bence Jones protein.
   b. Hypercalcemia also plays a role in renal decompensation.
4. Recurrent infections
   a. Secondary to deprivation of normal immunoglobulins; therefore, humoral immunity is affected
   b. **Most common cause of death**—up to 70% of patients die of infection (lung or urinary tract most common)
5. Amyloidosis—develops in 10% of patients (usually clinically insignificant)

C. Diagnosis

1. Serum and urine protein electrophoresis
   a. Monoclonal spike due to a malignant clone of plasma cells synthesizing a single Ig (usually IgG) called a monoclonal protein (M-protein)
   b. Serum monoclonal protein is present in 85% of patients, and 75% have a urine monoclonal protein.
2. Plain radiographs detect lytic bone lesions. An MRI may be needed to detect lesions not apparent on plain films.
3. Bone marrow biopsy reveals at least 10% abnormal plasma cells.
4. Other laboratory findings
   a. Hypercalcemia (due to bone destruction)
   b. Increased total protein in serum due to paraproteins in blood (hyperglobulinemia)
   c. Peripheral smear—RBCs are in **rouleaux formation**, which resembles a stack of poker chips. The hyperglobulinemia causes the RBCs to stick together (see Color Figure 9-4).
   d. Substantially elevated ESR
   e. Urine—large amounts of free light chains called **Bence Jones** protein
   f. Leukopenia, thrombocytopenia, and anemia may be present, especially in advanced disease.

D. Treatment

1. Treatment is usually reserved for patients with symptoms or advanced disease. Indications for treatment include hypercalcemia, bone pain, and spinal cord compression.
2. Systemic chemotherapy—preferred initial treatment (alkylating agents)
3. Radiation therapy—if no response to chemotherapy and if disabling pain is present
4. Transplantation—Autologous peripheral blood stem cell transplantation is preferred over bone marrow transplantation. *chemo* -

Waldenström's Macroglobulinemia

- Malignant proliferation of plasmacytoid lymphocytes. These cells produce IgM paraprotein, which is very large and causes hyperviscosity of the blood.
- Diagnosis: IgM >5 g/dL; Bence Jones proteinuria in 10% of cases; **absence of bone lesions**
- Clinical features: lymphadenopathy, splenomegaly, anemia, abnormal bleeding, and hyperviscosity syndrome (due to elevated IgM)
- There is no definitive cure. Use chemotherapy and plasmapheresis for hyperviscosity syndromes.

 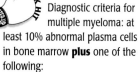
Diagnostic criteria for multiple myeloma: at least 10% abnormal plasma cells in bone marrow **plus** one of the following:
- M-protein in the serum
- M-protein in the urine
- Lytic bone lesions (well-defined radiolucencies on radiographs)—predominantly found in the skull and axial skeleton

Almost all patients with multiple myeloma have an M-protein in either the serum or urine.

- Radiographs show punched-out lytic lesions, osteoporosis, or fractures in 75% of patients with multiple myeloma.
- Osteolytic lesions are secondary to the release of osteoclast-activating factor by the neoplastic plasma cells.

Multiple myeloma has a poor prognosis with a median survival of only 2 to 4 years with treatment, and only a few months without treatment. The 5-year survival rate is about 10%.

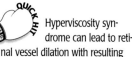
Hyperviscosity syndrome can lead to retinal vessel dilation with resulting hemorrhage and possible blindness.

410-313-7275

Monoclonal Gammopathy of Undetermined Significance (MGUS)

- Common in the elderly (up to 10% in patients >75 years of age)
- Usually asymptomatic
- Diagnosis: IgG spike <3.5 g; less than 10% plasma cells in bone marrow; Bence Jones proteinuria <1 g/24 hours
- Fewer than 20% develop multiple myeloma in 10 to 15 years.
- No specific treatment is necessary, just close observation.

LYMPHOMAS

Hodgkin's Disease

A. General characteristics

1. Bimodal age distribution: X_1 = 15 to 30 years of age; X_2 = >50 years of age
2. Lymph node histology divides the disease into four subtypes.
   a. Lymphocyte predominance (10% to 20%)—few Reed Sternberg cells and many B cells
   b. Nodular sclerosis (40% to 60%)—occurs more frequently in women; bands of collagen envelope pools of Reed Sternberg cells
   c. Mixed cellularity (20% to 40%)—large numbers of Reed Sternberg cells in a pleomorphic background
   d. Lymphocyte depletion (1% to 10%)—lacking in mix of reactive cells; associated with the worst prognosis
3. Staging is based on physical examination, CT scan (chest, abdomen, pelvis), and bone marrow biopsy. **Ann Arbor staging system:**
   a. Stages
      - Stage I: confined to single lymph node
      - Stage II: involvement of two or more lymph nodes but confined to same side of diaphragm
      - Stage III: both sides of diaphragm involved
      - Stage IV: dissemination of disease to extralymphatic sites
   b. Suffixes
      - A: No symptoms
      - B: Fever, weight loss, night sweats (presence of these constitutional symptoms worsens the prognosis)

B. Clinical features

1. Most common symptom is a painless lymphadenopathy
2. Supraclavicular, cervical, axillary, mediastinal lymph nodes
3. Spreads by continuity from one lymph node to adjacent lymph nodes
4. Other presentations may or may not be present, including B symptoms (fever, night sweats, weight loss), pruritus, and cough (secondary to mediastinal lymph node involvement).

C. Diagnosis

1. Lymph node biopsy—The presence of <u>**Reed Sternberg cells**</u> is required to make the diagnosis.
   a. Neoplastic, large cell with two or more nuclei; look like owl's eyes
   b. Usually B-cell phenotype
   c. Reed Sternberg cells may be found in other neoplasms.
2. Presence of inflammatory cell infiltrates—This distinguishes Hodgkin's lymphoma from non-Hodgkin's lymphoma (NHL). The inflammatory cells present are reactive to the Reed Sternberg cells. These include plasma cells, eosinophils, fibroblasts, and T and B lymphocytes.
3. CXR and CT scan (chest, abdomen)—to detect lymph node involvement
4. Bone marrow biopsy—to evaluate bone marrow involvement

- Lymphomas are cancers of the lymphatic system. There are two types: Hodgkin's disease and NHL.
- Lymphadenopathy is usually the first finding in lymphomas.

The histologic type does not greatly influence the prognosis of Hodgkin's disease (with the exception of the lymphocyte-depleted type, which has the worst prognosis). Treatment is effective in most patients with the other histologic types of Hodgkin's disease.

5. Laboratory findings—leukocytosis, eosinophilia; level of ESR elevation sometimes corresponds with disease activity

D. Treatment consists mainly of chemotherapy and radiation therapy to the involved field.

1. Stages I, II, and IIIA can be treated with radiotherapy alone. However, some physicians advocate the use of chemotherapy in these patients as well.

2. Stages IIIB and IV require chemotherapy.

Non-Hodgkin's Lymphoma (NHL)

A. General characteristics

1. NHL occurs with the malignant transformation and growth of B or T lymphocytes or their precursors in the lymphatic system.
   a. The type of lymphocyte involved and its level of differentiation determines the course of the disease and its prognosis.
   b. B-cell lymphomas account for 85% of all cases; T-cell lymphomas account for 15% of all cases.
   c. The disease usually starts in lymph nodes and may spread to blood and bone marrow.

2. NHL is twice as common as Hodgkin's disease. At presentation, patients with NHL tend to have more advanced disease than patients with Hodgkin's disease.

3. The etiology of NHL is still unknown.

4. NHL is the sixth most common cause of cancer-related death in the United States. The mean age of onset varies with subtype. There is an increased overall incidence with increasing age.

5. Risk factors for NHL
   a. HIV/AIDS
   b. Immunosuppression—e.g., organ transplant recipients
   c. History of certain viral infections (e.g., EBV, HTLV-1)
   d. History of *Helicobacter pylori* gastritis (risk of primary associated gastric lymphoma)
   e. Autoimmune disease—e.g., Hashimoto's thyroiditis or Sjögren's syndrome (risk of mucosa-associated lymphoid tissue [MALT])

6. Classification
   a. There are more than 20 different subtypes of NHL.
   b. There are multiple classification systems. The Working Classification system is probably the most common and classifies according to histologic grade: **low grade** (or indolent), **intermediate grade**, and **high grade** (see Table 9-6).

B. Clinical features

1. Lymphadenopathy—sometimes the only manifestation of disease
   a. Lymph nodes are usually painless, firm, and mobile.
   b. Enlargement of lymph nodes is often rapid.
   c. Supraclavicular, cervical, and axillary nodes are involved most often.

2. B symptoms—less common than in Hodgkin's lymphoma

3. Hepatosplenomegaly, abdominal pain, or fullness

4. Recurrent infections, symptoms of anemia or thrombocytopenia—due to bone marrow involvement

5. Various other findings are possible, e.g., superior vena cava obstruction, respiratory involvement, bone pain.

C. Diagnosis

1. Lymph node biopsy—for definitive diagnosis. **Any lymph node >1 cm present for more than 4 weeks that cannot be attributed to infection should be biopsied.**

2. Other tests that may help in diagnosis
   a. CXR—may reveal hilar or mediastinal adenopathy

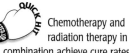
Chemotherapy and radiation therapy in combination achieve cure rates of over 70% in Hodgkin's disease.

 Key epidemiological associations with NHL
- Burkitt's lymphoma in regions of Africa
- Patients with HIV and HIV-associated lymphomas
- Adult T-cell lymphoma in Japan and the Caribbean

It is beyond the scope of this chapter to give a detailed account of each specific type of NHL. Focus on the general clinical presentations as well as certain commonly tested pathologic features—see highlighted points in Table 9-6.

 Staging NHL—Stages I-IV depend on the extent of disease.
- **Stage I**—single lymph node involved (or one extralymphatic site)
- **Stage II**—two or more lymph nodes on the same side of the diaphragm (or localized involvement of one lymph node region and a contiguous extralymphatic site)
- **Stage III**—lymph node involvement on both sides of the diaphragm
- **Stage IV**—disseminated involvement of one or more extralymphatic organs with or without lymph node involvement

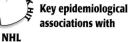

TABLE 9-6 Non-Hodgkin's Lymphomas

Grade[a]	Type[a]	Key Features	Prognosis
Indolent or low-grade	Small lymphocytic lymphoma	• **Closely related to CLL;** more common in elderly patients • **Indolent course**	• Eventually results in widespread lymph node involvement with dissemination to liver, spleen, and bone marrow
	Follicular, predominantly small, cleaved-cell lymphoma	• **Most common form of NHL** • Mean age of onset is 55 • May transform into diffuse, large cell; associated with translocation: t(14;18) • Indolent course • **Presents with painless, peripheral lymphadenopathy**	• Most patients with localized disease can be cured with radiotherapy, but only 15% of patients do have localized disease. • Median survival is approximately 10 years.
Intermediate	Diffuse, large-cell lymphoma	• Predominantly B-cell origin • Middle-aged and elderly patients • **Locally invasive; presents as large extranodal mass**	• 85% cure rate with CHOP therapy
High-grade	Lymphoblastic lymphoma	• **T-cell lymphoma;** more common in children • **May progress to T-ALL** • 50% of patients have B symptoms	• **Aggressive with rapid dissemination,** but may respond to combination chemotherapy
	Burkitt's (small non–cleaved-cell) lymphoma	• **B-cell lymphoma;** more common in children • Two types: African and American; the African variety involves facial bone and jaw, whereas the American variety often involves abdominal organs (hepatomegaly, abdominal masses, lymphadenopathy) • **African variety linked with EBV infection** • **Associated with specific translocation: t(8;14)**	• Grave prognosis unless treated very aggressively with chemotherapy • Treatment may cure 50% to 60% of patients.
Miscellaneous lymphomas	Mycosis fungoides	• T-cell lymphoma of the skin • Presents with **eczematoid skin lesions** that progress to generalized erythroderma • **Cribriform shape of lymphocytes** • Disseminate to lymph nodes, blood, and other organs	• Depends on degree of dissemination (<2 years if dissemination has occurred) • Potentially curable (with radiation, topical chemotherapy) if limited to skin
	Sézary syndrome	Involves skin as well as blood stream	
	HIV-associated lymphomas	Not a discrete entity: usually Burkitt's or diffuse, large-cell lymphoma	• Very poor prognosis

[a]Not all types for each grade are included in this table.

b. CT scan (chest, abdomen, pelvis)—to determine extent of disease spread and patient's response to treatment
c. Serum LDH and β_2 microglobulin are indirect indicators of tumor burden.
d. If alkaline phosphatase is elevated, bone or liver involvement is likely.
e. If liver function tests or bilirubin is elevated, liver involvement is likely.
f. CBC
g. Serum electrolytes, renal function tests
h. Bone marrow biopsy

D. Treatment

1. This varies depending on the stage and subtype of NHL. There is not always a standard treatment for a given type of NHL.
2. Indolent forms of NHL are not curable, but have a 5-year survival rate of 75%. These patients are treated in a variety of ways, depending on the patient's age, comorbidities, stage of disease, and wishes, as follows.
   a. Observation
   b. Chemotherapy (single-agent or combination)
   c. Radiation therapy
3. Intermediate and high-grade NHLs may be curable with aggressive treatments, but if complete remission is not achieved, survival is usually less than 2 years. In general, aggressive forms are treated with multiple regimens of combination chemotherapy (e.g., CHOP [see Quick Hit]) and radiation therapy.
4. Very-high-dose chemotherapy with bone marrow transplantation is a last resort.

LEUKEMIAS

Acute Leukemias

A. General characteristics

1. Two types
   a. Acute myelogenous leukemia (AML)
      • Neoplasm of myelogenous progenitor cells
      • AML occurs mostly in adults (accounts for 80% of adult acute leukemias).
      • Risk factors include exposure to radiation, myeloproliferative syndromes, Down's syndrome, and chemotherapy (e.g., alkylating agents).
      • Response to therapy is not as favorable as in acute lymphoblastic leukemia.
   b. Acute lymphoblastic leukemia (ALL)
      • ALL is a neoplasm of early lymphocytic precursors. Histology reveals a predominance of lymphoblasts.
      • **ALL is the most common malignancy in children under age 15 in the United States.**
      • It is the leukemia most responsive to therapy.
      • Poor prognostic indicators are as follows: age <2 or >9; WBC >10^5/mm^3; and/or CNS involvement.
      • Presence of any of the following is associated with an increased risk for CNS involvement: B-cell phenotype, increased LDH, rapid leukemic cell proliferation.
2. Many patients with acute leukemias can be cured if they are treated aggressively. However, the most aggressive acute leukemias can be fatal within months.

B. Clinical features

1. Anemia and associated symptoms
2. Increased risk of bacterial infections (due to neutropenia)

• Low-grade lymphomas—Cure is rare. Median survival is 5 to 7 years.
• Intermediate-grade lymphomas—Fifty percent of patients can be cured with aggressive therapy. Median survival is about 2 years.
• High-grade lymphomas—Up to 70% can be cured with aggressive therapy. Median survival without treatment is a few months.

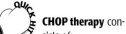

CHOP therapy consists of:
• **C**yclophosphamide
• **H**ydroxydaunomycin (doxorubicin)
• **O**ncovin (vincristine)
• **P**rednisone

Acute leukemias account for 60% of all leukemias, 25% are CLL and 15% are CML.

General evaluation in patients with leukemias (acute or chronic)
Evaluate the patient for:
• Evidence of infection
• Evidence of bleeding or easy bruising
• Lymphadenopathy, hepatosplenomegaly
• Signs of anemia
• Fatigue, weight loss

Box 9-5 Leukemias

• Leukemias are characterized by neoplastic proliferation of abnormal WBCs. As these abnormal WBCs accumulate, they interfere with the production of normal WBCs, as well as the production of erythrocytes and platelets, resulting in anemia and thrombocytopenia.
• Leukemias are classified in two ways.
  • The type of WBC affected
    • If granulocytes or monocytes are affected, myelogenous leukemia is present.
    • If lymphocytes are affected, lymphocytic leukemia is present.
  • The maturity of cells affected and the rapidity of disease progression
    • Acute leukemias are characterized by rapid progression and affect immature cells (i.e., immature cells proliferate before maturation).
    • Chronic leukemias progress slowly and affect mature cells.

a. Pneumonia, urinary tract infection, cellulitis, pharyngitis, esophagitis
b. Associated with high morbidity and mortality; potentially life-threatening
3. Abnormal mucosal or cutaneous bleeding (due to thrombocytopenia)—e.g., epistaxis, bleeding at puncture sites, petechiae, ecchymosis
4. Splenomegaly, hepatomegaly, lymphadenopathy
5. Bone and joint pain (invasion of periosteum)
6. CNS involvement—diffuse or focal neurologic dysfunction (e.g., meningitis, seizures)
7. Testicular involvement (ALL)
8. Anterior mediastinal mass (T-cell ALL)
9. Skin nodules (AML)

C. Diagnosis
1. Laboratory findings
   a. The WBC count is variable (from 1,000/mm^3 to 100,000/mm^3). There are significant numbers of blast cells (immature cells) in peripheral blood.
   b. Anemia
   c. Thrombocytopenia—monitor platelet counts regularly
   d. Granulocytopenia—puts the patient at high risk for infection
   e. Electrolyte disturbances (hyperuricemia, hyperkalemia, hyperphosphatemia)
2. Bone marrow biopsy is required for diagnosis—replacement of marrow by blasts

D. Treatment
1. Treatment of emergencies
   a. Blood cultures, antibiotics for infections
   b. Blood transfusion for anemia and platelet transfusion for bleeding, if necessary
2. Aggressive, combination chemotherapy in high doses for several weeks is appropriate to obtain remission (i.e., absent leukemic cells in bone marrow). Once remission occurs, maintenance therapy is used for months or years to prevent recurrence.
   a. ALL: More than 75% of children with ALL achieve complete remission (compared with 30% to 40% of adults). Relapses, when they occur, usually respond to treatment. With aggressive therapy, survival rates in children can be up to 15 years or longer. Up to 50% of patients are cured.
   b. AML: This is more difficult to treat and does not respond as well to chemotherapy. Survival rates are considerably lower despite intensive treatment. Bone marrow transplantation gives the best chance of remission or cure.
3. Bone marrow transplantation

Chronic Lymphocytic Leukemia (CLL)

A. General characteristics
1. CLL is the most common leukemia that occurs after age 50. Most patients with CLL are >60 years of age. It is the most common leukemia in the Western world.
2. The cause is unknown.
3. Monoclonal proliferation of lymphocytes that are morphologically mature but functionally defective (i.e., they do not differentiate into antibody-manufacturing plasma cells).
4. In general, this is the least aggressive type of leukemia, and CLL patients survive longer than those with acute leukemias or chronic myeloid leukemia (CML). The course is variable, but typically follows a prolonged indolent course. Many patients die of other causes.

B. Clinical features
1. Usually asymptomatic; CLL may be discovered on a routine CBC (lymphocytosis)
2. Generalized painless lymphadenopathy (lymph nodes are nontender), splenomegaly

QUICK HIT
Auer rods (granules and eosinophilic rods inside malignant cells) are present in AML but not ALL.

QUICK HIT
Tumor lysis syndrome
• This is a potential complication of chemotherapy seen in acute leukemia and high-grade NHL.
• Rapid cell death with release of intracellular contents causes hyperkalemia, hyperphosphatemia, and hyperuricemia.
• Treat as a medical emergency.

3. Frequent respiratory or skin infections due to immune deficiency
4. In more advanced disease: fatigue, weight loss, pallor, skin rashes, easy bruising, bone tenderness, and/or abdominal pain

C. Diagnosis
1. Laboratory findings
   a. CBC—WBC: 50,000 to 200,000
   b. Anemia, thrombocytopenia, and neutropenia are common.
   c. Peripheral blood smear is often diagnostic.
      • Absolute lymphocytosis—Almost all of the WBCs are mature, small lymphocytes.
      • Presence of **smudge cells**—leukemic cells that are "beaten up" in the blood.
2. Bone marrow biopsy—presence of infiltrating leukemic cells in bone marrow

D. Treatment
1. Chemotherapy has little effect on overall survival, but is given for symptomatic relief and reduction of infection. <u>Patients are often observed until symptoms develop.</u>
2. Fludarabine and chlorambucil have been shown to be of some benefit.

Autoimmune hemolytic anemias can be seen in patients with CML. The course of CML is more aggressive than CLL.

Chronic Myeloid Leukemia (CML)

A. General characteristics
1. Neoplastic, clonal proliferation of myeloid stem cells
2. Patients are usually older than 40 years of age.
3. CML follows an indolent (chronic) course for many years before it transforms to acute leukemia. The end point of the disease course is usually an acute phase (or **blast crisis**), which is an accelerated phase of blast and promyelocyte production.
4. It is associated with translocation t(9, 22), the Philadelphia chromosome—present in more than 90% of patients. Note that patients without the Philadelphia chromosome have shorter survival times and respond more poorly to treatment.
5. Survival is unpredictable, but the average is 3 years.

Remember that the cells of the myeloid line are <u>erythrocytes, granulocytes, and platelets.</u>

B. Clinical features
1. **Usually asymptomatic at time of diagnosis**—discovered on routine blood work
2. Constitutional symptoms—fevers, night sweats, anorexia, weight loss
3. Recurrent infections, easy bruising/bleeding, symptoms of anemia
4. Splenomegaly, hepatomegaly, lymphadenopathy

C. Diagnosis
1. Laboratory findings
   a. Marked leukocytosis—WBCs from 50,000 to 200,000 with a left shift toward granulocytes
   b. Small numbers of <u>blasts and promyelocytes</u>
   c. Eosinophilia
   d. Peripheral smear—leukemic cells in the peripheral blood: myelocytes, metamyelocytes, bands, and segmented forms
   e. Decreased leukocyte alkaline phosphatase activity
   f. Thrombocytosis
   g. Bone marrow biopsy: leukemic cells

Differentiating benign leukemoid reaction from CML leukemoid reaction
• Usually no splenomegaly
• Increased leukocyte alkaline phosphatase
• History of a precipitating event (e.g., infection) CML
• Opposite to the above findings

D. Treatment
1. Chemotherapy may control symptoms before the acute phase develops, but this is a progressive disease with no cure. The blast crisis is usually terminal—high-dose chemotherapy may be used to return the disease to the chronic phase.
2. An alkylating agent or an antimetabolite is used to treat the chronic phase.
3. Bone marrow or stem cell transplantation may be appropriate during the chronic phase because most cases eventually advance to an acute phase.

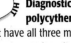

Diagnostic criteria for polycythemia vera
Must have all three major criteria or any two major criteria **plus** any two minor criteria:
Major criteria
• Elevated RBC mass (men >36 L/kg; women >32 L/kg)
• Arterial oxygen saturation >92%
• Splenomegaly
Minor criteria
• Thrombocytosis (platelet count >400 × 10⁹/L)
• Leukocytosis >12 × 10⁹/L
• Leukocyte alkaline phosphatase >100 (no fever or infection)
• Serum vitamin B₁₂ >900 pg/mL

Hyperviscosity and elevated total blood volume in polycythemia vera account for most of the clinical findings.

Thrombotic and hemorrhagic complications in polycythemia vera can be life-threatening.

MYELOPROLIFERATIVE DISORDERS

Polycythemia Vera

A. General characteristics
1. Malignant clonal proliferation of hematopoietic stem cells leading to excessive erythrocyte production
2. The increase in RBC mass occurs independent of erythropoietin.
3. The median survival with treatment is about 9 to 14 years.

B. Clinical features
1. Symptoms due to hyperviscosity: headache, dizziness, weakness, pruritus, visual impairment, dyspnea
2. **Thrombotic phenomena**—DVT, CVA, myocardial infarction, portal vein thrombosis
3. **Bleeding**—GI or genitourinary bleeding, ecchymoses, epistaxis
4. Splenomegaly, hepatomegaly
5. HTN

C. Diagnosis
1. Rule out causes of secondary polycythemia (e.g., hypoxemia, carbon monoxide exposure)
2. CBC
   a. **Elevated RBC count, hemoglobin, hematocrit (usually >50)**
   b. Thrombocytosis, leukocytosis may be present
3. Serum erythropoietin levels are reduced.
4. Elevated vitamin B₁₂ level
5. Hyperuricemia is common.
6. Bone marrow biopsy confirms the diagnosis.

D. Treatment
1. Repeated phlebotomy to lower hematocrit
2. Myelosuppression with hydroxyurea or recombinant interferon alfa (rIFN-α)

Myelodysplastic Syndromes

A. General characteristics
1. Myelodysplastic syndromes are a class of acquired clonal blood disorders. They are characterized by ineffective hematopoiesis, with apoptosis of myeloid precursors. The result is pancytopenia, despite a normal or hypercellular bone marrow.
2. They occur more commonly in elderly patients, and are slightly more common in men.
3. Causes
   a. Usually idiopathic
   b. Exposure to radiation, immunosuppressive agents, and certain toxins are known risk factors for development of myelodysplastic syndromes.
4. They are classified into subtypes according to findings on bone marrow biopsy and peripheral smear.
5. The prognosis, although variable, is generally poor and the end result is often progression to acute leukemia.

Clinical features in myelodysplastic syndromes are due to bone marrow failure and mimic those of aplastic anemia.

B. Clinical features
1. They are often asymptomatic in the early stages. Pancytopenia may be an incidental finding on a routine blood test.
2. They may present with manifestations of anemia, thrombocytopenia, or neutropenia.

C. Diagnosis
1. Bone marrow biopsy typically shows dysplastic marrow cells with blasts or ringed sideroblasts.

2. CBC with peripheral smear shows the following:
   a. Normal or mildly elevated MCV
   b. Low reticulocyte count
   c. Other abnormalities may include **Howell-Jolly bodies**, basophilic stippling, nucleated RBCs, hypolobulated neutrophilic nuclei, and large, agranular platelets.
3. Cytogenic studies often reveal chromosomal abnormalities or mutated oncogenes.

D. Treatment

1. Treatment is mainly supportive.
   a. RBC and platelet transfusions are the mainstays of treatment.
   b. Erythropoietin may help to reduce the number of blood transfusions necessary.
   c. Granulocyte colony-stimulating factor can be an effective adjunctive treatment for neutropenic patients.
   d. Vitamin supplementation, particularly with vitamins B_6, B_{12}, and folate, is important given the large turnover of marrow cells.
2. Pharmacologic therapies have variable results.
   a. Immunosuppressive agents
   b. Chemotherapy
   c. Androgenic steroids
3. Bone marrow transplantation is the only potential cure.

Essential Thrombocytosis

- Defined as platelet count $>600,000/mm^3$
- Reactive thrombocytosis (due to infection, inflammation, bleeding, and so on) and other myeloproliferative disorders must be excluded.
- It is primarily manifested by thrombosis (e.g., CVA), or paradoxically and less frequently, bleeding (due to defective platelet function). It is a disease with high morbidity but low mortality.
- Other findings may include splenomegaly, pseudohyperkalemia, and elevated bleeding time. Erythromelalgia is burning pain and erythema of the extremities due to microvascular occlusions.
- Peripheral smear shows hypogranular, abnormally-shaped platelets.
- Bone marrow biopsy shows an increased number of megakaryocytes.
- Treatment usually involves antiplatelet agents such as anagrelide and low-dose aspirin. Hydroxyurea is sometimes used for severe thrombocytosis.

Agnogenic Myeloid Metaplasia With Myelofibrosis

- This condition refers to fibrosis of the bone marrow resulting in pancytopenia and extramedullary hematopoiesis.
- Not surprisingly, massive splenomegaly is usually present. Other manifestations are secondary to pancytopenia—e.g., fatigue, bleeding, infection.
- **Teardrop cells on peripheral smear are a hallmark feature.** Large, abnormal platelets and immature myeloid cells are also present.
- Bone marrow aspirate shows marrow fibrosis—if severe enough, it may be a "dry tap."
- The prognosis is poor. Patients often progress to having AML, or may die of bleeding or infection.
- Treatment is primarily supportive, involving multiple blood transfusions, erythropoietin, and sometimes splenectomy for palliative relief of painful splenomegaly.
- Bone marrow transplantation is sometimes appropriate.

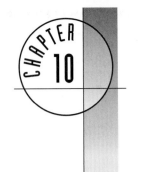

Infectious Diseases

INFECTIONS OF THE UPPER AND LOWER RESPIRATORY TRACTS

Pneumonia

A. General characteristics

1. There are two types of pneumonia: community-acquired and nosocomial.

   a. Community-acquired pneumonia (CAP) *4 days.*
   - Occurs in the community or within the first 72 hours of hospitalization
   - Can be typical or atypical *xhemolytic*
   - **Most common bacterial pathogen is** *Streptococcus pneumoniae*

   b. Nosocomial pneumonia *4 days.*
   - Occurs during hospitalization after first 72 hours
   - **Most common bacterial pathogens are gram-negative rods and *Staphylococcus aureus*** *Klebsiella, E. coli*

2. There are two recommended methods of prevention.

   a. Influenza vaccine—give yearly to people at increased risk for complications and to health care workers *to prevent 2° bacterial infection.*

   b. Pneumococcal vaccine—for patients >65 years and for younger people at high risk (e.g., those with heart disease, sickle cell disease, pulmonary disease, diabetes, or alcoholic cirrhosis, or asplenic individuals)

B. Typical CAP

1. Common agents
   a. *S. pneumoniae* (60%)
   b. *Haemophilus influenzae* (15%)
   c. Aerobic gram-negative rods (6% to 10%)—*Klebsiella* (and other Enterobacteriaceae) *alcoholics.*
   d. *S. aureus* (2% to 10%)

2. Clinical features
   a. Symptoms
   - Acute onset of fever and shaking chills
   - Cough productive of thick, purulent sputum
   - Pleuritic chest pain (suggests pleural effusion)
   - Dyspnea
   b. Signs
   - Tachycardia, tachypnea
   - Late inspiratory crackles, bronchial breath sounds, increased tactile and vocal fremitus, dullness on percussion
   - Pleural friction rub (associated with pleural effusion)

3. Chest radiograph (CXR)
   a. Lobar consolidation
   b. Multilobar consolidation indicates very serious illness.

- "Classic" CAP presents with a sudden chill followed by fever, pleuritic pain, and productive cough.
- The "atypical pneumonia" syndrome, associated with *Mycoplasma* or *Chlamydia* infection, often begins with a sore throat and headache followed by a nonproductive cough and dyspnea.

can't stain in intracellular organism

Most cases of CAP result from aspiration of oropharyngeal secretions because the majority of organisms that cause CAP are **normal inhabitants of the pharynx.**

S. pneumoniae accounts for up to 66% of all cases of bacteremic pneumonia, followed by *H. influenzae*, influenza virus, and *Legionella* spp.

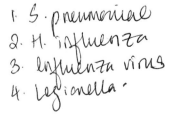

1. *S. pneumoniae*
2. *H. influenza*
3. *Influenza virus*
4. *Legionella*.

> **Box 10-1 General Approach to Diagnosis of Community-Acquired Pneumonia (CAP)**
>
> The first task is to **differentiate lower respiratory tract infection from the other causes of cough and from upper respiratory infection.**
> - If nasal discharge, sore throat, or ear pain predominates, upper respiratory infection is likely.
> - Once lower tract infection is suspected, the next task is to differentiate between pneumonia and acute bronchitis. Unfortunately, clinical features (cough, sputum, fever, dyspnea) are not reliable in differentiating between the two.
> - CXR is the only reasonable method of differentiating between pneumonia and acute bronchitis.

✱ Only way to differentiate b/n pneumonia and acute bronchitis — is CXR.

C. Atypical CAP

1. Common agents
   a. *Mycoplasma pneumoniae* (most common)
   b. *Chlamydia pneumoniae*
   c. *Chlamydia psittaci*
   d. *Coxiella burnetii* (Q fever)
   e. *Legionella* spp.
   f. Viruses: influenza virus (A and B), adenoviruses, parainfluenza virus, RSV *↝ in children*
2. Clinical features
   a. Symptoms
      - Insidious onset—headache, sore throat, fatigue, myalgias
      - Dry cough (no sputum production)
      - Fevers (chills are uncommon)
   b. Signs
      - Pulse–temperature dissociation—normal pulse in the setting of high fever is suggestive of atypical CAP.
      - Wheezing, rhonchi, crackles
   c. CXR
      - Diffuse reticulonodular infiltrates
      - Absent or minimal consolidation

D. Diagnosis

1. PA and lateral CXR required to confirm the diagnosis
   a. Considered sensitive—If CXR findings are not suggestive of pneumonia, do not treat the patient with antibiotics.
   b. After treatment, changes evident on CXR usually lag behind the clinical response (up to 6 weeks).
2. Pretreatment expectorated sputum for Gram stain and culture—low sensitivity and specificity, but still worthwhile tests because antimicrobial resistance is an increasing problem
   a. Sputum Gram stain—try to obtain in all patients
      - Commonly contaminated with oral secretions
      - A good specimen has a sensitivity of 60% and specificity of 85% for identifying gram-positive cocci in chains (*S. pneumoniae*).

 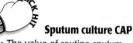
QUICK HIT
Studies have shown that if vital signs are entirely normal, the probability of pneumonia in outpatients is less than 1%.

QUICK HIT
Sputum culture CAP
- The value of routine sputum collection for Gram stain and culture is controversial. The Infectious Disease Society of America has recently advocated performing sputum Gram stain and culture in all patients hospitalized with CAP.
- A good sputum specimen has >25 PMNs and <10 epithelial cells per low-power field.

> **Box 10-2 Pneumonia Pearls**
>
> - In alcoholics, think of *Klebsiella pneumonia;* In immigrants, think of TB
> - In nursing home residents, consider a nosocomial pathogen and predilection for the upper lobes (e.g., *Pseudomonas*).
> - HIV-positive patients are at risk for *Pneumocystis carinii* and *Mycobacterium tuberculosis*, but are still more likely to have a typical infectious agent.
> - *Legionella* pneumonia is common in organ transplant recipients, patients with renal failure, patients with chronic lung disease, and smokers. *Legionella* pneumonia is rare in healthy children and young adults.

FIGURE
10-1 Chest PA (**A**) and lateral (**B**) radiographs: Right lower lobe pneumonia (straight arrows). On the PA radiograph, the right cardiac border is clearly visible, and the right hemidiaphragm is partially silhouetted (double straight arrows). These findings indicate that the infiltrate is posterior or in the right lower lobe as confirmed on the lateral radiograph (straight arrows).

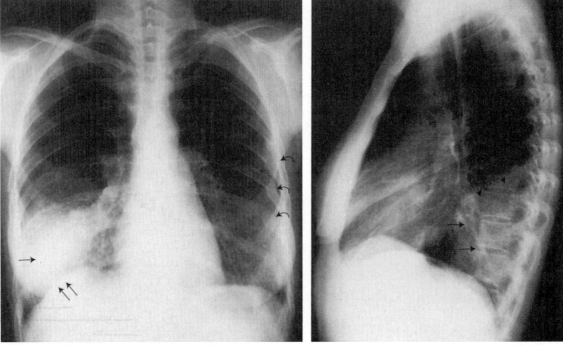

A   **B**

(From Erkonen WE, Smith WL. Radiology 101: The Basics and Fundamentals of Imaging. Philadelphia: Lippincott Williams & Wilkins, 1998:110, Figure 6-54A and B.)

The following steps are appropriate in patients admitted to the hospital with suspected pneumonia:
• CXR (PA and lateral)
• Laboratory tests—CBC and differential, BUN, creatinine, glucose, electrolytes
• O₂ saturation *Pulse Ox*
• Two pretreatment blood cultures
• Gram stain and culture of sputum
• Antibiotic therapy —›

CAP

b. Sputum culture—try to obtain in all patients requiring hospitalization
   • Specificity is improved if the predominant organism growing on the culture media correlates with the Gram stain.
3. Special stains of the sputum in selected cases
   a. Acid-fast stain (*Mycobacterium* spp.) if tuberculosis is suspected
   b. Silver stain (fungi, *Pneumocystis carinii*) for HIV/immunocompromised patients
4. Urinary antigen assay for *Legionella* in selected patients
   a. This test is very sensitive.
   b. The antigen persists in the urine for weeks (even after treatment has been started).
5. Consider two pretreatment blood cultures from different sites.

E. Treatment

1. Decision to hospitalize
   a. **The decision to hospitalize or treat as an outpatient is probably the most important decision to be made.**
   b. Patients are stratified into five classes based on severity (see Table 10-1). The Pneumonia Severity Index can serve as a general guideline, but clinical judgment is critical in making this decision.
2. Antimicrobial therapy
   a. Because the specific cause is usually not determined on initial evaluation, empiric therapy is often required.
   b. For outpatients
      • In people younger than 60 years of age, the most common organisms are *S. pneumoniae*, *Mycoplasma*, *Chlamydia*, and *Legionella*. Macrolides or

TABLE 10-1 **Pneumonia Severity Index**	
Patient Characteristic	**Points**
Demographics	
Male	+Age (yr)
Female	+Age (yr) − 10
Nursing home resident	+10
Comorbid illness	
Neoplastic disease	+30
Liver disease	+20
Congestive heart failure	+10
Cerebrovascular disease	+10
Renal failure	+10
Physical examination	
Altered mental status	+20
Respiratory rate >30	+20
Systolic BP <90	+20
Temp <95°F or >104°F	+15
Heart rate >125	+10
Laboratory and radiographic findings	
Arterial pH <7.35	+30
BUN >64	+20
Sodium <130	+20
Glucose >250	+10
Hematocrit <30%	+10
Partial pressure of arterial oxygen <60 or oxygen saturation <90%	+10
Pleural effusion	+10

ADD TOTAL POINTS FOR RISK ASSESSMENT:

Total Points	Risk	Risk Class	%Mortality	Treat as:
No predictors	Low	I	0.1	Outpatient
≤70	Low	II	0.6	Outpatient
71–90	Low	III	2.8	Inpatient (briefly)
91–130	Moderate	IV	8.2	Inpatient
>130	High	V	29.2	Inpatient

Adapted from Fine MJ, Auble TE, Yealy DM, et al. A prediction rule to identify low-risk patients with community-acquired pneumonia. N Engl J Med 1997;336:243–250.

[handwritten margin notes: "Any changes in vital." "Pneumonia severity index." "Outpatient younger ① Macrolide / Doxycycline or ② Fluoroquinolone. older. Cephalosporins."]

doxycycline cover all of these organisms and are the first-line treatment. Fluoroquinolones are alternative agents. Penicillins or cephalosporins do not cover the atypical organisms in this age group.

- In older adults and patients with comorbidities (more likely to have typical CAP), a second- or third-generation cephalosporin is the first-line treatment. Alternatives include amoxicillin/clavulanic acid, second-generation

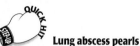

Quick HIT

Pleural effusion is common in patients with pneumonia. Progression to empyema (infected, loculated pleural fluid) requires chest tube drainage.

Quick HIT

Lung abscess pearls
- The dependent zones of the lungs are most likely to be infected by aspirated contents—the posterior segments of the upper lobes and superior segments of lower lobes.
- Aspirated material is more likely to affect the right lung due to the angle of the right main stem bronchus from the trachea.

macrolides, and fluoroquinolones with adequate pneumococcal coverage (e.g., levofloxacin, moxifloxacin).

   c. For hospitalized patients, a fluoroquinolone alone or a third-generation cephalosporin plus a macrolide is appropriate.

F. Complications

1. Pleural effusion ("parapneumonic effusions")—See Chapter 2.
   a. Can be seen in more than 50% of patients with CAP on routine CXR. Empyema is infrequent in these patients.
   b. Most of these effusions have an uncomplicated course and resolve with treatment of the pneumonia with antibiotics.
   c. Thoracentesis should be performed if the effusion is significant (>1 cm on lateral decubitus film). Send fluid for Gram stain, culture, pH, cell count, determination of glucose, protein, and LDH levels.
2. Pleural empyema occurs in 1% to 2% of all cases of CAP (up to 7% of hospitalized patients with CAP). See Chapter 2.
3. Acute respiratory failure may occur if the pneumonia is severe.

Lung Abscess

A. General characteristics

1. Abscess in the lung parenchyma results when infected lung tissue becomes necrotic and forms suppurative cavitary lesions. The typical case is aspiration of oropharyngeal contents or food, with resulting pneumonia and necrosis.
2. By definition, a lung abscess is formed by one or more cavities, each >2 cm in diameter.
3. Lung abscesses can be complications of the following:
   a. Aspiration of organisms
   b. Acute necrotizing pneumonia (gram-negative rods)
   c. Hematogenous spread of infection from distant site
   d. Direct inoculation with contiguous spread
4. Microbiologic causes are mainly bacteria that colonize the oropharynx.
   a. Oral anaerobes: *Prevotella, Peptostreptococcus, Fusobacterium, Bacteroides* spp.
   b. Other bacteria: *S. aureus, S. pneumoniae,* and aerobic gram-negative bacilli
5. Epidemiology/risk factors
   a. The main risk factor is predisposition to aspiration. This may be seen in patients with alcoholism, drug addition, CVA, seizure disorders, general anesthesia, or a nasogastric or endotracheal tube.
   b. Poor dental hygiene increases the content of oral anaerobes.
   c. Edentulous patients are **less** likely to aspirate oropharyngeal secretions.

B. Clinical features

1. The majority of cases have an indolent onset; some present more acutely.
2. Common symptoms and signs
   a. Cough—Foul-smelling sputum is consistent with anaerobic infection. It sometimes is blood-tinged.
   b. Shortness of breath
   c. Fever, chills
   d. Constitutional symptoms: fatigue, malaise, weight loss

C. Diagnosis

1. CXR
   a. This reveals thick-walled cavitation with air-fluid levels.
   b. Look for abscess in dependent, poorly ventilated lobes.
2. CT scan may be necessary to differentiate between abscess and empyema.
3. Sputum Gram stain and culture has low sensitivity and specificity.
4. Consider obtaining cultures via bronchoscopy or transtracheal aspiration rather than simple expectoration to avoid contamination with oral flora.

D. Treatment

1. Hospitalization is often required if lung abscess is found. Postural drainage should be performed.
2. Antimicrobial therapy
   a. Antibiotic regimens include coverage for the following:
      - Gram-positive cocci—ampicillin or amoxicillin/clavulanic acid, ampicillin/sulbactam, or vancomycin for *S. aureus*
      - Anaerobes—clindamycin or metronidazole
      - If gram-negative organisms are suspected, add a fluoroquinolone or ceftazidime.
   b. Continue antibiotics until the cavity is gone or until CXR findings have improved considerably—this may take months!

Gram(+) - Zosyn/Vancomycin
Anaerobes - clindamycin/ metronidazole.
Gram(-) - fluoroquinolone/ ceftazidime
↓ pseudomonas.

Tuberculosis (TB)

A. General characteristics

1. Microbiology
   a. Most commonly caused by *Mycobacterium tuberculosis* *intracellular aerobic.*
   b. Mycobacteria are acid-fast bacilli (AFB)—considered slow-growing but hardy organisms
   c. Inhibited by the cellular arm of the immune system
2. Transmission
   a. Transmission occurs via inhalation of aerosolized droplets containing the active organism.
   b. Only those people with active TB are contagious (e.g., by coughing, sneezing).
   c. People with primary TB are not contagious.
3. Pathophysiology
   a. Primary TB
      - Bacilli are inhaled and deposited into the lung, then ingested by alveolar macrophages.
      - Surviving organisms multiply and disseminate via lymphatics and the blood-stream. Granulomas form and "wall off" the mycobacteria. The granulomas in oxygen-rich areas, such as the lungs, allow these organisms to remain viable (they are aerobes). After the resolution of the primary infection, the organism remains dormant within the granuloma.
      - An insult to the immune system may activate the TB at any time.
      - Only 5% to 10% of individuals with primary TB will develop active disease in their lifetime.
   b. Secondary TB (reactivation)
      - Occurs when the host's immunity is weakened—e.g., HIV infection, malignancy, immunosuppressants, substance abuse, poor nutrition
      - Usually manifests in the most oxygenated portions of the lungs—the apical/posterior segments
      - Produces clinical manifestations of TB
      - Can be complicated by hematogenous or lymphatic spread, resulting in miliary TB
   c. Extrapulmonary TB
      - Individuals with impaired immunity may not be able to contain the bacteria at either the primary or the secondary stage of the infection.
      - This may result in active disease throughout the body.
      - It is common in patients with HIV because their cellular immunity is impaired.

infection + granuloma.

reactivation due to immunocompromise ↓ in immune system ↓ symptoms of TB and are active and contagious

QUICK HIT Tuberculosis is the most common cause of death due to infection worldwide.

B. Clinical features

1. Primary TB
   a. **Usually asymptomatic**
   b. Pleural effusion may develop.
   c. If the immune response is incomplete, the pulmonary and constitutional symptoms of TB may develop. This is known as progressive primary TB.

2. Secondary (active) TB
   a. Constitutional symptoms—fever, night sweats, weight loss, and malaise are common.
   b. Cough progresses from dry cough to purulent sputum. Hemoptysis suggests advanced TB.
   c. Apical rales may be present on examination.
3. Extrapulmonary TB
   a. May involve any organ. The lymph nodes, pleura, genitourinary tract, spine, intestine, and meninges are some of the common sites of infection.
   b. Miliary TB refers to hematogenous dissemination of the tubercle bacilli.
      • May be due to a reactivation of dormant, disseminated foci or a new infection
      • Also common in patients with HIV
      • May present with organomegaly, reticulonodular infiltrates on CXR, and choroidal tubercles in the eye

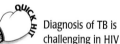

Radiographic findings in primary TB
• Ghon's complex: calcified primary focus
• Ranke's complex: calcified primary focus and calcified hilar lymph node

C. Diagnosis
1. Must have a high index of suspicion, depending on patient's risk factors and presentation
2. CXR
   a. Classic findings are **upper lobe infiltrates with cavitations.**
   b. Other possible findings
      • Pleural effusion(s)
      • *Ghon's complex* and *Ranke's complex*: evidence of healed primary TB
      • Atypical findings common in immunocompromised patients
3. Sputum studies
   a. Definitive diagnosis is made by sputum culture—growth of *M. tuberculosis.*
   b. Obtain three morning sputum specimens—culture takes 4 to 8 weeks.
   c. PCR can detect specific mycobacterial DNA more rapidly.
   d. Diagnosis is sometimes made by finding AFB on microscopic examination, but this is not definitive because other mycobacteria may colonize airways.
4. Tuberculin skin test
   a. Tuberculin skin test is a screening test to detect those who may have been exposed to TB. It is not for diagnosis of active TB, but rather of latent (primary) TB.
   b. Inject PPD into the volar aspect of forearm. Measure the amount of induration 48 to 72 hours later.
   c. The result is positive if induration ≥15 mm.
   d. In certain high-risk populations (e.g., those who live in high-prevalence areas, the homeless, prisoners, health care workers, nursing home residents), 10 mm of induration is considered positive.
   e. For patients with HIV, close contacts of patients with active TB, or those with radiographic evidence of primary TB, induration of 5 mm is positive.

Diagnosis of TB is challenging in HIV patients because:
• PPD skin test result is negative.
• Patients have "atypical" CXR findings.
• Sputum smears are more likely to be negative.
• Granuloma formation may not be present in the late stages.

• For a positive TB exposure and a positive PPD test (but no active disease), treatment is INH only.
• If the patient has active TB, multiagent therapy indicated.

D. Treatment
1. Patients with active TB must be isolated until sputum is negative for AFB.
2. First-line therapy is a four-drug regimen: isoniazid (INH), rifampin, pyrazinamide, and ethambutol or streptomycin.
3. The initial treatment regimen consists of 2 months of treatment with the four-drug regimen. After this initial 2-month phase, a phase of 4 months is recommended using INH and rifampin.
4. Prophylactic treatment for latent (primary) TB consists of 9 months of INH **after** active TB has been excluded (negative CXR, sputum, or both).

Influenza
• Orthomyxovirus is transmitted via respiratory droplets, typically occurring in winter months.
• Antigenic types A and B are responsible for the clinical syndrome known as the "flu."

[handwritten margin notes:]
3 AFB test
if low risk - 15mm is positive
living in prevalent area, prisoners, homeless, health care workers etc → 10mm is (+)
HIV, close contact w/ TB patients etc → 5mm is (+)

- Annual epidemics are due to minor genetic ~~reassortment~~ [*recombination*] and usually are not life-threatening except in the very young, the very old, the immunocompromised, and hosts with significant medical comorbidities.
- Rarely occurring pandemics are due to major genetic recombination [*reassortment*] and are often fatal, even in young, otherwise healthy hosts.

ex. Bird flu, H1N1 (Swine flu)

- Clinical findings are a rapid onset of fever, chills, malaise, headache, nonproductive cough, and sore throat. Nausea may also be present.
- Treatment is largely supportive. Amantadine or rimantadine decrease the duration of symptoms. Only give antibiotics for secondary bacterial infections. (See Chapter 12 for vaccination recommendations.)

oseltamivir - neuraminidase inhibitor: tamiflu.

INFECTIONS OF THE CENTRAL NERVOUS SYSTEM

Meningitis

A. General characteristics

1. This refers to inflammation of the meningeal membranes that envelop the brain and spinal cord. It is usually associated with infectious causes, but noninfectious causes (such as medications, SLE, sarcoidosis, and carcinomatosis) also exist.
2. Pathophysiology
   a. Infectious agents frequently colonize the nasopharynx and respiratory tract.
   b. These pathogens typically enter the CNS via one of the following:
      - Invasion of the bloodstream, which leads to hematogenous seeding of CNS
      - Retrograde transport along cranial (e.g., olfactory) or peripheral nerves
      - Contiguous spread from sinusitis, otitis media, surgery, or trauma
3. Can be classified as acute or chronic, depending on onset of symptoms
   a. Acute meningitis—onset within hours to days
   b. Chronic meningitis—onset within weeks to months; commonly caused by mycobacteria, fungi, Lyme disease, or parasites
4. Another important distinction is bacterial versus aseptic (described below)
5. Acute bacterial meningitis
   a. Causes
      - Neonates—Group B streptococci > *Escherichia coli* > *Listeria monocytogenes*
      - Children >3 months—*Neisseria meningitidis* > *Streptococcus pneumoniae* > *H. influenzae*
      - Adults (ages 18 to 50)—*S. pneumoniae* > *N. meningitidis* > *H. influenzae*
      - Elderly (>50)—*S. pneumoniae* > *N. meningitidis* > *L. monocytogenes*
      - Immunocompromised—*L. monocytogenes* > gram-negative bacilli > *S. pneumoniae*
   b. Complications
      - Seizures, coma, brain abscess, subdural empyema, DIC, respiratory arrest
      - Permanent sequelae—deafness, brain damage, hydrocephalus
6. Aseptic meningitis
   a. Aseptic meningitis is caused by a variety of nonbacterial pathogens, frequently viruses such as enterovirus and HSV. It can also be caused by certain bacteria, parasites, and fungi.
   b. **It may be difficult to distinguish clinically from acute bacterial meningitis. If there is uncertainty in diagnosis, treat for acute bacterial meningitis.**
   c. It is associated with a better prognosis than acute bacterial meningitis.

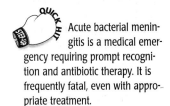

Acute bacterial meningitis is a medical emergency requiring prompt recognition and antibiotic therapy. It is frequently fatal, even with appropriate treatment.

B. Clinical features

1. Symptoms (any of the following may be present)
   a. Headache (may be more severe when lying down)
   b. Fevers
   c. Nausea and vomiting
   d. Stiff, painful neck
   e. Malaise

f. Photophobia

g. Alteration in mental status (confusion, lethargy, even coma)

2. Signs (any of the following may be present)

a. Nuchal rigidity: stiff neck, with resistance to flexion of spine (may be absent)

b. Rashes
   - Maculopapular rash with petechiae—purpura is classic for *N. meningitidis*
   - Vesicular lesions in varicella or HSV

c. Increased ICP and its manifestations—e.g., papilledema, seizures

d. Cranial nerve palsies

e. *Kerning's sign*—inability to fully extend knees when patient is supine with hips flexed (90°)
   - Caused by irritation of the meninges
   - Only present in approximately half of patients with bacterial meningitis

f. *Brudzinski's sign*—flexion of legs and thighs that is brought on by passive flexion of neck for same reason as above; also present in only half of patients with bacterial meningitis

Acute bacterial meningitis (clinical features)

Characteristic triad includes:
- Fever
- Nuchal rigidity
- Change in mental status

C. Diagnosis (see Table 10-2)

1. CSF examination (LP)—Perform this if meningitis is a possible diagnosis unless there is evidence of a space-occupying lesion. Also note the opening pressure.

a. Examine the CSF. Cloudy CSF is consistent with a pyogenic leukocytosis.

b. CSF should be sent for the following: cell count, chemistry (e.g., protein, glucose), Gram stain, culture (including AFB), and cryptococcal antigen or India ink.

c. Bacterial meningitis—pyogenic inflammatory response in CSF
   - Elevated WBC count—PMNs predominate
   - Low glucose
   - High protein
   - Gram stain—positive in 75% to 80% of patients with bacterial meningitis

d. Aseptic meningitis—nonpyogenic inflammatory response in CSF
   - There is an increase in mononuclear cells. Typically a lymphocytic pleocytosis is present.
   - Protein is normal or slightly elevated.
   - Glucose is usually normal.
   - CSF may be completely normal.

2. CT scan of the head is recommended before performing an LP if there are focal neurologic signs or if there is evidence of a space-occupying lesion with elevations in ICP.

3. Obtain blood cultures before antibiotics are given.

D. Treatment

1. Bacterial meningitis

a. Empiric antibiotic therapy—Start immediately after LP is performed. If a CT scan must be performed or if there are anticipated delays in LP, give antibiotics first.

TABLE 10-2 CSF Findings in Bacterial Versus Aseptic Meningitis

	Normal	Bacterial Meningitis	Aseptic Meningitis
WBC count (cells/mm³)	<5	>1,000 (1,000 to 20,000)	<1,000
WBC differential	All lymphocytes or monocytes; no PMNs	Mostly PMNs	Mostly lymphocytes and monocytes
Glucose (mg/dL)	50 to 75	Low	Normal
Protein (mg/dL)	<60	High	Moderate elevation

TABLE 10-3 **Empiric Treatment for Acute Bacterial Meningitis**

Age or Risk Factor	Likely Etiology	Empiric Treatment
Infants (<3 mo)	Group B streptococci, *Escherichia coli*, *Klebsiella* spp., *Listeria monocytogenes*	Cefotaxime + ampicillin + vancomycin (aminoglycoside if <4 weeks)
3 mo to 50 yr	*Neisseria meningitidis*, *Streptococcus pneumoniae*, *Haemophilus influenzae*	Ceftriaxone or cefotaxime + vancomycin
>50 yr	*S. pneumoniae*, *N. meningitidis*, *L. monocytogenes*	Ceftriaxone or cefotaxime + vancomycin + ampicillin
Impaired cellular immunity (e.g., HIV)	*S. pneumoniae*, *N. meningitidis*, *L. monocytogenes*, aerobic gram-negative bacilli (including *Pseudomonas aeruginosa*)	Ceftazidime + ampicillin + vancomycin

[handwritten note: Add ampicillin for the risk groups for L. monocytogenes]

b. Intravenous (IV) antibiotics
  • Initiate immediately if the CSF is cloudy or if bacterial infection is suspected.
  • Begin empiric therapy according to the patient's age (see Table 10-3).
  • Modify treatment as appropriate based on Gram stain, culture, and sensitivity findings.
c. Steroids—if cerebral edema is present
d. Vaccination
  • Vaccinate all adults >65 years for *S. pneumoniae*
  • Vaccinate asplenic patients for *S. pneumoniae*, *N. meningitidis*, and *H. influenzae* (organisms with capsules)
  • Vaccinate immunocompromised patients for meningococcus
e. Prophylaxis (e.g., rifampin or ceftriaxone)—For all close contacts of patients with meningococcus, give 1 dose of IM ceftriaxone.
2. Aseptic meningitis
  a. No specific therapy other than supportive care is required. The disease is self-limited.
  b. Analgesics and fever reduction may be appropriate.

Encephalitis

A. General characteristics
1. Encephalitis is a diffuse inflammation of the brain parenchyma and is often seen simultaneously with meningitis.
2. It is usually viral in origin. Nonviral causes, however, must also be considered.
  a. Viral causes
    • Herpes (HSV-1)
    • Arbovirus—e.g., Eastern equine encephalitis, West Nile virus
    • Enterovirus—e.g., polio
    • Less common causes—e.g., measles, mumps, EBV, CMV, VZV, rabies, and prion diseases such as Creutzfeldt-Jakob disease
  b. Nonviral infectious causes
    • Toxoplasmosis
    • Cerebral aspergillosis
  c. Noninfectious causes
    • Metabolic encephalopathies
    • T-cell lymphoma

3. Risk factors
   a. AIDS—patients with AIDS are especially at risk for toxoplasmosis when the CD4 count is <200
   b. Other forms of immunosuppression
   c. Travel in underdeveloped countries
   d. Exposure to insect (e.g., mosquito) vector in endemic areas
   e. Exposure to certain wild animals (e.g., bats) in an endemic area for rabies
4. The overall mortality associated with viral encephalitis is approximately 10%.

B. Clinical features
1. Patients often have a prodrome of headache, malaise, and myalgias.
2. Within hours to days, patients become more acutely ill.
3. Patients frequently have signs and symptoms of meningitis (e.g., headache, fever, photophobia, nuchal rigidity).
4. In addition, patients have altered sensorium, possibly including confusion, delirium, disorientation, and behavior abnormalities.
5. Focal neurologic findings (e.g., hemiparesis, aphasia, cranial nerve lesions) and seizures may also be present.

C. Diagnosis
1. Routine laboratory tests (to rule out nonviral causes) include CXR, urine and blood cultures, urine toxicology screen, and serum chemistries.
2. Perform an LP to examine CSF, unless the patient has signs of significantly increased ICP.
   a. Lymphocytosis (>5 WBC/μL) with normal glucose is consistent with viral encephalitis (similar CSF as in viral meningitis). CSF cultures are usually negative.
   b. CSF PCR is the most specific and sensitive test for diagnosing many various viral encephalitides, including HSV-1, CMV, EBV, and VZV.
3. MRI of the brain is the imaging study of choice.
   a. Can rule out focal neurologic causes, such as an abscess
   b. Increased areas of T2 signal in the frontotemporal localization are consistent with HSV encephalitis
4. EEG can be helpful in diagnosing HSV-1 encephalitis—it would show unilateral or bilateral temporal lobe discharges.
5. Brain biopsy is indicated in an acutely ill patient with a focal, enhancing lesion on MRI without a clear diagnosis.

D. Treatment
1. Supportive care, mechanical ventilation if necessary
2. Antiviral therapy
   a. There is no specific antiviral therapy for most causes of viral encephalitis.
   b. HSV encephalitis—acyclovir for 2 to 3 weeks
   c. CMV encephalitis—ganciclovir or foscarnet
3. Management of possible complications
   a. Seizures—require anticonvulsant therapy
   b. Cerebral edema—Treatment may include hyperventilation, osmotic diuresis, and steroids. *mannitol*

Brain Abscess
A. General characteristics
1. By definition, is focal and involves the brain parenchyma
2. Can manifest as a sequela of the following:
   a. Ear, nose, or throat infection—e.g., sinusitis, otitis media
   b. Cranial trauma, brain surgery
   c. Pyogenic lung infection (with hematogenous spread)
   d. Dental infection

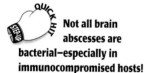

Differential diagnosis in patients with fever and altered mental status:
Infection
- Sepsis, UTI/urosepsis, pneumonia, bacterial meningitis, intracranial abscess, subdural empyema

Medication/drugs
- Neuroleptic malignant syndrome (haloperidol, phenothiazines)
- Delirium tremens

Metabolic
- Thyroid storm

Not all brain abscesses are bacterial—especially in immunocompromised hosts!
- *Toxoplasma gondii* and fungi in patients with AIDS
- *Candida* spp., *Aspergillus* spp., or zygomycosis in neutropenic patients

3. Common microbial etiologies
   a. *Streptococcus* spp. (*S. intermedius*)—sinusitis
   b. *S. aureus*—posttraumatic, postoperative infection
   c. Anaerobes—chronic otitis media and chronic pulmonary disease; frequently polymicrobial

B. Risk factors: In addition to those listed above, include AIDS, neutropenia, bone marrow transplantation, bacterial meningitis

C. Clinical features
1. These are mainly due to mass effect rather than systemic infection: headache (most common symptom), change in mental status, seizures, nausea, vomiting, and nuchal rigidity may be seen. **Note that fever and chills may be absent.**
2. With progression, intracranial abscess may cause an increasing mass effect.

↑ ICP

D. Diagnosis
1. CT scan—typically shows focal, low-density mass with peripheral enhancement and variable degree of surrounding edema
2. MRI—may result in earlier diagnosis and is overall a better imaging study
3. Aspiration or surgical excision—is diagnostic (obtaining cultures) and therapeutic

E. Treatment
1. May involve IV antibiotics, surgical drainage, and/or glucocorticoids, depending on size of abscess and presence of mass effect
2. Specific antibiotic guidelines
   a. Broad-spectrum antibiotics if bacterial cause is unknown
   b. Parenteral antibiotics for at least 4 to 6 weeks
   c. A common regimen is penicillin G plus chloramphenicol or metronidazole (if anaerobe is suspected).
   d. Add nafcillin if *S. aureus* is suspected; vancomycin for MRSA.

Penicillin G + (chloramphenicol/ metronidazole if anaerobe suspected)

INFECTIONS OF THE GASTROINTESTINAL TRACT (SEE ALSO CHAPTER 3)

Viral Hepatitis

A. General characteristics
1. Hepatitis simply means inflammation of the liver. There are many noninfectious types of hepatitis, such as alcoholic hepatitis, drug-induced hepatitis, and autoimmune hepatitis, and numerous hereditary diseases that can cause hepatitis.
2. Causes of viral hepatitis
   a. There are five well-understood, main categories of viral hepatitis: hepatitis A, B, C, D, and E. Hepatitis viruses are often abbreviated by their type (i.e., HAV is hepatitis A virus, HBV is hepatitis B virus, and so forth.)
   b. Other viruses that can cause one form or another of hepatitis are EBV, CMV, and HSV. These are not commonly associated with hepatitis in immunocompetent patients.
3. Transmission varies depending on the specific virus.
   a. Hepatitis A and E are transmitted via the fecal–oral route and are more prevalent in developing countries.
   b. Hepatitis E is particularly prevalent in India, Pakistan, southeast Asia, and parts of Africa.
   c. **Hepatitis B is transmitted parenterally or sexually.** Perinatal transmission is also possible and is a significant health issue in parts of Africa and Asia.
   d. Hepatitis D requires the outer envelope of the Hb$_s$Ag for replication and therefore can only be transmitted as a coinfection with HBV, or as a superinfection in a chronic HBV carrier.

- **Hepatitis B** is associated with polyarteritis nodosa (PAN).
- **Hepatitis C** is associated with cryoglobulinemia.

Box **10-3** **Hepatitis Serology**

Hepatitis A
- Hepatitis A antibody (anti-HAV)
  - Anti-HAV is detectable during acute infection and persists for life, so its presence does not distinguish between active disease and immunity. IgM-specific antibody denotes acute infection.

Hepatitis B
- Hepatitis B surface antigen (HB$_s$Ag)
  - Present in acute or chronic infection
  - Detectable as early as 1 to 2 weeks after infection
  - It persists in chronic hepatitis regardless of whether symptoms are present. If virus is cleared, then HB$_s$Ag is undetectable.
- Hepatitis B e antigen (HB$_e$Ag)
  - Reflects active viral replication, and presence indicates infectivity
  - Appears shortly after HB$_s$Ag
- Anti-HB$_s$Ag antibody (anti-HBs)
  - Present after vaccination or after clearance of HB$_s$Ag—usually detectable 1 to 3 months after infection
  - In most cases, presence of anti-HBs indicates immunity to HBV
- Hepatitis B core antibody (anti-HBc)
  - Assay of IgM and IgG combined
  - Useful because it may be the only serological marker of HBV infection during the "window period" in which HB$_s$Ag is disappearing, but anti-HB$_s$Ag is not yet detectable
  - Does not distinguish between acute and chronic infection, and presence does not indicate immunity
- Viral load
  - HBV DNA measured by PCR; if it persists for more than 6 weeks, patient is likely to develop chronic disease

Hepatitis C
- Hepatitis C antibody
  - Key marker of HCV infection
  - Sometimes not detectable until months after infection, so its absence does not rule out infection
- Viral load: HCV RNA measured by PCR
  - Detectable 1 to 2 weeks after infection—more sensitive than HCV antibody

Hepatitis D
- Hepatitis D antibody (anti-HDV)
  - Presence indicates HDV superinfection ·
  - The antibody may not be present in acute illness, so repeat testing may be necessary.

---

   e. **The main route of transmission for hepatitis C is parenteral**, and it is there-
      fore more prevalent in IV drug users. Sexual or perinatal transmission is not
      common.
   f. **Hepatitis B, C, and D are the types that can progress to chronic disease.**

B. Clinical features
   1. Classified as acute (<6 months of liver inflammation) or chronic (>6 months of
      persistent liver inflammation)
   2. Acute hepatitis has a wide spectrum of clinical presentations, ranging from virtu-
      ally asymptomatic to fulminant liver failure.
      a. General clinical features
         - Jaundice—Look first in the sclera, because this may be the first place jaundice
           can be detected, especially in black patients.
         - Dark-colored urine may be present (due to conjugated hyperbilirubinemia).
         - RUQ pain
         - Nausea and vomiting
         - Fever and malaise
         - Hepatomegaly may also be present.
      b. In severe cases, acute hepatitis may result in liver failure and its complications.
         This is known as fulminant hepatitis (uncommon) and may be life-threatening. It
         occurs more commonly in hepatitis B, D, and E than in other types. Complica-
         tions include:

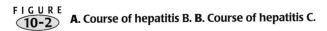

FIGURE 10-2 A. Course of hepatitis B. B. Course of hepatitis C.

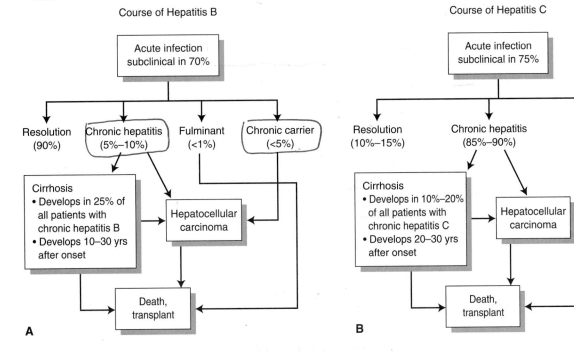

A

B

- Hepatic encephalopathy—Look for **asterixis** and **palmar erythema**.
- Hepatorenal syndrome
- Bleeding diathesis—This occurs only when liver function is very compromised.

c. Sometimes acute hepatitis may only present with transient flu-like symptoms such as fever, myalgias, and malaise.

d. Acute HBV may also present with a serum sickness–like illness.

e. Hepatitis C typically does not cause significant **acute** illness. *usually subclinical presentation*

3. Chronic hepatitis also has a wide variety of presentations. Some patients are asymptomatic ("chronic carriers") and may only present with late complications of hepatitis, such as cirrhosis or hepatic cell carcinoma (HCC).

a. Chronic hepatitis occurs after acute hepatitis in 1% to 10% of patients with HBV and >80% patients with HCV.

b. It is categorized based on the grade of inflammation, the stage of fibrosis, and the etiology of disease.

c. The risk of developing cirrhosis or HCC is 25% to 40% in patients with chronic HBV and 10% to 25% in patients with chronic HCV.

HCC - 25% - 40% in HBV
HCC - 10% - 25% in HCV

C. Diagnosis

1. Serum serology—The presence of serum antigens and immunoglobulins is the most important factor for diagnosing viral hepatitis. These are helpful for determining the acuity or chronicity of illness as well as adequate immunity (see Box 10-3).

2. PCR is used to detect viral RNA to diagnose HCV.

3. LFTs—Elevation of serum transaminases is not diagnostic, but LFTs are helpful.

a. ALT (SGPT) is typically elevated more than AST (SGOT) for all forms of viral hepatitis (the opposite of alcoholic hepatitis).

b. In acute hepatitis, ALT is usually >1,000. It is generally not as high as in drug-induced hepatitis.

c. In chronic HBV, ALT can also be >1,000, but this varies. In chronic HCV, ALT is generally lower than this.

D. Treatment

1. Active (vaccine) and passive (immunoglobulin) immunization are available for both hepatitis A and B. It is the standard of care for infants and health care workers to be vaccinated for HBV (see Chapter 12).

QUICK HIT Generally, HAV and HEV cause a more mild form of hepatitis and do not become chronic.

QUICK HIT If transaminases are markedly elevated (>500), think of acute viral hepatitis, shock liver, or drug-induced hepatitis.

2. Travelers often receive vaccinations for HAV. [Passive immunization can be given for people who are exposed to the virus.]
3. Treatment for hepatitis A and E is supportive.
4. Chronic HBV—Treat with interferon (IFN)-α. Alternatively, treat with lamivudine (nucleoside analog). *anti- reverse transcriptase able used abacavir.*
5. Chronic HCV—Treat with IFN-α and ribavirin.
6. Consider liver transplantation in advanced disease, although recurrence can occur after transplantation.

Botulism

A. General characteristics

1. Results from ingestion of **preformed toxins** produced by spores of *Clostridium botulinum*. Improperly stored food (e.g., home-canned foods) can be contaminated with these spores. Toxins can be inactivated by cooking food at high temperatures (e.g., 100°C [212°F] for 10 minutes).
2. Wound contamination is another source.

B. Clinical features

1. The severity of illness ranges widely, from mild, self-limiting symptoms, to rapidly fatal disease.
2. Abdominal cramps, nausea, vomiting, and diarrhea are common.
3. **The hallmark clinical manifestation is symmetric, descending flaccid paralysis.** It starts with dry mouth, diplopia, and/or dysarthria. Paralysis of limb musculature occurs later. *anti- cholinergic*

C. Diagnosis

1. The definitive diagnosis is identification of toxin in serum, stool, or gastric contents (bioassay).
2. Identifying *C. botulinum* alone in food is not a reliable diagnostic indicator.

D. Treatment

1. Admit the patient and observe respiratory status closely. Gastric lavage is helpful only within several hours after ingestion of suspected food.
2. If suspicion of botulism is high, administer antitoxin (toxoid) as soon as laboratory specimens are obtained (do not wait for the results).
3. For contaminated wounds (in addition to above)—wound cleansing and penicillin

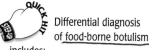

QUICK HIT

Differential diagnosis of food-borne botulism includes:
• Guillain-Barré syndrome—characteristically ascending paralysis, but one variety (Fischer) can be descending
• Eaton-Lambert syndrome
• Myasthenia gravis—EMG studies differentiate
• Diphtheria
• Tick paralysis

Botulism Rx:
① If time of indigestion in near past → gastric lavage.
② administer antitoxin.

Intra-abdominal Abscess

• Causes include spontaneous bacterial peritonitis, pelvic infection (e.g., tubo-ovarian abscess), pancreatitis, perforation of the GI tract, and osteomyelitis of the vertebral bodies with extension into the retroperitoneal cavity.
• Usually polymicrobial in origin
• Diagnose using CT scan or ultrasound.
• Treatment typically involves drainage of the abscess. *percutaneous*
• The antibiotic regimen should include broad coverage against gram-negative rods, enterococci, and anaerobes. *Ciprofloxacin and metronidazole.*

INFECTIONS OF THE GENITOURINARY TRACT

Lower Urinary Tract Infections

A. General characteristics

1. Urinary tract infections (UTIs) are much more common in women than in men. Up to 33% of all women experience a UTI in their lifetime. The most common UTI is uncomplicated acute cystitis.
2. The majority of UTIs are caused by ascending infection from the urethra.

3. Common organisms
   a. *E. coli* (most common)—causes 80% of cases
   b. Other organisms—*Staphylococcus saprophyticus, Enterococcus, Klebsiella, Proteus* spp., *Pseudomonas, Enterobacter*, and yeast (such as *Candida* spp.)

[handwritten: ↓ alkaline pH.]

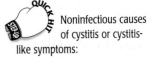

QUICK HIT More than 90% of uncomplicated UTIs are caused by *E. coli, S. saprophyticus*, and *Enterococcus* spp. A small percentage is caused by *Proteus, Klebsiella, Enterobacter*, and *Pseudomonas*.

B. Risk factors

1. Female gender—greater risk due to the shorter female urethra and vaginal colonization of bacteria
2. Sexual intercourse
   a. Often the trigger of a UTI in women, thus the term "honeymoon cystitis"
   b. Use of diaphragms and spermicides increases risk further (alters vaginal colonization)
3. Pregnancy
4. Indwelling urinary catheters—risk factor for hospitalized patients
5. Personal history of recurrent UTIs
6. Host-dependent factors—increase risk for recurrent or complicated UTIs
   a. Diabetes—diabetic patients are at risk for upper UTI
   b. Patients with spinal cord injury
   c. Immunocompromised state
   d. Any structural or functional abnormality that impedes urinary flow (e.g., incomplete voiding, neurogenic bladder, BPH, vesicourethral reflux, calculi)
7. Male risk factors
   a. Uncircumcised males are at higher risk due to bacterial colonization of the foreskin
   b. Anal intercourse
   c. Vaginal intercourse with a female colonized with uropathogens

C. Clinical features

1. Dysuria—commonly expressed as burning on urination
2. Frequency
3. Urgency
4. Suprapubic tenderness
5. Gross hematuria is sometimes present
6. **In lower UTIs, fever is characteristically absent.**

QUICK HIT Noninfectious causes of cystitis or cystitis-like symptoms:
- Cytotoxic agents—e.g., cyclophosphamide
- Radiation to the pelvis
- Dysfunctional voiding
- Interstitial cystitis

D. Diagnosis

1. Dipstick urinalysis
   a. Positive urine leukocyte esterase test—rapid screen for pyuria
   b. Positive nitrite test for presence of bacteria (gram-negative)
   c. Combining the above two tests yields a sensitivity of 85% and specificity of 75%.

[handwritten: need both bacteriuria and pyuria]

2. Urinalysis (clean-catch midstream specimen)
   a. Adequacy of collection
      - The presence of epithelial (squamous) cells indicates vulvar or urethral contamination.
      - If contamination is suspected, perform a straight catheterization of the bladder.
   b. Criteria for UTI
      - Bacteriuria: >1 organism per oil-immersion field. Bacteriuria without WBCs may reflect contamination and is not a reliable indicator of infection.
      - Pyuria: >8 WBC/HPF
   c. Other findings—Hematuria and mild proteinuria may be present.
3. Urine Gram stain
   - A count of >10^5 organisms/mL represents significant bacteriuria.
   - It is 90% sensitive and 88% specific.
4. Urine culture
   a. Confirms the diagnosis (high specificity)
   b. Traditional criteria: ≥10^5 CFU/mL of urine from a clean-catch sample; misses up to one-third of UTIs
   c. Colony counts as low as 10^2 to 10^4 CFU/mL are adequate for diagnosis if clinical symptoms are present.

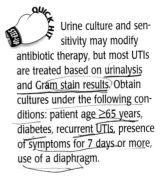

QUICK HIT Urine culture and sensitivity may modify antibiotic therapy, but most UTIs are treated based on urinalysis and Gram stain results. Obtain cultures under the following conditions: patient age ≥65 years, diabetes, recurrent UTIs, presence of symptoms for 7 days or more, use of a diaphragm.

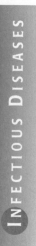

INFECTIOUS DISEASES

5. Blood cultures—only indicated if patient is ill and urosepsis is suspected
6. IVP, cystoscopy, and excretory urography are not recommended unless structural abnormalities or obstruction is suspected.

E. Complications

1. Complicated UTI
   a. Any UTI that spreads beyond the bladder (e.g., pyelonephritis, prostatitis, urosepsis)—risk factors for upper UTI: pregnancy, diabetes, and vesicoureteral reflux
   b. Any UTI caused by structural abnormalities, metabolic disorder, or neurologic dysfunction
2. UTI during pregnancy—increased risk of preterm labor, low birth weight, and other complications, especially in advanced pregnancy
3. Recurrent infections
   a. Usually due to infection with new organism, but sometimes is a relapse due to unsuccessful treatment of the original organism
   b. Risk factors include impaired host defenses, pregnancy, vesicourethral reflux, and sexual intercourse in women.
   c. Generally the consequences are not significant unless the patient is at risk for upper UTI.

F. Treatment

1. Acute uncomplicated cystitis—i.e., nonpregnant women
   a. Use empiric treatment with oral TMP/SMX (Bactrim) for 3 days. If the resistance rate to TMP/SMX is high in the community (or if the patient is sulfa-allergic), use of a fluoroquinolone (ciprofloxacin) for 3 days is appropriate.
   b. Amoxicillin is a less popular alternative due to increasing antimicrobial resistance.
   c. The most cost-effective treatment duration is 3 days. Single-dose treatments have a higher recurrence rate, and 7-day treatments are associated with higher rates of side effects.
   d. Treat presumptively for pyelonephritis if the condition fails to respond to a short course of antibiotics.
   e. Phenazopyridine (Pyridium) is a urinary analgesic; it can be given for 1 to 3 days for dysuria.
2. Pregnant women with UTI
   a. Treat with ampicillin, amoxicillin, or oral cephalosporins for 7 to 10 days.
   b. Avoid fluoroquinolones (can cause fetal arthropathy)
3. UTIs in men
   a. Treat as with uncomplicated cystitis in women, except for 7 days.
   b. Perform a urologic workup if there are complications or recurrences, or if initial treatment fails.
4. Recurrent infections
   a. If relapse occurs within 2 weeks of cessation of treatment, continue treatment for 2 more weeks and obtain a urine culture.
   b. Otherwise treat as for uncomplicated cystitis. If the patient has more than two UTIs per year, give chemoprophylaxis.
      - Single dose of TMP/SMX after intercourse or at first signs of symptoms
      - Alternative low-dose prophylactic antibiotics, e.g., low-dose TMP/SMX, for 6 months ; Nitrofurantoin.

[Handwritten margin note:]
Uncomplicated UTIs
① Women - Rx for 3 days
② Men - Rx for 7 days
③ Pregnant ladies - Rx w/ ampicillin for 7/10 days.

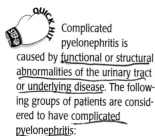

Pyelonephritis

A. General characteristics

1. Pyelonephritis is an infection of the upper urinary tract.
   a. It is usually caused by ascending spread from the bladder to the kidney.
   b. Uncomplicated pyelonephritis is limited to the renal pyelocalyceal–medullary region.
   c. Vesicoureteral reflux facilitates this ascending spread. See above for other risk factors.

2. Organisms
   a. *E. coli* (most frequent cause)
   b. Other gram-negative bacteria include *Proteus*, *Klebsiella*, *Enterobacter*, and *Pseudomonas* spp.
   c. Gram-positive bacteria (less common) include *Enterococcus faecalis* and *S. aureus*.
3. Complications (unusual)
   a. Sepsis occurs in 10% to 25% of patients with pyelonephritis. May lead to shock.
   b. Emphysematous pyelonephritis—caused by gas-producing bacteria in diabetic patients
   c. Chronic pyelonephritis and scarring of the kidneys—rare unless underlying renal disease exists

B. Clinical features

1. Symptoms
   a. Fever, chills
   b. Flank pain
   c. Symptoms of cystitis (may or may not be present)
   d. Nausea, vomiting, and diarrhea (sometimes present)
2. Signs
   a. Fever with tachycardia
   b. Patients generally appear more ill than patients with cystitis
   c. Costovertebral angle tenderness—unilateral or bilateral
   d. Abdominal tenderness may be present on examination.

C. Diagnosis

1. Urinalysis
   a. Look for pyuria, bacteriuria, and leukocyte casts. *WBC casts.*
   b. As in cystitis, hematuria and mild proteinuria may be present.
2. Urine cultures—obtain in all patients with suspected pyelonephritis
3. Blood cultures—obtain in ill-appearing patients and all hospitalized patients
4. CBC—leukocytosis with left shift
5. Renal function—This is usually preserved. Impairment is usually reversible, especially with intravenous fluids.
6. Imaging studies—Perform these if treatment fails or in any patient with complicated pyelonephritis. Consider renal ultrasound, CT, IVP, or retrograde ureterogram.

D. Treatment

1. For uncomplicated pyelonephritis
   a. Use outpatient treatment if the patient can take oral antibiotics. Treat based on Gram stain:
      • TMP/SMX or a fluoroquinolone for 10 to 14 days is effective for most gram-negative rods.
      • Amoxicillin is appropriate for gram-positive cocci (enterococci, *S. saprophyticus*).
      • A single dose of ceftriaxone or gentamicin is often given initially before starting oral treatment.
   b. Repeat urine culture 2 to 4 days after cessation of therapy.
   c. If symptoms fail to resolve within 48 hours, adjust treatment based on urine culture.
   d. Failure to respond to appropriate antimicrobial therapy suggests a functional or structural abnormality; perform a urologic investigation.
2. If the patient is very ill, elderly, pregnant, unable to tolerate oral medication, or has significant comorbidities, or if urosepsis is suspected
   a. Hospitalize the patient and give IV fluids.
   b. Treat with antibiotics.
      • Start with parenteral antibiotics (broad-spectrum)—ampicillin plus gentamicin or ciprofloxacin are common initial choices.

- If blood cultures are negative, treat with IV antibiotics until the patient is afebrile for 24 hours, then give oral antibiotics to complete a 14- to 21-day course.
- If blood cultures are positive (urosepsis), treat with intravenous antibiotics for 2 to 3 weeks.

3. For recurrent pyelonephritis
   a. If relapse is due to the same organism despite appropriate treatment, treat for 6 weeks.
   b. If relapse is due to a new organism, treat with appropriate therapy for 2 weeks.

Prostatitis — gram negative organisms.

A. General characteristics

1. Acute bacterial prostatitis
   a. Less common than chronic bacterial prostatitis
   b. Occurs more commonly in younger men
   c. Pathophysiology
      - Ascending infection from the urethra and reflux of infected urine
      - May occur after urinary catheterization
      - Other causes—direct or lymphatic spread from the rectum
      - Hematogenous spread (rare)
   d. Gram-negative organisms predominate, e.g., *E. coli*, *Klebsiella*, *Proteus*, *Pseudomonas*, *Enterobacter*, and *Serratia* spp.
2. Chronic bacterial prostatitis
   a. More common than acute bacterial prostatitis; true prevalence is difficult to determine because many cases are asymptomatic and are diagnosed incidentally
   b. It most commonly affects men 40 to 70 years of age.
   c. It has the same routes of infection as acute bacterial prostatitis. It may develop from acute bacterial prostatitis.
   d. Organisms are similar to those in acute prostatitis.

B. Clinical features

1. Acute prostatitis
   a. Fever, chills—Patients may appear toxic.
   b. Irritative voiding symptoms—Dysuria, frequency, and urgency are common.
   c. Perineal pain, low back pain, and urinary retention may be present as well.
2. Chronic prostatitis
   a. Patients may be asymptomatic. Patients do not appear ill. Fever is uncommon.
   b. Patients frequently have recurrent UTIs with irritative voiding and/or obstructive urinary symptoms.
   c. There is dull, poorly localized pain in the lower back, perineal, scrotal, or suprapubic region.

C. Diagnosis

1. DRE—There is a boggy, exquisitely tender prostate in acute disease. In chronic disease, prostate is enlarged and usually nontender.
2. Urinalysis—Numerous (sheets of) WBCs are present in acute bacterial prostatitis.
3. Urine cultures—almost always positive in acute prostatitis
4. Chronic prostatitis—The presence of WBCs in expressed prostatic secretions suggests diagnosis. Urine cultures may be positive (chronic bacterial prostatitis) or negative (nonbacterial prostatitis).
5. Obtain CBC and blood cultures if patient appears toxic or if sepsis is suspected.

D. Treatment

1. Acute prostatitis
   a. If it is severe and the patient appears toxic, hospitalize the patient and initiate IV antibiotics.

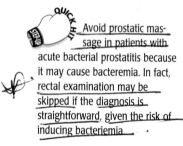

Acute versus chronic prostatitis
- Acute prostatitis is a more serious condition than chronic prostatitis, and urgent treatment is necessary.
- Acute prostatitis is much more obvious clinically (fever, exquisitely tender prostate), whereas chronic prostatitis is difficult to diagnose because the prostate may not be tender and findings are variable.

Avoid prostatic massage in patients with acute bacterial prostatitis because it may cause bacteremia. In fact, rectal examination may be skipped if the diagnosis is straightforward, given the risk of inducing bacteriemia.

b. If it is mild, treat on an outpatient basis with antibiotics—TMP/SMX or a fluoroquinolone and doxycycline. Treat for 4 to 6 weeks.

c. The patient usually responds to therapy.

2. Chronic prostatitis

a. Treat with a fluoroquinolone. For chronic bacterial prostatitis, a prolonged course is recommended but does not guarantee complete eradication.

b. It is very difficult to treat. Recurrences are common.

SEXUALLY TRANSMITTED DISEASES (STDs)

Genital Warts (See Color Figure 10-1)

- These are caused by HPV.
- They are the **most common STD.**
- See Chapter 11, Common Dermatologic Problems, Inflammatory, Allergic, and Autoimmune Skin Conditions, Warts.

Chlamydia

A. General characteristics

1. **Chlamydia is the most common bacterial STD.** The organism is an intracellular pathogen.

2. Many patients are coinfected with gonorrhea (up to 40% of women and 20% of men).

3. The incubation period is 1 to 3 weeks.

B. Clinical features

1. Many cases are asymptomatic (80% of women, 50% of men).

2. Men who are symptomatic may have any of the following: dysuria, purulent urethral discharge, scrotal pain and swelling, and fever.

3. Women who are symptomatic may have purulent urethral discharge, intermenstrual or postcoital bleeding, and dysuria.

C. Diagnosis

1. Diagnostic tests include culture, enzyme immunoassay, and molecular tests such as PCR. Serologic tests are not used for *Chlamydia.*

2. Molecular diagnostic tests are replacing culture as the screening test of choice due to higher sensitivity.

3. Sexually active adolescents (particularly females) should be screened for chlamydial infection even if they are asymptomatic.

D. Treatment

1. Azithromycin (oral one dose) or doxycycline (oral for 7 days)

2. Treat all sexual partners.

Gonorrhea

A. General characteristics

1. The responsible organism is *Neisseria gonorrhoeae* (a gram-negative, intracellular diplococcal organism).

2. Gonorrhea is usually asymptomatic in women but symptomatic in men. Therefore, complications occur more often in women due to undetected disease.

3. It is almost always transmitted sexually (except with neonatal transmission).

4. Coinfection with *Chlamydia trachomatis* occurs in 30% of patients (more common in women).

B. Clinical features

1. Men

a. Gonorrhea is asymptomatic in up to 10% of carriers. These asymptomatic carriers can still transmit the disease.

 Recurrent exacerbations are common in chronic prostatitis if not treated adequately. Recurrent UTI is very common in these patients.

Eighty percent of cases of Reiter's syndrome are associated with chlamydial infection.

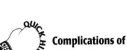 Chlamydia infection is a risk factor for cervical cancer, especially when there is a history of multiple infections.

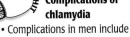 **Complications of chlamydia**
- Complications in men include epididymitis and proctitis.
- Complications in women include pelvic inflammatory disease, salpingitis, tubo-ovarian abscess, ectopic pregnancy, and Fitz-Hugh-Curtis syndrome. **Chlamydia is a leading cause of infertility in women due to tubal scarring.**

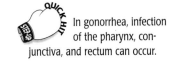 In gonorrhea, infection of the pharynx, conjunctiva, and rectum can occur.

b. Most men have symptoms involving the urethra—e.g., purulent discharge, dysuria, erythema and edema of urethral meatus, and frequency of urination.

2. Women
   a. **Most women are asymptomatic or have few symptoms.**
   b. Women may have symptoms of cervicitis or urethritis—e.g., purulent discharge, dysuria, intermenstrual bleeding, and dyspareunia.

3. Disseminated gonococcal infection (occurs in 1% to 2% of cases; more common in women)—possible findings:
   a. Fever, arthralgias, tenosynovitis (of hands and feet)
   b. Migratory polyarthritis/septic arthritis, endocarditis, or even meningitis
   c. Skin rash (usually on distal extremities)

C. Diagnosis

1. Gram stain of urethral discharge showing organisms within leukocytes is highly specific for gonorrhea.
2. Obtain cultures in all cases—in men from the urethra; in women from the endocervix. May treat empirically because culture results take 1 to 2 days to return.
3. Consider testing for syphilis and HIV.
4. Obtain blood cultures if disease has disseminated.

D. Treatment

1. Ceftriaxone (IM, one dose) is preferred because it is also effective against syphilis. Other options are oral cefixime, ciprofloxacin, or ofloxacin.
2. Also give azithromycin (one dose) or doxycycline (for 7 days) to cover coexistent chlamydial infection.
3. If disseminated, hospitalize the patient and initiate ceftriaxone (IV or IM for 7 days).

HIV and AIDS

A. General characteristics

1. Pathophysiology
   a. The most common virus associated with HIV is the HIV type 1 human retrovirus.
   b. The virus attaches to the surface of CD4+ T lymphocytes (targets of HIV-1); it enters the cell and uncoats, and its RNA is transcribed to DNA by reverse transcriptase.
   c. Billions of viral particles are produced each day by activated CD4 cells. When the virus enters the lytic stage of infection, CD4 cells are destroyed. It is the depletion of the body's arsenal of CD4 cells that weakens the **cellular immunity** of the host.
2. Transmission is usually sexual or parenteral. Other than semen and blood, fluids that transmit the disease are breast milk and vaginal fluid.
3. Mortality is usually secondary to opportunistic infection, wasting, or cancer.
4. High-risk individuals: homosexual or bisexual men, IV drug abusers, blood transfusion recipients before 1985 (before widespread screening of donor blood), heterosexual contacts of HIV-positive individuals, unborn and newborn babies of mothers who are HIV-positive

B. Clinical features

1. Primary infection
   a. A mononucleosis-like syndrome about 2 to 4 weeks after exposure to HIV. Duration of the illness is brief (3 days to 2 weeks).
   b. Symptoms include fever, sweats, malaise, lethargy, headaches, arthralgias/myalgias, diarrhea, sore throat, lymphadenopathy, and a truncal maculopapular rash.
2. Asymptomatic infection (seropositive, but no clinical evidence of HIV infection)
   a. CD4 counts are normal ($>500/mm^3$).
   b. Longest phase (lasts 4 to 7 years, but varies widely, especially with treatment)
3. Symptomatic HIV infection (pre-AIDS)
   a. First evidence of immune system dysfunction
   b. Without treatment, this phase lasts about 1 to 3 years.

QUICK HIT

Gonorrheal complications
• Pelvic inflammatory disease, with possible infertility and chronic pelvic pain
• Epididymitis, prostatitis (uncommon)
• Salpingitis, tubo-ovarian abscess
• Fitz-Hugh-Curtis syndrome (perihepatitis)–RUQ pain; elevated LFTs
• Disseminated gonococcal infection

QUICK HIT

It is important (but often difficult) to identify patients with primary HIV infection because of the benefits of early antiretroviral therapy. A high index of suspicion is necessary.

Box 10-4 HIV Serology

CD4 Cell Count
- It is the best indicator of the status of the immune system and of the risk for opportunistic infections and disease progression.
- It is used to determine when to initiate antiretroviral therapy and PCP prophylaxis. It is also useful in assessing the response to antiretroviral therapy.
- If untreated (no retroviral therapy), the CD4-cell count decreases at an average rate of about 50 per year.
- If >500, the immune system is essentially normal. HIV-related infection or illness is unlikely.
- If 200 to 500, there is an increased risk of HIV-related problems, such as herpes zoster, TB, lymphoma, bacterial pneumonias, and Kaposi's sarcoma. However, many patients are asymptomatic at these CD4 levels.
- Most opportunistic infections occur when the CD4 count falls below 200.

Viral Load (HIV-1 RNA Levels)
- Used to assess response to and adequacy of antiretroviral therapy; provides complementary prognostic information to the CD4+ count
- If the viral load is still >50 after about 4 months of treatment, modification in the regimen may be needed.
- Do not stop antiretroviral therapy even if viral loads are undetectable for years. Latently infected cells can lead to reappearance of viral RNA once therapy is stopped.
- Measure the plasma HIV RNA levels and the CD4-cell count at the time of diagnosis and every 3 to 4 months thereafter.

---

c. The following frequently appear.
- Persistent generalized lymphadenopathy
- Localized fungal infections (e.g., on fingernails, toes, mouth)
- Recalcitrant vaginal yeast and trichomonal infections in women
- Oral hairy leukoplakia on the tongue
- Skin manifestations that include seborrheic dermatitis, psoriasis exacerbations, molluscum, and warts
- Constitutional symptoms (night sweats, weight loss, and diarrhea)

4. AIDS
   a. Marked immune suppression leads to disseminated opportunistic infections and malignancies.
   b. CD4 count is <200 cells/mm^3.
   c. Pulmonary, GI, neurologic, cutaneous, and systemic symptoms are common (see Table 10-4).

C. Diagnosis

1. Diagnosis of HIV infection
   a. Enzyme-linked immunosorbent assay (ELISA) method
      - Screening test for detecting antibody to HIV; becomes positive 1 to 12 weeks after infection
      - A negative ELISA essentially excludes HIV (99% sensitive) as long as the patient has not had a subsequent exposure before testing (before seroconversion).
      - If positive, Western blot test should be performed for confirmation.
   b. Western blot test is a specific test used to confirm a positive result on an ELISA test.
2. Diagnosis of AIDS
   a. Depends principally on the identification of an indicator condition or on finding in an HIV-1–seropositive patient a CD4-cell count lower than 200.
   b. There are many indicator conditions (**AIDS-defining illnesses**). (See Table 10-5)

D. Treatment

1. Antiretroviral therapy
   a. Indications
      - Symptomatic patients regardless of CD4 count
      - Asymptomatic patients with CD4 count <500

The course of HIV varies considerably from patient to patient. However, the typical course can be divided into the following four phases: primary infection, asymptomatic infection, symptomatic infection, and full-blown AIDS.

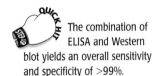
The combination of ELISA and Western blot yields an overall sensitivity and specificity of >99%.

	TABLE 10-4	**Clinical Manifestation of AIDS**

System	Condition	Comments
Pulmonary	Community-acquired bacterial pneumonia	Recurrent bacterial pneumonia (two or more episodes per year) is 20 times more common in HIV-1 patients with low CD4-cell counts (<200/mm³) than in those with normal counts.
	PCP	• Seventy percent of patients acquire PCP at some point; often the initial opportunistic infection establishes the diagnosis of AIDS. • **Leading cause of death in patients with AIDS** • **Occurs when CD4 count is ≤200** • Clinical findings: fever, nonproductive cough, shortness of breath (with exertion at first, then occurring at rest) • CXR: diffuse interstitial infiltrates; negative radiographs in 10% to 15% of patients with PCP • Treatment: TMP-SMX (PO or IV) for 3 weeks; steroid therapy if patient is hypoxic or has elevated A-a gradient • Prophylaxis: Oral TMP-SMX, 1 dose daily, is recommended.
	Tuberculosis	Negative PPD test results are frequent among AIDS patients due to immunosuppression.
	Other infections	• CMV or MAC: **increased risk when the CD4 count <50** • *Cryptococcus neoformans, Histoplasma capsulatum*, neoplasms (Kaposi's sarcoma)
Nervous system	AIDS dementia	• Progressive process in 33% of patients • Early stages: subtle impairment of recent memory and other cognitive deficits • Later stages: changes in mental status, aphasia, motor abnormalities
	Toxoplasmosis	• Usually a reactivation of latent infection of *Toxoplasmosis gondii* • Symptoms both of a mass lesion (discrete deficits, headache) and of encephalitis (fever, altered mental status) • CT scan or MRI shows characteristic findings: multiple (more than three) **contrast-enhanced mass lesions in the basal ganglia and subcortical white matter.**
	Cryptococcal meningitis	• Diagnosed by identifying organisms in CSF by cryptococcal antigen, culture, or **staining with India ink** • Treat with amphotericin B for 10 to 14 days. Follow this with 8 to 10 weeks of oral fluconazole. Lifelong maintenance therapy with fluconazole is indicated.
	Other CNS infections	Bacterial meningitis, histoplasmosis, CMV, progressive multifocal leukoencephalopathy (PML), HSV, neurosyphilis, TB
	Noninfectious CNS diseases	CNS lymphoma, CVA, metabolic encephalopathies
Gastrointestinal	Diarrhea	Most common GI complaint; caused by a variety of pathogens (*Escherichia coli, Shigella, Salmonella, Campylobacter*, CMV, *Giardia, Cryptosporidium, Isospora belli, Mycobacterium avium-intracellulare*). Antibiotic therapy is also a common cause.
	Oral lesions	Oral thrush (candidiasis), HSV or CMV (ulcers), oral hairy leukoplakia (EBV infection), Kaposi's sarcoma
	Esophageal involvement	Candidiasis is most common cause of dysphagia; also CMV and HSV—**seen with CD4 counts <100**
	Anorectal disease	Proctitis—*Neisseria gonorrhoeae, Chlamydia trachomatis*, syphilis, HSV
Dermatologic	Kaposi's sarcoma	• More common in homosexual men than in other groups • Painless, raised brown-black or purple papules (common sites: face, chest, genitals, oral cavity) • Widespread dissemination can occur.
	Infections	HSV infections, molluscum contagiosum, secondary syphilis, warts, shingles, and many other skin conditions/infections occur with higher frequency.
Miscellaneous	CMV infection	• Common cause of serious opportunistic viral disease • Disseminated disease is common and usually involves the GI or pulmonary systems. • Most important manifestation is retinitis—unilateral visual loss that can become bilateral if untreated (seen in 5% to 10% of AIDS patients) • Colitis and esophagitis are other findings. • Treat with ganciclovir or foscarnet.

(continued)

TABLE 10-4	Clinical Manifestation of AIDS *(Continued)*	
System	**Condition**	**Comments**
	Mycobacterium avium complex (MAC)	• Most common opportunistic bacterial infection in AIDS patients • MAC causes disseminated disease in 50% of AIDS patients. • Diarrhea and weight loss are constitutional symptoms.
	HIV-1 wasting syndrome	Profound involuntary loss of more than 10% of body weight in conjunction with **either** of the following: • Chronic diarrhea (two or more stools per day for more than 1 mo) • Fever and persistent weakness for a similar period in the absence of another cause
	Malignancies	• Kaposi's sarcoma • Non-Hodgkin's lymphoma—rapidly growing mass lesion in CNS • Primary CNS lymphoma

b. Triple-drug regimens known as HAART: To target and prevent HIV replication at three different points along the replication process, use two nucleoside reverse transcriptase inhibitors and either of the following:
  • A nonnucleoside reverse transcriptase inhibitor
  • A protease inhibitor

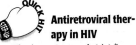

Antiretroviral therapy in HIV
• The importance of strict (i.e., 100%) adherence to the triple-drug regimen cannot be overemphasized, because even minor deviations may result in drug resistance.
• Do not initiate triple-drug therapy in a patient who is not willing or able to fully comply with the prescribed regimen.

TABLE 10-5	AIDS Indicator Diseases
Candidiasis, invasive
Cervical cancer, invasive
Coccidioidomycosis, extrapulmonary
Cryptococcosis, extrapulmonary
Cryptosporidiosis of >1 month duration
Cytomegalovirus disease outside lymphoreticular system
Encephalopathy, HIV-related
Herpes simplex infection of >1 month duration or visceral herpes simplex
Salmonella bacteremia, recurrent
Histoplasmosis, extrapulmonary
Isosporiasis of >1 month duration
Kaposi's sarcoma
Lymphoma: primary central nervous system, immunoblastic, or Burkitt's
Mycobacterial disease, disseminated or extrapulmonary
Mycobacterium tuberculosis infection
PCP
Pneumonia, recurrent (more than one episode in 1 year)
Progressive multifocal leukoencephalopathy
Toxoplasmosis, cerebral
Wasting syndrome due to HIV

Modified from Stoller JK, Ahmad M, Longworth DL. The Cleveland Clinic Intensive Review of Internal Medicine. 3rd Ed. Philadelphia: Lippincott Williams & Wilkins, 2002:188, Table 15.6.

c. Monitor the response to treatment using plasma HIV RNA load—the goal is to reduce the viral load to undetectable levels.

d. It is generally recommended that HAART therapy be continued in pregnant patients with HIV.

2. Opportunistic infection prophylaxis
   a. *P. carinii*
      • If the CD4-cell count is ≤200 or the patient has a history of oropharyngeal candidiasis, start *P. carinii* pneumonia (PCP) prophylaxis.
      • TMP/SMX is the preferred agent. *if allergic to sulfa primethamine + clindamycin*
   b. TB
      • Screen all patients with a yearly PPD test.
      • Prescribe isoniazid plus pyridoxine if the patient has positive PPD.
   c. Atypical mycobacteria—*Mycobacterium avium complex* (MAC)
      • Start prophylaxis when CD4 cell count is <100.
      • Clarithromycin and azithromycin are prophylactic agents.
   d. Toxoplasmosis
      • Give this to patients with CD4 count <100
      • TMP/SMX is the preferred agent.
3. Vaccination (**no live-virus vaccines!**)
   a. Pneumococcal polysaccharide vaccine (Pneumovax)—every 5 to 6 years
   b. Influenza vaccine—yearly
   c. Hepatitis B vaccine (if not already antibody-positive) (See Chapter 12.)

[handwritten margin note: prophalyxis for PCP <500 } TMP-SMX TOXO <100 } MAC <100 - azithro]

Herpes Simplex

A. General characteristics

1. There are two types of herpes simplex virus (HSV): HSV-1 and HSV-2. Both are very prevalent in the general population.
   a. HSV-1 is typically associated with lesions of the oropharynx.
   b. HSV-2 is associated with lesions of the genitalia (see Table 10-6).
   c. Both viruses, however, can cause either genital or oral lesions.
2. Pathophysiology: After inoculation, the HSV replicates in the dermis and epidermis, then travels via sensory nerves up to the dorsal root ganglia. It resides as a latent infection in the dorsal root ganglia, where it can be reactivated at any time and reach the skin through peripheral nerves.
3. Transmission
   a. HSV is transmitted by contact with people who have active ulcerations or shedding of virus from mucous membranes. HSV-1 is typically associated with transmission through nonsexual personal contact (e.g., kissing), and HSV-2 through sexual contact.
   b. Most people acquire HSV-1 in childhood, and more than 80% of adults have been infected with HSV-1.
   c. The incidence of HSV-2 has increased in recent years.
   d. Episodes of genital herpes frequently may be asymptomatic or may produce symptoms that often go unrecognized. Virus is still shed, and the infected person is contagious.
   e. Contracting one form of herpes confers some degree of cross-immunity, rendering primary infection with the other form of herpes less severe.
   f. Infection with genital herpes is associated with an increased risk of contracting HIV.

B. Clinical features

1. HSV-1
   a. Primary infection is usually asymptomatic and often goes unnoticed.
   b. When symptomatic, primary infection is associated with systemic manifestations (e.g., fevers, malaise) as well as oral lesions (described below).

   c. Oral lesions involve groups of vesicles on patches of erythematous skin. Herpes labialis (cold sores) are most common on the lips (usually painful, heal in 2 to 6 weeks).

   d. HSV-1 is associated with Bell's palsy as well.

2. HSV-2

   a. Primary infection results in more severe and prolonged symptoms, lasting up to 3 weeks in duration.

   b. Recurrent episodes are milder and of shorter duration, usually resolving within 10 days. There is also a decrease in the frequency of episodes over time.

   c. Constitutional symptoms (e.g., fever, headache, malaise) often present in primary infection.

   d. HSV-2 presents with painful genital vesicles or pustules (see Color Figure 10-1). Other findings are tender inguinal lymphadenopathy and vaginal and/or urethral discharge.

3. Disseminated HSV

   a. Usually limited to immunocompromised patients

   b. May result in encephalitis, meningitis, keratitis, chorioretinitis, pneumonitis, and esophagitis

   c. Rarely, pregnant women may develop disseminated HSV, which can be fatal to the mother and fetus.

4. Neonatal HSV (vertical transmission at time of delivery) is associated with congenital malformations, intrauterine growth retardation (IUGR), chorioamnionitis, and even neonatal death.

5. Ocular disease—Either form of herpes simplex can cause keratitis, blepharitis, and keratoconjunctivitis.

C. Diagnosis

1. The diagnosis can be made clinically when characteristic lesions are recognized.

2. If there is uncertainty, perform the following tests to confirm the diagnosis.

   a. Tzanck smear—quickest test
      • Perform by swabbing the base of the ulcer and staining with Wright's stain.
      • This shows multinucleated giant cells. It does not differentiate between HSV and VZV.

   b. **Culture of HSV is the gold standard of diagnosis**
      • Perform by swabbing the base of the ulcer.
      • Results are available within 2 to 3 days.

   c. Direct fluorescent assay and ELISA
      • 80% sensitive
      • Results available within minutes to hours

D. Treatment

1. There is no cure available for either type of herpes simplex. Antiviral treatment provides symptomatic relief and reduces the duration of symptoms (see below).

2. Mucocutaneous disease

   a. Treat with oral and/or topical acyclovir for 7 to 10 days.

   b. Valacyclovir and famciclovir have better bioavailability.

   c. Oral acyclovir may be given as prophylaxis for patients with frequent recurrences.

   d. Foscarnet may be given for resistant disease in immunocompromised patients.

3. Disseminated HSV warrants hospital admission. Treat with parenteral acyclovir.

Syphilis

A. General characteristics

1. It is caused by *Treponema pallidum* spirochetes and transmitted by **direct sexual contact** with infectious lesions.

2. It is a systemic illness with four stages (see below). The late stages can be prevented by early treatment.

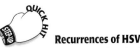

Recurrences of HSV
• Recurrences are associated with the following: stress, fever, infection, and sun exposure.
• Recurrent episodes tend to become shorter in duration and less frequent over time.

Herpetic whitlow
• HSV infection of the finger caused by inoculation into open skin surface. Common in healthcare workers.
• Painful vesicular lesions erupt at the fingertip.
• It may cause fever and axillary lymphadenopathy.
• Treat with acyclovir. Do not mistake for paronychia. Incision and drainage should NOT be done for herpetic whitlow.

I & D.

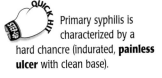

Primary syphilis is characterized by a hard chancre (indurated, **painless ulcer** with clean base).

B. Clinical features

1. Primary stage
   a. **Chancre**—a **painless**, crater-like lesion that appears on the genitalia 3 to 4 weeks after exposure (see Color Figure 10-2)
   b. Heals in 14 weeks, even without therapy
   c. Highly infectious—Anyone who touches the lesion can transmit the infection.
2. Secondary stage
   a. This may develop 4 to 8 weeks after the chancre has healed. **A maculopapular rash is the most characteristic finding in this stage.**
   b. Other possible manifestations: flu-like illness, aseptic meningitis, hepatitis
   c. Patients are contagious during this stage.
   d. About one-third of untreated patients with secondary syphilis develop latent syphilis.
3. Latent stage
   a. Latent stage is defined as the presence of positive serologic test results in the absence of clinical signs or symptoms. Two-thirds of these patients remain asymptomatic; one-third develop tertiary syphilis.
   b. It is called early latent syphilis if serology has been positive for <1 year. During this time, the patient may relapse back to the secondary phase.
   c. It is called late latent syphilis if serology has been positive for >1 year. Patients are not contagious during this time and do not have any symptoms of the disease.
4. Tertiary stage
   a. One-third of untreated syphilis patients in the latent phase enter this stage.
   b. It occurs years after the development of the primary infection (up to 40 years later).
   c. Major manifestations include cardiovascular syphilis, neurosyphilis, and gummas (subcutaneous granulomas).
   d. Neurosyphilis is characterized by dementia, personality changes, and **tabes dorsalis** (posterior column degeneration).
   e. It is very rare nowadays due to treatment with penicillin.

C. Diagnosis

1. Darkfield microscopy (definitive diagnostic test)—examines a sample of the chancre with visualization of spirochetes
2. Serologic tests (most commonly used tests)
   a. Nontreponemal tests—RPR, VDRL (most commonly used)
      • High sensitivity—ideal for screening
      • Specificity is only around 70%. If positive, confirmation is necessary with the specific treponemal tests.
   b. Treponemal tests—FTA-ABS, MHA-TP
      • More specific than nontreponemal tests
      • Not for screening, just for confirmation of a positive nontreponemal test
3. All patients should be tested for HIV infection.

D. Treatment

1. Antibiotics are effective in early syphilis but less so in late syphilis.
2. Benzathine penicillin g (one dose IM) is the preferred agent. If the patient is allergic to penicillin, give oral antibiotics (doxycycline, tetracycline) for 2 weeks.
3. If the patient has late latent syphilis or tertiary syphilis, give penicillin in three doses IM once per week.
4. Repeat nontreponemal tests every 3 months to ensure adequate response to treatment. Titers should decrease fourfold within 6 months. If they do not, that may signal treatment failure or reinfection.

Chancroid

- Caused by *Haemophilus ducreyi*, a gram-negative rod
- Transmission through sexual contact
- Incubation period of 2 to 10 days

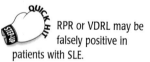

Most common presentations for syphilis include:
• Genital lesion (chancre)
• Inguinal lymphadenopathy
• Maculopapular rash of secondary syphilis

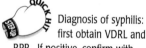

Diagnosis of syphilis: first obtain VDRL and RPR. If positive, confirm with FTA-ABS.

RPR or VDRL may be falsely positive in patients with SLE.

TABLE 10-6 **Clinical Manifestations of Genital Ulcers With Regional Lymphadenopathy**

Genital Lesions	Incubation (Days)	Type	Pain	Number	Duration
Primary syphilis	3–90	Clean ulcer, raised	No	Usually single	3–6 weeks
Primary herpes simplex virus	1–26	Grouped papules, vesicles, pustules, ulcers	Yes	Often multiple	1–3 weeks
Chancroid	1–21	Purulent ulcer, shaggy border	Yes	Single in men, multiple in women	Progressive
Lymphogranuloma venereum	3–21	Papule, vesicle, ulcer	No	Usually single	Few days
Granuloma inguinale	8–80	Nodules, coalescing granulomatous ulcers	No	Single or multiple	Progressive

Inguinal Adenopathy	Onset	Pain	Type	Frequency	Constitutional Symptoms
Primary syphilis	Same time	No	Firm	80%, 70% bilateral	Absent
Primary herpes simplex virus	Same time	Yes	Firm	80%, usually bilateral	Common
Chancroid	Same time	Yes	Fluctuant, may fistulize	50%–65%, usually unilateral	Uncommon
Lymphogranuloma venereum	2–6 weeks later	Yes	Indurated, fluctuant, may fistulize	Unilateral, one-third bilateral	Common
Granuloma inguinale	Variable	—	Suppurating pseudobuboe	10%	1%–5%

From Stoller JK, Ahmad M, Longworth DL. The Cleveland Clinic Intensive Review of Internal Medicine. 3rd Ed. Philadelphia: Lippincott Williams & Wilkins, 2002:168, Table 14.3.

- There are no systemic findings. Disseminated infection does not occur.
- Clinical features: **painful genital ulcer(s)** that can be deep with ragged borders and with a purulent base (see Color Figure 10-3); unilateral tender inguinal lymphadenopathy ("buboes") that appears 1 to 2 weeks after ulcer
- Diagnosis is made clinically. Rule out syphilis and HSV and consider testing for HIV. No serologic tests are available, and culture of the organism is not practical because it requires special media that are not widely available.
- Treatment options include azithromycin (oral, one dose), ceftriaxone (IM, one dose), or an oral course of azithromycin, erythromycin, or ciprofloxacin.
- With treatment, most ulcers resolve in 1 or 2 weeks.

Diagnosis of chancroid
- Painful genital ulcer(s)
- Tender lymphadenopathy
- Syphilis ruled out (negative, dark-field examination for *Treponema pallidum* and negative serologic tests)
- HSV ruled out based on clinical presentation or negative culture for HSV

Lymphogranuloma venereum

- A sexually transmitted disease **caused by *C. trachomatis***
- Clinical features—painless ulcer at the site of inoculation that may go unnoticed. A few weeks later, tender inguinal lymphadenopathy (usually unilateral) and constitutional symptoms develop.
- If untreated, proctocolitis may develop with perianal fissures and rectal stricture; obstruction of lymphatics may lead to elephantiasis of genitals.
- Diagnosis is made by serologic tests (complement fixation, immunofluorescence).
- The treatment is doxycycline (oral for 21 days).

Pediculosis Pubis (Pubic Lice)

- Pediculosis pubis (pubic lice or "crabs") is a common STD caused by *Phthirus pubis* (the pubic or crab louse).

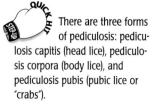

There are three forms of pediculosis: pediculosis capitis (head lice), pediculosis corpora (body lice), and pediculosis pubis (pubic lice or "crabs").

- It can be transmitted through sexual contact, clothing, or towels.
- **Severe pruritus** in the genital region is characteristic. Other hairy areas of the body can be involved.
- Diagnosis is made by examination of hair under microscope (or possibly with the naked eye)—identification of adult lice or nits.
- Treat with permethrin 1% shampoo (Elimite)—apply to all hairy regions from neck down and wash off after several hours. Sexual partner(s) should also be treated. Combs, clothes, and bed linens should be washed thoroughly.

WOUND AND SOFT TISSUE INFECTIONS

Cellulitis

A. General characteristics

1. Cellulitis is an inflammatory condition of **skin and subcutaneous tissue.**
2. It is caused by a wide variety of bacteria, the most common being group A strepto-cocci or *S. aureus*.
3. **Likely bacterial pathogens are based on patient histories.** Bacteria gain entry through breaks in the skin: IV catheters, incisions, immersion in water, and bites or wounds. Venous stasis diseases, lymphedema, and diabetic ulcers also are associated with cellulitis (see Table 10-7).
4. If untreated, cellulitis may lead to potentially life-threatening bacteremia.

B. Clinical features

1. Classic findings of inflammation: erythema, warmth, pain, swelling
2. Fever (may or may not be present)

C. Diagnosis

1. The diagnosis is essentially clinical.
2. Obtain blood cultures if the patient has a fever.
3. Obtain tissue cultures if there is a wound, ulcer, or site of infection.
4. Obtain imaging (plain film, MRI) if there is suspicion of deeper infection.

D. Treatment

1. Base treatment on suspected pathogens from the patient history. Most patients require parenteral antibiotic therapy.
2. Treat with a staphylococcal penicillin (e.g., oxacillin, nafcillin) or a cephalosporin (e.g., cefazolin).
3. Continue IV antibiotics until signs of infection improve. Follow up with oral antibiotics for 2 weeks.

Erysipelas

- Erysipelas is a cellulitis that is usually confined to the dermis and lymphatics.
- It is usually caused by group A streptococci (other forms of streptococci less commonly).
- The classic presentation is a well-demarcated, fiery red, painful lesion, most commonly on the lower extremities and the face. High fever and chills may be present.
- Predisposing factors include lymphatic obstruction (e.g., after radical mastectomy), local trauma or abscess, fungal infections, diabetes mellitus, and alcoholism.

QUICK HIT

Patients with cellulitis are predisposed to recurrences in the same area because of damage that occurs to the local lymphatic vessels.

QUICK HIT

Spread to the face is a worrisome complication of cellulitis, and any evidence of orbital involvement is a medical emergency requiring urgent evaluation by an ophthalmologist.

> **Box 10-5 Differentiating Deep Vein Thrombosis (DVT) From Cellulitis**
>
> - Like cellulitis, acute DVT also presents with erythema, warmth, and tenderness in the affected extremity.
> - Inflammation in DVT is usually restricted to the posterior calf.
> - Because Homans' sign and the palpation of venous cords are not sensitive in detecting DVT, venous Doppler must sometimes be performed to differentiate between cellulitis and acute DVT.

TABLE 10-7	Common Pathogens in Cellulitis
Means of Bacterial Invasion	**Likely Pathogen**
Local trauma, breaks in skin	Group A Streptococcus *(Streptococcus pyogenes)*
Wounds, abscesses	*Staphylococcus aureus*
Immersion in water	*Pseudomonas aeruginosa, Aeromonas hydrophila, Vibrio vulnificus*
Acute sinusitis	*Haemophilus influenzae*

- Complications include sepsis, local spread to subcutaneous tissues, and necrotizing fasciitis.
- Treatment for uncomplicated cases is IM or oral penicillin or erythromycin; otherwise treat as for cellulitis.
- Unfortunately, erysipelas has a high rate of recurrence.

Necrotizing Fasciitis

- Necrotizing fasciitis is a life-threatening infection of deep soft tissues that rapidly tracks along fascial planes.
- Common bacterial causes include *Streptococcus pyogenes* and *Clostridium perfringens*.
- Risk factors include recent surgery, diabetes, trauma, and IV drug use.
- Clinical features may include fever and pain out of proportion to appearance of skin in early stages, so a high index of suspicion is important. Extension of infection leads to thrombosis of microcirculation, resulting in tissue necrosis, discoloration, crepitus, and cutaneous anesthesia.
- It may rapidly progress to sepsis, TSS, and multiorgan failure.
- Antibacterial treatment alone is not sufficient. **Rapid surgical exploration and excision of devitalized tissue is an absolute necessity!**
- Broad-spectrum parenteral antimicrobial therapy is warranted.

Lymphadenitis

- This is inflammation of a lymph node (single or multiple) usually caused by local skin or soft tissue bacterial infection (often hemolytic streptococci and staphylococci).
- It presents with fever, tender lymphadenopathy of regional lymph nodes, and red streaking of skin from the wound or area of cellulitis.
- Complications include thrombosis of adjacent veins, sepsis, and even death if untreated.
- Helpful diagnostic studies include blood and wound cultures.
- It usually responds well to treatment. Treat with appropriate antibiotics (penicillin G, antistaphylococcal penicillin, or cephalosporin) and warm compresses. Wound drainage may ultimately be necessary.

Tetanus

A. General characteristics
1. Causes
   a. It is caused by neurotoxins produced by spores of *Clostridium tetani*, a gram-positive anaerobic bacillus.
   b. *C. tetani* proliferates and produces its exotoxin in contaminated wounds. The exotoxin blocks inhibitory transmitters at the neuromuscular junction.
2. Patients at risk are those who have incomplete or no tetanus immunization (see Chapter 12).

B. Clinical features
1. The classic and earliest symptom is hypertonicity and contractions of the masseter muscles, resulting in *trismus*, or "lockjaw."
2. Progresses to severe, generalized muscle contractions including:

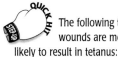
The following types of wounds are most likely to result in tetanus:
- Wounds contaminated with dirt, feces, or saliva
- Wounds with necrotic tissue
- Deep-puncture wounds

The incubation period for tetanus ranges from about 2 days to 2 weeks. The onset of symptoms is characteristically gradual (1 to 7 days).

TABLE 10-8	Guide to Tetanus Immunization in Wound Management			
	Clean, Minor Wounds		**Other Wounds**	
History of Immunization (Td Doses)	**Td**	**TIG**	**Td**	**TIG**
≥3 known Td Doses	No	No	No	No
<3 doses, unknown status, or >10 yr since last booster	Yes	No	Yes	Yes

TD, tetanus/diphtheria toxoid; TIG, tetanus immune globulin.

    a. *Risus sardonicus*—grin due to contraction of facial muscles
    b. *Opisthotonos*—arched back due to contraction of back muscles
  3. Sympathetic hyperactivity

C. Diagnosis
  1. The diagnosis is mainly clinical.
  2. Obtain wound cultures, but they are not a reliable means of diagnosis.

D. Treatment
  1. Admit the patient to the ICU and provide respiratory support if necessary. Give diazepam for tetany.
  2. Neutralize unbound toxin with passive immunization—give a single IM dose of tetanus immune globulin (TIG).
  3. Provide active immunization with tetanus/diphtheria toxoid (Td).
  4. Thoroughly clean and débride any wounds with tissue necrosis.
  5. Give antibiotics (metronidazole or penicillin G), although efficacy is somewhat controversial.

INFECTIONS OF THE BONES AND JOINTS

Osteomyelitis

A. General characteristics
  1. Osteomyelitis refers to inflammatory destruction of bone due to infection.
  2. There are two main categories of osteomyelitis.
    a. Hematogenous osteomyelitis (most common in children)—occurs secondary to sepsis
    b. Direct spread of bacteria from any of the following:
      • An adjacent infection (e.g., infected diabetic foot ulcer, decubitus ulcer)
      • Trauma (e.g., **open fractures**)
      • Vascular insufficiency (e.g., peripheral vascular disease)
  3. The most common microorganisms causing osteomyelitis are *S. aureus* and coagulase-negative staphylococci.
  4. Osteomyelitis can involve any bone. Common locations include long bones (tibia, humerus, femur), foot and ankle, and vertebral bodies.

B. Risk factors (for complications or chronic osteomyelitis)
  1. Open fractures
  2. Diabetes mellitus (causes predisposition to infection and peripheral vascular disease)
  3. Use of illicit IV drugs
  4. Sepsis

C. Clinical features
  1. Pain over the involved area of bone is the most common finding.
  2. Localized erythema, warmth, or swelling may be present.

Common bugs in osteomyelitis
• Catheter septicemia: *S. aureus*
• Prosthetic joint: coagulase-negative staphylococci
• Diabetic foot ulcer: polymicrobial organisms
• Nosocomial infections: *Pseudomonas* spp.
• IV drug abuse, neutropenia: fungal species, *Pseudomonas* spp.
• Sickle cell disease: *Salmonella* spp.

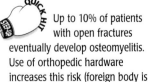

Up to 10% of patients with open fractures eventually develop osteomyelitis. Use of orthopedic hardware increases this risk (foreign body is the site of bacterial colonization).

3. Systemic symptoms (e.g., fever, headache, fatigue) may be present, but are inconsistent findings.
4. A draining sinus tract through the skin may form in chronic disease.

D. Diagnosis

1. WBC count—may or may not be elevated and is not useful for diagnosis
2. ESR and CRP
   a. These are fairly nonspecific, but if these markers of inflammation are elevated in the appropriate clinical setting, seriously consider a diagnosis of osteomyelitis. However, a normal ESR and CRP do not exclude the diagnosis.
   b. **Both ESR and CRP are very useful in monitoring the response to therapy.**
3. **Needle aspiration** of infected bone or bone biopsy (obtained in operating room)—**most direct and accurate means of diagnosis.** Culture results can determine the specific antibiotic therapy.
4. Plain radiography
   a. The earliest radiographic changes (periosteal thickening or elevation) are not evident for at least 10 days.
   b. Lytic lesions are only apparent in advanced disease.
5. Radionucleotide bone scans—usually positive within 2 to 3 days of infection, but are relatively nonspecific (can be positive in metastatic bone disease, trauma, or overlying soft tissue inflammation)
6. MRI is generally the most effective imaging study for diagnosing osteomyelitis and assessing the extent of disease process.

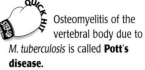

QUICK HIT
Osteomyelitis of the vertebral body due to *M. tuberculosis* is called **Pott's disease.**

E. Treatment: Give IV antibiotics for extended periods (4 to 6 weeks). Initiate antibiotic therapy only after the microbial etiology is narrowed based on data from cultures. General guidelines:

1. Empiric therapy requires penicillinase-resistant penicillin (e.g., oxacillin) or a first-generation cephalosporin (e.g., cefazolin).
2. Add an aminoglycoside and possibly a β-lactam antibiotic if there is a possibility of infection with a gram-negative organism.
3. Surgical debridement of infected necrotic bone is an important aspect of treatment.

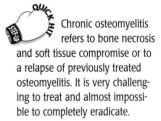

QUICK HIT
Chronic osteomyelitis refers to bone necrosis and soft tissue compromise or to a relapse of previously treated osteomyelitis. It is very challenging to treat and almost impossible to completely eradicate.

Acute Infectious Arthritis

A. General characteristics

1. Acute infectious arthritis occurs when microorganisms (usually bacteria) invade the joint space (not bone itself), where they release endotoxins and trigger cytokine release and neutrophil infiltration. These inflammatory reactions ultimately lead to erosion and destruction of the joint.
2. Pathogenesis—Microorganisms penetrate the joint via the following mechanisms:
   a. Hematogenous spread—most common route
   b. Contiguous spread from another locus of infection, e.g., osteomyelitis, abscess, or cellulitis

---

Box 10-6 Gonococcal Arthritis

- This presents with acute monoarthritis or oligoarthritis, and often progresses within days in a migratory or additive pattern.
- Knees, wrists, hands, and ankles are the most commonly involved.
- Tenosynovitis is often present in the hands and feet.
- Fever, chills, and rash (macules, papules, and/or pustules) are signs of disseminated gonococcal infection. If the patient has disseminated gonococcal infection, admit to the hospital.
- After the joint is initially aspirated, repeated aspiration is unnecessary (unlike in other causes of septic arthritis), and antibiotics alone usually lead to improvement. Treat presumptively for chlamydial infection (e.g., with doxycycline).
- Consider testing for HIV and syphilis. Educate the patient about the risks of sexual practices.

c. Traumatic injury to joint
d. Iatrogenic, e.g., from arthrocentesis, arthroscopy
3. Microbiology
a. The most common offender is bacteria.
b. Acute bacterial arthritis can be caused by any of the following.
- **S. aureus is the most common agent overall in adults and children.** Various streptococcal species are also frequently involved.
- An important gram-negative agent is N. gonorrhoeae. **Gonococcal arthritis is the most common cause of acute infectious arthritis in young, sexually active adults.**
- Consider gram-negative organisms such as *Pseudomonas aeruginosa* or *Salmonella* spp. if there is a history of sickle cell disease, immunodeficiency, or IV drug abuse.
4. Other risk factors for acute infectious arthritis
a. Prior joint damage (e.g., rheumatoid arthritis)
b. Joint prosthesis
c. Diabetes mellitus

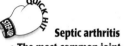

QUICK HIT

If patient has a painless range of motion of involved joint, septic arthritis is very unlikely, even in presence of erythema. Micromotion of joint causes severe pain in septic arthritis.

QUICK HIT

Septic arthritis
- **The most common joint affected is the knee.** The hip, wrist, shoulder, and ankle may also be involved.
- Patients with immunosuppression or connective tissue diseases may have polyarticular arthritis (and a worse prognosis).

B. Clinical features

1. The joint is swollen, warm, and painful.
a. **The range of motion (active or passive) is very limited.**
b. An effusion can be palpated.
2. Constitutional symptoms such as fever, chills, and malaise are common.

C. Diagnosis

1. **Perform a joint aspiration ("tap") and analysis of synovial fluid in all patients suspected of having a septic joint.** Order the following studies on aspirated synovial fluid.
a. WBC count with differential—usually >50,000 WBCs/mm^3 with >80% PMNs—the most helpful test
b. Gram stain of fluid—positive in approximately 75% of gram-positive cases, but only 30% to 50% of gram-negative cases
c. Culture—aerobic and anaerobic
d. Crystal analysis—Keep in mind that acute gout may present like septic arthritis.
e. PCR of synovial fluid—This may be useful if gonococcal arthritis is suspected but Gram stain and cultures are negative.
2. Blood cultures are positive in >50% of all cases (frequently negative in gonococcal arthritis).
3. Other laboratory abnormalities
a. Leukocytosis—present in about half of patients with a septic joint

TABLE 10-9 Medical Treatment of Acute Bacterial Arthritis

Adult (Relatively Healthy): Treat for *Staphylococcus aureus*	Patient Is Immunocompromised or Has Significant Risk Factors for Gram-Negative Arthritis	Young Adult With History and Presentation Consistent With Gonococcal Arthritis
Parenteral, β-lactamase resistant penicillin (e.g., oxacillin) or first-generation cephalosporin × 4 weeks	Parenteral, broad-spectrum antibiotics (with gram-negative coverage) (e.g., a third-generation cephalosporin or aminoglycoside) × 3–4 weeks	Parenteral, third-generation cephalosporin (e.g., ceftriaxone) until there is clinical improvement
Treat with vancomycin if MRSA is suspected.	For pseudomonal infection, use aminoglycoside + extended-spectrum penicillin.	Switch to an oral agent with gram-negative coverage (e.g., ciprofloxacin × 10 days) once there is clinical improvement.

b. Elevated ESR—elevated in up to 90% of patients with septic joint

c. Elevated CRP—useful in monitoring clinical improvement

4. Imaging studies

   a. Plain radiographs—generally not useful unless joint damage is severe

   b. CT or MRI—helpful if the sacroiliac or facet joints are involved

5. Obtain cultures from appropriate mucosal surfaces (e.g., genitourinary tract) if gonococcal arthritis is suspected.

D. Treatment

1. Prompt antibiotic treatment

   a. Do not delay in initiating antimicrobial therapy when acute infectious arthritis is suspected.

   b. If the Gram stain result is negative but acute bacterial arthritis is still suspected, treat empirically based on the clinical scenario (see Table 10-9) until culture and sensitivity results are available.

2. Drainage

   a. Daily aspiration of affected joint as long as effusion persists is one treatment option. However, surgical drainage is recommended to prevent further damage to the articular cartilage that occurs with persistent infectious process. Certain joints are amenable to arthroscopic drainage (shoulder, knee) whereas others are not (hip, wrist, elbow, ankle) and should be opened.

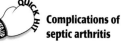

Complications of septic arthritis

- Destruction of joint and surrounding structures (e.g., ligaments, tendons), leading to stiffness, pain, and loss of function
- Avascular necrosis (if hip is involved)
- Sepsis

ZOONOSES AND ARTHROPOD-BORNE DISEASES

Lyme Disease

A. General characteristics

1. Three major endemic areas in the United States

   a. <u>Northeastern</u> seaboard (from Maine to Maryland)

   b. <u>Midwest</u> (north central states—e.g., Minnesota, Wisconsin)

   c. <u>West coast</u> (Northern California)

2. Incubation period is 3 to 32 days

3. Transmission cycle

   a. Caused by spirochete *Borrelia burgdorferi*

   b. Transmitted by ticks—commonly the deer tick *Ixodidae scapularis*

   c. The tick is hosted by white-footed mice (immature ticks), white-tailed deer (mature ticks), and brief and unfortunate encounters with humans.

Lyme disease is the most common vector-borne illness in the United States. The peak incidence is in summer months. It is associated with outdoor activities in wooded areas (e.g., hiking, camping).

- Patients with tick bites should be followed up closely for the appearance of erythema migrans, but the majority of tick bites do not result in infection.
- A vaccine against *B. burgdorferi* has been developed but was taken off the market due to lack of use in the medical community.

B. Clinical features

1. Stage 1—early, localized infection

   a. **Erythema migrans** is the hallmark skin lesion at site of the tick bite. Characteristically it is a large, painless, well-demarcated target-shaped lesion, commonly seen on the thigh, groin, or axilla (see Color Figure 10-4).

   b. Multiple lesions signify that hematogenous spread has occurred (see below).

Box 10-7 Lyme Serology

- IgM antibodies peak 3 to 6 weeks after the onset of symptoms. If a few months have passed since the onset of disease, IgM levels are basically worthless.
- IgG antibodies slowly increase and remain elevated in patients with disseminated illness. If a patient has had Lyme disease in the past and now has symptoms consistent with new illness, IgG levels will not indicate whether the infection is acute or chronic.
- Patients with a history of distant Lyme disease may have elevated IgG levels despite adequate antibiotic treatment.
- IgG antibodies cross-react with *Treponema pallidum,* but patients with Lyme disease will not have a positive VDRL.

2. Stage 2—early, disseminated infection
   a. Infection spreads via lymphatics and the bloodstream within days to weeks after the onset of erythema migrans.
   b. Clinical features: intermittent flu-like symptoms, headaches, neck stiffness, fever/chills, fatigue, malaise, musculoskeletal pain
   c. After several weeks, about 15% of patients develop one or several of the following (usually resolve within several months):
      • Meningitis (Brudzinski's and Kerning's signs negative)
      • Encephalitis
      • Cranial neuritis (often bilateral facial nerve palsy)
      • Encephalitis
      • Peripheral radiculoneuropathy (motor or sensory)
   d. Within weeks to months of onset of symptoms, about 8% will have cardiac manifestations (e.g., AV block, pericarditis, carditis). These usually only last for several weeks, but recurrence is not uncommon.
3. Stage 3—late, persistent infection (months to years after initial infection)
   a. Arthritis—This occurs in 60% of untreated patients; it typically affects the large joints (especially knees). Chronic arthritis will develop in some patients.
   b. Chronic CNS disease—subacute, mild encephalitis, transverse myelitis, or axonal polyneuropathy.
   c. Acrodermatitis chronica atrophicans (a rare skin lesion)—reddish-purple plaques and nodules on the extensor surfaces of the legs.

C. Diagnosis

1. Clinical diagnosis—In early, localized disease, documented erythema migrans in a patient with a history of tick exposure in an endemic area obviates the need for laboratory confirmation. Treat empirically.
2. **Serologic studies—most important tests to confirm a clinical suspicion of Lyme disease**
   a. ELISA is used to detect serum IgM and IgG antibodies during the first month of illness.
   b. Western blot is used to confirm positive or equivocal results.

D. Treatment

1. Early localized disease
   a. If it is confined to the skin, 10 days of antibiotic therapy is adequate.
   b. If there is any evidence of spread beyond the skin, extend treatment to 20 to 30 days.
   c. For early Lyme disease
      • Oral doxycycline (for 21 days)—contraindicated in pregnant women and in children ≤12 years of age
      • Amoxicillin and cefuroxime are alternative agents.
      • Erythromycin may be given to pregnant patients with penicillin allergies.
2. Treatment of complications such as facial nerve palsy, arthritis, or cardiac disease is prolonged antibiotic therapy (30 to 60 days). For meningitis or other CNS complications, treat with IV antibiotics for 4 weeks.

Early treatment with antibiotics is extremely important because later sequelae of disease can usually be prevented. Treatment in later stages is usually effective, but recovery may be delayed.

Rocky Mountain Spotted Fever

A. General characteristics

1. Caused by the intracellular bacteria *Rickettsia rickettsii.*
2. Ticks feeding on various mammals serve as vectors for disease transmission.
3. The major endemic areas include the southeastern, midwestern, and western United States. Peak incidence is in the spring and summer months due to increased outdoor activity.
4. Pathophysiology of disease
   a. Organisms enter the host cells via tick bites, multiply in the vascular endothelium, and spread to different layers of the vasculature.

b. Damage to the vascular endothelium results in increased vascular permeability, activation of complement, microhemorrhages, and microinfarcts.

B. Clinical features

1. The onset of symptoms is typically 1 week after the tick bite.
2. It classically presents with a sudden onset of fever, chills, malaise, nausea, vomiting, myalgias, photophobia, and headache.
3. Papular rash usually appears after 4 to 5 days of fever. **Rash starts peripherally (wrists, forearms, palms, ankles, and soles) but then spreads centrally** (to the rest of the limbs, trunk, and face). It becomes maculopapular, and eventually petechial.
4. It may lead to interstitial pneumonitis.

C. Diagnosis

1. Diagnosis is primarily clinical. Laboratory abnormalities may include elevated liver enzymes and thrombocytopenia.
2. Acute and convalescent serology and immunofluorescent staining of skin biopsy are confirmatory tests.

D. Treatment

1. Doxycycline—usually given for 7 days; given intravenously (IV) if the patient is vomiting
2. CNS manifestations or pregnant patients—give chloramphenicol

Malaria

A. General characteristics

1. A protozoal infection caused by one of four organisms
   a. *Plasmodium falciparum*
   b. *Plasmodium ovale*
   c. *Plasmodium vivax*
   d. *Plasmodium malariae*
2. Prevalent in tropical climates, parts of Africa and the Middle East
3. Transmitted via mosquito bite in endemic areas

B. Clinical features

1. Symptoms may include fever and chills, myalgias, headache, nausea, vomiting, and diarrhea.
2. Fever pattern varies depending on cause
   a. *P. falciparum*—fever is usually constant
   b. *P. ovale* and *P. vivax*—fever usually spikes every 48 hours
   c. *P. malariae*—fever usually spikes every 72 hours

C. Diagnosis

1. Identify organism on peripheral blood smear
2. Blood smear must have **Giemsa stain**

D. Treatment

1. Use chloroquine phosphate unless resistance is suspected. In many countries, chloroquine resistance is so prevalent that it should be assumed.
2. If chloroquine resistance is suspected, give quinine sulfate and tetracycline. Alternative agents are atovaquone-proguanil and mefloquine.
3. *P. falciparum* infection may require IV quinidine and doxycycline.
4. Relapses can occur in *P. vivax* and *P. ovale* infection as a result of dormant hypnozoites in the liver. Add a 2-week regimen of primaquine phosphate for these types of malarial infection. → to eradicate the dormant form.
5. Prophylaxis is important for travelers to endemic regions. Mefloquine is the agent of choice in chloroquine-resistant areas. Chloroquine can be used in areas where chloroquine resistance has not been reported.

QUICK HIT — The onset of illness in malaria usually occurs weeks to months after infection, but it is dependent on the specific cause.

QUICK HIT — *P. falciparum* infection is by far the most serious and life-threatening cause of malaria.

Rabies

A. General characteristics
1. A devastating, deadly viral encephalitis
2. Contracted from a bite or scratch by an infected animal; infection from a corneal transplant has been documented as well
3. More prevalent in developing countries where rabies vaccination of animals is not widespread

B. Clinical features
1. The incubation period typically ranges from 30 to 90 days, but varies considerably.
2. Once symptoms are present, rabies is almost invariably fatal.
3. Symptoms (in progressive order)
   a. Pain at site of bite
   b. Prodromal symptoms of sore throat, fatigue, headache, nausea, and/or vomiting
   c. Encephalitis—Confusion, combativeness, hyperactivity, fever, and seizures may be present.
   d. Hydrophobia—inability to drink, laryngeal spasm with drinking, hyper-salivation ("foaming at mouth"), usually progresses to coma and death
   e. Some patients may present with ascending paralysis.

C. Diagnosis
1. Virus or viral antigen can be identified in infected tissue. Virus can be isolated in saliva as well.
2. Four-fold increase in serum antibody titers
3. Identification of **Negri bodies** histologically
4. PCR detection of virus RNA

D. Treatment (postexposure management)
1. Clean the wound thoroughly with soap.
2. For wild animal bites (e.g., bat or raccoon), the animal should be captured if possible, destroyed, and sent to a laboratory for immunofluorescence of brain tissue.
3. If a patient was bitten by a healthy dog or cat in an endemic area, the animal should be captured and observed for 10 days. If there is no change in the animal's condition, then it most likely does not have rabies.
4. For known rabies exposure, both of the following should be performed.
   a. Passive immunization—Administer the human rabies immunoglobulin to patients, into the wound as well in the gluteal region.
   b. Active immunization—Administer the antirabies vaccine in three IM doses into the deltoid or thigh over a 28-day period.

QUICK HIT

Pre-exposure prophylaxis—Rabies vaccine is available for at-risk individuals (e.g., those with potential occupational exposure, such as veterinarians, wildlife officials, and laboratory workers).

Other Zoonoses

• Table 10-10 covers leptospirosis, ehrlichiosis, tularemia, Q fever, and cat scratch fever.

COMMON FUNGAL INFECTIONS

Candidiasis

A. General characteristics
1. *Candida* species are oval, budding yeasts known for their formation of hyphae and long pseudohyphae. They normally colonize humans, and it is the overgrowth of these organisms that results in the clinical pathology of candidiasis.
2. *Candida albicans* is the most common cause of candidiasis.
3. Risk factors for candidiasis
   a. Antibiotic therapy
   b. Diabetes mellitus

TABLE 10-10 Other Zoonoses and Arthropod-Borne Diseases

Disease	Organism	Transmission	Reservoir	Clinical Findings	Diagnosis	Treatment
Leptospirosis	*Leptospira* spp. (spirochetes)	Contaminated water	Rodents, farm animals	**Anicteric:** rash, LAN,* ↑ LFTs **Icteric:** renal and/or liver failure, vasculitis, vascular collapse	Isolation of organism in blood or urine CTX*	Oral antibiotics: tetracycline or doxycycline; if severe, IV penicillin G
Ehrlichiosis	*Ehrlichia* spp. (intracellular, gram-negative bacteria)	Tick bite	Deer	Fever, chills, malaise ± rash **Complications:** renal failure, GI bleeding	Clinical; confirm by serology	Oral tetracycline or doxycycline ± 1 week
Tularemia	*Francisella tularensis* (small gram-negative bacillus)	Tick bite, animal bites, handling carcass	Rabbits, other rodents	Fever, headache, nausea; ulcer at site of tick bite; painful LAN	Isolation of organism in blood or wound CTX	IM streptomycin or gentamicin
Q fever	*Coxiella burnetii* (gram-negative organism)	Blood, ingestion of infected milk, inhalation	Farm animals	**Acute:** constitutional symptoms, nausea, vomiting **Chronic:** endocarditis **Chronic:** rifampin	Serology; CXR—multiple opacities in acute illness	**Acute:** doxycycline or fluoroquinolone
Cat scratch disease	*Bartonella henselae* (gram-negative bacillus)	Scratch from a flea-infested cat	Cats, fleas	LAN or lymphadenitis; systemic symptoms rare	Serology, clinical	Usually self-limited; if severe, oral doxy cycline or ciprofloxacin

*LAN, lymphadenopathy; CTX, culture.

c. Immunosuppressive therapy

d. Immunocompromised hosts (increased risk for both mucocutaneous and systemic candidiasis)

B. Clinical features

1. Typical presentation is the mucocutaneous growth. The most common affected areas are:

   a. Vagina—"yeast infection"
   - This results in a thick, white, "cottage cheese–like" vaginal discharge.
   - The discharge characteristically is painless but does cause pruritus.

   b. Mouth, oropharynx—"thrush"
   - This causes thick, white plaques that adhere to the oral mucosa.
   - Usually painless
   - Unexplained oral thrush should raise suspicion of HIV infection.

   c. Cutaneous candidiasis
   - This causes erythematous, eroded patches with "satellite lesions" (see Color Figure 10-5).
   - It is more common in obese diabetic patients; it appears in skin folds, underneath breasts, and in macerated skin areas.

   d. GI tract—e.g., esophagus
   - Candida esophagitis may cause significant odynophagia.
   - It may also be asymptomatic.

2. Disseminated or invasive disease may occur in immunocompromised hosts. Manifestations include sepsis/septic shock, meningitis, and multiple abscesses in various organs.

C. Diagnosis
1. Mucocutaneous candidiasis diagnosis is primarily clinical; KOH preparation demonstrates yeast.
2. Invasive candidiasis is diagnosed by blood or tissue culture.

D. Treatment
1. Remove indwelling catheters or central lines.
2. Acceptable treatments for oropharyngeal candidiasis
   a. Clotrimazole troches (dissolve in the mouth) five times per day
   b. Nystatin mouthwash ("swish and swallow") three to five times per day; only for oral candidiasis
   c. Oral ketoconazole or fluconazole for esophagitis
3. Vaginal candidiasis—miconazole or clotrimazole cream
4. Cutaneous candidiasis—oral nystatin powder, keeping skin dry
5. For systemic candidiasis, use amphotericin B or fluconazole. New, alternative antifungal agents include voriconazole and caspofungin.

Aspergillus

A. General characteristics
1. *Aspergillus* spp. spores are found everywhere in the environment. Typically disease occurs when spores are inhaled into the lung.
2. There are three main types of clinical syndromes associated with *Aspergillus* (see clinical features below).
3. Invasive aspergillosis is usually limited to severely immunocompromised patients. It should be considered in any immunocompromised patient with fever and respiratory distress despite use of broad-spectrum antibiotics.

B. Clinical features
1. Allergic bronchopulmonary aspergillosis
   a. A type I hypersensitivity reaction to *Aspergillus*
   b. It presents with **asthma and eosinophilia**. Recurrent exacerbations are common.
2. Pulmonary aspergilloma
   a. Pulmonary aspergilloma is caused by inhalation of spores into the lung. Patients with a history of sarcoidosis, histoplasmosis, tuberculosis, and bronchiectasis are at risk.
   b. It presents with chronic cough; hemoptysis may be present as well.
   c. It may resolve spontaneously or invade locally.
3. Invasive aspergillosis
   a. This occurs when hyphae invade the lung vasculature, resulting in thrombosis and infarction.
   b. Hosts are typically at-risk patients with acute leukemia, transplant recipients, and patients with advanced AIDS.
   c. It usually presents with acute onset of fever, cough, respiratory distress, and diffuse, bilateral pulmonary infiltrates.
   d. It is transmitted via hematogenous dissemination, and may invade the sinuses, orbits, and brain.

C. Diagnosis
1. CXR reveals a dense pulmonary consolidation and sometimes a **fungus ball**.
2. Definitive diagnosis of invasive aspergillosis is by tissue biopsy, but diagnosis is presumed when *Aspergillus* is isolated from the sputum of a severely immunocompromised/neutropenic patient with clinical symptoms.
3. Blood cultures are usually not helpful because they are rarely positive.

D. Treatment
1. For allergic bronchopulmonary aspergillosis, patients should avoid exposure to *Aspergillus*; corticosteroids may be beneficial.

2. For pulmonary aspergilloma, patients with massive hemoptysis may require a lung lobectomy.
3. For invasive aspergillosis, treat with IV amphotericin B, voriconazole, or caspofungin.
4. Suspicion of head or brain involvement warrants prompt evaluation (imaging studies). Surgery may be required.

Cryptococcosis

A. General characteristics
1. Caused by *Cryptococcus neoformans*, a budding, round yeast with a thick polysaccharide capsule
2. Associated with pigeon droppings
3. Most commonly seen in patients with advanced AIDS
4. Infection is due to inhalation of fungus into lungs. Hematogenous spread may involve the brain and meninges.

B. Clinical features
1. CNS disease—meningitis or meningoencephalitis; brain abscess is also possible
   a. CNS disease is a life-threatening condition that requires aggressive treatment (see below). It should always be on the differential diagnosis of an HIV-positive patient with a fever and headache. If untreated, it is almost invariably fatal.
   b. Symptoms include fever, headache, irritability, dizziness, confusion, and possibly seizures. The onset may be insidious.
2. Isolated pulmonary infection may also occur.

C. Diagnosis
1. LP is absolutely essential if meningitis is suspected.
   a. Latex agglutination detects cryptococcal antigen in the CSF.
   b. India ink smear shows encapsulated yeasts.
2. Tissue biopsy is characterized by **lack of inflammatory response**.
3. The organism may also be present in urine and blood.

D. Treatment
1. Use amphotericin B with flucytosine for approximately 2 weeks, followed by oral fluconazole.
2. The duration of therapy varies depending on follow-up CSF cultures.

Other Fungal Infections

• Table 10-11 covers blastomycosis, histoplasmosis, coccidioidomycosis, and sporotrichosis.

COMMON PARASITIC INFECTIONS

• Table 10-12 covers cryptosporidiosis, amebiasis, giardiasis, ascariasis, hookworm, pinworm (enterobiasis), tapeworm, and schistosomiasis.

FEVER AND SEPSIS

Fever of Unknown Origin (FUO)

A. General characteristics
1. Defining FUO
   a. Classically defined as having the following necessary criteria:
      • Fever >38.3°C (101°F)
      • Continuing "on several occasions" for at least 3 weeks
      • No diagnosis over this time period despite 1 week of inpatient workup.

TABLE 10-11 **Other Important Fungal Infections**

Infection	Organism	Transmission	Findings	Diagnosis	Treatment
Blastomycosis	*Blastomyces dermatitidis* (dimorphic fungus)	Inhalation of spores from the environment	Disseminated infection → chronic, indolent disease: constitutional symptoms, LAN, pneumonia	CTX from urine, sputum, body fluids	PO itraconazole × 6–12 mo Amphotericin B for meningitis
Histoplasmosis	*Histoplasma capsulatum* (dimorphic fungus with septate hyphae)	Exposure to bird/bat droppings (endemic in Ohio and Mississippi River valleys)	Flu-like symptoms, erythema nodosum, hepatosplenomegaly	Demonstration of yeast in body fluids or skin	PO itraconazole; amphotericin B for severe infection or ↓ immunocompromised host
Coccidioidomycosis	*Coccidioses immitis* (dimorphic fungus)	Inhalation of spores	Asymptomatic or nonspecific respiratory symptoms Dissemination → focal CNS findings	Visualization of fungus in fluids or skin	PO fluconazole or itraconazole × 6 mo IV amphotericin B for severe infection or ↓ immunocompromised host
Sporotrichosis	*Sporothrix schenckii* (dimorphic, cigarshaped yeast)	Invasion of skin by thorn or other plant material Keyword: gardening	Lymphocutaneous form: hard, subcutaneous nodules → ulcerate and drain Disseminated form: pneumonia, meningitis	Visualization of yeast in tissue or body fluids or serology	Potassium iodide × 1–2 mo or itraconazole × 3–6 mo Disseminated: amphotericin B

LAN, lymphadenopathy; CTX, culture.

b. Because of changes in medical practice, this definition has been altered: Three outpatient visits now substitute for 1 week in the hospital.
2. Causes
   a. Infection—most common cause
      • TB and other mycobacterial infection
      • Occult abscesses, e.g., hepatic, retroperitoneal
      • UTI/complicated UTI
      • Endocarditis
      • Sinusitis
      • HIV
      • Infectious mononucleosis and other viruses
      • Malaria and other parasitic infections
   b. Occult neoplasms are the second most common cause, particularly:
      • Lymphoma (especially Hodgkin's lymphoma)
      • Leukemia
   c. Collagen vascular disease
      • SLE
      • Still's disease
      • PAN
      • Temporal arteritis
      • Polymyalgia rheumatica
   d. Other causes (in no particular order)
      • Granulomatous disease, e.g., sarcoidosis, Crohn's disease

TABLE 10-12 Important Parasitic Infections

Infection	Organism	Transmission/Life Cycle	Findings	Diagnosis	Treatment
Cryptosporidiosis	Cryptosporidium spp. (spore-forming protozoa)	Fecal–oral route	Watery diarrhea ↓ Severe diarrhea in an immuno-compromised host	Stool sample: see oocytes	Supportive care
Amebiasis	Entamoeba histolytica (protozoan)	Fecal–oral route Contaminated water/food, anal–oral sexual contact	Bloody diarrhea, tenesmus, abdominal pain ± liver abscess	Stool sample: see trophozoites	Iodoquinol or paromomycin Metronidazole for liver abscess
Giardiasis	Giardia lamblia (protozoan)	Fecal–oral route (as in amebiasis) Hints: daycare, camping	Watery diarrhea Chronic infection; weight loss	Stool sample: see cysts or trophozoites	Metronidazole
Ascariasis	Ascaris lumbricoides (roundworms = nematodes)	Ingestion of food or water contaminated by human feces	Varies: no symptoms, postprandial abdominal pain, or vomiting Heavy worm burden: bowel, pancreatic duct or common bile duct obstruction	Stool sample: see eggs or adult worms	Albendazole, mebendazole, or pyrantel pamoate
Hookworm	Ancylostoma duodenale or Necator Americanus (roundworm)	Larvae invade skin → travel to lung → coughed and swallowed → reside in intestine	Usually no symptoms Cough, anemia, malabsorption, weight loss, eosinophilia	Stool sample: see adult worms	Mebendazole or pyrantel pamoate
Enterobiasis (pinworm)	Enterobius vermicularis (roundworm)	Fecal–oral route (self-infection with anus–hand–mouth contact) Common in children	Perianal pruritus, worse at night	"Tape test": see eggs on tape after it is placed near the anus	Mebendazole or pyrantel pamoate
Tapeworm (cestodes)	Taenia saginata (beef), Taenia solium (pork), Diphyllobothrium latum (fish)	Eating raw or undercooked meat	Usually asymptomatic Possible nausea, abdominal pain, weight loss Fish tapeworm: vitamin B_{12} deficiency	Tape test For D. l atum, stool sample (see eggs)	Praziquantel; vitamin B_{12} if deficient
Schistosomiasis (trematodes)	Schistosoma mansoni, S. haematobium, S. japonicum	Penetration of human skin (in contaminated fresh water) → migrate to lungs → to portal vein → to venules of mesentery, bladder, or ureters	S. mansoni and S. japonicum: fever, diarrhea (acute) → liver fibrosis, portal HTN (chronic) S. haematobium: urinary tract granulomas → bladder polyps and fibrosis, dysuria	Demonstration of eggs in urine or feces	Praziquantel

- Drug fevers, e.g., sulfonamides, penicillin, quinidine, barbiturates, "diet pills" (with phenolphthalein)
- Pulmonary embolism
- Hemolytic anemia
- Familial Mediterranean fever
- Gout
- Subacute thyroiditis
- Factitious illnesses

QUICK HIT

Persistence of fever in the ICU, despite antimicrobial therapy, should raise the index of suspicion for:
- Fungal infection
- Antimicrobial resistance
- Infections requiring surgical intervention—e.g., occult abscess, wound necrosis
- Drug fever

QUICK HIT

FUO is obviously a term of exclusion, and is not itself a diagnosis. In patients with persistent unexplained fevers, continue diagnostic testing until the cause is found.

B. Clinical features

1. Manifestations that **may** accompany fever but are not specific to any specific entity
   a. Chills—ironic sensation of cold, often with shivering
   b. Rigors—severe form of chills with pronounced shivering and chattering of teeth
   c. Night sweats
   d. Change in mental status—especially at extremes of age
2. Look for systemic manifestations of some of the more common causes of FUO, e.g., skin changes, constitutional symptoms, anemia, weight loss.

C. Diagnosis

1. Careful history and physical examination—with attention to medications, travel, immune system competency, and review of systems
2. Laboratory tests
   a. CBC with differential
   b. Urinalysis
   c. Cultures of blood, sputum, CSF, urine, and stool when indicated by clinical presentation
   d. Analysis and culture of abnormal fluid collections (e.g., joint, pleural)
   e. Complement assay
   f. PPD when TB is on the differential
   g. Other laboratory values: LFTs, ESR, ANA, rheumatoid factor, TSH
3. Imaging studies
   a. CXR, CT scan of the chest and abdomen—to detect tumors and abscesses
   b. Tagged WBC scan—sometimes helpful
   c. MRI, ultrasound, and echocardiogram may be appropriate, depending on the clinical situation.
4. Invasive diagnostic procedures—biopsy of lymph node, bone marrow, or other tissue when there is a high suspicion of tumor or abscess
5. Observation is sometimes necessary to make a diagnosis.

D. Treatment

1. Antibiotics and corticosteroids may mask the patterns of fever response. Base empiric treatment with antibiotics on the severity of illness.

Box 10-8   Approach to Fever

- There is no uniformly accepted definition, but most sources define fever as body temperature >37.5°C (99.5°F) measured by a modern oral thermometer.
- Measurement—Readings obtained using rectal thermometers are slightly higher than oral or axillary thermometer readings.
- Hyperthermia versus fever
  - Hyperthermia is an elevation in body temperature not caused by "raising the thermostat"—i.e., no change in the hypothalamic set-point.
  - Hyperthermia is usually caused by the inability of the body to dissipate heat.
  - Causes of hyperthermia include neuroleptic malignant syndrome, malignant hyperthermia, and heat stroke.
  - Hyperthermia does not respond to antipyretics, but rather to external cooling measures (e.g., ice, fans) and medications specific to the cause (e.g., dantrolene for malignant hyperthermia).
  - Fever occurs when there is an elevation in the hypothalamic set-point. It is a natural response to an inflammatory process.
  - Fever usually responds to antipyretics.
- Treat a fever with antipyretics when:
  - The fever is really hyperthermia.
  - The fever is dangerously high: >41°C (>105°F).
  - The patient is pregnant.
  - There is significant cardiopulmonary disease (increased oxygen demand may cause ischemia).
  - The patient wants symptomatic relief (chills, myalgias).

2. If the patient is not acutely ill, observation alone may be all that is necessary to arrive at a specific diagnosis.

3. In some cases of FUO, fevers may resolve spontaneously without ever being diagnosed.

4. The sense of urgency in determining the cause of the fevers should be in proportion to the severity of illness and the host's immune status.

Toxic Shock Syndrome (TSS)

A. General characteristics

1. TSS is most commonly associated with menstruating women and tampon use, but can occur in patients of all ages, male and female.

2. Other risk factors include surgical wounds, burns, and infected insect bites.

3. It is caused by an enterotoxin of *S. aureus*, or less frequently an exotoxin of group A *Streptococcus*. **Note that it is the toxin rather than the bacteria that causes the pathology associated with TSS.**

B. Clinical features

1. The onset of symptoms is characteristically abrupt.

2. Symptoms may include:
   a. Flu-like symptoms: high fevers, headache, myalgias
   b. Diffuse macular, erythematous rash
   c. Hyperemic mucus membranes, "strawberry tongue"
   d. Warm skin due to peripheral vasodilation (see Chapter 1, Shock)
   e. Hypotension
   f. Nausea, vomiting, and diarrhea may also be present.

3. By definition, there must be involvement of at least three organ systems, which may include:
   a. GI—nausea, vomiting, and diarrhea; elevations of aminotransferases
   b. Renal—elevations of BUN and/or creatine, pyuria
   c. Hematologic—thrombocytopenia
   d. Musculoskeletal—elevations of creatine kinase levels
   e. CNS—confusion, disorientation (must be present when fever is absent)

4. Multisystem organ dysfunction or failure may occur.

5. During the convalescent phase of illness, the **rash usually desquamates over the palms and soles.**

- The mortality rate for menstrual-related TSS is now <2% but is slightly higher (8%) for non–menstrual-related TSS.
- Previous TSS does **not** confer immunity. If fact, patients with a history of TSS are at greater risk for recurrent TSS.

C. Diagnosis

1. A high index of clinical suspicion is important.

2. Blood cultures are often negative.

3. Cultures may be taken from the suspected source, but the diagnosis is primarily clinical.

D. Treatment

1. Hemodynamic stabilization should be the first concern and may require aggressive fluids and even vasopressors.

2. The source of toxin (e.g., tampon) should be removed immediately. Wounds may require drainage or debridement.

3. Give antistaphylococcal therapy, such as nafcillin, oxacillin, or vancomycin, in a very ill patient. Clindamycin is sometimes used as adjunctive therapy.

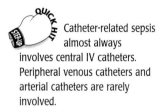

Catheter-related sepsis almost always involves central IV catheters. Peripheral venous catheters and arterial catheters are rarely involved.

Catheter-Related Sepsis

- Central venous catheters are a common cause of fever and sepsis in the hospital, especially in the ICU.
- The most common organisms are *S. aureus* and *S. epidermidis*.
- Risk factors for catheter-related sepsis are emergent placement, femoral lines, and prolonged indwelling of the line.

INFECTIOUS DISEASES

TABLE 10-13	Common Organisms in Various Infections	
Pneumonia	Community-acquired	
	Typical	*Streptococcus pneumoniae, H. influenzae, Moraxella catarrhalis*
	Atypical	*Mycoplasma* spp., *Chlamydia* spp., *Legionella* spp.
	Nosocomial	*Staphylococcus aureus*, gram-negative rods
	Aspiration pneumonia	Oral anaerobes, gram-negative rods, *S. aureus*
Urinary tract infection		*E. coli, S. saprophyticus, Enterococcus, Klebsiella, Proteus* spp., *Pseudomonas, Enterobacter*, yeast (*Candida* spp.)
Osteomyelitis, septic arthritis		*S. aureus, S. epidermidis, Streptococcus* spp., gram-negative rods
		Consider *Neisseria gonorrhoeae* in septic arthritis in adolescent
Skin/soft tissue	Surgical wound	*S. aureus*, gram-negative rods
	Diabetic ulcer	*S. aureus*, gram-negative rods, anaerobes
	Intravenous catheter site	*S. aureus, S. epidermidis*
	Cellulitis	*S. aureus*, group A streptococci
	Necrotizing fasciitis	*Clostridium perfringens*, group A streptococci
Upper respiratory	Pharyngitis	Viral, group A streptococci
	Acute bronchitis	Viral
	Acute sinusitis	Viral, *S. pneumoniae, H. influenzae, M. catarrhalis*
	Chronic sinusitis	*S. aureus*, anaerobes
Endocarditis	Subacute	*Streptococcus viridans*
	Acute	IV drug abuser: *S. aureus*, gram-negative rods, *Enterococcus* spp., yeast
		Prosthetic valve: *S. epidermidis*
Gastroenteritis		Viral, *Salmonella, Shigella, E. coli, Clostridium botulinum, Giardia, Helicobacter* spp., *Campylobacter*
Intra-abdominal		*Enterococcus, Bacteroides fragilis, E. coli*
Meningitis		See Table 10-6.

- Neutropenia is defined by absolute neutrophil count (ANC) <1,500/mm³ (ANC: combination of bands and mature neutrophils).
- ANC <500/mm³ corresponds to a severely increased risk of infection.

- Only half of all patients with catheter-related sepsis have clinical evidence of infection **at the site of insertion** (i.e., erythema, purulence). Therefore, a high index of suspicion is required.
- If you suspect catheter-related sepsis, promptly remove the catheter and send the tip for culture. This alone typically leads to resolution of fever and a decrease in leukocytosis. Antibiotics are usually initiated. Narrow the spectrum once the organism is identified.

Neutropenic Fever

- Common causes include bone marrow failure (e.g., due to toxins, drugs), bone marrow invasion (e.g., from hematologic malignancy, metastatic cancer), and peripheral causes (e.g., hypersplenism, SLE, AIDS). Isolated neutropenia (agranulocytosis) is commonly caused by drug reactions.
- Because neutropenia severely compromises the patient's ability to mount an inflammatory response, fever may be the only manifestation of a raging infection.
- The most common infections seen in neutropenic individuals are septicemia, cellulitis, and pneumonia.
- Obtain the following for any neutropenic patient with a fever: CXR, PAN culture (blood, urine, sputum, line tips, wound), CBC, complete metabolic panel.

- Place the patient on reverse isolation precautions (positive-pressure room, masks and strict handwashing for those entering the patient's room).
- Give broad-spectrum antibacterial agents immediately after cultures are drawn.
- If fever persists beyond 4 to 5 days despite broad-spectrum antibacterial therapy, give antifungal agents, such as IV amphotericin B. Consider G-CSF.

MISCELLANEOUS INFECTIONS

Infectious Mononucleosis

A. General characteristics

1. Caused by the EBV (rarely by CMV)
2. It is most commonly seen in adolescents and young adults, especially college students and military recruits (but may occur at any age). Infected children often experience milder symptoms.
3. Transmission
   a. The usual mode of transmission is through infected saliva (e.g., kissing, sharing food)
   b. Most adults (90%) have been infected with EBV and are carriers.
   c. One infection usually confers lifelong immunity.
   d. The incubation period is typically 2 to 5 weeks.

B. Clinical features

1. Symptoms
   a. Fever—Temperatures may be as high as 40°C (104°F); fever usually resolves within 2 weeks.
   b. Sore throat
   c. Malaise, myalgias, weakness—may linger for several months
2. Signs
   a. Lymphadenopathy—This is found in >90% of patients. Tonsillar or cervical (especially posterior cervical) lymph nodes may be quite enlarged, painful, and tender.
   b. Pharyngeal erythema and/or exudate—frequently present
   c. Splenomegaly—present in half of patients
   d. Maculopapular rash—present in approximately 15% of patients, but much higher if ampicillin is given
   e. Hepatomegaly—in 10% of cases
   f. Palatal petechiae and eyelid (periorbital) edema—may occur in a minority of cases

C. Diagnosis

1. Serology
   a. Monospot test—for detection of heterophile antibody
      - Heterophile antibodies are positive within 4 weeks of infection with EBV mononucleosis and are undetectable by 6 months. Thus, a positive monospot test indicates acute infection with EBV mononucleosis.
      - Heterophile antibodies do not form in CMV mononucleosis.
      - Rapid heterophile tests are highly sensitive and specific, particularly in adolescents.
   b. EBV-specific antibody testing—Perform in cases in which diagnosis is not straightforward (usually done by indirect immunofluorescence microscopy or by ELISA)
2. Peripheral blood smear—usually reveals lymphocytic leukocytosis with large, atypical lymphocytes
3. Throat culture—perform if pharyngitis is present to rule out a secondary infection with β-hemolytic streptococci

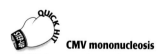

CMV mononucleosis
- Most commonly seen in sexually active adolescents/young adults
- Characterized by fevers, chills, fatigue, headaches, and frequently, splenomegaly
- Cervical lymphadenopathy and pharyngitis usually absent
- Negative for heterophile antibodies

D. Complications

1. Hepatitis
2. Neurologic complications (rare): meningoencephalitis, Guillain-Barré syndrome, Bell's palsy
3. Splenic rupture
4. Thrombocytopenia, hemolytic anemia
5. Upper airway obstruction due to lymphadenopathy

E. Treatment

1. Generally, no specific treatment is indicated (or available) as most people recover completely within 3 to 4 months. Supportive care includes:
   a. Rest, fluids
   b. Avoidance of strenuous activities until splenomegaly resolves to prevent splenic rupture
   c. Analgesics to reduce temperature and pharyngeal pain
2. Give a short course of glucocorticoids if there is airway compromise. Glucocorticoids have also been effective in patients with thrombocytopenia or hemolytic anemia.

CHAPTER 11

Diseases of the Skin and Hypersensitivity Disorders

COMMON DERMATOLOGIC PROBLEMS

INFLAMMATORY, ALLERGIC, AND AUTOIMMUNE SKIN CONDITIONS

Acne Vulgaris

A. General characteristics

1. Acne vulgaris an inflammatory condition of the skin that is most prevalent during adolescence.
2. Severe acne is more common in men than in women due to higher levels of circulating androgens.
3. Pathogenesis
   a. Obstruction of sebaceous follicles (by sebum) leads to the proliferation of *Propionibacterium acnes* (an anaerobic bacterium) in the sebum.
   b. This obstruction can lead to either noninflammatory comedones ("pimples"), or, if severe, inflammatory papules or pustules.
   c. Both noninflammatory and inflammatory lesions are present in most patients with acne.
4. Risk factors are male sex, puberty, Cushing's syndrome, oily complexion, androgens (due to any cause), and medications.
5. Classification
   a. Obstructive acne: closed comedones (whiteheads) or open comedones (blackheads)
   b. Inflammatory acne: Lesions progress from papules/pustules to nodules, then to cysts, then scars.

B. Treatment

1. General guidelines
   a. Instruct patient to: keep affected area clean (vigorous washing is unnecessary); reduce or discontinue acne-promoting agents (certain make-up, creams, oils, steroids, androgens).
   b. It takes about 6 weeks to notice the effects of medications (skin may get worse before it gets better). Start with one drug to assess its efficacy.
2. Mild to moderate acne
   a. Begin with topical benzoyl peroxide (2.5%)—should be applied once or twice daily. It destroys acne-causing bacteria and prevents plugging of pores by drying the skin.
   b. Add topical retinoids if the above fails. They cause peeling of the skin, which prevents clogging of pores.
   c. Add topical erythromycin or topical clindamycin—both act to suppress *P. acnes.*

QUICK HIT

- There is no proven link between acne and diet (e.g., chocolate, fatty foods).
- Oral contraceptives (especially some of the newer oral contraceptive pills) help some women with acne.

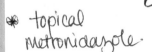

Do not give systemic antibiotics unless the patient is already on topical benzoyl peroxide, topical tretinoin, and topical antibiotics and the response is inadequate.

✱ *topical metronidazole.*

3. Moderate to severe nodular pustular acne
   a. Prescribe systemic antibiotic therapy: tetracycline, minocycline, doxycycline, erythromycin, clindamycin, and TMP-SMX.
   b. Add oral retinoids (e.g., isotretinoin) for severe cystic acne that is not responsive to the above treatments. Oral retinoids are teratogenic.

Rosacea

- A chronic condition resulting in reddening of the face (mainly the forehead, nose, and cheeks)
- Mostly affects Caucasian women between 30 and 50 years of age
- The most common skin findings include erythema, telangiectasia, papules, and pustules with redness, typically affecting the face. Unlike acne vulgaris, there are no comedones (see Color Figure 11-1).
- In severe cases, skin can become thickened and greasy—on the nose, it creates a bulbous appearance; this is called rhinophyma (mostly seen in men).
- Symptoms may be reduced by avoiding alcoholic or hot beverages, as well as extremes of temperature, and by reducing emotional stressors.
- Treatment: Topical metronidazole (gel form) is effective and is applied twice per day for several months. Systemic antibiotics (e.g., tetracycline) are used for maintenance therapy. If the patient does not experience an appropriate response, prescribe isotretinoin for daily use.

Seborrheic Dermatitis — *caused by yeast & inflammation*

A. General characteristics
1. A chronic, idiopathic, inflammatory skin disorder
2. Very common problem (affects 5% of the population), especially in patients with oily skin
3. Exacerbating factors: anxiety, stress, fatigue, hormonal factors
4. Common locations: scalp (dandruff), hairline, behind ears, external ear canal, folds of skin around nose, eyebrows, armpits, under breasts, groin area (skin folds)
5. May be complicated by secondary bacterial infection.

Seborrheic dermatitis is a chronic condition with no cure. Therapy may be needed indefinitely for control of symptoms.

B. Clinical features
1. Mild cases manifest as dandruff
2. Scaly patches with surrounding areas of mild to moderate erythema (see Color Figure 11-2)
3. Usually asymptomatic, but pruritus can occur

C. Treatment
1. Sunlight exposure often helps.
2. Dandruff shampoo (over-the-counter) is usually adequate.
3. Topical ketoconazole (to decrease yeast count on skin) has been found to be effective.
4. Topical corticosteroids are appropriate in severe cases.

Contact Dermatitis

A. General characteristics
1. There are two forms of contact dermatitis: irritant and allergic.
2. Irritant contact dermatitis (more common than allergic type) results from a chemical or physical insult to the skin (e.g., contact with detergents, acids, or alkalis, or from frequent hand washing).
   a. A previous sensitizing event is not needed to produce the rash (i.e., it is not an immunologic reaction).

b. The rash begins shortly after exposure to the irritant (in contrast to the allergic type, which begins several hours to a few days later).

3. Allergic contact dermatitis is **a delayed-type hypersensitivity reaction.**

a. No history of atopy is necessary for allergic contact dermatitis to occur. It can occur in anyone.

b. Sensitization of the skin occurs 1 to 2 weeks after the first exposure to the allergen. Subsequent exposure leads to dermatitis hours to days after the reexposure. Therefore, dermatitis develops only in patients who have already been sensitized to the allergen. Common allergens include poison ivy, oak, and sumac; iodine; nickel; rubber; topical medications (e.g., neomycin, topical anesthetics); and cosmetics.

B. Clinical features

1. The appearance of the rash depends on the stage.

a. Acute stage: erythematous papules and vesicles with oozing (see Color Figure 11-3); edema may be present

b. Chronic stage: crusting, thickening, and scaling; lichenification

2. The rash is usually very pruritic.

3. The interval between exposure and appearance of the rash varies, but is usually from several hours to as long as 4 to 5 days.

C. Diagnosis

1. Diagnosis is usually made clinically based on history and examination.

2. Patch testing (to identify the allergen that caused the allergic reaction) is indicated in any of the following cases.

a. The diagnosis is in doubt.

b. The rash does not respond to treatment.

c. The rash recurs.

D. Treatment

1. Avoid the contact allergen!

2. Apply cool tap water compresses.

3. Apply topical corticosteroids.

4. Prescribe systemic corticosteroids (e.g., prednisone, 1 mg/kg/day) for severe cases. Continue for 10 to 14 days and then taper.

Pityriasis Rosea

- Papulosquamous eruption—Initially, "*herald patches*" that resemble a ring worm (multiple round/oval patches) appear, and then a generalized rash with multiple oval-shaped lesions appears. The rash is classically described as having a Christmas tree–type appearance (see Color Figure 11-4).

- It is **not** contagious and is possibly related to herpes type 7.

- It is common on the trunk and upper arms and thighs, and is usually not found on the face. Pruritus is often present, and varies in severity.

- It spontaneously remits within a few (6 to 8) weeks without treatment. There is no treatment other than antihistamines for pruritus. Recurrences are rare.

Erythema Nodosum

- Erythema nodosum appears as painful, red, subcutaneous, elevated nodules, typically located over the anterior aspect of the tibia (less commonly on the trunk or arms) (see Color Figure 11-5). It is self-limited and usually resolves within a few weeks. Low-grade fever, malaise, and joint pain may precede the rash.

- It is much more common in women (especially young women) than in men.

- Many causes: *Streptococcus* infection, sarcoidosis, inflammatory bowel disease, fungal infections, pregnancy, medications (e.g., oral contraceptives, sulfa drugs, amiodarone, antibiotics), syphilis, tuberculosis; many cases are idiopathic

QUICK HIT
Do not confuse allergic contact dermatitis with any of the following.
- Irritant contact dermatitis—Rash is usually identical to that seen in allergic contact dermatitis except the rash begins very soon after exposure.
- Atopic dermatitis—Onset is in infancy or childhood.
- Seborrheic dermatitis
- Psoriasis

- Perform the following to help determine the underlying condition: chest radiograph (for sarcoidosis, tuberculosis); VDRL (serologic test for syphilis); CBC, erythrocyte sedimentation rate, and cultures, as appropriate. Skin biopsy may be helpful.
- Treat the underlying condition, if known.
- Prescribe bed rest, leg elevation, NSAIDs, and heat for symptoms. Potassium iodide may help.

Erythema Multiforme (EM)

- EM is an inflammatory skin condition characterized by erythematous macules/papules that resemble target lesions ("**bull's-eye lesions**") that can become bullous (see Color Figure 11-6).
- Skin lesions may be pruritic and painful.
- EM can be caused by medications and may follow an infection by HSV. Many cases are idiopathic. EM due to HSV infection can recur.
- Medications implicated include sulfa drugs (most common), penicillin and other antibiotics, phenytoin, allopurinol, and barbiturates.
- If initiated early when the first symptom of HSV infection appear, acyclovir can help to prevent HSV-associated EM. For recurrent and debilitating EM, acyclovir may be given prophylactically for prolonged periods.
- Antihistamines or analgesics for symptomatic relief.

Stevens-Johnson Syndrome and Toxic Epidermal Necrolysis

- No precise definition exists, but Stevens-Johnson syndrome (SJS) is considered the most severe form of EM. Toxic epidermal necrolysis (TEN) is considered to be the most severe form of SJS.
- In SJS and TEN, skin involvement is extensive and severe, with possible detachment of areas of epidermis.
- The eyes and mouth may also be involved.
- Systemic manifestations include fever, difficulty eating, renal failure, and sepsis.
- **Potentially life-threatening** (mortality rate is 5% for SJS and 30% for TEN)
- Half of all cases are due to medications (e.g., sulfa drugs, penicillins, barbiturates, phenytoin, allopurinol, carbamazepine, vancomycin, rifampin). In many cases, no specific cause is identified.
- Admit patient to an ICU. Withdraw the suspected medication; aggressive rehydration and symptomatic management.

Lichen Planus

- Chronic, inflammatory lesions of unknown etiology
- (4 Ps): Pruritic, polygonal, purple, flat-topped papules
- Most commonly seen on wrists, shins, oral mucosa, and genitalia
- Treat with glucocorticoids.

Bullous Pemphigoid

- Multiple subepithelial blisters on abdomen, groin, and extremities
- Elderly people are most commonly affected.
- Blisters are less easily ruptured than in pemphigus vulgaris.
- Autoimmune condition; no malignant potential but may be persistent
- Treat with systemic glucocorticoids with or without azathioprine.

Pemphigus Vulgaris

- Autoimmune blistering condition resulting in loss of normal adhesion between cells (acantholysis)
- Starts in oral mucosa; may become generalized

- Blisters rupture, leaving painful erosions.
- Most commonly affects elderly people, **often fatal if untreated**
- Treat with systemic glucocorticoids and other immunosuppressants.

SKIN CONDITIONS RELATED TO MICROBIAL INFECTION

Warts

A. General characteristics

1. Warts are caused by HPV and are transmitted via skin-to-skin contact. For genital warts, transmission is via intimate sexual contact.
2. Types
   a. **The common wart (*Verruca vulgaris*)—most common type**
      - May occur anywhere, but the most common sites include elbows, knees, fingers, and palms
      - Appearance: flesh-colored or whitish with a hyperkeratotic surface
   b. The flat wart (*Verruca plana*)
      - Common sites include the chin/face, dorsum of hands, and legs.
      - Appears flesh-colored with smooth papules and a flat surface
   c. The plantar wart (*Verruca plantaris*)
      - Solitary or multiple warts found on the plantar side of the foot; can cause foot pain if located on pressure areas (e.g., metatarsal head, heel)
      - Appearance: flesh-colored with a rough, hyperkeratotic surface
   d. Anogenital wart (*Condyloma acuminatum*)
      - **Most common STD**, commonly associated with HPV 6 and 11 (see Color Figure 11-7)
      - HPV (types 16, 18) infection can lead to cervical cancer in women (Pap smear is important).
      - Appearance: single or multiple soft, fleshy growths on the genitalia, perineum, and anus

B. Clinical features

1. Most warts are asymptomatic unless "bumped." Plantar warts can be painful during walking.
2. Some warts may bleed.
3. Warts are unsightly and can be disfiguring.

C. Treatment

1. Freezing lesion with liquid nitrogen (applied on a cotton swab)—multiple treatments may be necessary
2. Salicylic acid (Compound W)—applied daily for several weeks
3. 5-FU cream or retinoic acid cream for flat warts
4. Surgical excision or laser therapy
5. Podophyllin for genital warts

Molluscum Contagiosum

- A common, self-limited viral infection caused by a poxvirus; common in sexually active young adults and in children
- It manifests as small papules (2 to 5 mm) with central umbilication. Lesions are asymptomatic. In HIV-positive patients, lesions can be extensive (see Color Figure 11-8).
- It is transmitted via skin-to-skin contact (sexual contact can lead to genital involvement) and is **highly contagious.**
- It persists up to 6 months, but spontaneously regresses with time. In immunosuppressed individuals (HIV-positive patients), the lesions can progress to grow quite large and often are refractory to treatment.
- Multiple treatment modalities are effective (e.g., curettage, drops containing podophyllin and cantharidin, cryosurgery), but scarring is always a risk.

Most warts disappear spontaneously within 1 to 2 years. However, if the condition is left untreated, more warts can appear.

Warts can be recurrent and may require multiple treatments (despite the method of therapy chosen).

Herpes Zoster (Shingles)

A. General characteristics

1. Caused by reactivation of varicella-zoster virus, which remains dormant in the dorsal root ganglia and is reactivated in times of stress, infection, or illness; only occurs in those who have previously had chickenpox

2. It is typically seen in patients over 50 years of age. In patients less than 50 years of age, suspect an immunosuppressed state.

3. Contagious when open vesicles present and only for those who have never had chickenpox or are immunocompromised (or newborns). Zoster is not as contagious as chickenpox.

B. Clinical features

1. **Severe pain and rash in a dermatomal distribution.** Pain comes before the rash. Rash is characterized by grouped vesicles on an erythematous base. If severe, low-grade fever and malaise may be present.

2. The most common sites of involvement are the thorax (most cases) and trigeminal distribution (especially ophthalmic division). Affected sites can also include other cranial nerves, as well as arms and legs (see Color Figure 11-9).

3. Rarely life threatening, even if dissemination occurs. Herpes zoster is more severe, however, in immunocompromised patients.

C. Treatment

1. Keep the lesions clean and dry.

2. Prescribe analgesics for pain relief (aspirin or acetaminophen; codeine if needed). In severe cases, administer a local injection of triamcinolone in lidocaine.

3. Prescribe antiviral agents (acyclovir, famciclovir, valacyclovir) to reduce the pain, decrease the length of illness, and reduce the risk of postherpetic neuralgia.

4. The use of corticosteroids to decrease the incidence of postherpetic neuralgia remains controversial.

Dermatophytes

- Dermatophytes are superficial fungi that infect cutaneous epithelium, nails, and hair.
- The three main genera of dermatophytes are *Trichophyton, Microsporum,* and *Epidermophyton.*
- Important dermatophyte infections are covered in Table 11-1.
- Scrape lesions and use KOH preparation to visualize the fungus.

Scabies

A. General characteristics

1. Caused by the human skin mite *Sarcoptes scabiei* var *hominis*

2. Highly contagious—transmitted via skin-to-skin contact or through towels, bed linens, or clothes

3. Pathogenesis—The mites tunnel into the epidermis, lay eggs, and deposit feces (called scybala). A delayed type IV hypersensitivity reaction develops toward the mites, eggs, and feces, causing intense pruritus.

4. Common locations
   a. Fingers, interdigital areas, and wrists
   b. Elbows, feet, ankles, penis, scrotum, buttocks, and axillae
   c. Head, neck, palms, and soles are typically spared (except in infants, the elderly, or immunosuppressed people)

B. Clinical features

1. Severe pruritus—This is often the most severe during the night. The head and neck are usually spared.

QUICK HIT

Complications of zoster
- Postherpetic neuralgia
- Occurs most frequently in patients older than 50 years
- Manifests as excruciating pain that persists after the lesions have cleared, and does not respond to analgesics
- Can be chronic and debilitating
- Uveitis
- Dissemination
- Meningoencephalitis, deafness

QUICK HIT

Treat tinea capitis and onychomycosis with oral antifungal agents. Others are treated with topical antifungals.

TABLE 11-1 **Important Dermatophyte Infections**

Fungal Infection	Location	Age Group	Findings	Diagnosis	First-Line Treatment
Tinea corporis ("ringworm")	Body/trunk	All ages	Pinkish, annular lesions	Direct microscopy: visualization of hyphae from skin scrapings with KOH preparation	Topical antifungals (e.g., ketoconazole, miconazole)
Tinea capitis	Scalp	Children	Areas of scaling with hair loss ± pruritus	• Direct microscopy • Wood's lamp: if hairs fluoresce, *Microsporum* spp. is the cause. If not, *Trichophyton* spp is the cause	Oral griseofulvin (antifungal)
Tinea unguium (onychomycosis)	Nails	Elderly people	Thick, opacified nails	Direct microscopy (nail scrapings)	Oral griseofulvin (antifungal)
Tinea pedis ("athlete's foot")	Feet—web spaces of toes	Young adults	Scaling, erythema, pruritus	Direct microscopy	Topical antifungals, good foot hygiene
Tinea cruris ("jock itch")	Groin, inner thighs	Adults: males > females	Areas of scaling, erythema: spares scrotum	Direct microscopy	Topical antifungals, good hygiene

2. Burrows—Linear marks (several millimeters in length) represent the tunneled path of the mite. There is typically a dark dot at one end, representing the female mite.
3. Scratching may lead to excoriations.
4. Eczematous plaques, crusted papules, or secondary bacterial infection may develop (see Color Figure 11-10).

QUICK HIT Suspect scabies in any patient who has persistent, generalized, severe pruritus.

C. Diagnosis
1. Look for characteristic burrows on hands, wrists, and ankles, and in the genital region.
2. Confirm the diagnosis by scraping the burrow with a scalpel and examining it under a microscope to detect the presence of mites, ova, or scybala.

D. Treatment
1. Specific medications
   a. Permethrin 5% cream (Elimite)
      • First-line treatment; causes paralysis of the parasite (acts on nerve cell membrane)
      • Should be applied to **every area of the body** (head to toe), even under fingernails and toenails, around the genital area, and in the cleft of the buttocks.
      • Patients should leave cream on overnight (>8 to 10 hours) and wash it off the next morning.
   b. Lindane (γ-benzene-hexachloride) lotion
      • Alternative treatment
      • Contraindicated in children under 2 years of age, as well as in pregnant or lactating women
2. General recommendations
   a. Treat all close contacts of the patient simultaneously (even if asymptomatic) with permethrin 5% cream.
   b. The patient is no longer contagious after one treatment, although pruritus may continue for a few weeks as dead mites are shed from the skin. Use topical corticosteroids and oral antihistamines to control pruritus during this time.
   c. Thoroughly wash all underwear and bed linens.

DISEASES OF THE SKIN AND HYPERSENSITIVITY DISORDERS

PRECANCEROUS AND CANCEROUS DISEASES OF THE SKIN

Actinic Keratosis (Also Called Solar Keratosis)

- Small, rough, scaly lesions due to prolonged and repeated sun exposure (see Color Figure 11-11)
- Most commonly seen in fair-skinned people. Lesions are typically on the face.
- Prevention: Advise patients to avoid excessive sun exposure and to use sunscreen.
- Although the risk of malignancy is low, biopsy is still recommended for hyperkeratotic actinic keratosis lesions to exclude squamous cell carcinoma (SCC).
- Treatment options include surgical removal (scraping), freezing with liquid nitrogen, or application of topical 5-FU for multiple lesions (destroys sun-damaged skin cells).

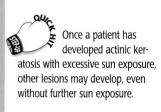

Once a patient has developed actinic keratosis with excessive sun exposure, other lesions may develop, even without further sun exposure.

Basal Cell Carcinoma (BCC)

- **BCC is the most common skin cancer** (accounts for 60% to 75% of all skin cancers).
- It arises from the basal layer of cells in the epidermis.
- The most important risk factor is sun exposure.
- It occurs most frequently in fair-skinned individuals who burn easily and involves sun-exposed areas, such as the head and neck (the nose is the most common site).
- The classic appearance is a pearly, smooth papule with rolled edges and surface telangiectases (3 Ps: pearly, pink, papule) (see Color Figure 11-12).
- Metastasis is extremely rare, but can be locally destructive.
- Surgical resection is curative.

Squamous Cell Carcinoma (SCC)

- SCC is less common than BCC. (SCC accounts for less than 20% of all skin cancers.)
- It arises from epidermal cells undergoing keratinization.
- Sunlight exposure is the most important risk factor. Chronic skin damage and immunosuppressive therapy are also risk factors.
- It is typically described as a crusting, ulcerated nodule or erosion (see Color Figure 11-13).
- The likelihood of metastasis is higher than with BCC, but much lower than with melanoma.
- The prognosis is excellent if it is completely excised (95% cure rate). Lymph node involvement, however, carries a poor prognosis.

Marjolin's ulcer: a squamous cell carcinoma arising from a chronic wound (tends to be very aggressive)

Melanoma

A. General characteristics

1. Most aggressive form of skin cancer and **the number one cause of death due to skin cancer**
2. Increasing incidence worldwide
3. Risk factors
   a. Fair complexion; primarily affects Caucasian patients, especially those with any of the following:
      - Inability to tan
      - Easily sunburned
      - Red hair and/or freckles
      - Numerous moles
   b. Sun exposure, especially for:
      - Patients with a history of severe sunburn before age 14
      - Patients living in a sunny climate
   c. Family history of melanoma (e.g., first-degree relative)
   d. Genodermatoses (e.g., xeroderma pigmentosa)
   e. Increasing age

f. Large numbers of nevi (moles)
- Although most melanomas arise de novo, they may arise from preexisting nevi in up to 50% of cases.
- Any change in a nevus is concerning because it may indicate malignancy or malignant transformation. Look for color change, bleeding, ulceration, or a papule arising from the center of an existing nevus.

g. Dysplastic nevus syndrome
- Numerous, atypical moles—These tend to be large with indistinct borders and variations in color. The chances of **a single** dysplastic nevus becoming a melanoma are small.
- If dysplastic nevus syndrome **and** a family history of melanoma are present, the risk of developing melanoma approaches 100%.

h. Giant congenital nevi—The risk of melanoma is about 5% to 8%. Prophylactic excision is recommended.

4. Growth phases
a. Radial (initial) growth phase
- Growth is predominantly lateral within the epidermis.
- There is a good prognosis with surgical resection because metastasis is unlikely.
b. Vertical (later) phase
- Growth extends into the reticular dermis or beyond.
- Lymphatic or hematogenous metastasis may occur.
- **Depth of invasion is the most important indicator of prognosis.**

B. Clinical features

1. A melanoma may present with some or all of the following features.
a. **A**symmetry
b. **B**order irregularity
c. **C**olor variegation—ranging from pink to blue to black
d. **D**iameter greater than 6 mm
e. **E**levation—typically has a raised surface (see Color Figure 11-14)
2. Changing mole—most common presentation of melanoma
3. The most common site is the back.
4. Advanced lesions often present with itching and bleeding.

C. Diagnosis

1. Excision biopsy is the standard of care for diagnosis of any suspicious lesion.
a. Shave biopsy and punch biopsy are less accurate than excision biopsy in assessing the depth of invasion.
b. Acceptable skin margins are 1 to 3 cm for most lesions, as determined by depth of invasion.
2. Lymph node dissection is appropriate if nodes are palpable.

D. Treatment

1. Early detection is the most important way to prevent death, because prognosis is directly related to depth of invasion.
2. Perform lymph node dissection if nodes are involved. This is controversial because of risk of lymphedema and the little benefit gained in patients with distant metastasis.

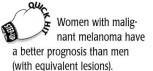 Women with malignant melanoma have a better prognosis than men (with equivalent lesions).

 Spitz nevi
- Well-circumscribed, raised lesion commonly confused with melanoma; color varies
- Complete excision is recommended.

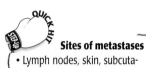 **Sites of metastases**
- Lymph nodes, skin, subcutaneous (59%)
- Lung (36%)
- Liver (20%)
- Brain (20%)—common cause of death
- Bone (17%)
- GI tract (7%)

Box 11-1 Stages of Decubitus Ulcers

- Stage 1: skin is intact; nonblanching erythema, signs of impending ulceration may be present
- Stage 2: partial-thickness skin loss—epidermis and varying amounts of dermis (abrasion, blister, superficial ulcer or crater)
- Stage 3: full-thickness skin loss—extends into subcutaneous tissue, but not through underlying fascia
- Stage 4: full-thickness skin loss—extends into muscle, bone, joints, tendons; severe tissue necrosis is present; osteomyelitis, pathologic fractures, sinus tracts may be present

Decubitus Ulcers

- Decubitus ulcers are also called pressure sores. They result from necrosis of tissue that becomes ischemic and ulcerates, and they are caused by prolonged pressure from the weight of the patient.
- Risk factors include immobilization for any reason, peripheral vascular disease, and dementia. Those at increased risk include debilitated or paraplegic people, nursing home residents, and people with neurologic disorders.
- They typically occur over bony prominences. The sacrum, greater tuberosity, and ischial tuberosity are the most common sites. Other sites include the calcaneus, malleoli occiput, elbows, and back.
- If unrecognized and untreated, tissue can become necrotic and secondary bacterial infection can occur: cellulitis, osteomyelitis, sepsis, necrotizing fasciitis, gangrene, tetanus, and wound botulism are all potential consequences.
- Prevention is most important; patients should be turned and repositioned every 2 hours. Special mattresses and beds are designed to reduce local tissue pressure by distributing it more evenly.
- Treatment
  - Local wound care (e.g., for more superficial ulcers)
  - Wet-to-dry dressings or wound gel for deeper ulcers
  - Surgical débridement of necrotic tissue
  - Antibiotics if evidence of infection (e.g., surrounding cellulitis)

Psoriasis

A. General characteristics

1. Psoriasis is due to abnormal (markedly accelerated) proliferation of skin cells. Because of this, the skin does not have time to mature normally. This leads to defective keratinization, which causes the scaling.
2. The cause is unknown, but genetics are believed to be important.
3. This is a chronic condition characterized by exacerbations and remissions—it improves during the summer (sun exposure) and worsens in the winter (dries skin).
4. Trauma to the skin in any form (e.g., infection, abrasion) can cause exacerbations, as can psychosocial stress.
5. Up to three-fourths of patients have somewhat localized disease (<20% to 25% of body surface area). Nevertheless, clinical features vary, and some patients have generalized skin involvement.
6. **Less than 10% of patients develop psoriatic arthritis** (see Chapter 6).

B. Clinical features

1. Well-demarcated, erythematous papules or plaques that are covered by a thick, *silvery scaling*; pruritus is often present (see Color Figure 11-15).
2. *Auspitz's sign*—Removal of the scale causes pinpoint bleeding.
3. It can involve any part of the body, but the most common areas are the extensor surfaces of extremities (knees, elbows), scalp, intergluteal cleft, palms, and soles.
4. Pitting of the surface of nails, or onycholysis (distal separation of the nail from the nail bed)

C. Treatment

1. Topical therapy
   a. Corticosteroids are the most commonly prescribed first-line agents, but they have adverse side effects with prolonged use.
   b. Calcipotriene is a vitamin D derivative that has become a first- or second-line agent. It is very effective in most patients.

c. Tars have an unpleasant odor, so they are less desirable to use. Patients should use tars for 4 to 6 weeks before expecting to see a benefit. Tars are more effective in combination therapy and are associated with an 80% to 90% remission rate.

d. Other options include tazarotene (a vitamin A derivative) and anthralin.

e. Combination therapy (e.g., steroids and calcipotriene) is more effective than either agent alone.

2. Systemic treatment is indicated in patients with severe psoriasis. Options include:

a. Immune-modulating therapy—e.g., methotrexate, infliximab, cyclosporine

b. Photochemotherapy

c. Acitretin (a systemic retinoid)

d. Acitretin plus phototherapy

QUICK HIT

There is no cure for psoriasis, but the disease can be managed.

Seborrheic Keratosis

• These are very common skin lesions that begin to appear after age 30. Hereditary— they probably are autosomal dominant, and are harmless growths with no malignant potential.

• There is no association with sunlight.

• They can be located anywhere, but are common on the face and trunk. They increase in number with time, and some patients have many of them.

• They are slightly elevated plaques, gradually turning darker in color, and appear as if they were "stuck" on the skin (see Color Figure 11-16).

• Treatment is not necessary and is only for cosmetic reasons: liquid nitrogen cryotherapy or curettage is effective and easily performed in the office setting.

Vitiligo

• Chronic, depigmenting condition due to unknown cause; hereditary component is suspected

• Sharply demarcated areas of skin become amelanotic—most common on the face

• Associated with diabetes mellitus, hypothyroidism, pernicious anemia, and Addison's disease   *autoimmune*

• Topical glucocorticoids and photochemotherapy are used to promote repigmentation with varying degrees of success.

ALLERGIC REACTIONS

Urticaria (Hives)

• Urticaria is caused by the release of mediators from mast cells, with a resultant increase in vascular permeability. There are different types of urticaria.

• Urticaria can be precipitated by foods, drugs, latex allergy, animal dander, pollen, dust, plants, an infection, or cold/heat. It can also be idiopathic.

• Findings—edematous wheals (hives) that are fleeting in nature, i.e., they disappear within hours only to return in another location. They blanch with pressure, and may cause intense pruritus or stinging. Lesions get worse with scratching (see Color Figure 11-17).

• Treatment involves removal of the offending agent. Antihistamines are effective for symptomatic relief. Systemic corticosteroids may help in more severe cases.

Box 11-2   Types of Hypersensitivity Reactions

• **Type I:** IgE-mediated: e.g., anaphylaxis, asthma
• **Type II:** IgG- (or IgM-) and cytotoxic cell-mediated: e.g., Goodpasture's disease, pemphigus vulgaris
• **Type III:** antigen–antibody complexes: e.g., SLE, Arthus reaction, serum sickness
• **Type IV:** T-cell–mediated (delayed hypersensitivity): e.g., allergic contact dermatitis, tuberculosis, transplant rejection

---

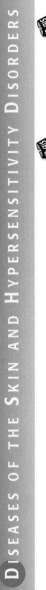

QUICK HIT

Hereditary angioedema: autosomal dominant condition caused by C1 esterase inhibitor deficiency, characterized by recurrent episodes of angioedema; can be life-threatening

QUICK HIT

Angioedema usually resolves in a few days, but can persist longer in some cases. (Although the swelling at any one spot resolves in a few days, the swelling can move from one location to another.)

Angioedema

- The mechanism is similar to that in urticaria, though angioedema occurs deeper in the skin (i.e., fluid extravasation occurs in deeper layers of skin/subcutaneous tissue). Angioedema and urticaria can occur simultaneously or independently.
- Angioedema can be caused by any of the precipitants of urticaria. ACE inhibitors are a specific cause of angioedema (reaction usually occurs within 1 week of initiating the drug).
- Unlike urticaria, which can occur anywhere, angioedema usually affects the eyelids, lips and tongue, genitalia, hands, or feet.
- Angioedema is characterized by localized edema of deep subcutaneous tissue, resulting in nonpitting, puffy skin with firm swelling that is more tender and "burning" than pruritic (because there are fewer mast cells/sensory nerve endings in deeper tissues) (see Color Figure 11-18).
- **Severe angioedema can lead to potentially life-threatening airway obstruction.**
- Angioedema can even involve the GI tract, causing nausea/vomiting and abdominal pain (can be so severe as to mimic acute abdomen).
- Treatment is similar to treatment of urticaria. Give SC epinephrine for laryngeal edema or bronchospasm.

Drug Allergy

- An adverse drug reaction is not necessarily an allergic drug reaction. Adverse drug reactions include drug side effects, drug–drug interactions, drug toxicity and associated illnesses, and drug allergy. Most cases of adverse drug reactions are **not** related to allergy (only 10% have a true allergic basis).
- Many patients who state they are "allergic" to a medication believe themselves to be allergic because they have been incorrectly labeled without direct immunologic evidence. However, given the serious risks of a true drug allergy, one should avoid the suspected medication.
- All four types of hypersensitivity reactions may serve as the underlying mechanism of drug allergies. In many cases, however, the mechanism is unknown.
- β-Lactam antibiotics (penicillins), aspirin, NSAIDs, and sulfa drugs account for more than 80% of all cases of drug allergy. Other drugs implicated include insulin, local anesthetics, ACE inhibitors, and radiocontrast agents.
- Drug-induced hypersensitivity reactions can affect multiple organ systems and can manifest in a variety of forms, including:
  - **Dermatologic eruptions** (most common)—e.g., urticaria or angioedema, allergic contact dermatitis, EM-like eruptions, erythema nodosum
  - **Pulmonary findings**—e.g., asthma, pneumonitis
  - **Renal manifestations**—e.g., interstitial nephritis, nephrotic syndrome
  - **Hematologic manifestations**—e.g., thrombocytopenia, hemolytic anemia, eosinophilia, agranulocytosis
- If a drug allergy is suspected, inquire about any recent changes in the patient's medications. **Allergic reactions typically appear within 1 month of initiating the drug.** It is uncommon for a drug reaction to occur within less than 1 week of initiating the drug.
- Treatment: Discontinue the drug (if known). Give antihistamines for symptomatic relief. Treat as for anaphylaxis if severe.

Food Allergy

- Adverse food reactions can be due to true food allergies, food poisoning, metabolic conditions (e.g., lactose intolerance, phenylketonuria), malabsorption syndromes (e.g., celiac disease), or preexisting illnesses (e.g., ulcer).
- As with drug allergies, people generally tend to believe they are allergic to a food based on an adverse reaction even when they may not have a true food allergy.

- Hypersensitivity reactions to foods are usually due to immunoglobulin (Ig) E-mediated reactions to food and/or additives.
- The most common foods responsible include eggs, peanuts, milk, soy, tree nuts, shellfish, wheat, chocolate, legumes, and some fruits (e.g., kiwi). There are others, and preservatives or additives may be responsible. The cause may never be found.
- Food allergy reactions have the following effects.
  - **Dermatologic manifestations (most common)**—e.g., pruritus, erythema, urticaria, angioedema
  - **GI manifestations (second-most common)**—e.g., nausea, vomiting, abdominal cramps, diarrhea
  - **Anaphylactic reactions**—can affect the respiratory system and can be fatal
  - **Cutaneous manifestations**—e.g., angioedema, urticaria
- Treatment for mild reactions is supportive, with administration of antihistamines to lessen symptoms. If the reaction is more severe, treat as for anaphylaxis. Avoid the offending agent.

Insect Sting Allergy

- Insects responsible include yellow jackets, honeybees, wasps, and yellow and bald-faced hornets.
- Local (**nonallergic**) reaction is localized swelling, pain, pruritus, and redness, all of which subside in several hours. This is the normal reaction to an insect sting.
- Large local (**allergic**) reaction is marked swelling and erythema over a large area around the sting site. **Can be confused with cellulitis.** It may last for several days, and sometimes presents with mild, systemic manifestations (malaise, nausea). Prescribe antihistamines and analgesics for symptoms (short course of prednisone for severe cases).
- Anaphylaxis may occur and can be fatal.
- Treatment: ice and oral antihistamines for mild local reactions; if severe, treat as for anaphylaxis

Anaphylaxis

- Most severe form of allergy—This is a systemic allergic reaction (usually a type I IgE reaction) that may be life-threatening.
- It occurs within seconds to minutes after exposure to antigen. Numerous causes have been identified, including foods (**most common cause**), medications, radiocontrast agents, blood products, venoms (e.g., from snakes), insect stings, latex, hormones, ragweed/molds, and various chemicals.
- It can progress within seconds to minutes to a life-threatening situation characterized by shock or respiratory compromise (airway obstruction, vascular collapse).
- Typically, the initial findings are cutaneous, followed by respiratory symptoms.
- Treatment of anaphylaxis
  - ABCs—Secure the airway; intubation may be necessary.
  - Give epinephrine immediately. Give IV if severe (1:10,000), SC if less severe (1:1,000).
  - Give antihistamines (both H$_1$ and H$_2$ blockers) and corticosteroids as well (although they have a minimal effect in hyperacute condition).
  - Supportive care—IV fluids, oxygen

distributive shock

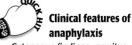

Clinical features of anaphylaxis
- Cutaneous findings—pruritus, erythema, urticaria, angioedema
- Respiratory findings—dyspnea, respiratory distress, asphyxia
- Cardiovascular findings—hypotension, shock, arrhythmias
- GI findings—abdominal pain, nausea/vomiting, severe diarrhea

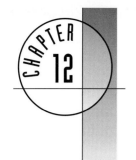

Ambulatory Medicine

AMBULATORY MEDICINE

CARDIOVASCULAR DISEASES

Hypertension (HTN)

A. General characteristics

1. **Essential HTN (i.e., there is no identifiable cause) applies to more than 95% of cases of HTN.**
2. Secondary HTN has many identifiable causes
   a. **Renal/renovascular disease—renal artery stenosis (most common cause of secondary HTN),** chronic renal failure, polycystic kidneys
   b. Endocrine causes—hyperaldosteronism, thyroid or parathyroid disease, Cushing's syndrome, pheochromocytoma, hyperthyroidism, acromegaly
   c. Medications—oral contraceptives, decongestants, estrogen, appetite suppressants, chronic steroids, tricyclic antidepressants (TCAs), nonsteroidal anti-inflammatory drugs (NSAIDs)
   d. Coarctation of the aorta — ↑ BP–upper extremities
   e. Cocaine, other stimulants
   f. Sleep apnea

B. Risk factors

1. Age—Both systolic and diastolic BP increase with age.
2. Gender—more common in men (gap narrows over age 60); men have higher complication rates
3. Race—It is twice as common in African-American patients as in Caucasian patients; African-American patients have higher complication rates (stroke, renal failure, heart disease).
4. Obesity, sedentary lifestyle
5. Family history
6. Increased sodium intake—This correlates with increased prevalence in large populations, although not in individuals; individual susceptibility to the effects of high salt intake varies.
7. Alcohol—Intake of more than 2 oz (8 oz of wine or 24 oz of beer) per day is associated with HTN.

C. Complications

1. **The major complications of HTN are cardiac complications (coronary artery disease [CAD], CHF with left ventricular hypertrophy [LVH]), stroke, and renal failure.** These account for the majority of deaths associated with untreated HTN.
2. HTN has effects on the following organs (target organ damage):
   a. Cardiovascular system
      • Effects on the heart are most important. **HTN is a major risk factor for CAD,** with resultant angina and MI.
      • **CHF is a common end-result of untreated HTN as LVH occurs.**
      • Most deaths due to HTN are ultimately due to MI or CHF.

Handwritten margin note:
Renalvascular HTN
→ elderly due to atherosclerosis
→ fibromuscular dx of the renal artery in young women.

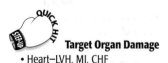

Birth control pills are the most common secondary cause of HTN in young women

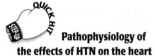

Pathophysiology of the effects of HTN on the heart
• Increased systemic vascular resistance (afterload) → concentric LVH → decreased LV function. As a result, the chamber dilates → symptoms and signs of heart failure.
• HTN accelerates atherosclerosis, leading to a higher incidence of CAD (as well as peripheral vascular disease and stroke).

Target Organ Damage
• Heart–LVH, MI, CHF
• Brain–stroke, TIA
• Chronic kidney disease
• Peripheral vascular disease
• Retinopathy

TABLE 12-1 Classification and Management of Hypertension

Classification	Systolic BP (mm Hg)		Diastolic BP (mm Hg)	Recommended Management
Normal	<120	and	<80	No Treatment
Prehypertension	120–139	and	80–89	Lifestyle modification
Stage I	140–159	or	90–99	Lifestyle modification, drug therapy
Stage II	≥160	or	≥100	Lifestyle modification and drug therapy (2-drug combination for most)

Modified from Chobanian et al. The seventh report of the Joint National Committee on Prevention, Detection, Evaluation and Treatment of High Blood Pressure: The JNC VII report. JAMA 2003;289:2560–2572.

- HTN predisposes the patient to peripheral vascular disease (PVD).
- HTN is associated with increased incidence of **aortic dissection**.

b. Eyes (retinal changes)
- Early changes—Arteriovenous nicking (discontinuity in the retinal vein secondary to thickened arterial walls) and cotton wool spots (infarction of the nerve fiber layer in the retina) can cause visual disturbances and scotomata (see Color Figure 12-1).
- More serious disease—hemorrhages and exudates
- **Papilledema**—an ominous finding seen with severely elevated BP

c. CNS
- Increased incidence of **intracerebral hemorrhage**
- Increased incidence of other stroke subtypes as well (transient ischemic attacks [TIAs], ischemic stroke, and lacunar stroke)
- Hypertensive encephalopathy when BP is severely elevated (uncommon)

d. Kidney
- Arteriosclerosis of afferent and efferent arterioles and glomerulus—called nephrosclerosis
- Decreased GFR and dysfunction of tubules—with eventual **renal failure**

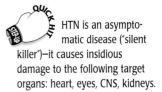 HTN is an asymptomatic disease ("silent killer")—it causes insidious damage to the following target organs: heart, eyes, CNS, kidneys.

D. Diagnosis

1. BP measurement
   a. Unless the patient has severe HTN or evidence of end-organ damage, never diagnose hypertension on the basis of one BP reading. Establish the diagnosis on the basis of at least two readings over a span of 4 or more weeks.
   b. Observe the following to obtain an accurate BP reading.
   - The arm should be at heart level, and the patient should be seated comfortably.
   - Have the patient sit quietly for at least 5 minutes before measuring BP.
   - Make sure the patient has not ingested caffeine or smoked cigarettes in the past 30 minutes (both elevate BP temporarily).
   - Use a cuff of adequate size (a cuff that is too small can falsely elevate BP readings). The bladder within the cuff should encircle at least 80% of the arm.

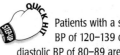 Patients with a systolic BP of 120–139 or a diastolic BP of 80–89 are considered prehypertensive and require lifestyle modifications to prevent cardiovascular disease.

2. Order the following laboratory tests to evaluate target organ damage and assess overall cardiovascular risk.
   a. Urinalysis
   b. Chemistry panel: serum K+, BUN, Cr } check renal function.
   c. Fasting glucose (if patient is diabetic, check for microalbuminuria)
   d. Lipid panel
   e. ECG
3. If the history and physical examination (H & P) or laboratory tests suggest a secondary cause of hypertension, order appropriate tests.

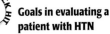 **Goals in evaluating a patient with HTN**
- Look for secondary causes (may be treatable).
- Assess damage to target organs (heart, kidneys, eyes, CNS).
- Assess overall cardiovascular risk.
- Make therapeutic decisions based on above.

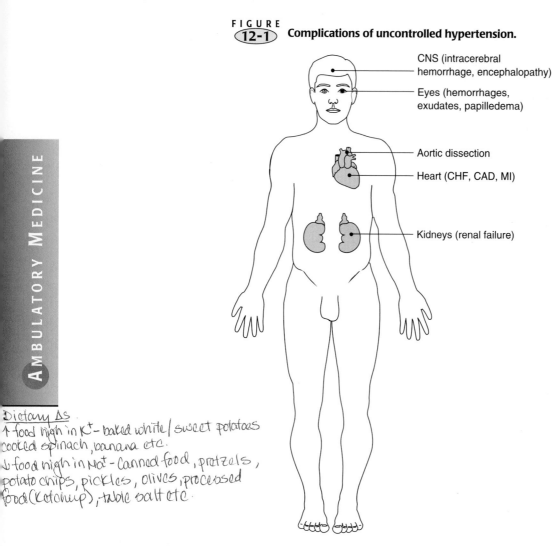

FIGURE
12-1 **Complications of uncontrolled hypertension.**

CNS (intracerebral hemorrhage, encephalopathy)

Eyes (hemorrhages, exudates, papilledema)

Aortic dissection

Heart (CHF, CAD, MI)

Kidneys (renal failure)

Dietary ∆s
↑ food high in K⁺ - baked white/sweet potatoes
cooked spinach, banana etc.
↓ food high in Na⁺ - Canned food, pretzels,
potato chips, pickles, olives, processed
food (Ketchup), table salt etc.

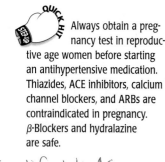

Always obtain a pregnancy test in reproductive age women before starting an antihypertensive medication. Thiazides, ACE inhibitors, calcium channel blockers, and ARBs are contraindicated in pregnancy. β-Blockers and hydralazine are safe.

① Tx - lifestyle ∆s
② diuretics
③ β-blockers
④ Vasodilators (always use w/
   β-blockers to
   prevent tachycardia)
⑤ ACE Inhibitors/ARBs

E. Treatment

1. Lifestyle changes—Advise patients to do the following, as appropriate.
   a. Reduce salt intake. Reduction in dietary salt has been shown to reduce BP. Recommend either a no-added-salt diet (4 g sodium/day) or a low-sodium diet (2 g/day).
   b. Lose weight. Weight loss lowers BP significantly. In patients with central obesity (who often have coexisting diabetes, hyperlipidemia, and other risk factors), weight loss is particularly important because multiple risk factors are reduced concomitantly.
   c. Avoid excessive alcohol consumption. Alcohol has a pressor action, and excessive use can increase BP.
   d. Exercise regularly. Regular aerobic exercise can lower BP (and reduces overall cardiovascular risk).
   e. Follow a low-saturated-fat diet rich in fruits, vegetables, and low-fat dairy products. Such a diet has been shown to lower BP.
   f. Stop unnecessary medications that may contribute to HTN.
   g. Engage in appropriate stress management practices.
2. Pharmacologic treatment (seven classes of drugs)
   a. Thiazide diuretics *(Hydrochlorthiazide)*
      • Because "salt-sensitive" HTN is more common in African-American patients, diuretics are the best initial choice in African-American patients. However, if an African-American patient has diabetes, an ACE inhibitor is still the initial agent of choice.

- Check serum potassium regularly (hypokalemia can be exacerbated by high salt intake).
b. β-blockers—decrease HR and cardiac output and decrease renin release
c. ACE inhibitors
  - Inhibit the renin-angiotensin-aldosterone system and inhibit bradykinin degradation
  - **Preferred in all diabetic patients** because of their protective effect on kidneys
d. Angiotensin II receptor blockers (ARBs)
  - Also inhibit renin-angiotensin-aldosterone system
  - Recent studies suggest that ARBs have the same beneficial effects on the kidney in diabetic patients as ACE inhibitors.
e. Calcium channel blockers—cause vasodilation of arteriolar vasculature
f. β-blockers ⍺₁ blockers
  - Work by decreasing arteriolar resistance
  - May be of benefit if the patient has concurrent benign prostatic hyperplasia (BPH)
g. Vasodilators (hydralazine and minoxidil)—not commonly used; typically given in combination with β-blockers and diuretics to patients with refractory HTN

3. General principles of treatment
a. BP should be lowered to <140/90 mm Hg, with 135/85 mm Hg the **minimum** goal in people with diabetes or renal insufficiency. The ideal goal is to lower BP to <120/80, but this is not always practical or well tolerated by the patient.
b. Drug treatment is often lifelong. However, patients with very mild HTN may be able to be weaned off medication if their BP can be lowered and controlled with nonpharmacologic measures. However, these patients need frequent BP checks.
c. **β-blockers and thiazide diuretics have been shown to reduce mortality and morbidity and are the most common initial choices.** ACE inhibitors are also a good choice, especially in diabetics.
d. If the patient's response to one agent is not adequate, change to another first-line agent of a different class before adding a second agent.
e. Choose thiazide diuretics as either the first or second drug because they enhance the effectiveness of all of the other antihypertensive agents.
f. If a patient's response is still inadequate with two agents, consider a third agent.
g. When to start treatment
  - The decision of when to start pharmacologic treatment is based on the patient's total cardiovascular risk, not just the elevation in BP.
  - For any level of BP elevation, the presence of cardiovascular risk factors and/or comorbid conditions dramatically accelerates the risk from HTN, and therefore modifies the treatment plan. Estimation of overall risk depends on **cardiovascular risk factors** and **clinical risk factors** (see Box 12-1).

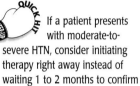 If a patient presents with moderate-to-severe HTN, consider initiating therapy right away instead of waiting 1 to 2 months to confirm diagnosis and start treatment.

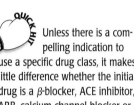 Unless there is a compelling indication to use a specific drug class, it makes little difference whether the initial drug is a β-blocker, ACE inhibitor, ARB, calcium channel blocker or diuretic.

 Treatment with ACE inhibitors and ARBs is associated with decreased risk of new-onset diabetes in patients with HTN.

 Most patients eventually need more than one drug to attain goal BP (especially diabetics, obese patients and those with renal failure)

TABLE 12-2	Side Effects of Antihypertensive Medications
Medication	**Side Effects**
Thiazide diuretics	**Hypokalemia,** hyperuricemia, hyperglycemia, elevation of cholesterol and triglyceride levels, metabolic alkalosis, hyperuricemia, hypomagnesemia
β-blockers	Bradycardia, bronchospasm, sleep disturbances (insomnia), fatigue, may increase TGs and decrease HDL, depression, sedation, may mask hypoglycemic symptoms in diabetic patients on insulin
ACE inhibitors	Acute renal failure, hyperkalemia, dry cough angioedema, skin rash, altered sense of taste, contraindicated in pregnancy

---

Box 12-1 Risk Factors for Coronary Artery Disease (CAD) in Evaluation of Patients With Hyperlipidemia

- Current cigarette smoking (dose-dependent risk)
- Hypertension
- Diabetes mellitus
- Low HDL cholesterol (<35 mg/dL); high HDL (>60 mg/dL) is a negative risk factor (subtract 1 from total)
- Age
  - Male: >45 years of age
  - Female: >55 years of age
- Male gender—if you count as a risk factor, do not count age
- Family history of **premature** CAD
  - MI/sudden death in male first-degree relative <55 years of age
  - MI/sudden death in female first-degree relative <65 years of age

---

Hyperlipidemias

A. General characteristics

1. Hyperlipidemia is one of the most important (and modifiable) risk factors for CAD. It causes accelerated atherosclerosis.
2. Hyperlipidemia may be a primary disorder, such as a familial dyslipidemia syndrome, or secondary to another cause.
3. Classification of dyslipidemia syndromes—Types IIA, IIB, and IV account for over 80% of all of familial dyslipidemias (see Table 12-3).
4. Secondary causes of hyperlipidemia
   a. Endocrine disorders—hypothyroidism, DM, Cushing's syndrome
   b. Renal disorders—nephrotic syndrome, uremia
   c. Chronic liver disease
   d. Medications—glucocorticoids, estrogen, thiazide diuretics, β-blockers
   e. Pregnancy
5. Risk factors
   a. Diet
      - Saturated fatty acids and cholesterol cause elevation in LDL and total cholesterol.

 Cardiovascular risk factors: smoking, diabetes, hypercholesterolemia, age over 60, family history, male sex (higher than for female only until menopause)
Clinical risk factors: presence of CAD, PVD, or prior MI; any manifestations of target organ disease–LVH, retinopathy, nephropathy; stroke or TIA

If "white coat hypertension" is suspected, there are two options for determining whether the increased BP persists outside the office.
- 24-hour ambulatory blood pressure monitoring is the most effective.
- Home blood pressure monitoring is an alternative.

All people should be screened with fasting lipid profile every 5 years starting at age 20. Earlier and more frequent screening is recommended for a strong family history and/or obesity.

Ambulatory Medicine

TABLE 12-3 Dyslipidemia Syndromes

Class	Name	Lipoprotein Elevated	Treatment
Type I	Exogenous hyperlipidemia	Chylomicrons	Diet
Type IIa	Familial hypercholesterolemia	LDL	Statins Niacin Cholestyramine
Type IIb	Combined hyperlipoproteinemia	LDL + VLDL	Statins Niacin Gemfibrozil
Type III	Familial dysbetalipoproteinemia	IDL	Gemfibrozil Niacin
Type IV	Endogenous hyperlipidemia	VLDL	Niacin Gemfibrozil Statins
Type V	Familial hypertriglyceridemia	VLDL + chylomicrons	Niacin Gemfibrozil

IDL , intermediate density lipoprotein.

- High-calorie diets do not increase LDL or cholesterol levels (are "neutral") but do increase triglyceride (TG) levels.
- Alcohol increases TG levels and HDL levels but does not affect total cholesterol levels.
b. Age—Cholesterol levels increase with age until approximately age 65. The increase is greatest during early adulthood—about 2 mg/dL per year.
c. Inactive lifestyle, abdominal obesity
d. Family history of hyperlipidemia
e. Gender—Men generally have higher cholesterol levels than do women; when women reach menopause, cholesterol levels then equalize and may even be higher in women than in men.
f. Medications
- Thiazides—Increase LDL, total cholesterol, TG (VLDL) levels
- β-blockers (propranolol)—Increase TGs (VLDL) and lower HDL levels
- Estrogens—TG levels may further increase in patients with hypertriglyceridemia.
- Corticosteroids and HIV protease inhibitors can elevate serum lipids.
g. Genetic mutations that predispose to the most severe hyperlipidemias
h. Secondary causes of dyslipidemia (see above)
6. Role of lipids in CAD risk
a. LDL cholesterol
- Accounts for two-thirds of total cholesterol. **CAD risk is primarily due to the LDL component** because LDL is thought to be the most atherogenic of all lipoproteins.
- Levels above 160 mg/dL significantly increase CAD risk.
- LDL cholesterol is not directly measured. It is calculated as follows: LDL = total cholesterol − HDL − TG/5.
b. Total cholesterol
- Levels less than 200 mg/dL are desirable. However, levels between 160 and 200 may still be associated with an increased risk of CAD.
- The risk of CAD increases sharply when total cholesterol is above 240 mg/dL.
c. HDL cholesterol
- Its protective effect (removes excess cholesterol from arterial walls) is at least as strong as the atherogenic effect of LDL.
- For every 10 mg/dL increase in HDL levels, CAD risk decreases by 50%.
- Low HDL (<35 mg/dL) is a major independent risk factor for CAD.
- High HDL (>60 mg/dL) is a "negative" risk factor (counteracts one risk factor).
d. **The total cholesterol-to-HDL ratio**—The lower the total cholesterol-to-HDL ratio, the lower the risk of CAD.
- Ratio of 5.0 is average (standard) risk.
- Ratio of 10 is double the risk.
- Ratio of 20 is triple the risk.
- Ratio of <4.5 is desirable.
e. Triglycerides—The importance of elevated TGs to CAD risk is controversial.

B. Clinical features

1. Most patients are asymptomatic.
2. The following may be manifestations of severe hyperlipidemia.
   a. *Xanthelasma*—yellow plaques on eyelids

TABLE 12-4 Threshold Levels for Hyperlipidemia

	Ideal (mg/dL)	Borderline (mg/dL)	High (mg/dL)
Total cholesterol	<200	200–240	>240
LDL	<130	130–160	>160
Triglycerides	<125	125–250	>250

TABLE 12-5 **Therapy for Hyperlipidemia**

Risk Category	LDL Goal	Initiate Lifestyle Changes	Consider Drug Therapy
CHD or CHD risk equivalents*	<100 mg/dL	100 mg/dL (All pts regardless of LDL)	130 mg/dL
No CHD but >2 risk factors	<130 mg/dL	130 mg/dL (All pts regardless of LDL)	130 mg/dL
No CHD but 2 risk factors	<130 mg/dL	130 mg/dL	160 mg/dL
No CHD and 0-1 risk factors	<160 mg/dL	160 mg/dL	190 mg/dL

*CHD risk equivalents include DM, PVD, CAD, AAA

Modified from Grundy SM, et al. Implications of recent clinical trials for the National Cholesterol Education Program Adult Treatment Panel III guidelines. Circulation 2004;110:227–239.

AMBULATORY MEDICINE

> **QUICK HIT**
>
> **Estrogen replacement therapy in postmenopausal women**
> Recent HERS trial showed no benefit of hormone replacement therapy on cardiovascular outcomes in women with established CHD. However, the study did not address the issue in women without CHD. The results are somewhat controversial.

> **QUICK HIT**
>
> Statins and fibrates can induce transient elevation in serum transaminases. LFT must be monitored.

> **QUICK HIT**
>
> Statins have been shown to significantly reduce rates of MI, stroke, and coronary and all-cause mortality in prospective placebo-controlled trials.

> **QUICK HIT**
>
> Potency of HMG CoA reductase inhibitors ("statins") increases in the following order (cost increases with potency): fluvastatin (Lescol) < lovastatin (Mevacor) and pravastatin (Pravachol) < simvastatin (Zocor) and atorvastatin (Lipitor).

   b. *Xanthoma*—hard, yellowish masses found on tendons (finger extensors, Achilles tendon, plantar tendons)
3. Pancreatitis can occur with severe hypertriglyceridemia.

C. Diagnosis

1. Lipid screening (see Health Maintenance section)—Measure total cholesterol and HDL levels (nonfasting is acceptable). If either is abnormal, then order a full fasting lipid profile.
2. A full fasting lipid profile includes TG levels and calculation of LDL levels.
3. Consider checking laboratory tests to exclude secondary causes of hyperlipidemia.
   a. TSH (hypothyroidism)
   b. LFTs (chronic liver disease)
   c. BUN and Cr, urinary proteins (nephrotic syndrome)
   d. Glucose levels (diabetes)

D. Treatment

1. General guidelines
   a. The long-term goal is to reduce coronary heart disease (CHD) risk. The short-term goal is to reduce LDL levels.
   b. If the patient has no established CHD, the target LDL level is <130 mg/dL.
   c. If the patient has established CHD or is diabetic, the target LDL level is <100 mg/dL.
2. Therapy for high LDL cholesterol
   a. Dietary therapy is the initial measure. Lowering fat intake (especially saturated fats) reduces serum cholesterol more than lowering cholesterol intake. Foods rich in omega-3 fatty acids (such as fish) are particularly beneficial. With an intensive diet, LDL can be reduced by an average of 10%, as follows: <30% of total calories from fat; with fewer than 10% from saturated fat; <300 mg/day of cholesterol.
   b. Exercise and weight loss—reduce risk of CAD
      • Exercise increases HDL and reduces other CAD risk factors by lowering BP and enhancing the efficiency of peripheral oxygen extraction.
      • Weight loss reduces myocardial work as well as the risk of diabetes.
   c. Drug therapy—See Table 12-6. Available agents include HMG CoA reductase inhibitors (statins), niacin, bile-acid sequestrants, and gemfibrozil.
   d. **When to initiate therapy**—See Table 12-5.
3. Therapy for high TG levels
   a. TG levels >500 mg/dL should be treated with medication.
      • Niacin is the first-line drug for hypertriglyceridemia.
      • Gemfibrozil also lowers TGs effectively.

TABLE 12-6	**Drug Therapy for Hyperlipidemia**		
Drug	**Effects**	**Comments**	**Side Effects**
HMG CoA reductase inhibitors (statins)	Lower LDL levels (most potent for lowering LDL) Minimal effect on HDL and TG levels	Have been shown to reduce mortality from cardiovascular events and significantly reduce total mortality Drugs of choice for lowering LDL	Monitor LFTs (monthly for first 3 months, then every 3–6 months). Harmless elevation in muscle enzymes (CPK) may occur.
Niacin	Lowers TG levels Lowers LDL levels Increases HDL levels	Do not use in diabetic patients (may worsen glycemic control) Most potent agent for increasing HDL levels and lowering TG levels Second-line agent for lowering LDL	Flushing effect (cutaneous flushing of face/arms; pruritus may be present) Check LFTs and CPK levels as with statin drugs.
Bile acid–binding resins (cholestyramine, colestipol)	Lowers LDL **Increases** TG levels	Effective when used in combination with statins or niacin to treat severe disease in high-risk patients Third-line agent for lowering LDL	Adverse GI side effects, poorly tolerated
Fibrates (gemfibrozil)	Lower VLDL and TG Increase HDL	Can be used if the above fail	GI side effects (mild) Mild abnormalities in LFTs Gynecomastia, gallstones, weight gain, and myopathies are other side effects.
CPK=creatine phosphokinase.			

b. TG levels <500 mg/dL can be managed with weight loss, diet, and exercise. Weight loss should be the primary goal. Initiate drug therapy if weight reduction is insufficient or not feasible.

HEADACHE

Tension Headache

A. General characteristics
1. Cause is unknown; may be similar to that of migraines (see below)
2. Usually worsens throughout the day; precipitants include anxiety, depression, and stress
3. Mild migraine can easily be confused with tension headache and vice versa.

B. Clinical features
1. Pain is steady, aching, "viselike," and encircles the entire head (tight band-like pain around the head).
   a. Usually generalized, but may be the most intense around the neck or back of head
   b. Can be accompanied by tender muscles (posterior cervical, temporal, frontal)
2. Tightness in posterior neck muscles

C. Treatment
1. Attempt to find the causal factor(s). Evaluate the patient for possible depression or anxiety. Stress reduction is important.
2. NSAIDs, acetaminophen, and aspirin are the standard treatment for mild/moderate headaches.
3. If headaches are severe, medications that are used for migraines may be appropriate, given the difficulty in distinguishing between these two entities.

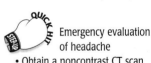

Emergency evaluation of headache
- Obtain a noncontrast CT scan to first rule out any type of intracranial bleed.
- However, small bleeds (subarachnoid hemorrhage) may be missed by CT scan, so a lumbar puncture may be necessary.

Cluster Headaches

A. General characteristics
1. Very rare—thought by some to be a variant of migraine headache
2. Usually occurs in middle-aged men
3. Subtypes
   a. Episodic cluster headaches (90% of all cases)—last 2 to 3 months, with remissions of months to years
   b. Chronic cluster headaches (10% of all cases)—last 1 to 2 years; headaches do not remit

B. Clinical features
1. Excruciating periorbital pain ("behind the eye")—**almost always unilateral**
2. Cluster headache is described as a "deep, burning, searing, or stabbing pain." Pain may be so severe that the patient may even become suicidal.
3. Accompanied by ipsilateral lacrimation, facial flushing, nasal stuffiness/discharge
4. Usually begins a few hours after the patient goes to bed and lasts for 30 to 90 minutes; awakens patient from sleep (but daytime cluster headaches also occur)
5. Attacks occur nightly for 2 to 3 months and then disappear. Remissions may last from several months to several years.
6. Worse with alcohol and sleep

C. Treatment
1. Acute attacks
   a. **Sumatriptan** (Imitrex) is the drug of choice.
   b. **O_2 inhalation** is also beneficial.
   c. The combination of sumatriptan and O_2 therapy is very effective, and narcotics are not usually necessary.
2. Prophylaxis
   a. Of all headache types, cluster headaches are the most responsive to prophylactic treatment. Offer all patients prophylactic medication. **Verapamil** taken daily is the drug of choice.
   b. Ergotamine, methysergide, lithium, and corticosteroids (prednisone) are alternative agents.
   c. These agents cause resolution (or marked reduction) of the number of headaches within 1 week.

Migraine

A. General characteristics
1. An inherited disorder (probably an autosomal dominant trait with incomplete penetrance)
2. The pathogenesis is not clearly defined, but serotonin depletion plays a major role.

Box 12-2   Differential Diagnosis of Headache

- Primary headache syndromes: migraines, cluster headache, tension headache
- Secondary causes of headache ("VOMIT")
  - **V**ascular—subarachnoid hemorrhage, subdural hematoma, epidural hematoma, intraparenchymal hemorrhage, temporal arteritis
  - **O**ther causes—malignant HTN, pseudomotor cerebri, postlumbar puncture, pheochromocytoma
  - **M**edication/drug related—nitrates, alcohol withdrawal, chronic analgesic use/abuse
  - **I**nfection—meningitis, encephalitis, cerebral abscess, sinusitis, herpes zoster, fever
  - **T**umor

3. More common in women than men; more common in those with a family history; typically occurs one to two times per month
4. Types
   a. Migraine with aura (15% of cases)—"classic migraine." Aura is usually visual (flashing lights, scotomata, visual distortions), but can be neurologic (sensory disturbances, hemiparesis, dysphasia).
   b. Migraine without aura (85% of cases)—"common migraine"
   c. Menstrual migraine
      • Occurs between 2 days before menstruation and the last day of menses; linked to estrogen withdrawal
      • Treatment is similar to that of nonmenstrual migraine except that estrogen supplementation is sometimes added.
   d. Status migrainous—lasts over 72 hours and does not resolve spontaneously
5. The following can provoke a migraine:
   a. Hormonal alteration (menstruation)
   b. Stress, anxiety
   c. Sleeping disturbances (lack of sleep)
   d. Certain drugs/foods: chocolate, cheese, alcohol, smoking, oral contraceptive pills
   e. Weather changes and other environmental factors

B. Clinical features

1. Prodromal phase (occurs in 30% of patients)
   a. Consists of symptoms of excitation or inhibition of the CNS: elation, excitability, increased appetite and craving for certain foods (especially sweets); alternatively, depression, irritability, sleepiness, and fatigue may be manifested.
   b. May precede the actual migraine attack by up to 24 hours
2. Severe, throbbing, unilateral headache (not always on the same side)
   a. Lasts 4 to 72 hours
   b. At times, it may be generalized over the entire head and may last for days if not treated.
   c. Pain is aggravated by coughing, physical activity, or bending down.
   d. Variable pain quality: "throbbing" or "dull and achy"
3. Other symptoms include nausea and vomiting (in as many as 90% of cases), photophobia, and increased sensitivity to smell.

C. Treatment

1. Acute attacks of migraine
   a. If migraines are mild, analgesics such as NSAIDs or acetaminophen may be effective. If they are not effective, try either dihydroergotamine (DHE) or a triptan.
   b. DHE—a serotonin (5-HT1) receptor agonist
      • This is highly effective in terminating the pain of migraines. It is available for SC, IM, IV, or nasal administration.
      • Contraindications: CAD, pregnancy, TIAs, PVD, sepsis
   c. Sumatriptan—a more selective 5-HT1 receptor agonist than DHE or other triptans
      • Acts rapidly (within 1 hour) and is highly effective
      • Should not be used more than once or twice per week
      • Contraindications: CAD, uncontrolled HTN, basilar artery migraine, hemiplegic migraine, use of MAOI, SSRI, or lithium
   d. If none of the available migraine medications work, it is unlikely that the patient is suffering from a migraine headache.
2. Prophylaxis (must be taken daily)
   a. Consider prophylaxis for patients with weekly episodes that are interfering with activities. Before initiating prophylactic medications, the patient should make attempts to avoid any known precipitants of the migraines.

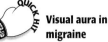

Visual aura in migraine
• The classic presentation is a bilateral homonymous scotoma. Bright, flashing, crescent-shaped images with jagged edges often appear on a page, obscuring the underlying print. The aura usually lasts 10 to 20 minutes.
• A patient may have isolated visual migraines (as above) without headaches.

Many patients who are labeled as having migraines actually have **rebound analgesic headaches**. These occur more frequently (every 1 to 2 days) than migraines. These headaches do **not** respond to drugs used to treat migraines. Wean patient from analgesics. Do not use narcotics!

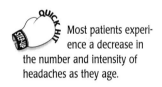

Most patients experience a decrease in the number and intensity of headaches as they age.

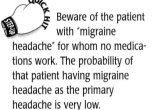

Beware of the patient with "migraine headache" for whom no medications work. The probability of that patient having migraine headache as the primary headache is very low.

AMBULATORY MEDICINE

    b. First-line agents include TCAs (amitriptyline) and propranolol (β-blocker).
    c. Second-line agents include verapamil (calcium channel blocker), valproic acid (anticonvulsant), and methysergide.
    d. NSAIDs are effective for menstrual migraines.

UPPER RESPIRATORY DISEASES

Cough

A. General characteristics

1. Cough can be divided into acute (less than 3 weeks duration) and chronic (more than 3 weeks duration).
2. If the cause is benign, cough usually resolves in a few weeks. If a cough lasts for longer than 1 month, further investigation is appropriate.
3. Causes
    a. Conditions that are usually associated with other symptoms and signs
      • Upper respiratory infections (URIs)—This is probably the most common cause of acute cough.
      • Pulmonary disease—pneumonia, chronic obstructive pulmonary disease (COPD), pulmonary fibrosis, lung cancer, asthma, lung abscess, tuberculosis
      • CHF with pulmonary edema
    b. Isolated cough in patients with normal chest radiograph
      • Smoking
      • Postnasal drip—may be caused by URIs (viral infections), rhinitis (allergic or nonallergic), chronic sinusitis, or airborne irritants
      • Gastroesophageal reflux disease (GERD)—especially if nocturnal cough (when lying flat, reflux worsens due to position and decreased lower esophageal sphincter (LES) tone)
      • Asthma—cough may be only symptom in 5% of cases
      • ACE inhibitors—may cause a dry cough (due to bradykinin production)

B. Diagnosis

1. Usually no tests are indicated in a patient with acute cough.
2. CXR is indicated only if a pulmonary cause is suspected, if the patient has hemoptysis, or if the patient has a chronic cough. It also may be appropriate in a long-term smoker in whom COPD or lung cancer is a possibility.
3. CBC if infection is suspected
4. Pulmonary function testing if asthma is suspected or if cause is unclear in a patient with chronic cough
5. Bronchoscopy (if there is no diagnosis after above workup) to look for tumor, foreign body, or tracheal web

C. Treatment

1. Treat the underlying cause, if known.
2. Smoking cessation, if smoking is the cause
3. Postnasal drip—Treat this with a first-generation antihistamine/decongestant preparation. If sinusitis is also present, consider antibiotics. For allergic rhinitis, consider a nonsedating long-acting oral antihistamine (loratadine). ✓Claritin.
4. Nonspecific antitussive treatment
    a. Unnecessary in most cases, because cough usually resolves with specific treatment of the cause
    b. May be helpful in the following situations
      • If cause is unknown (and thus specific therapy cannot be given)
      • If specific therapy is not effective
      • If cough serves no useful purpose such as clearing excessive sputum production or secretions

---

Handwritten margin note:
3 MC causes of cough
- post nasal drip
- Asthma/COPD
- GERD

Postnasal drip
The mucosal receptors in the pharynx and larynx are stimulated by secretions of the nose and sinuses that drain into the hypopharynx.

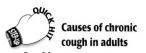

Causes of chronic cough in adults
• **Smoking**
• Postnasal drip
• GERD
• Asthma

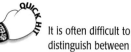

It is often difficult to distinguish between a viral and a bacterial infection.

Common Features of Viral Versus Bacterial URIs

Feature	Viral	Bacterial
Rhinorrhea	X	–
Myalgias	X	–
Headache	X	–
Fever	X	X
Cough	X	X
Yellow sputum	–	X

Handwritten note: what color is the sputum?

   c. Medications
   - Codeine
   - Dextromethorphan
   - Benzonatate (Tessalon Perles) capsules
   d. Agents used to improve the effectiveness of antitussive medications include expectorants such as guaifenesin and water.

Acute Bronchitis

A. General characteristics
1. Viruses account for the majority of cases.
2. Laboratory tests are not indicated. Only obtain a chest radiograph if you suspect pneumonia; there is no infiltrate or consolidation in acute bronchitis (presence of fever, tachypnea, crackles, egophony on auscultation, or dullness to percussion suggests pneumonia).

B. Clinical features
1. **Cough (with or without sputum) is the predominant symptom**—it lasts 1 to 2 weeks. In a significant number of patients, the cough may last for 1 month or longer.
2. Chest discomfort and shortness of breath may be present.
3. Fever may or may not be present.

[handwritten margin note: Cough suppressants – Codeine – Dextromethorphan – Benzonatate.]

C. Treatment
1. Antibiotics are usually **not** necessary—most cases are viral.
2. Cough suppressants (codeine-containing cough medications) are effective for symptomatic relief.
3. Bronchodilators (albuterol) may relieve symptoms.

The Common Cold

A. General characteristics
1. The "common cold" is the most common upper respiratory tract infection. Children are more frequently affected than adults. Susceptibility depends on pre-existing antibody levels.
2. Caused by viruses (identification of virus is not important)
   a. Rhinoviruses are the most common (at least 50% of cases)—there are more than 100 antigenic serotypes, so reinfection with another serotype can lead to symptoms (no cross-immunity among the serotypes).
   b. Other viruses include coronavirus, parainfluenza viruses (types A, B, and C), adenovirus, coxsackievirus, and RSV.
3. **Hand-to-hand transmission** is the most common route.
4. Complications include secondary bacterial infection (bacterial sinusitis or pneumonia). These secondary infections (especially pneumonia) are very rare.
5. Most resolve within 1 week, but symptoms may last up to 10 to 14 days.

[handwritten note: 1–2 wks]

B. Clinical features
1. Rhinorrhea, sore throat, malaise, nonproductive cough, nasal congestion
2. Fever is uncommon in adults (suggests a bacterial complication or influenza), but is not unusual in children.

C. Treatment (symptomatic)
1. Adequate hydration
   a. Loosens secretions and prevents airway obstruction
   b. Can be achieved by increasing fluid intake and inhaling steam

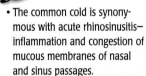

- The common cold is synonymous with acute rhinosinusitis—inflammation and congestion of mucous membranes of nasal and sinus passages.
- In most cases, it is very difficult to distinguish between the common cold (viral rhinosinusitis) and acute bacterial sinusitis on the basis of clinical features.
- Sneezing/rhinorrhea, nasal discharge (whether clear, purulent, or colored), nasal obstruction, and facial pain/headaches occur in both.

[handwritten note: Common Cold.]

Many of the symptoms seen with the common cold are also seen in influenza, but are more severe in the latter. Fever, headache, myalgias, and malaise are much more pronounced with influenza.

2. Rest and analgesics (aspirin, acetaminophen, ibuprofen)—for relief of malaise, headache, fever, aches
3. Cough suppressant (dextromethorphan, codeine)
4. Nasal decongestant spray (Neo-Synephrine) for less than 3 days
5. Oral first-generation antihistamines for rhinorrhea/sneezing

Sinusitis

A. General characteristics

1. There is inflammation of the lining of the paranasal sinuses, often due to infection. Mucosal edema obstructs the sinus openings (ostia), trapping sinus secretions.
2. Most cases of acute sinusitis occur as a complication of the common cold or other URIs. (However, fewer than 1% of URIs lead to acute sinusitis.) May also be caused by nasal obstruction due to polyps, deviated septum, or foreign body.
3. Classification
   a. Acute bacterial sinusitis—usually due to *Streptococcus pneumoniae*, *Haemophilus influenzae*, or anaerobes
   b. Other types: viral, fungal, or allergic
4. The most common sinuses involved are the <u>maxillary sinuses</u>.

B. Clinical features

1. Acute sinusitis
   a. Nasal stuffiness, purulent nasal discharge, cough
   b. Sinus pain or pressure (location depends on which sinus is involved)—pain worsens with percussion or bending head down
      • Maxillary sinusitis (most common)—pain over the cheeks that **may mimic pain of dental caries**
      • Frontal sinusitis—pain in the lower forehead
      • Ethmoid sinusitis—retro-orbital pain, or pain in the upper lateral aspect of the nose
   c. Fever in 50% of cases
2. <u>Chronic sinusitis</u>
   a. Nasal congestion, postnasal discharge
   b. Pain and headache are usually mild or absent; fever is uncommon
   c. By definition, symptoms should be present <u>for at least 2 to 3 months.</u>
   d. In addition to the organisms listed for acute sinusitis, patients with a history of multiple sinus infections (and courses of antibiotics) are at risk for infection with *Staphylococcus aureus* and gram-negative rods. because of resistance.

C. Diagnosis

1. Diagnosis is based on clinical findings. Consider acute bacterial sinusitis if a patient has a cold for more than 8 to 10 days or has prolonged nasal congestion.
2. Physical examination
   a. Look for purulent discharge draining from one of the turbinates.
   b. Perform transillumination of maxillary sinuses (note impaired light transmission)—The room must be completely dark with a strong light source.
   c. Palpate over the sinuses for tenderness (not a reliable finding).
3. Imaging studies—usually not indicated in routine community-acquired infections
   a. Conventional sinus radiographs—Look for air-fluid levels in acute disease.
   b. <u>A CT scan (coronal view) is superior to a plain radiograph.</u> It should be performed in complicated disease or if surgery is being planned.

D. Complications

1. Mucocele, polyps
2. Orbital cellulitis—usually originating from ethmoid sinusitis

QUICK HIT Sinusitis is usually self-limited, but **can be associated with high morbidity.** It can be life-threatening if the infection spreads to bone or to the CNS.

QUICK HIT If a patient has a cold beyond 8 to 10 days, or if the cold symptoms improve and then worsen after a few days ("double-sickening"), consider acute bacterial sinusitis (may be a secondary bacterial infection after a primary viral illness).

QUICK HIT Treat with antibiotics and decongestants for 1 to 2 weeks, depending on severity. If there is no improvement after 2 weeks of therapy, then sinus films and a penicillinase-resistant antibiotic are appropriate. Consider ENT consultation. Because of the anatomic difficulties in drainage, the course of acute sinusitis takes longer to resolve than other URIs.

3. Osteomyelitis of the frontal bones or maxilla
4. Cavernous sinus thrombosis (rare)
5. Very rare: epidural abscess, subdural empyema, meningitis, and brain abscess—due to contiguous spread through bone or via venous channels

E. Treatment
1. Acute purulent sinusitis
   a. General measures/advice for the patient
      - Saline nasal spray aids drainage.
      - Avoid smoke and other environmental pollutants.
   b. Decongestants (pseudoephedrine or oxymetazoline)
      - **Facilitate sinus drainage** and relieve congestion
      - Available in both topical and systemic preparations
      - Give for no more than 3 to 5 days
   c. Antibiotics
      - Amoxicillin, amoxicillin-clavulanate, TMP/SMX, levofloxacin, moxifloxacin, and cefuroxime are good choices.
   d. Antihistamines
      - Reserve for patients with allergies; use discriminately because of the "drying effect"
      - Loratadine (Claritin), fexofenadine (Allegra), chlorpheniramine (Chlor-Trimeton)
   e. Nasal steroids (fluticasone, beclomethasone)—may be worth a trial if sinusitis is secondary to allergic rhinitis or if there is concurrent allergic rhinitis
2. Chronic sinusitis
   a. Treat with a broad-spectrum penicillinase-resistant antibiotic.
   b. Refer to an otolaryngologist—endoscopic drainage may be necessary.

 Antihistamines have a drying effect (making secretions thicker) and can sometimes worsen congestion. If this occurs, avoid decongestants with antihistamines.

Laryngitis

- Usually viral in origin; may also be caused by *Moraxella catarrhalis* and *H. influenzae*
- Common cause of hoarseness; cough may be present along with other URI symptoms
- Typically self-limiting
- Patient should rest voice until laryngitis resolves to avoid formation of vocal nodules

Sore Throat

A. General characteristics
1. Causes of sore throat
   a. Viruses are by far the most common cause (adenovirus, parainfluenza and rhinovirus, Epstein-Barr virus, herpes simplex)
   b. **The main concern is infection with group A β-hemolytic streptococcus due to the possibility of rheumatic fever.**
   c. Other organisms
      - Chlamydia, mycoplasma
      - Gonococci (oral sex)
      - *Corynebacterium diphtheriae*—pseudomembrane covering pharynx
      - *Candida albicans* (if immunosuppressed, on antibiotics, or severely ill)
2. Viral versus bacterial infection—often difficult to distinguish, but if patient has a cough and runny nose, virus is more likely

Think of the following if a patient has a sore throat:
- Viral infection
- Tonsillitis (usually bacterial)
- **Strep throat**
- Mononucleosis

B. Diagnosis
1. Throat culture—takes 24 hours, but is more accurate than rapid strep test
2. Rapid strep test—results within 1 hour, but will not indicate whether sore throat is caused by a bacterium other than *Streptococcus* or a virus
3. If mononucleosis is suspected, obtain the appropriate blood tests (Monospot).

Only 50% of patients with pharyngeal exudates have strep throat, and only 50% of patients with strep throat have exudates.

C. Treatment
1. If strep throat—penicillin for 10 days (erythromycin if patient has penicillin allergy)
2. If viral—symptomatic treatment (see below)
3. If mononucleosis—advise rest and acetaminophen/ibuprofen for symptoms
4. Symptomatic treatment of sore throat
   a. Acetaminophen or ibuprofen
   b. Gargling with warm salt water
   c. Use of a humidifier
   d. Sucking on throat lozenges, hard candy, flavored frozen desserts (such as Popsicles)

GASTROINTESTINAL DISEASES

Dyspepsia

A. General characteristics
1. "Dyspepsia" refers to a spectrum of epigastric symptoms, including heartburn, "indigestion," bloating, and epigastric pain/discomfort.
2. Dyspepsia is extremely common, and sometimes is confused with angina.
3. Etiology
   a. GI causes—**peptic ulcer disease (PUD)**, **GERD**, **nonulcer dyspepsia (functional dyspepsia)**, **gastritis**, hepatobiliary disease (cholecystitis, biliary colic), malignancy (gastric, esophageal), pancreatic disease (pancreatitis, pseudocyst, cancer), esophageal spasm, hiatal hernia
   b. Other causes include lactose intolerance, malabsorption, DM (gastroparesis), and irritable bowel syndrome (IBS).

B. Diagnosis
1. Base the decision to perform tests on clinical presentation and response to empiric therapy.
2. **Endoscopy** is the test of choice for evaluation of dyspepsia.
   a. It can identify an esophageal stricture or ulcer, cancer, and reflux esophagitis.
   b. It should **not** be routinely performed in all patients with dyspepsia. Some general indications include:
      • Patients with alarming symptoms—weight loss, anemia, dysphagia, or obstructive symptoms
      • Patients >45 to 50 years of age with new-onset dyspepsia
      • Patients with recurrent vomiting or any evidence of upper GI bleeding
      • Patients who do not respond to empiric therapy (see below)
      • Patients with signs of complications of PUD
      • Patients with recurrent symptoms
      • Patients with evidence of systemic illness
3. Noninvasive testing for *Helicobacter pylori*
   a. If positive, treat empirically for *H. pylori*.
   b. If negative, PUD is unlikely and the patient likely has either GERD or nonulcer dyspepsia (treat empirically—see below).

C. Treatment
1. Treat the cause if known.
2. Advise the patient to:
   a. Avoid alcohol, caffeine, and other foods that irritate the stomach
   b. Stop smoking
   c. Raise the head of the bed when sleeping
   d. Avoid eating before sleeping

Most cases (up to 90%) of dyspepsia/heartburn are due to PUD, GERD, gastritis, or nonulcer dyspepsia.

Nonulcer dyspepsia
• A diagnosis of exclusion after appropriate tests (including endoscopy) do not reveal a specific cause.
• Dyspepsia symptoms must be present for at least 4 weeks to make the diagnosis of nonulcer dyspepsia.

3. Use antacids; use an H_2 blocker, sucralfate, or a proton pump inhibitor (PPI) if antacids fail. Endoscopy is indicated if all of these fail to relieve symptoms.
4. Eradication of *H. pylori* infection—See Chapter 3.

Gastroesophageal Reflux Disease (GERD)

A. General characteristics

1. GERD is a multifactorial problem. Inappropriate relaxation of the lower esophageal sphincter (LES) (**decreased LES tone**) is the primary mechanism, leading to retrograde flow of stomach contents into the esophagus. Other factors that may contribute include:
   a. Decreased esophageal motility to clear refluxed fluid
   b. A gastric outlet obstruction
   c. **A hiatal hernia (common finding in patients with GERD)**
   d. Dietary factors (e.g., alcohol, tobacco, chocolate, high-fat foods, coffee)—may decrease LES pressure and exacerbate the condition
2. GERD is a very common condition. Its prevalence increases with age.

B. Clinical features

1. **Heartburn, dyspepsia**
   a. Retrosternal pain/burning shortly after eating (especially after large meals)
   b. Exacerbated by lying down after meals
   c. **May mimic cardiac chest pain** (which may lead to unnecessary workup for ischemic heart disease)
2. Regurgitation
3. Waterbrash—reflex salivary hypersecretion
4. Cough—due to either aspiration of refluxed material or a reflex triggered by acid reflux into the lower esophagus
5. Hoarseness, sore throat, feeling a lump in the throat
6. Early satiety, postprandial nausea/vomiting

 If GERD is associated with dysphagia, this suggests the development of **peptic stricture.** Alternatively, a motility disorder or cancer may be present.

C. Diagnosis

1. **Endoscopy with biopsy**—the test of choice
   a. This is indicated if cancer or a complication of GERD is suspected.
   b. A biopsy should also be performed to assess changes in esophageal mucosa.
2. Upper GI series (barium contrast study)—This is only helpful in identifying complications of GERD (strictures/ulcerations), but cannot diagnose GERD itself.
3. 24-hour pH monitoring in the lower esophagus—This is the most sensitive and specific test for GERD. It is the gold standard, but is usually unnecessary.
4. Esophageal manometry—Use if a motility disorder is suspected.

Diagnostic tests are usually not necessary for typical, uncomplicated cases of GERD, and therapy can be initiated. Tests are indicated in atypical, complicated, or persistent cases (despite treatment). Endoscopy should be performed if worrisome symptoms (anemia, weight loss, or dysphagia) are present.

D. Complications

1. Erosive esophagitis—These patients are at high risk of developing complications such as stricture, ulcer, or Barrett's esophagus. These patients are candidates for long-term PPI therapy (see below).
2. Peptic stricture
   a. Consists of fibrotic rings that narrow the lumen and obstruct the passage of food
   b. Presents with dysphagia; may mimic esophageal cancer
   c. EGD can confirm the diagnosis. Dilation should be performed.
3. Esophageal ulcer—possible cause of upper GI bleeding
4. Barrett's esophagus—occurs in 10% of patients with chronic reflux
   a. The normal, stratified, squamous epithelium of the distal esophagus is replaced by columnar epithelium. Dysplastic changes may occur, with risk of adenocarcinoma.

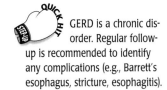 GERD is a chronic disorder. Regular follow-up is recommended to identify any complications (e.g., Barrett's esophagus, stricture, esophagitis).

    b. Patients who have had symptomatic GERD for at least 5 years (and can undergo surgery if cancer is found) should be screened for the possibility of Barrett's esophagus.

    c. Endoscopy with biopsy is required. If the patient has documented Barrett's esophagus without any dysplastic changes, periodic surveillance is appropriate (every 3 years or so).

    d. Medical treatment: long-term PPIs

  5. Recurrent pneumonia (due to recurrent pulmonary aspiration)—The cytologic aspirate finding on bronchoscopy that can diagnose aspiration of gastric contents is **lipid-laden macrophages** (from phagocytosis of fat).

  6. Pitting of dental enamel (dental erosion); gingivitis

  7. Laryngitis, pharyngitis

E. Treatment

  1. Initial treatment (phase I):

    a. Behavior modification—diet (avoid fatty foods, coffee, alcohol, orange juice, chocolate; avoid large meals before bedtime); sleep with trunk of body elevated; stop smoking

    b. Antacids—after meals and at bedtime

  2. Phase II—add an H_2 blocker—can be used instead of or in addition to antacids

  3. Phase III—switch to a PPI—use if above treatments fail to resolve symptoms or in patients with erosive esophagitis

  4. Phase IV—Add a promotility agent, such as metoclopramide (a dopamine blocker), which is most commonly used, or bethanechol (a cholinergic agonist).

  5. Phase V

    a. Combination therapy

      • H_2 blocker plus promotility agent

      • PPI plus promotility agent

    b. Increased dose of H_2 blocker or PPI

  6. Phase VI—antireflux surgery for severe or resistant cases

    a. Indications for surgery

      • Intractability (failure of medical treatment)

      • Respiratory problems due to reflux and aspiration of gastric contents

      • Severe esophageal injury (ulcer, hemorrhage, stricture, Barrett's esophagus)

    b. Types of surgery

      • Nissen fundoplication (may be done open or laparoscopically)—procedure of choice for a patient with normal esophageal motility

      • Partial fundoplication—when esophageal motility is poor

    c. Outcome of surgery—Excellent results have been reported.

Diarrhea

A. General characteristics

  1. Most cases of diarrhea are acute, benign, and self-limited. Some cases are chronic and may be associated with underlying disease.

Box 12-3 **Diarrhea Pearls**

• Acute diarrhea is usually due to infection (virus, bacteria, and parasite) or medications.

• If nausea and vomiting are present, suspect viral gastroenteritis or food poisoning.

• If food poisoning is the cause, diarrhea appears within hours of the meal.

• Remember that occult blood in the stool **may** be present in all types of acute infectious diarrhea, but it is much less common to have gross blood.

• A finding of fever and blood together is typical of infection with *Shigella, Campylobacter, Salmonella* (may also be without blood), enterohemorrhagic *Escherichia coli.*

• No fever and no blood is typical of infection with viruses (rotavirus, Norwalk virus), enterotoxic *E. coli,* and food poisoning (*Staphylococcus aureus, Clostridium perfringens*).

2. Acute diarrhea is diarrhea that lasts less than 2 to 3 weeks; chronic diarrhea lasts more than 4 weeks.

3. Most common cause of acute diarrhea is viral infection (rotavirus and the Norwalk virus are the most common). Most severe forms of acute diarrhea are due to bacterial infections (*Shigella*, *Escherichia coli*, *Salmonella*, *Campylobacter*, *Clostridium perfringens*, *Clostridium difficile*). Protozoa that may cause diarrhea include *Giardia lamblia*, *Entamoeba histolytica*, and *Cryptosporidium*.

4. Elderly and immunocompromised patients (e.g., with HIV, transplantation patients) are vulnerable to diarrheal illnesses due to impaired immunity. In patients with HIV, diarrhea can be caused by *Mycobacterium avium-intracellulare*, *Cryptosporidium*, *Cyclospora*, or CMV.

B. Causes

1. Acute diarrhea
   a. **Infection**—viruses most common (viral gastroenteritis), followed by bacteria, then parasites
   b. **Medications**
      - Antibiotics (most common cause)—Antibiotic-associated diarrhea is caused by *C. difficile* toxin in 25% of cases (see Chapter 3).
      - Others include laxatives, prokinetic agents (cisapride), antacids, digitalis, colchicine, antibiotics, alcohol, magnesium-containing antacids, and chemotherapeutic agents.
   c. Malabsorption—e.g., lactose intolerance
   d. Ischemic bowel in elderly patients with history of PVD and bloody diarrhea, along with abdominal pain
   e. Intestinal tumors (very rare)

2. Chronic diarrhea
   a. IBS (most common cause, but is a diagnosis of exclusion)
   b. Inflammatory bowel disease (IBD)
   c. Medications—see above
   d. Infection—see above, bacterial enterocolitis (*Shigella*, *Salmonella*, *Campylobacter*, enteroinvasive *E. coli*)
   e. Colon cancer
   f. Diverticulitis
   g. Malabsorption syndromes—pancreatic insufficiency, celiac disease, short bowel syndrome, ischemic bowel, bacterial overgrowth
   h. Postsurgical (e.g., gastrectomy, vagotomy)
   i. Endocrine causes (hyperthyroidism, Addison's disease, diabetes, gastrinoma, VIPoma)
   j. Fecal impaction—because only liquid stool can pass around the impaction
   k. Laxative abuse (factitious diarrhea)
   l. Immunocompromised patients with acute infectious diarrhea

C. Diagnosis

1. Laboratory tests are usually unnecessary in acute diarrhea.
2. Some indications for diagnostic studies

Box 12-4 Important Parts of the History in a Patient With Diarrhea

- Is the stool bloody or melanotic?
- Are there any other symptoms (e.g., fever, abdominal pain, vomiting)?
- Is there anyone in the family or group with a similar illness?
- Has there been any recent travel outside the United States, or any hiking trips? (parasitic infections)
- Are symptoms linked to ingestion of certain foods (e.g., milk)?
- Are there any medical problems (e.g., AIDS, hyperthyroidism)?
- Have there been recent changes in medications (e.g., antibiotics within the past few weeks)?

FIGURE
(12-2) **Approach to the patient with acute diarrhea.**

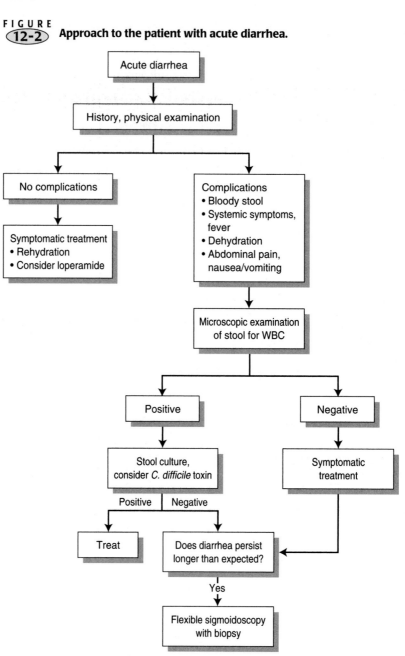

(Adapted from Humes DH, Dont HL, Gardner LB, et al. Kelley's Textbook of Internal Medicine. 4th Ed. Philadelphia: Lippincott Williams & Wilkins, 2000:748, Figure 99.1.)

QUICK HIT
Assess volume status (dehydration is a concern), perform an abdominal examination, and check stool for occult blood in patients with diarrhea. In mild to moderate cases of acute diarrhea, further workup is unnecessary.

   a. Chronic diarrhea or diarrhea that is prolonged
   b. Severe illness or high fever
   c. Presence of blood in the stool/high suspicion for IBD
   d. Severe abdominal pain
   e. Immunodeficiency
   f. Signs of volume depletion
3. Laboratory tests to order
   a. CBC—look for anemia, WBC elevation
   b. Stool sample—for presence of fecal leukocytes
     • If fecal leukocytes are absent, there is no need to order stool cultures because they are unlikely to grow pathogenic organisms (unless invasive bacterial enteritis is suspected or the patient has bloody diarrhea).
     • If fecal leukocytes are present and the patient has moderate to severe diarrhea, send stool for culture or *C. difficile* toxin assay or treat empirically with an antibiotic.

- Fecal leukocytes are present in *Campylobacter, Salmonella, Shigella,* enteroinvasive *E. coli* infection, and *C. difficile*; absent in staphylococcal or clostridial food poisoning; and absent in viral gastroenteritis.

c. Stool sample—Test three samples for presence of ova and parasites. Order this if a parasite is suspected. For *Giardia*, order enzyme-linked immunosorbent assay test for antigen.

d. Bacterial stool culture
  - This has low sensitivity (and is an expensive test), and usually does not affect treatment or outcome.
  - It should not be ordered routinely. Some indications include: if invasive bacterial enteritis is suspected, if the patient has moderate to severe illness or fever, if the patient requires hospitalization, and if the stool sample is positive for fecal leukocytes.
  - Most laboratory tests examine stool culture for only three organisms: *Shigella, Salmonella,* and *Campylobacter.*

e. Stool sample—Measure for *C. difficile* toxin if the patient has been treated with antibiotics recently. Note that this test has a false-negative rate of 10%. Treat the patient empirically even before laboratory results are back if the suspicion is high.

f. Colonoscopy/flexible sigmoidoscopy—may be considered for patients with blood in the stool or for patients with chronic diarrhea for which a cause cannot be identified.

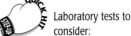

Laboratory tests to consider:
- Stool WBCs
- Stool for ova and parasites
- Stool culture
- Stool for *C. difficile* culture
- Stool for *C. difficile* toxin assay
- Stool for *Giardia* antigen

Salmonella, Campylobacter, Shigella, and enteroinvasive *E. coli* cause diarrhea with fecal leukocytes and often blood.

The most common electrolyte/acid-base abnormality seen with severe diarrhea is **metabolic acidosis** and **hypokalemia.**

D. Treatment

1. Acute diarrhea is typically self-limited and does not require hospitalization. However, consider hospitalization for any of the following reasons.
   a. Dehydration (especially in elderly patients)
   b. Patients initially unable to tolerate or hold down PO fluids
   c. Bloody diarrhea (with profuse or brisk bleeding)
   d. High fever, toxic appearance
2. The identification of the specific agent responsible for acute infectious diarrhea is not critical with regard to treatment. Treat the diarrhea according to the patient's medical history and clinical condition.
3. Specific therapy
   a. Rehydrate; monitor electrolytes and replace if necessary
   b. Treat the underlying cause (e.g., stop or change medication, advise a lactose-free diet). Consider a trial of NPO status to see if diarrhea stops.
   c. Consider antibiotics. Use of antibiotics in **infectious** diarrhea has been shown to decrease the duration of illness by 24 hours (regardless of the etiologic agent). Therefore, consider a 5-day course of ciprofloxacin in patients who have moderate to severe disease. Antibiotics are definitely recommended in the following situations:
      - Patient has high fever, bloody stools, or severe diarrhea—quinolones are appropriate
      - Stool culture grows one of the pathogenic organisms (see Table 12-7)
      - Patient has traveler's diarrhea
      - *C. difficile* infection—metronidazole
4. Loperamide (Imodium) is an antidiarrheal agent that should only be given if diarrhea is mild to moderate and is not recommended in patients with fever or with blood in their stool.

Constipation

A. Causes

1. Diet—lack of fiber
2. Medications—anticholinergic drugs (antipsychotics), antidepressants, **narcotic analgesics**, iron, calcium-channel blockers, aluminum- or calcium-containing antacids, laxative abuse and dependence

TABLE 12-7 Common Pathogens Responsible for Acute Infectious Diarrhea

Pathogen	Symptoms	Fever?	Fecal Leukocytes	Duration of Illness	Transmission	Comments
Acute viral gastroenteritis (rotavirus, Norwalk virus)	**Myalgias, malaise,** headache, watery diarrhea, abdominal pain, **nausea/ vomiting**	Possible, low-grade	No	48–72 hours, symptoms may linger for up to 1 week	Fecal-oral route	Most common cause of acute diarrhea in the United States Look for similar illness in family members.
Salmonella	Abdominal pain, diarrhea, nausea and vomiting	Possible	Yes	Resolves within 1 week (rarely longer)	Food (domestic fowl and their eggs—most common); fecal-oral route as well	Symptoms appear 24–48 hours after ingesting food. No treatment is required except in immuno-compromised patients or in cases of enteric fever (caused by *Salmonella typhi*)—rare in the United States. Ciprofloxacin (Cipro) is the preferred agent.
Shigella	Diarrhea, abdominal pain, **tenesmus;** nausea, vomiting less common	Possible	Yes	Resolves within 1 week (4–5 days)	Fecal-oral route more common than food	Treat with TMP/SMX (Bactrim).
Staphylococcus food poisoning	Abdominal pain, nausea and vomiting, diarrhea	No	No	**Within 24 hours**	Food (e.g., ham, poultry, potato salad, any food containing mayonnaise)	Exposed people become ill **within 1–6 hours** (e.g., after a picnic). Can be quite severe and may require hospitalization
Campylobacter jejuni	Headache, fatigue followed by diarrhea and abdominal pain	Yes	Yes	Less than 1 week	Fecal-oral route more common than food	Most common cause of acute bacterial diarrhea. Can be severe: blood appears in stool in 50% of cases. Treat with erythromycin. Relapses may occur.
Clostridium perfringens	Diarrhea; **crampy abdominal pain is prominent;** vomiting and fever are rare	No	No	Within 24 hours	Food	Illness begins soon after ingesting food (within 12–24 hours).
Enterotoxic *E. coli*	Watery diarrhea, nausea, abdominal pain	No	No	Few days	Food	Self-limiting disease is common in developing countries. (Travelers are often susceptible.)
E. coli 0157:H7	Bloody diarrhea; patient can appear very sick	Yes	Yes		Food (undercooked meat, raw milk)	Hemorrhagic colitis that is usually self-limited, but has been associated with hemolytic-uremic syndrome and thrombotic thrombocytopenic purpura

(continued)

TABLE 12-7		Common Pathogens Responsible for Acute Infectious Diarrhea *(Continued)*				
Pathogen	**Symptoms**	**Fever?**	**Fecal Leukocytes**	**Duration of Illness**	**Transmission**	**Comments**
Giardiasis	Watery, foul-smelling diarrhea; abdominal bloating	No	No	5–7 days, sometimes longer	Fecal-oral route, food, or contaminated water	Treat with metronidazole; can become chronic
Vibrio cholera	Voluminous diarrhea ("rice water" stools), abdominal pain, vomiting	Low-grade	No			Rare in the United States, but common in developing countries

3. IBS
4. Obstruction—colorectal cancer (Always keep this in mind!), anal stricture, hemorrhoids, anal fissure
5. Ileus, pseudo-obstruction
6. Anorectal problems—hemorrhoids, fissures
7. Endocrine/metabolic causes—hypothyroidism, hypercalcemia, hypokalemia, uremia, dehydration
8. Neuromuscular disorders—Parkinson's disease, multiple sclerosis, CNS lesions, scleroderma, DM (autonomic neuropathy)
9. Congenital disorders—Hirschsprung's disease

B. Diagnosis
1. Laboratory tests that **may** be necessary include TSH, serum calcium levels, CBC (if colon cancer is suspected), and electrolytes (if obstruction is suspected).
2. Always attempt to rule out obstruction.
   a. If H & P is suggestive of obstruction, order abdominal films.
   b. Consider flexible sigmoidoscopy in select cases (if an obstructing colorectal mass is suspected).
3. A rectal examination may help identify fissures, hemorrhoids, fecal impaction, or masses.
4. If no cause is found after the above measures, and conservative treatment does not help, more specialized tests are available—e.g., radiopaque marker transit study, anorectal motility study.

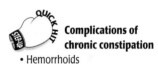

Complications of chronic constipation
• Hemorrhoids
• Rectal prolapse
• Anal fissures
• Fecal impaction

C. Treatment
1. Diet and behavioral modification are the most important aspects of treatment. Advise the patient to:
   a. Increase physical activity
   b. Eat high-fiber foods
   c. Increase fluid intake
2. Use an enema, such as a disposable Fleet enema, for temporary relief if no bowel movement occurs despite the above measures or if the patient is bedridden.
3. If obstruction is present, urgent surgery consultation is indicated.

Irritable Bowel Syndrome (IBS)

A. General characteristics
1. IBS refers to an idiopathic disorder associated with an intrinsic bowel motility dysfunction (abnormal resting activity of GI tract) that affects 10% to 15% of all adults.
2. Common associated findings include depression, anxiety, and somatization. Psychiatric symptoms often precede bowel symptoms. **Symptoms are exacerbated by stress and irritants in the intestinal lumen.**

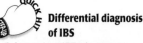

Differential diagnosis of IBS

Colon cancer, IBD, drugs, mesenteric ischemia, celiac disease, ischemic colitis, giardiasis, pseudo-obstruction, depression, somatization, intermittent sigmoid volvulus, megacolon, bacterial overgrowth syndrome, endometriosis

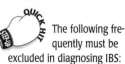

The following frequently must be excluded in diagnosing IBS:
- Obstruction (plain abdominal film)
- Inflammatory bowel disease
- Lactose or sorbitol intolerance
- Malignancy (in older patients or those with family history)—colonoscopy, occult blood in stool

3. All laboratory test results are normal, and no mucosal lesions are found on sigmoidoscopy. IBS is a benign condition and has a favorable long-term prognosis.
4. Symptoms should be present for **at least 3 months** to diagnose IBS.

B. Clinical features
1. Change in frequency/consistency of stool—diarrhea, constipation (or alternating diarrhea and constipation)
2. Cramping abdominal pain (relieved by defecation)—location varies widely, but sigmoid colon is the common location of pain
3. Bloating or feeling of abdominal distention

C. Diagnosis
1. This is a clinical diagnosis, and a diagnosis of exclusion.
2. Initial tests that may help exclude other causes include CBC, renal panel, fecal occult blood test, stool examination for ova and parasites, erythrocyte sedimentation rate, and possibly a flexible sigmoidoscopy. Order these tests only if there is suspicion of other causes for the symptoms.

D. Treatment
1. Usually, no specific treatment is necessary. Manage the symptoms below as indicated.
   a. Diarrhea—diphenoxylate, loperamide
   b. Constipation—Colace, psyllium, cisapride
2. The following may help: avoid dairy products, avoid excessive caffeine.
3. Tegaserod maleate (Zelnorm) is a serotonin agonist recently introduced for the treatment of IBS. In a short-term study, it improved abdominal pain, bloating, and constipation in women.

Nausea and Vomiting

A. General characteristics
1. The most common causes are viral gastroenteritis and food poisoning. However, other more emergent diseases must be kept in mind.
2. Many of the conditions listed below present with other prominent symptoms (e.g., abdominal pain, diarrhea, fever) in addition to nausea/vomiting.

B. Causes
1. Pregnancy
2. Metabolic
   a. Diabetic ketoacidosis
   b. Addisonian crisis
   c. Uremia
   d. Electrolyte disturbance—hypercalcemia, hypokalemia
   e. Hyperthyroidism
3. GI
   a. Gastroenteritis
      • Viral (most common)
      • Food poisoning (e.g., *Salmonella*, *Shigella*)
      • Cholera
   b. PUD
   c. GERD
   d. Gastric retention—gastroparesis (diabetic patients), gastric outlet obstruction
   e. Intestinal obstruction (small bowel obstruction or pseudo-obstruction), ileus
   f. Peritonitis
4. Acute visceral conditions—pancreatitis, appendicitis, pyelonephritis, cholecystitis, cholangitis
5. Neurologic—increased intracranial pressure, vestibular disturbance (vertigo), migraine headache

6. Acute MI
7. Drugs (medications, toxins)
   a. Chemotherapy medications (cisplatin especially)
   b. Digitalis toxicity
   c. NSAIDs, aspirin
   d. Narcotics
   e. Antibiotics (erythromycin)
   f. Excessive alcohol intake (after binge drinking and morning-after hangover)
8. Miscellaneous—motion sickness, systemic illness, radiation therapy, postoperatively
9. Psychiatric—eating disorder (bulimia, anorexia nervosa), anxiety

C. Approach

1. Questions to ask when taking the history: Ask about recent food intake (Unusual foods? Time of onset of vomiting in relation to food intake? Did anyone else eat that food?). Are symptoms related to meals? Ask about medications and recent changes/additions. Is there a history of abdominal surgery (obstruction) or recent surgery? Are there family members with similar illness?
2. Define the vomitus
   a. Bilious—obstruction is distal to ampulla of Vater
   b. Feculent—distal intestinal obstruction, bacterial overgrowth, gastrocolic fistula
   c. Vomiting of undigested food—esophageal problem more likely (achalasia, stricture, diverticulum)
   d. Projectile vomiting—increased intracranial pressure or pyloric stenosis
   e. Coffee-ground material or blood—GI bleeding
3. Accompanying symptoms
   a. Diarrhea and fever point to an infectious process (gastroenteritis).
   b. Abdominal pain points to obstruction, acute inflammatory conditions (e.g., peritonitis, cholecystitis)
   c. Headache, visual disturbances, and other neurologic findings point to increased intracranial or intraocular pressure (IOP).

D. Diagnosis

1. Order routine laboratory tests such as CBC, electrolytes, glucose levels, LFTs, if appropriate, based on history and examination findings.
2. Order a pregnancy test in women of child-bearing age.
3. Abdominal films—Order upright and supine films in patients with acute vomiting if obstruction or perforation is suspected.
4. Order other diagnostic tests depending on clinical findings (e.g., upper GI endoscopy for ulcer disease or outlet obstruction, ultrasound for biliary disease, CT scan of head for neurologic findings).
5. In at least 50% of patients, the above tests do not reveal a cause. Special tests for GI motility may be indicated if there is suspicion of a motility disorder.

E. Treatment

1. Most causes are self-limiting. If vomiting is severe it may cause dehydration, requiring hospitalization.
2. Assess hydration status—Fluid replacement is the first step in management; use 1/2 NS with potassium replacement.

F. Identify the underlying cause (e.g., diabetic ketoacidosis, obstruction) if possible and treat accordingly.

G. For symptomatic relief of nausea/vomiting

1. Prochlorperazine (Compazine) and promethazine (Phenergan) are commonly used.
2. Follow a liquid diet (liquid is cleared from the stomach more quickly than solids).
3. Avoid large meals and fatty meals.
4. Nasogastric suction may improve symptoms.

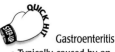

Gastroenteritis
- Typically caused by an enterovirus, and is seen in groups among family members, colleagues, and so on.
- Diarrhea is often present as well, but may appear later.

Possible complications of severe or prolonged vomiting
- Fluid/electrolytes: dehydration, metabolic alkalosis, hypokalemia
- Dental caries
- Aspiration pneumonitis
- GI: Mallory-Weiss tears, Boerhaave's syndrome, Mallory-Weiss syndrome

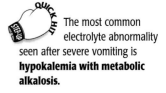

The most common electrolyte abnormality seen after severe vomiting is **hypokalemia with metabolic alkalosis.**

Hemorrhoids

A. General characteristics

1. Varicose veins of anus and rectum
2. Two types
   a. External hemorrhoids—dilated veins arising from inferior hemorrhoidal plexus; distal to dentate line (sensate area)
   b. Internal hemorrhoids—dilated submucosal veins of superior rectal plexus; above dentate line (insensate area)

B. Risk factors

1. Constipation/straining
2. Pregnancy
3. Portal HTN
4. Obesity
5. Prolonged sitting (especially truck drivers and pilots) or prolonged standing
6. Anal intercourse

C. Clinical features

1. Bleeding and rectal prolapse (main symptoms)
   a. Bright red blood per rectum
   b. This is usually harmless, but look for iron deficiency anemia (rare). Occult rectal bleeding should prompt an investigation into more serious causes and should never be attributed to hemorrhoids until other conditions are ruled out.
   c. Bleeding is usually painless.
2. External hemorrhoids are usually asymptomatic unless thrombosed, in which case they present as sudden painful swelling (may ulcerate, bleed). Pain lasts for several days, and then gradually subsides. The response to surgery is rapid.
3. Internal hemorrhoids usually do not cause pain. A mass is present when they prolapse.

D. Treatment

1. General measures to ease symptoms
   a. Sitz bath
   b. Application of ice packs to anal area and bed rest
   c. Stool softeners to reduce strain
   d. High-fiber, high-fluid diet
   e. Topical steroids
2. Rubber band ligation for internal hemorrhoids—rubber bands applied to hemorrhoidal bundle(s) leads to necrosis and sloughing of lesion
3. Surgical (hemorrhoidectomy)—Perform surgery if the condition does not respond to conservative methods, or if severe prolapse, strangulation, very large anal tags, or fissure is present. Surgery can be performed in an ambulatory setting.

MUSCULOSKELETAL PROBLEMS

Low Back Pain

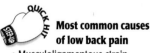

Most common causes of low back pain
- Musculoligamentous strain
- Degenerative disc disease
- Facet arthritis

A. Causes

1. Musculoligamentous strain
   a. This is a tear/strain of muscle fibers/ligaments in the paraspinal muscles around the iliac crest/lower lumbar regions. The resultant bleeding and spasm can cause tenderness in the region.
   b. The patient usually recalls an episode of bending/twisting or of the back "giving way" when lifting a heavy object, with immediate onset of pain.
   c. Radiation of pain occurs across the low back (often to buttock/upper thigh to knee level posteriorly). Pain typically does not radiate distal to the knee because no nerve root injury has occurred.

2. Lumbar disc herniation
   a. Nucleus pulposus (inner portion of intervertebral disc) extrudes through the annulus fibrosis (outer portion) and impinges on nerve roots, causing lower extremity radiculopathy.
   b. Ninety-five percent occur at L5-S1 or L4-L5 levels.
   c. Low back pain/stiffness and radiculopathy are main clinical findings.
   d. Radiculopathy is due to compression of nerve root by extruded disc.
      - **Sciatica is a term used to refer to pain along course of the sciatic nerve.**
      - Neurologic deficits may be present, depending on the extent/duration of nerve root compression.
3. Degenerative disc disease (osteoarthritis)
   a. Common cause of chronic low back pain
   b. In addition to low back pain, disc space narrowing and osteophytes can cause compression of nerve roots, causing lower extremity radiculopathy as well.
4. Lumbar spinal stenosis (narrowing of spinal canal)
   a. May be acquired (due to **degenerative changes**, iatrogenic causes, posttraumatic) or congenital (achondroplasia or idiopathic); most cases are acquired and due to advanced degenerative changes that narrow the canal.
   b. Pain is caused by activity and relieved by rest or spinal flexion (**neurogenic claudication**). Spine flexion increases size of spinal canal.
   c. Symptoms: low back pain, sciatica (involving one or both legs), **decreased ambulatory capacity**
5. Vertebral compression fracture
   a. Acute back pain caused by a minor stress in elderly patients; pain is at the level of fracture with local radiation across the back and around the trunk (rarely into legs)
   b. In normal bone, this fracture requires severe flexion-compression trauma. In elderly patients with osteoporosis, compression fractures can occur with minimal or no trauma.
   c. Multiple compression fractures can lead to severe kyphosis.
   d. Kyphoplasty (injection of cement into vertebral body) is effective for pain relief and prevention of deformity (kyphosis).
   e. Spontaneous vertebral body collapse, or pathologic fracture, is most commonly seen in the following patients:
      - Elderly patients with severe osteoporosis
      - Patients on long-term steroid therapy
      - Cancer patients with lytic bony metastases, or multiple myeloma.
6. Neoplasms
   a. The most common spinal tumor is metastatic carcinoma—common primary neoplasms that metastasize to spine include breast, lung, prostate, kidney, and thyroid
   b. Night pain is characteristic and is a worrisome complaint.
   c. On MRI, neoplasms classically do not involve the disc space (as opposed to infection).
7. Infection (vertebral osteomyelitis)
   a. Possible sources include UTI, skin abscess, indwelling catheter, and IV drug abuse.
   b. On MRI, infection involves the disc space.
   c. Complications
      - Epidural abscess develops in the context of bacteremia or osteomyelitis. If not promptly treated, it can compromise the blood supply to the spinal cord, with rapid progression to motor and sensory deficits. In presence of neurologic symptoms, this is a surgical emergency.
      - Compression fracture with collapse of vertebral body.
8. Ankylosing spondylitis and other spondyloarthropathies (see Chapter 6)
9. Cauda equina syndrome
   a. Occurs after spinal trauma or central lumbosacral disc herniations, which compresses multiple S1, S2, S3, S4 nerve roots

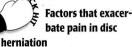

Factors that exacerbate pain in disc herniation
- Maneuvers that increase intraspinal pressure, such as coughing or sneezing
- Forward flexion–sitting, driving, or lifting: worsens leg pain

Patients with spinal stenosis have leg pain on back extension–pain worsens with standing or walking (relief with bending or sitting).

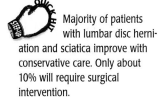

Majority of patients with lumbar disc herniation and sciatica improve with conservative care. Only about 10% will require surgical intervention.

[handwritten margin note] Epidural abscess + neurologic symptoms = surgical emergency.

Pathology in other organ systems cause back pain and should be ruled out:
- Vascular disease (aortic aneurysm, aortic dissection)
- Pancreatic disease
- Urologic disease (prostate infection, renal calculi)
- Gynecologic/obstetric disease (endometriosis, ectopic pregnancy, pelvic inflammatory disease)

Major segmental innervation of the lower limb
- Hip flexion–L2
- Knee extension–L3
- Ankle dorsiflexion–L4 and L5
- Great toe dorsiflexion–L5
- Ankle plantar flexion–S1

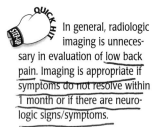

In general, radiologic imaging is unnecessary in evaluation of low back pain. Imaging is appropriate if symptoms do not resolve within 1 month or if there are neurologic signs/symptoms.

b. Clinical features
  - Bilateral sciatica, saddle anesthesia over buttocks/perineum
  - Low back pain, lower extremity weakness
  - Bowel or bladder dysfunction—frequency, retention, incontinence
  - Impotence, perianal anesthesia, lax anal sphincter

c. Immediate MRI is indicated to identify any lesions that can be treated surgically. Cauda equina syndrome is a surgical emergency.

10. Spinal deformity (kyphosis, scoliosis)

11. Spondylolisthesis—forward slipping of the cephalad vertebra on the caudad vertebra. In adults, this is usually due to advanced degenerative changes in disc and facet joints that have progressed to instability.

B. Back examination

1. Observe posture and gait, and check for asymmetry and spinal curvature.

2. Note the range of motion in the lumbosacral region (extension, flexion, rotation, side-bending).

3. Palpate for focal tenderness in the spine (tumor, fracture, infection, disk herniation) or sacroiliac joint tenderness.

4. Perform a complete neurologic examination motor examination (also grade muscle strength from 0 to 5).

5. Straight leg raising test
   a. Sensitive test for nerve root compression. If a compressed L5 or S1 nerve root is stretched, radicular pain is produced.
   b. The test result is positive if radiculopathy is reproduced when the leg is elevated 30° to 60° with the patient supine. The earlier the onset of pain (i.e., at a lower elevation), the more specific the result and the greater the severity of disk herniation.
   c. Contralateral leg pain produced by straight-leg raising is more specific for a herniated disc.

6. Neurologic examination
   a. Tests for L4 root function
      - Ankle dorsiflexion, sensation anteromedial leg
      - Patellar tendon reflex (knee jerk)
   b. Tests for L5 root function
      - **Dorsiflexion of the ankle and big toe against resistance**
      - Sensation along lateral shin and dorsum of foot
   c. Tests for S1 root function
      - Ankle plantar flexion (gastrocnemius muscle)
      - Ankle deep tendon reflexes (Achilles reflex)
      - Sensation lateral foot and heel
   d. Reflex examination
      - Patella or knee jerk—L4
      - Hamstring—L5
      - Achilles or ankle—S1
   e. Sensory examination

C. Diagnosis

1. Plain films of the lumbar spine are not indicated in all patients with low back pain. Most cases resolve with rest and NSAIDs. If symptoms persist for longer than 3 to 4 weeks, radiographs are appropriate. If compression fracture, infection or tumor are suspected, radiographs should be obtained immediately.

2. MRI is indicated if patient has failed a course of conservative treatment (rest, physical therapy, NSAIDs) for at least 3 months. Patients with neurologic signs or symptoms should have an MRI sooner, depending on severity and acuteness of clinical findings.

Handwritten notes:
① Gait and symmetry
② check all four movements
③ Straight leg test to reproduce the pain
④ local tenderness/sacroiliac joint tenderness.

D. Treatment

1. Most patients with **acute** low back pain with or without radiculopathy are best managed conservatively with NSAIDs, brief period of rest, and judicious use of narcotic analgesics and muscle relaxants if necessary. Patients should be advised to continue ordinary activities within the limits permitted by pain. The acute pain lasts for several days.

2. If neurologic deficits present, a more aggressive approach is indicated. An MRI should be obtained, and if nerve root or spinal cord compression is present, evaluation by a spine specialist is recommended.

3. Most patients with **chronic** low back pain with or without radiculopathy are treated conservatively (with physical therapy, NSAIDs, epidural steroid injections).
   - Physical therapy is focused on trunk stabilization exercises and aerobic conditioning.
   - If these measures fail and symptoms persist for several months, surgery can be considered depending on findings on imaging studies and degree of disability. In general, outcomes from surgery are more predictable and successful when surgery is done for radiculopathy (to decompress nerve roots) than for low back pain per se.

It is helpful to differentiate patients with predominantly low back pain from those with predominantly leg pain. When conservative treatment has failed, surgery is often effective for leg pain, but results for low back pain are less predictable.

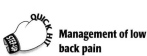
Management of low back pain
Avoid prolonged inactivity (leads to deconditioning). In the first week, attempt a walking routine (20 minutes, three times per day, interspersed with bed rest).

Knee Pain

A. Causes

1. Osteoarthritis—most common cause of knee pain in older patients (see below)

2. Patellofemoral pain—very common cause of anterior knee pain; worse with climbing and descending stairs. Physical therapy aimed at quadriceps/hamstrings rehabilitation (stretching/strengthening) is very effective.

3. Degeneration or tear of a meniscus—Meniscus tear may be due to a specific injury or secondary to degenerative process (the latter being a common cause of knee pain in older patients). Key features include recurrent knee effusions, tenderness along medial or lateral joint lines, and positive McMurray test. If no arthritic changes present, surgery (arthroscopic meniscectomy or repair) is effective. Surgery is less effective when concomitant arthritic changes are present and results are less predictable.

4. Rheumatoid arthritis, psoriatic arthritis, SLE

5. Acute monoarticular arthritis—septic arthritis, disseminated gonorrhea, gout, pseudogout, rheumatic fever, seronegative spondyloarthropathy, Lyme disease

6. Osteochondritis dissecans (OCD)—an area of necrotic bone and degenerative changes in the overlying cartilage. The bone/cartilage piece may separate from the underlying bone and become a loose body in the joint, causing symptoms of pain, catching, and popping. Treatment options are limited. If loose fragment in joint, arthroscopic removal of fragment is indicated.

7. Osgood-Schlatter disease in adolescents—resolves with skeletal maturity

8. Baker's cyst—caused by intra-articular pathology (e.g., meniscus tear)
   a. Rupture can cause pain/swelling, and if it extends into the calf, may mimic thrombophlebitis or acute deep venous thrombosis.
   b. Ultrasound may help in diagnosis.
   c. It is more common in patients with rheumatoid disease or osteoarthritis.
   d. Majority resolve spontaneously.

9. Patellar tendinitis ("jumper's knee")
   a. Common cause of anterior knee pain (at inferior pole of patella)
   b. Running and jumping sports—an "overuse" injury
   c. Treatment is activity modification and quadriceps/hamstring rehabilitation (stretching/strengthening program).

B. Diagnosis

1. Radiographs—if degenerative disease is suspected or if there is a history of trauma or acute injury

2. MRI—if any ligamentous instability is apparent or a meniscus tear is suspected

> **Box** 12-5 **Causes of Arthritis**
>
> - Osteoarthritis (most common cause)
> - Systemic immune disease: rheumatoid arthritis, SLE, IBD, seronegative spondyloarthropathies
> - Crystal disease: gout, pseudogout
> - Infectious: septic arthritis, Lyme disease
> - Trauma
> - Charcot joint (diabetes)
> - Pediatric orthopaedic conditions such as congenital hip dysplasia, Legg-Calve-Perthes disease, slipped capital femoral epiphysis
> - Hematologic: sickle cell disease (avascular necrosis of femoral head), hemophilia (recurrent hemarthrosis)
> - Deposition diseases: Wilson's disease, hemochromatosis

3. Knee aspiration ("tap")—Use this for analysis of synovial fluid if septic joint is suspected. In general, synovial fluid examination is recommended for monoarticular joint swelling. It may relieve symptoms.

Ankle Sprains

A. General characteristics
1. The lateral side of ankle consists of three ligaments: anterior talofibular ligament (ATFL), calcaneofibular ligament (CFL), and posterior talofibular ligament. The ATFL is most commonly injured.
2. The medial side ligaments (deltoid ligament) are typically not injured in a classic inversion ankle sprain.
3. Classification into three grades is based on severity.
   a. Grade 1: partial rupture of ATFL
   b. Grade 2: complete rupture of ATFL and partial rupture of CFL
   c. Grade 3: complete rupture of both ATFL and CFL

B. Diagnosis
1. Patients typically have tenderness directly over the injured ligament. ATFL is located just at the anterior tip of the distal fibula.
2. Ankle radiographs are not necessary if the following conditions are met (Ottawa rules):
   a. Patient is able to walk four steps at time of injury and at time of evaluation
   b. There is no bony tenderness over distal 6 cm of either malleolus.

C. Treatment
1. Rest, ice, compression, elevation (RICE) in the acute period, then controlled pain-free range of motion exercises with gradual return to weight bearing
2. Physical therapy after the acute phase of swelling has subsided to regain full range of motion, strength, and proprioception. Physical therapy involves peroneal tendon strengthening and proprioceptive training.
3. Surgery is rarely necessary acutely, even for grade 3 sprains.
4. Chronic ankle instability (recurrent ankle sprains) needs further evaluation by an orthopaedic specialist.

Tendinitis and Bursitis

A. Tendinitis
1. Supraspinatus (rotator cuff) tendinitis—impingement syndrome (see Quick Hit)
   a. Most common cause of shoulder pain
   b. Pain occurs subacromially and on the lateral aspect of the shoulder with arm abduction; pain is poorly localized (difficult for patient to pinpoint) with an insidious onset. It is generally located over the lateral deltoid.

QUICK HIT

By following the Ottawa rules, unnecessary radiographs of the ankle are avoided and clinically significant fractures are not missed.

QUICK HIT

Treatment of all acute ankle sprains (even severe sprains) involves RICE and physical therapy. Surgery is rarely, if ever, needed acutely. Recurrent ankle sprains, however, require evaluation for possible surgery.

   c. This is seen in elderly patients (degeneration of tendons) and in young patients who do a lot of overhand lifting/throwing (sports or work-related).

   d. Pain may be referred to the lateral arm.

   e. If weakness is present on shoulder abduction, a rotator cuff tear should be suspected (MRI is best test for diagnosis of rotator cuff tear).

2. Lateral epicondylitis at the elbow ("tennis elbow")

   a. Caused by inflammation/degeneration of the extensor tendons of the forearm, which originate from the lateral epicondyle; results from excessive/repetitive supination/pronation

   b. Splinting the forearm (counterforce brace) is the initial treatment (do not splint or wrap the elbow itself).

   c. Physical therapy is often helpful—strengthening/stretching extensors of forearm.

   d. Injections are rarely used. Surgery is effective but only used if all conservative measures have been exhausted.

3. Medial epicondylitis ("golfer's elbow")

   a. Pain distal to medial epicondyle (origin of flexor muscles of the forearm)

   b. Exacerbated by wrist flexion; caused by overuse of the flexor pronator muscle group

4. De Quervain's disease

   a. Pain at the radial aspect of the wrist (especially with pinch gripping) in region of radial styloid; common for pain to radiate to elbow or into thumb

   b. Due to inflammation of the abductor pollicis longus and extensor pollicis brevis tendons

   c. Positive Finkelstein's test—Have the patient clench the thumb under the other fingers when making a fist. Then ulnarly deviate the wrist. The test is positive if pain is reproduced.

   d. Treatment is thumb spica splint and NSAIDs. Local cortisone injections can be helpful. Surgery done if conservative measures fail and is usually effective.

B. Bursitis

1. Olecranon bursitis—swelling (and perhaps pain) at point of elbow; spongy "bag of fluid" over olecranon (due to effusion into the olecranon bursa).

   a. Treatment is conservative.

   b. If infection is suspected, drainage may be necessary.

2. Trochanteric bursitis—This is a common cause of lateral hip pain. The greater trochanter is exquisitely painful on palpation.

   a. Treatment is NSAIDs and activity modification.

   b. Local cortisone injections can provide excellent relief.

Carpal Tunnel Syndrome

A. General characteristics

1. Caused by **median nerve compression** within the tight confines of the carpal tunnel, causing numbness and pain in median nerve distribution. If long-standing and severe, atrophy of thenar muscles may be seen.

2. Associated conditions include hypothyroidism, diabetes, repetitive use of hands in certain activities, pregnancy, recent trauma or fracture of the wrist.

B. Clinical features

1. Numbness, pain, or tingling in the **median nerve distribution**—usually worse at night; sometimes patient has pain/numbness along the entire arm (as far as the shoulder)

2. Muscle weakness and thenar atrophy may develop later.

C. Diagnosis

1. Physical examination

   a. **Tinel's sign**—tap over median nerve at wrist crease; causes paresthesias in median nerve distribution

Impingement syndrome
- Common cause of shoulder pain
- Due to impingement of greater tuberosity on acromion
- Pain with overhead activity
- May lead to rotator cuff pathology over time
- Steroid injections give temporary relief
- Surgery (acromioplasty) is very effective.

Differential diagnosis of hand numbness (as seen in carpal tunnel syndrome):
- Cervical radiculopathy (nerve root compression in the cervical spine)
- Peripheral neuropathy (diabetes)
- Median nerve compression in forearm

AMBULATORY MEDICINE

> **QUICK HIT**
> A negative Phalen's test or Tinel's sign does not exclude carpal tunnel syndrome.

   b. **Phalen's test**—palmar flexion of the wrist for 1 minute; causes paresthesias in median nerve distribution

2. Electromyography and nerve conduction velocity study
   a. For definitive diagnosis
   b. Indicated if diagnosis is not clear from clinical findings or if patient develops weakness or persistent symptoms

D. Treatment

1. Wrist splints (volar carpal splint) should be worn at night during sleep. The purpose is to prevent wrist flexion during sleep (which compresses the nerve).
2. Anti-inflammatory medications (NSAIDs)
3. Local corticosteroid injection—Relief can be long-term in some patients.
4. Surgical release is very effective. Consider this option for patients who have persistent symptoms or if the symptoms are limiting the patient's activities or quality of life.

Osteoarthritis

A. General characteristics

1. Osteoarthritis is characterized by **degeneration of cartilage** (due to wear and tear) and by hypertrophy of bone at the articular margins.
2. By age 65, more than 75% of the population has radiographic evidence of osteoarthritis in weight-bearing joints (hips, knees, lumbar spine).
3. Any joint can be affected, but weight-bearing joints are most commonly involved (hips, knees, cervical and lumbar spine).

B. Risk factors

1. Age—Patients age 65 or older are at greatly increased risk.
2. Obesity
3. Excessive joint loading (manual labor, athletes, etc.)
4. Trauma
   a. Repeated microtrauma—In many cases, a patient's occupation or athletic activities require repetitive motions (such as repeated knee bending) that predispose the patient to degenerative joint disease in later years.
   b. Macrotrauma (fractures, ligament injuries)
5. Genetic predisposition
6. Altered joint anatomy or instability (developmental hip dysplasia, dislocation due to trauma, rheumatoid arthritis, gout, pseudogout)
7. Deposition diseases cause chondrocyte injury, or make the cartilage more stiff (hemochromatosis, ochronosis, alkaptonuria, Wilson's disease, Gaucher's disease, gout, CPPD).
8. Hemophilia (hemarthroses)

> **QUICK HIT**
> The following can contribute to or exacerbate forces to the cartilage:
> • Compromised pain sensation or proprioception
> • Ligamental laxity
> • Falls of very short distances (because they do not provide ample opportunity for compensatory movements to decrease the impact load)

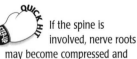

> **QUICK HIT**
> If the spine is involved, nerve roots may become compressed and lead to radicular pain.

C. Clinical features

1. Joint pain (often monoarticular)

Box   **12-6**   **Physical Examination for Knee Pain**

- Assess distortion of normal knee contours, irregular bony prominences at the joint margin.
- Determine presence of **effusion.**
- Check for **muscle atrophy.**
- Assess meniscal injury by McMurray and Apley tests.
- Determine **range of motion.**
- Test stability of collateral ligaments.
- Assess anterior cruciate ligament stability via Lachman test or anterior drawer test.
- Assess joint line tenderness (medial or lateral)—meniscus tear or osteoarthritis.
- Patellar grind test—Push down on the patella and ask the patient to raise his or her leg.

a. This is caused by movement of one joint surface against another (bone on bone) because of cartilage loss. There are no pain fibers in cartilage, so its insidious destruction over time goes unnoticed. Once it is completely worn out, the bones (which do have pain fibers) start rubbing against each other, producing the pain of osteoarthritis.

b. Deep, dull ache that is relieved with rest and worsened with activity

c. Insidious onset, with gradual progression over many years

2. Stiffness in the morning or after a period of inactivity

3. Limited range of motion (late stages) due to bony enlargement of joints (osteophytes), bony crepitus may be present.

4. No systemic symptoms; no erythema or warmth. Swelling may be present.

D. Diagnosis

1. Plain radiographs are the initial tests and should be obtained in all patients suspected of having osteoarthritis. Findings include:

a. **Joint space narrowing** (due to loss of cartilage)—key finding on radiographs

b. **Osteophytes**

c. **Sclerosis** of subchondral bony end-plates adjacent to diseased cartilage—most severe at points of maximum pressure

d. **Subchondral cysts**—occur as a result of increased transmission of intra-articular pressure to the subchondral bone

2. MRI of the spine if indicated (neurologic findings, before surgery)

E. Treatment

1. Nonpharmacologic treatment

a. Avoid activities that involve excessive use of the joint.

b. Weight loss is very important.

c. Physical therapy can be beneficial. Goals are to maintain range of motion and muscle strength. Swimming is an ideal exercise (involves minimal involvement of weight-bearing joints); avoid excessive walking.

d. Use canes or crutches to reduce weight on the joint.

2. Pharmacologic treatment

a. Acetaminophen is the first-line agent. NSAIDs are just as effective (but GI bleeding is a concern with long-term use).

b. Intra-articular injections of corticosteroids are very helpful, but more than three to four injections per year is not recommended. Patients may have up to 3 months of pain relief with each injection.

c. Viscosupplementation (series of three injections of hyaluronic acid given once a week)—Recent studies show good pain relief, but results are variable.

3. Surgery for serious disability

a. Total joint replacement may be performed if conservative therapy fails to control pain. It should be delayed as long as possible because a revision may be needed 15 to 20 years after surgery. Total hip and knee replacements are among the most successful procedures in orthopaedics with reliable pain relief.

b. Spine surgery may be performed for patients with severe disease, with intractable pain, or with neurologic sequelae (nerve root compression) if a prolonged period of nonoperative therapy fails.

• Surgical options include decompression (laminectomy) with or without spinal fusion, depending on the pathology.

• Total disc replacement is available but more evidence is needed regarding efficacy.

4. Nutritional products—glucosamine and chondroitin sulfate

a. Over-the-counter products that many patients claim to improve arthritis symptoms

b. Well-tolerated with no significant adverse effects

c. A number of studies have shown a decrease in pain, but evidence from randomized controlled trials is not as convincing.

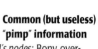 Radiographic findings in osteoarthritis: joint space narrowing, osteophytes, subchondral sclerosis, subchondral cysts

Common (but useless) "pimp" information
• *Bouchard's nodes:* Bony overgrowth and significant osteoarthritic changes (i.e., osteophytes) at the PIP joints
• *Heberden's nodes:* Bony overgrowth and significant osteoarthritic changes (i.e., osteophytes) at the DIP joints

 With osteoarthritis of the hips, the pain is in the **groin region** and sometimes radiates to the anterior thigh.

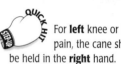 For **left** knee or hip pain, the cane should be held in the **right** hand.

FIGURE
(12-3) **A.** Right knee AP radiograph showing osteoarthritis. Note medial joint space narrowing, osteophyte formation (curved arrow), and irregular articular surfaces (straight arrow). **B.** Pelvic AP radiograph. Bilateral osteoarthritis of the hip. Note narrowing of hip joint spaces, osteophytes (curved arrows), and osteophytes in the lumbar spine (double curved arrows). Also note subchondral cysts and sclerosis of the femoral heads.

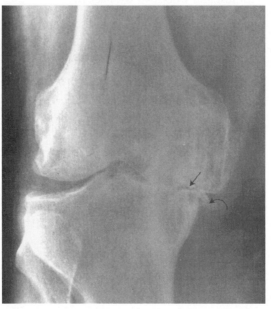

A

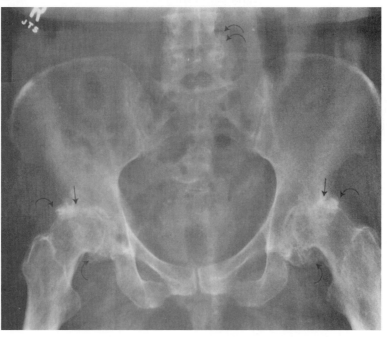

B

(**A** from Erkonen WE, Smith WL. Radiology 101: The Basics and Fundamentals of Imaging. Philadelphia: Lippincott Williams & Wilkins, 1998:287, Figure 11-72.)
(**B** from Erkonen WE, Smith WL. Radiology 101: The Basics and Fundamentals of Imaging. Philadelphia: Lippincott Williams & Wilkins, 1998:288, Figure 11-73A.)

Osteoporosis

A. General characteristics

1. Decreased bone mass/quality causes increased bone fragility and fracture risk. In osteoporosis, the bone mineral density is at least 2.5 standard deviations below that of young, normal individuals.

2. Mechanism: Failure to attain optimal (peak) bone mass before age 30, or rate of bone resorption exceeds rate of bone formation after peak bone mass is attained

3. Most osteoporotic patients are postmenopausal women and elderly men.

4. Classification
   a. Primary osteoporosis (two types that are impractical clinically)
      • Type I (most often in postmenopausal women 51 to 75 years of age)—excess loss of trabecular bone; vertebral compression fractures and Colles fractures are common
      • Type II (most often in men and women over 70 years of age)—equal loss of both cortical and trabecular bone; fractures of femoral neck, proximal humerus, and pelvis most common
   b. Secondary osteoporosis—An obvious cause is present, such as excess steroid therapy/Cushing's syndrome, immobilization, hyperthyroidism, long-term heparin, hypogonadism in men, and vitamin D deficiency.

It is often difficult to differentiate between primary and secondary osteoporosis, and the two may coexist. It is best to attempt to identify any predisposing conditions and eliminate them if possible.

B. Risk factors

1. Estrogen depletion
   a. Postmenopausal state—All women are estrogen-deficient after menopause; however, osteoporosis does not develop in all women.
   b. History of athletic amenorrhea, eating disorders, oligomenorrhea
   c. Early menopause
2. Female gender—Women have a lower peak bone mass and smaller vertebral end plates.
3. Calcium deficiency/vitamin D deficiency
4. Decreased peak bone mass
5. Heritable risk factors—family history, European or Asian ancestry, thinness/slight build
6. Decreased physical activity (prolonged immobility)
7. Endocrine—hypogonadism in men (with low testosterone), hyperthyroidism, vitamin D deficiency
8. Smoking and alcohol abuse
9. Medications—corticosteroids, prolonged heparin use

C. Clinical features

1. Vertebral body compression fractures (of the middle and lower thoracic and upper lumbar spine) are the most common.
   a. Result in pain and deformity, including kyphosis and lumbar lordosis
   b. Severe back pain after minor trauma
   c. Restricted spinal movement, loss of height
2. Colles fracture (distal radius fracture)—usually due to fall on outstretched hand; more common in postmenopausal women
3. Hip fractures—femoral neck, intertrochanteric fractures
4. Increased incidence of long bone fractures—humerus, femur, tibia

Some elderly patients have progressive kyphosis (hunchback deformity) because they have multiple vertebral compression fractures.

Osteoporosis is a "silent" disease. It is asymptomatic until a fracture occurs.

D. Diagnosis

1. DEXA scan is the gold standard.
   a. Very precise for measuring bone density
   b. Perform at menopause
   c. Take bone samples from the hip and the lumbar vertebrae. Compare the density of bone with a standard control, which is the bone density of a healthy 30-year-old person.
   d. Can range from normal to osteopenia to osteoporosis
2. Rule out secondary causes—check calcium, phosphorus, alkaline phosphatase, TSH, vitamin D, free PTH, creatinine, CBC.

E. Treatment

1. Inhibit bone resorption
   a. Bisphosphonates for treatment and prevention. They decrease osteoclastic activity (via binding to hydroxyapatite) and decrease the risk of fractures.

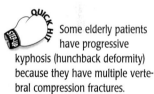

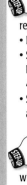

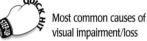

An exercise program with calcium and vitamin D supplements is the mainstay of the therapy for prevention or treatment of osteoporosis.

The **PROOF trial** showed the following regarding **calcitonin**:
• No effect at hip
• Shown to decrease risk of vertebral fractures by as much as 40%
• Slight increase in bone density at lumbar vertebrae

Recommend the following to all patients with osteoporosis:
• Daily calcium
• Daily vitamin D
• Weight-bearing exercise
• Smoking cessation

Most common causes of visual impairment/loss in developed countries:
• Diabetic retinopathy (most common cause in adults <65 years)
• ARMD (most common cause in adults >65 years)
• Cataracts
• Glaucoma

Age-related macular degeneration
• The "wet" form of ARMD can develop at any time, so patients with "dry" ARMD must be monitored closely.
• Supplements of certain vitamins containing antioxidants are thought to be beneficial, but a preventative or therapeutic effect has not been proven.
• **Ranibizumab (and several other related drugs), given as an intraocular injection,** has been shown to be effective in reducing the rate of visual loss due to "wet" ARMD.

• Alendronate—increases bone density by 5% to 6%
• Second-generation bisphosphonates (e.g., alendronate, risedronate) are more effective than first-generation agents (e.g., etidronate).
• Side effects include esophageal irritation and ulceration.
    b. Calcium supplements
    c. Vitamin D supplements
    d. Calcitonin (can be administered by nasal spray)—Long-term benefits are minimal, but it is useful as short-term therapy, especially in elderly female patients with vertebral compression fracture.
 2. Weight-bearing exercise to stimulate bone formation
 3. To prevent osteoporosis
    a. Reduce or eliminate modifiable risk factors (such as smoking and alcohol intake).
    b. Estrogen replacement therapy for perimenopausal and postmenopausal women
       • Estrogen suppresses bone resorption by osteoclasts
       • Has been shown to increase bone density by 2% to 3%
       • Reduction in hip, wrist, and vertebral fractures
    c. Raloxifene
       • Selective estrogen receptor modulator
       • Functions as estrogen agonist in some tissues and antagonist in others
       • Increases bone density by 1% to 2%
    d. Calcium supplementation
    e. Prevent injures.

DISEASES OF THE EYE

Age-Related Macular Degeneration (ARMD)

• Most common cause of vision loss in people over 65 years of age
• ARMD is characterized by loss of central vision (because the macula is affected). Blurred vision, distortion, and scotoma are common. Complete loss of vision almost never occurs. Peripheral vision is preserved.
• The main risk factor for ARMD is advanced age. Other risk factors are female gender, Caucasian race, smoking, HTN, and family history.
• Two categories: exudative ("wet") and nonexudative ("dry") macular degeneration
• Exudative ARMD is less common than nonexudative ARMD, but is responsible for most cases of severe vision loss. It causes sudden visual loss due to leakage of serous fluid into the retina, followed by abnormal vessel formation (neovascularization) under the retinal pigment epithelium.
• Nonexudative ARMD is characterized by atrophy and degeneration of the central retina. Yellowish-white deposits called **drusen** form under the pigment epithelium and can be seen with an ophthalmoscope.
• Effective treatment does not exist, although laser photocoagulation may reduce the risk of severe vision loss if there is subretinal neovascularization.

Glaucoma

A. General characteristics

 1. Glaucoma is **one of the most important causes of blindness worldwide**. It is a complex disease typically characterized by increased IOP, damage to the optic nerve, and irreversible vision loss.
 2. The pathogenesis of optic nerve damage in glaucoma is not fully understood. Ischemia may play a major role. Over time there is a loss of ganglion cells, leading to atrophy of the optic disc (and enlargement of the optic cup, called "**cupping**").
 4. There are many types of glaucoma, but they generally fall into the following two categories.
    a. Open-angle glaucoma—accounts for 90% of all cases
       • Characterized by impaired outflow of aqueous humor from the eye.
       • Absence of symptoms early in the course can lead to delay in diagnosis and "silent" progression.

b. Closed-angle glaucoma
- Acute angle-closure glaucoma—characterized by very rapid increase in IOP due to occlusion of the narrow angle and obstruction of outflow of aqueous humor
- **This is an ophthalmologic emergency that can lead to irreversible vision loss within hours if untreated.**
- May be precipitated by dilation of the iris in a patient with a pre-existing anatomically narrow anterior chamber angle

 Glaucoma is the most common cause of nonreversible blindness in African Americans.

B. Risk factors

1. Older age (over 50 years)
2. African-American race (increased incidence of open-angle glaucoma)
3. Asian or Eskimo ancestry (increased incidence of acute angle-closure glaucoma)
4. Family history of glaucoma
5. History of significant eye trauma or intraocular inflammation
6. Steroid medications

C. Clinical features

1. Open-angle glaucoma
   a. Painless, increased IOP (may be the only sign), characteristic changes in optic nerve
   b. Progressive and insidious visual field loss (usually sparing central vision until end-stage disease)
2. Closed-angle glaucoma
   a. Red, painful eye
   b. Sudden decrease in visual acuity (blurred vision), seeing "halos," markedly elevated IOP
   c. Nausea and vomiting (common), headache
   d. Involved pupil is dilated and nonreactive (in mid-dilation)

Patients with acute angle-closure glaucoma may have severe abdominal pain and nausea, and they are occasionally misdiagnosed as having an acute surgical abdomen (e.g., appendicitis).

D. Diagnosis

1. Tonometry measures IOP; should be performed regularly in patients with or at risk for glaucoma.
2. Ophthalmoscopy—Evaluate the optic nerve for glaucomatous damage.
3. Gonioscopy is used to visualize the anterior chamber and helps determine the cause of glaucoma. It requires skill to perform.
4. Visual field testing should be performed in all patients in whom glaucoma is suspected and regularly in everyone with glaucoma to monitor disease progression.

E. Treatment

1. Chronic open-angle glaucoma (in escalating order)
   a. Topical medications—Most patients are first treated topically with a β-blocker, α-agonist, carbonic anhydrase inhibitor, and/or prostaglandin analogue singly or in combination to reach the target pressure.
   b. Laser or surgical treatment for refractory cases
2. Acute angle-closure glaucoma
   a. An ophthalmic emergency—Refer to an ophthalmologist immediately. Emergently lower the IOP. Medical treatment includes pilocarpine drops, IV acetazolamide, and oral glycerin.
   b. Laser or surgical iridectomy is a definitive treatment.

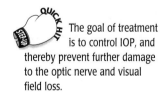 The goal of treatment is to control IOP, and thereby prevent further damage to the optic nerve and visual field loss.

Cataracts

- Opacifications of the natural lens of the eye: **Half of people over age 75 have cataracts** (see Color Figure 12-2).
- There is a **loss of visual acuity** that progresses slowly over many years. Patients may complain of glare and difficulty driving at night.
- Risk factors include old age, cigarette smoking, glucocorticoid use, prolonged UV radiation exposure, trauma, diabetes, Wilson's disease, Down syndrome, and certain metabolic diseases.

AMBULATORY MEDICINE

QUICK HIT
"Second sight"
- Some patients with cataracts become increasingly near-sighted and may no longer require reading glasses. This is referred to as "second sight."
- This phenomenon is due to increased refractive power of the lens of the eye caused by the cataract.

QUICK HIT
In general, steroid eye drops should be given by an ophthalmologist.

- Surgery is the definitive treatment and is very effective in restoring vision. It is indicated if visual loss is significant to the patient and interferes with daily or occupational activities. It involves extraction of the cataract with implantation of an artificial intraocular lens.

Red Eye

A. General characteristics

1. Many causes of red eye are benign, but the initial goal in evaluation should be to identify conditions that require referral (emergent or nonemergent) to an ophthalmologist.
2. Conjunctivitis is the most common cause of red eye, but always attempt to exclude other, more serious causes.
3. The following conditions require a referral to an ophthalmologist.
    a. Eye pain that does not respond to therapy
    b. Flashers, floaters, or a sudden decrease in visual acuity
    c. History of recent eye surgery—especially if infection is suspected
    d. Corneal opacification, corneal ulcer, or corneal foreign body that cannot be removed
    e. History of penetrating trauma or significant blunt trauma
    f. History of chemical exposure (especially alkali agents)
    g. Orbital cellulitis
4. Always check visual acuity, pupil size, and reactivity. Evert lids to look for a foreign body.

B. Differential diagnosis

1. Conjunctivitis—see below.
2. Subconjunctival hemorrhage
    a. Caused by rupture of small conjunctival vessels; usually induced by Valsalva maneuver (cough, straining with defecation, vomiting); trauma; or, less commonly, coagulopathies or HTN
    b. Causes focal unilateral blotchy redness of the conjunctiva (looks worse than it is)
    c. Usually self-limiting and resolves in a few weeks.
3. Keratoconjunctivitis sicca (dry eye)
    a. Very long differential diagnosis, including: medications (e.g., anticholinergics or antihistamines), autoimmune diseases (e.g., Sjögren's), CN V or VII lesions
    b. The eye may appear normal, or may be mildly injected.
    c. Patients may complain of a foreign body sensation.
    d. Treat with artificial tears during the day. Consider a lubricating ointment at night.
    e. Occlusion of the tear puncta to reduce the outflow of lacrimal fluid is often effective.
4. Acute angle-closure glaucoma (see above)—Consult an ophthalmologist immediately.
5. Blepharitis
    a. Inflammation of the eyelid; often associated with infection with *Staphylococcus* spp.
    b. Usually diagnosed by careful examination of the eyelid margins, which are red and often swollen with crusting that sticks to the lashes
    c. Treat with lid scrubs and warm compresses. Give topical antibiotics for severe cases.
6. Episcleritis
    a. Inflammation of vessels lining the episclera (the lining just beneath the conjunctiva)
    b. Thought to be an autoimmune process—may be seen with connective tissue diseases
    c. Causes redness, irritation, dull ache, and possible watery discharge
    d. The sclera may appear blotchy with areas of redness over the episcleral vessels.

    e. It is usually self-limited; NSAIDs may provide symptomatic relief.

    f. Refer the patient for evaluation by an ophthalmologist.

7. Scleritis

    a. Inflammation of the sclera is associated with systemic immunologic disease, such as rheumatoid arthritis.

    b. It causes significant eye pain (severe, deep pain). On examination, there is ocular redness and pain on palpation of the eyeball. It can cause visual impairment.

    c. Refer the patient for prompt evaluation by an ophthalmologist. Treatment involves topical and sometimes systemic corticosteroids.

9. Acute anterior uveitis (also known as iritis or iridocyclitis)

    a. Inflammation of the iris and ciliary body; more common in the young and middle-aged

    b. Associated with connective tissue diseases (e.g., sarcoidosis, ankylosing spondylitis, Reiter's syndrome, and IBD)

    c. Clinical findings: circumcorneal injection (redness most prominent around the cornea), blurred vision, pain and photophobia; constricted pupil compared with contralateral eye

    d. Refer the patient for prompt evaluation by an ophthalmologist.

10. Herpes simplex keratitis

    a. Caused by HSV-1; may present similarly to viral conjunctivitis, except usually unilateral

    b. Presents with ocular irritation and photophobia

    c. Look for classic dendrite on the cornea of fluorescein staining—**indicates a dendritic ulcer and can result in irreversible vision loss if untreated.**

    d. Warrants semiurgent ophthalmology referral

    e. Treat with topical antiviral eye drops. Consider oral acyclovir for severe or refractory disease.

Conjunctivitis

A. General characteristics

1. Conjunctivitis is the most common cause of red eye.

2. Conjunctivitis generally refers to inflammation of the transparent membrane that lines the inside of the eyelids (palpebral conjunctiva) and the globe (bulbar conjunctiva).

B. Causes

1. Viral conjunctivitis

    a. The **most common** form of conjunctivitis

    b. Adenovirus is the most frequently indicted etiology. Inquire about a recent history of URI, because this often precedes or simultaneously causes viral conjunctivitis.

    c. The patient will generally present with edema and hyperemia of one or both eyes, usually one followed by spread to the other in a few days. The eyelids may also be swollen. A watery discharge is frequently present.

    d. A palpable preauricular lymph node may be present.

    e. It is usually self-limited, but some patients develop membranous conjunctivitis that requires steroids.

2. Bacterial conjunctivitis

    a. Most commonly caused by *S. pneumoniae* but can also be caused by gram-negative organisms

    b. Rapid onset of irritation, hyperemia, and tearing with spread to the other eye in less than 2 days

    c. Characterized by a mucopurulent exudate with crusting

    d. Treat empirically with broad-spectrum antibiotics (see below), and advise strict personal hygiene. Sometimes conjunctival cultures are taken.

3. Chlamydial conjunctivitis—two important forms

QUICK HIT

Viral conjunctivitis is highly contagious! Patients should avoid any direct or indirect eye contact with others. Encourage strict personal hygiene and frequent handwashing. Clean all surfaces and equipment in contact with the patient as soon as the patient leaves the office.

> **Box 12-7 Do Not Send a Patient Home Who Has a Rapid Onset of Copious, Purulent Exudate!**
>
> - This is consistent with **hyperacute bacterial conjunctivitis,** caused by *Neisseria gonorrhoeae.*
> - The typical patient is a sexually active young adult.
> - Symptoms progress rapidly to severe redness, swelling, and pain.
> - **This warrants immediate attention from an ophthalmologist.**
> - If untreated, it can lead to corneal scarring and blindness.

> **QUICK HIT**
>
> When a patient presents with red and itchy eyes, tearing, and nasal congestion, think allergic conjunctivitis.

  a. Trachoma (caused by *Chlamydia trachomatis* serotypes A, B, and C)
     - Most common cause of blindness worldwide due to chronic scarring
     - Less common in developed countries
  b. Inclusion conjunctivitis (*C. trachomatis* serotypes D to K)
     - Mainly transmitted by genital-hand-eye contact in patients with the STD
     - Symptoms are similar to those of bacterial conjunctivitis
     - Typically does not lead to corneal scarring and blindness
4. Allergic conjunctivitis
  a. Very common in patients with atopic disease; usually seasonal
  b. It is typically characterized by redness, itching, tearing, and nasal conjunctivitis. Eyelid edema may also be present. It is typically bilateral.
5. Conjunctivitis secondary to irritants (e.g., contact lenses, chemicals, foreign bodies, dryness)

> **QUICK HIT**
>
> Wearing contact lenses overnight dramatically increases a person's risk for developing corneal infection and ulceration.

C. Clinical features
1. Redness and edema of the conjunctiva due to dilation of conjunctival vessels
2. Purulent discharge is suggestive of bacterial conjunctivitis. A watery discharge may be present in viral, allergic, and some forms of bacterial conjunctivitis.
3. May present with chemosis (a build-up of fluid under the bulbar conjunctiva, causing it to puff up away from the globe)
4. Ocular pain or vision loss is not usually present in uncomplicated cases.

D. Treatment
1. Viral conjunctivitis: cold compress, strict hand washing; topical antibiotics if bacterial superinfection is suspected
2. Bacterial conjunctivitis
  a. Acute—Use broad-spectrum topical antibiotics, e.g., erythromycin, ciprofloxacin, sulfacetamide. Therapy can be altered based on culture results.
  b. Hyperacute—Treat gonococcal conjunctivitis with a one-time dose of ceftriaxone, 1g IM, as well as topical therapy.
3. Chlamydial conjunctivitis
  a. Adults and adolescents—oral tetracycline, doxycycline, or erythromycin for 2 weeks
  b. Treat sexual partner(s) for STD.
4. Allergic conjunctivitis
  a. Remove the allergen, if possible. Advise the use of cold compresses.
  b. Treat with topical antihistamines or mast cell stabilizers.
  c. Systemic antihistamines can be effective as well.
  d. Topical NSAIDs may be a useful adjunct to treatment.

Amaurosis Fugax

- Presents with sudden, transient monocular loss of vision
- Due to embolization of cholesterol plaque from the carotid arterial system with retinal ischemia
- When reperfusion is established (spontaneously), vision returns.
- Order carotid ultrasonography and cardiac workup (e.g., lipid profile, ECG).

SLEEP DISORDERS

Obstructive Sleep Apnea (OSA)

A. General characteristics

1. Intermittent obstruction of the air flow (typically at the level of the oropharynx) produces periods of apnea during sleep.
2. Each apneic period is usually 20 to 30 seconds long (but may be longer) and results in hypoxia, which arouses the patient from sleep. This occurs multiple (sometimes hundreds of) times overnight.

B. Risk factors

1. Obesity (especially around the neck)—nonobese patients can also have OSA, however
2. Structural abnormalities—enlarged tonsils, uvula, soft palate; nasal polyps; hypertrophy of muscles in the pharynx; deviated septum; deep overbite with small chin
3. Family history
4. Alcohol and sedatives worsen the condition
5. Hypothyroidism (multifactorial)

C. Clinical features

1. Snoring
2. Daytime sleepiness due to disrupted nocturnal sleep
3. Personality changes, decreased intellectual function, decreased libido
4. Repeated oxygen desaturation and hypoxemia can lead to systemic and pulmonary HTN as well as cardiac arrhythmias.
5. Other features: morning headaches, polycythemia

D. Diagnosis: Polysomnography (overnight sleep study in a sleep laboratory) confirms the diagnosis.

E. Treatment

1. Mild to moderate OSA (<20 apneic episodes on polysomnogram with mild symptoms)
   a. Weight loss
   b. Avoid alcohol, sedatives
   c. Avoid supine position during sleep
2. Severe OSA (>20 apneic episodes with arterial oxygen desaturations)
   a. Nasal **continuous positive airway pressure** provides positive pressure, thus preventing occlusion of the upper pharynx. This is the preferred therapy for the majority of patients because it is noninvasive and has proven efficacy. It is poorly tolerated by some due to noise and discomfort.
   b. Uvulopalatopharyngoplasty—removal of redundant tissue in oropharynx to allow more air flow
   c. Tracheostomy is a last resort for those in whom all other therapies have failed or who have life-threatening OSA (severe hypoxemia or arrhythmias).

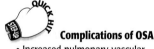

Complications of OSA
- Increased pulmonary vascular resistance (due to hypoxemia); over time, can lead to pulmonary HTN and eventually cor pulmonale (more likely if the patient is obese)
- Systemic HTN (due to increase in sympathetic tone)

Narcolepsy

- Inherited disorder (of variable penetrance) of REM sleep regulation (i.e., REM sleep involuntarily occurs at random and inappropriate times)
- Results in **excessive sleepiness** during the day
- Characterized by the following features:
  - Involuntary "sleep attacks" at any time of day (during any activity, including driving) that last several minutes
  - Cataplexy, which is loss of muscle tone that generally occurs with an intense emotional stimulus (e.g., laughter, anger)

- Sleep paralysis, in which patient cannot move when waking up
- Hypnagogic hallucinations that are vivid hallucinations (visual or auditory)—"dreams" while awake
- The disorder can range from mild to severe.
- Automobile accidents are a major problem.
- Treatment: methylphenidate (Ritalin); planned naps during the day may prevent sleep attacks

Insomnia

A. Causes

1. Acute or transient insomnia is usually due to psychological stress or travel over time zones ("jet lag").
2. Chronic causes
   a. Secondary insomnia accounts for over 90% of all cases.
      - Psychiatric conditions—depression, anxiety disorders, posttraumatic stress disorder, manic phase of bipolar disorder, schizophrenia, obsessive-compulsive disorder
      - Medications and substance abuse—alcohol, sedatives (with prolonged use, patients develop tolerance and withdrawal rebound insomnia), caffeine, β-blockers, stimulant drugs (amphetamines), decongestants, some SSRIs, nicotine
      - Medical problems—advanced COPD, renal failure, CHF, chronic pain
      - Other—fibromyalgia, chronic fatigue syndrome
   b. Primary insomnia is a diagnosis of exclusion. The DSM IV defines it as either of the following:
      - Difficulty initiating or maintaining sleep
      - Nonrestorative sleep that lasts for at least 1 month in the absence of other medical, psychiatric, or other sleep disorders, and that causes clinically significant distress and social or occupational impairment.
      - Patients worry excessively about not falling to sleep and become preoccupied with it. The cause is unknown.

B. Treatment

1. Treat the underlying cause, if found.
2. Consider a psychiatric evaluation if psychiatric causes or primary insomnia is suspected.
3. Use sedative-hypnotic medications sparingly and with caution for symptomatic relief. Use the smallest dose possible, and avoid use for longer than 2 to 3 weeks.

> **QUICK HIT**
>
> Questions to ask the patient with insomnia: sleep history, timing of insomnia, sleep habits

MISCELLANEOUS TOPICS

Hearing Loss/Impaired Hearing

A. General characteristics—two types of hearing loss

1. Conductive hearing loss
   a. Caused by lesions in the external or middle ear
   b. Interference with mechanical reception or amplification of sound, as occurs with disease of the auditory canal, tympanic membrane, or ossicles, creates conductive hearing loss.
2. Sensorineural hearing loss—due to lesions in the cochlea or CN VIII (auditory branch)

B. Causes

1. Conductive hearing loss
   a. External canal
      - Cerumen impaction—buildup obstructs the auditory canal (most common cause)

- Otitis externa
- Exostoses—bony outgrowths of external auditory canal related to repetitive exposure to cold water (e.g., scuba divers, swimmers)

b. Tympanic membrane perforation
- Usually due to trauma (direct or indirect)
- May be secondary to middle ear infection

c. Middle ear
- Any cause of middle ear effusion (fluid in middle ear interferes with sound conduction)—otitis media, allergic rhinitis
- Otosclerosis—bony fusion (immobilization) of the stapes to the oval window; an autosomal dominant condition (variable penetrance); corrected with surgery; rarely progresses to deafness
- Other—neoplasms, congenital malformation of the middle ear

2. Sensorineural hearing loss

a. Presbycusis (most common cause)
- Gradual, symmetric hearing loss associated with aging—most common cause of diminished hearing in elderly patients
- Pathology—degeneration of sensory cells and nerve fibers at the base of the cochlea
- Hearing loss is most marked at high frequencies with slow progression to lower frequencies.

b. Noise-induced hearing loss
- Chronic, prolonged exposure to sound levels >85 dB
- Hair cells in the organ of Corti are damaged.

c. Infection—viral or bacterial infection of cochlear structures or labyrinth

d. Drug-induced hearing loss
- Aminoglycoside antibiotics, furosemide, ethacrynic acid; cisplatin, quinidine
- Aspirin can cause tinnitus and reversible hearing impairment.

e. Injury to inner ear or cochlear nerve (e.g., skull fracture)

f. Congenital (TORCH infections)

g. Ménière's disease
- Fluctuating, unilateral hearing loss
- Sensorineural hearing loss (usually unilateral), sense of pressure/fullness in ear, tinnitus, vertigo
- Vertigo usually responds to dietary salt restriction and meclizine, but hearing loss is progressive

h. CNS causes—acoustic neuromas, meningitis, auditory nerve neuritis (multiple sclerosis, syphilis), meningioma

C. Clinical features

1. Conductive hearing loss
   a. Decreased perception of sound (especially for low-frequency sounds)
   b. Can hear loud noises well

2. Sensorineural hearing loss
   a. Difficulty hearing loud noises; shouting may exacerbate the problem (annoyed by loud speech)
   b. Can hear sounds, but has trouble deciphering words (poor speech discrimination)
   c. More difficulty with high-frequency sounds (doorbells, phones, child's voice, female voice)
   d. Tinnitus is often present.

D. Diagnosis

1. Whisper test—Ask the patient to repeat words whispered into the tested ear (mask the other ear).
2. An audiogram is an essential component of the evaluation.
3. MRI—in selected cases (e.g., if CNS tumor or multiple sclerosis is suspected)

Tympanic mimbane perforation
- History: pain, conductive hearing loss, tinnitus
- Examination: bleeding from the ear, clot in the meatus, visible tear in the tympanic membrane
- Ninety percent heal spontaneously within 6 weeks. Surgery is appropriate for larger perforations.

Hearing impairment
- History: medications; history of head trauma, infection (otitis media, otitis externa); noise exposure (occupational or recreational)
- Physical examination: inspect auditory canal (impacted cerumen, exostoses); examine tympanic membrane (inflammation, perforation, scarring); assess middle ear (fluid).

AMBULATORY MEDICINE

> **Box 12-8 Rinne and Weber Tests**
>
> - Conductive loss
>   - Abnormal Rinne test—bone conduction is better than air conduction
>   - Weber—**sound lateralizes to the affected side** (tuning fork is perceived more loudly in the ear with a conductive hearing loss)
> - Sensorineural loss
>   - Normal Rinne test—air conduction is better than bone conduction
>   - Weber—**sound lateralizes to the unaffected side**

E. Treatment

1. Cerumen impaction is best treated by irrigation after several days of softening with carbamide peroxide (Debrox) or triethanolamine (Cerumenex).
2. Conductive hearing loss
   a. Treat underlying cause
   b. Surgical techniques such as tympanoplasty (reconstructs middle ear) for patients with chronic otitis media; stapedectomy for otosclerosis
   c. Hearing aids
3. Sensorineural hearing loss
   a. Treat underlying cause
   b. Hearing aids
   c. Cochlear implants—transduce sounds to electrical energy, stimulates CN VIII

Urinary Incontinence

A. General characteristics

1. There are five major types of incontinence (urge, stress, overflow reflex, functional). Many patients have more than one type.
2. Male incontinence is usually due to benign prostatic hypertrophy (BPH) or neurologic disease. A urology evaluation is indicated in incontinent male patients.
3. Female incontinence is usually due to hormonal changes, pelvic floor dysfunction or laxity, or uninhibited bladder contractions (detrusor contractions) due to aging.

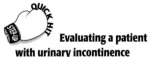

The most common cause of incontinence in elderly patients is urge incontinence. In **women <70 years** of age, the most common cause is stress incontinence.

B. Risk factors

1. Age—diminished size of bladder, earlier detrusor contractions, postmenopausal genitourinary atrophy
2. Recurrent urinary tract infections
3. Immobility, decreased mental status, dementia, stroke, Parkinson's disease, depression
4. DM, CHF
5. Multiparity, history of prolonged labor
6. Pelvic floor dysfunction in women, BPH and prostate cancer in men
7. Medications
   a. Diuretics increase bladder filling, increasing the episodes of incontinence.
   b. Anticholinergics and adrenergics cause urinary retention.
   c. β-blockers diminish sphincter tone.
   d. Calcium channel blockers and narcotics can decrease detrusor contraction.
   e. Alcohol, sedatives, hypnotics (depress mentation)

Evaluating a patient with urinary incontinence Inquire about the history of diabetes, multiple sclerosis, Parkinson's disease, stroke, spinal cord injury or disease, and pelvic surgery.

C. Types of urinary incontinence

1. Urge incontinence (also called detrusor instability)
   a. Most common type in elderly and nursing home patients
   b. Multiple causes (often idiopathic), including dementia, strokes, severe illness, Parkinson's disease
   c. Mechanism: Involuntary and uninhibited detrusor contractions result in involuntary loss of urine.

d. Clinical features: This is characterized by a sudden urge to urinate (e.g., patients are unable to make it to the bathroom), a loss of large volumes of urine with small postvoid residual, and nocturnal wetting.

e. Management: anticholinergic medications (oxybutynin), TCAs (imipramine), bladder retraining (behavioral therapy) to help regain control of voiding reflex that has been lost (goal is to increase the amount of time between voiding, "timed toileting")

2. Stress incontinence
   a. Occurs mostly in women (after multiple deliveries of children)
   b. Mechanism: Weakness of the pelvic diaphragm (pelvic floor) leads to loss of bladder support (with resultant hypermobility of the bladder neck). This causes the proximal urethra to descend below the pelvic floor so that an increase in intra-abdominal pressure is transmitted mostly to the bladder (instead of an equal transmission to the bladder and urethra).
   c. Clinical features: involuntary urine loss (only in spurts) during activities that increase intra-abdominal pressure (cough, laugh, sneeze, exercise); small postvoid volume
   d. Management: Kegel exercises (multiple contractions of pelvic floor muscles as if patient were interrupting flow of urine) to strengthen pelvic floor musculature; estrogen replacement therapy; use of a pessary; surgery (urethropexy to elevate the vesicourethral junction and return the hypermobile bladder neck to its original position)

3. Overflow incontinence
   a. Common in diabetic patients and patients with neurologic disorders
   b. Mechanism: Inadequate bladder contraction (due to impaired detrusor contractility) or a bladder outlet obstruction leads to urinary retention and subsequent overdistention of the bladder. Bladder pressure increases until it exceeds urethral resistance, and urine leakage occurs.
   c. Causes: neurogenic bladder (diabetic patients, lower motor neuron lesions), medications (anticholinergics, α-agonists, and epidural/spinal anesthetics), **obstruction to urine flow** (BPH, prostate cancer, urethral strictures, severe constipation with fecal impaction)
   d. Clinical features: nocturnal wetting, frequent loss of small amount of urine; large postvoid residual (usually exceeds 100 mL)
   e. Management (primarily medical): intermittent self-catheterization is best management; cholinergic agents (e.g., bethanechol) to increase bladder contractions; α-blockers (e.g., terazosin, doxazosin) to decrease sphincter resistance

4. Reflex incontinence
   a. Spinal cord injury is the most common cause. Other causes include multiple sclerosis, diabetes, tabes dorsalis, disc herniation, and spinal cord compression secondary to tumor.
   b. The patient cannot sense the need to urinate.

5. Functional incontinence—secondary to disabling and debilitating diseases

D. Diagnosis

1. Urinalysis (all patients)—to exclude infection and hematuria
2. Postvoid urine catheterization—Record the residual volume. Normal residual volume is less than 50 mL. A urine volume greater than 50 mL may indicate urinary obstruction or a hypotonic bladder.
3. Urine cultures—if dysuria and positive urinalysis
4. Renal function studies (BUN/Cr), glucose levels
5. Voiding record is useful—time, volume of episodes, record of oral intake, medications, associated activities
6. Perform further testing in carefully selected patients in whom the cause is not identified. Tests include cystometry, uroflow measurement/urethral pressure profile, imaging studies such as intravenous pyelogram, and voiding cystourethrogram, as needed.

- If urgency of urination is the prominent finding, suspect urge incontinence.
- If increased intra-abdominal pressure (cough, laugh) causes urine loss, suspect stress incontinence.

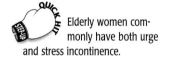

Elderly women commonly have both urge and stress incontinence.

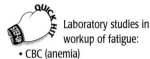

Laboratory studies in workup of fatigue:
- CBC (anemia)
- TSH (hypothyroidism)
- Fasting glucose (diabetes mellitus)
- BMP (electrolyte abnormalities)
- Urinalysis, BUN/creatinine (renal disease)
- LFT (liver disease)

Etiology of chronic fatigue
- Only 5% of cases are diagnosed as chronic fatigue syndrome.
- Most cases of chronic fatigue are due to depression, anxiety, or both (up to two thirds of cases).
- Between 20% and 25% of cases are idiopathic yet do not fit the criteria for chronic fatigue syndrome.
- Less than 5% are due to an unidentified medical illness.

Fatigue

A. General characteristics

1. Fatigue refers to a lack of energy or a sense of being tired—differentiate this from muscular weakness. It is not directly related to exertion.
2. Differential diagnosis
   a. Psychiatric causes—depression (most common cause); anxiety and somatization
   b. Endocrine causes—hypothyroidism, poorly controlled DM, apathetic hyperthyroidism of elderly patients, Addison's disease, hypopituitarism, hyperparathyroidism and other causes of hypercalcemia
   c. Hematologic/oncologic causes—severe anemia, occult malignancy (e.g., pancreatic carcinoma)
   d. Metabolic causes—chronic renal failure, hepatocellular failure
   e. Infectious diseases—mononucleosis, viral hepatitis, HIV, syphilis, hepatitis B and C, CMV, parasitic disease, tuberculosis and subacute bacterial endocarditis, Lyme disease
   f. Cardiopulmonary disease—OSA, CHF
   g. Medications—antihypertensive medications (clonidine, methyldopa), antidepressants (amitriptyline, doxepin, trazodone are more sedating), hypnotics, β-blockers, antihistamines, drug abuse/withdrawal
   h. Other causes: chronic fatigue syndrome, fibromyalgia, sleep disturbances (sleep apnea, narcolepsy, insomnia)
3. Chronic fatigue syndrome (CFS)
   a. CFS is profound fatigue for longer than 6 months that is not due to a medical or psychiatric disorder. More common in women.
   b. Cause is unknown. A flu-like illness may act as the triggering event, but infection has not been established as the proven cause. Other theories point to immunologic disturbance or endocrine dysfunction as possible causes.
   c. CFS is a diagnosis of exclusion—Rule out other causes before making a diagnosis of CFS.
   d. Most patients experience partial recovery within 2 years, but relapses can occur at any time.
   e. There are specific criteria for diagnosis. The key features include:
      - New or definite onset of unexplained fatigue, not alleviated by rest, not due to exertion, and significantly affecting quality of life.
      - Four or more of the following symptoms (for at least 6 months): diminished short-term memory or concentration, muscle pain, sore throat, tender lymph nodes, unrefreshing sleep, joint pain (without redness/swelling), headaches, postexertional malaise for longer than 24 hours.
   f. Depression is common in patients with CFS.

B. Diagnosis

1. Basic laboratory tests to exclude other causes—Consider CBC, LFTs, serum electrolytes, calcium, TSH, erythrocyte sedimentation rate, and HIV testing (if indicated).
2. Extensive testing other than the above is not indicated.

C. Treatment

1. Treat the underlying disorder, if known.
2. Treat CFS and patients with idiopathic fatigue as follows:
   a. Cognitive behavior therapy, including exercise, social, and psychological behavior modifications
   b. Antidepressants, as appropriate
   c. NSAIDs for relief of headache, arthralgias

Erectile Dysfunction

A. General characteristics

1. Erectile dysfunction is the recurring inability to achieve and maintain an erection sufficient for satisfactory sexual performance.

2. It is thought that up to half of all men in the United States between the ages of 40 and 70 have some form of erectile dysfunction. Prevalence increases with age.
3. Pathophysiology—once thought to be psychogenic in origin, it is now known that most cases (80%) are organic. A normal erection is largely dependent on the healthy penile and systemic vasculature.
4. Some cases of erectile dysfunction are psychogenic.

B. Risk factors

1. The most important risk factors are those that contribute to atherosclerosis (e.g., HTN, smoking, hyperlipidemia, diabetes).
2. Medications—antihypertensives (may indirectly lower intracavernosal pressure by virtue of lowering systemic BP)
3. Hematologic—sickle cell disease
4. History of pelvic surgery or perineal trauma
5. Alcohol abuse
6. Any cause of hypogonadism/low testosterone state, including hypo-thyroidism
7. Congenital penile curvature

C. Diagnosis

1. Detailed history and examination, including a digital rectal examination and neurologic examination. Assess for signs of PVD.
2. Laboratory tests—Obtain a CBC, chemistry panel, fasting glucose, and lipid profile. If there is hypogonadism or loss of libido, order serum testosterone, prolactin levels, and thyroid profile.
3. Nocturnal penile tumescence—If normal erections occur during sleep, a psychogenic cause is likely. If not, the cause is probably organic.
4. Consider vascular testing—evaluate arterial inflow and venous trapping of blood. Tests include intracavernosal injection of vasoactive substances, duplex ultrasound, and arteriography.
5. Psychologic testing may be appropriate in some cases.

D. Treatment

1. Treat the underlying cause. Address atherosclerotic risk factors.
2. Hormonal replacement (e.g., testosterone) in patients with hypogonadism
3. Sildenafil citrate (Viagra)—This is an oral phosphodiesterase inhibitor that promotes penile smooth muscle relaxation. It can be taken 30 to 60 minutes before anticipated intercourse. It is contraindicated with use of nitrates because together they can cause profound hypotension. There are other new drugs on the market, such as tadalafil.
4. Intracavernosal injections of vasoactive agents (patient learns to self-administer)
5. Vacuum constriction devices are rings placed around the base of the penis that enhance venous trapping of blood; they may interfere with ejaculation.
6. Psychologic therapy may be indicated to reduce performance anxiety and address underlying factors that may be causing or contributing to erectile dysfunction.

Alcoholism

A. General characteristics

1. Ten to fifteen percent of people have alcoholism (alcohol abuse or dependence). There is a **genetic component** to alcoholism—close relatives of alcoholics (especially sons) are at increased risk for alcoholism.
2. Screening for alcoholism—ask all patients about alcohol use. If alcoholism is suspected, use one of the following screening methods.
   a. CAGE (Any more than one positive answer may suggest alcohol abuse)
   • Cut down? (Have you ever felt the need to cut down on your drinking?)
   • Annoyed? (Have you ever felt annoyed by criticisms of your drinking?)
   • Guilty? (Have you ever felt guilty about drinking?)
   • Eye-opener? (Have you ever taken a morning eye-opener?)
   b. MAST (Michigan Alcoholism Screening Test) questionnaire—a 25-item questionnaire that also helps identify alcoholism

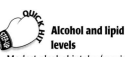

Alcohol and lipid levels

Modest alcohol intake (maximum of 1 to 2 drinks per day) is associated with an increase in HDL. On the other hand, alcohol use increases TG levels.

> **Box** 12-9 **Alcohol Withdrawal**
>
> - Features include tachycardia, sweating, anxiety, hallucinations
> - Goal is to prevent progression to delirium tremens (DT), which is a medical emergency (mortality rate, 20%). DT occurs in 5% of alcoholic withdrawals.
> - DT is delirium developing within a week of the last alcohol intake, usually 2 to 4 days after the last drink. DT is characterized by tactile hallucinations, visual hallucinations, confusion, sweating, increased tachycardia, and elevated BP.
> - Risk factors are pancreatitis, hepatitis, or other illness. DT is rare in healthy people.
> - Give benzodiazepines if withdrawal symptoms are present. Prevention of DT is the best treatment.
> - Diet is important in treatment (high in calorie, high in carbohydrates, multivitamins).

B. Complications

1. GI—gastritis, esophagitis, peptic ulcer disease, alcoholic liver disease (alcoholic hepatitis, cirrhosis, portal HTN), pancreatitis (acute and chronic), Mallory-Weiss tears
2. Cardiac—alcoholic cardiomyopathy, essential HTN (more than three drinks per day significantly increases BP)
3. CNS
   a. **Wernicke's encephalopathy**—often reversible
      - Caused by thiamine deficiency
      - Manifests as nystagmus, ataxia, ophthalmoplegia, confusion
   b. **Korsakoff's psychosis**—irreversible
      - Caused by thiamine deficiency
      - Alcohol-induced amnestic disorder
      - Mostly affects short-term memory; confabulation is common
4. Pulmonary—pneumonia, aspiration
5. Nutritional deficiencies (vitamins, minerals)—especially thiamine deficiency, hypomagnesemia, and folate deficiency
6. Peripheral neuropathy—due to thiamine deficiency
7. Sexual dysfunction—impotence, loss of libido
8. Psychiatric—depression, anxiety, insomnia
9. Increased risk of malignancy—esophagus, oral, liver, lung
10. Frequent falls, minor injuries, **motor vehicle accidents**

C. Treatment

1. Alcoholics Anonymous (AA) is the best treatment.
2. Disulfiram (Antabuse)—A few minutes after drinking alcohol, patient experiences shortness of breath, flushing, palpitations, tachycardia. If more alcohol is taken, headache and nausea/vomiting ensue. Symptoms last about 90 minutes. It is appropriate for short-term use and should not be taken chronically. Routine follow-up is important.
3. Naltrexone (Trexan)—This has been shown to improve abstinence rates. It reduces the craving for alcohol.
4. Drugs for withdrawal—benzodiazepines—best to use long-acting agents (diazepam)
5. Correction of fluid imbalance, vitamin supplementation (thiamine, folate, multivitamins)

Smoking

A. Health risks associated with cigarette smoking

1. Cardiovascular disease—CAD, acute MI, and stroke; there is a dose-dependent relationship between smoking and cardiovascular disease.
2. COPD risk increases with smoking in a dose-dependent manner.
3. Malignancy—Smoking increases the risk of cancer of the lungs, oral cavity, esophagus, larynx/pharynx, bladder, cervix, and pancreas.

QUICK HIT STEP-UP

Laboratory findings in alcoholics
- Anemia
- Macrocytic (most common)—due to folate deficiency
- Microcytic—due to GI bleeding
- LFTs: Increased GGT; AST–ALT ratio is 2:1
- Hypertriglyceridemia
- Hyperuricemia, hypocalcemia
- Thiamine deficiency
- Decreased testosterone level

AMBULATORY MEDICINE

4. PUD
5. Osteoporosis—decreases peak bone mass and increases the rate of bone loss
6. Premature skin aging
7. PVD, Buerger's disease
8. Adverse effects during pregnancy—Smoking increases risk of spontaneous abortion, fetal death, neonatal death, sudden infant death syndrome, and low birth weight.

B. Smoking cessation

1. Nicotine patch
   a. Quit rates are 2.5 times higher at 6 months than with placebo.
   b. Continuous nicotine delivery weans the patient from nicotine, and the dose is gradually decreased. There are no peaks or troughs as associated with smoking, so it eliminates nicotine withdrawal symptoms.
   c. The patch should be worn for 16 hours per day (should not be worn during sleep at night because it can cause headaches). The strongest dose (21-mg patch) is used for 1 month or so, then is gradually tapered to a lower dose (14-mg patch) for a few weeks, and finally to the lowest dose (7-mg patch) for a few weeks. Once the habit is broken, the patch use is stopped.
   d. **The patient should not continue to smoke while using the patch** (there have been case reports of MIs in these patients).
2. Nicotine chewing gum (4-mg and 2-mg gum)
   a. Gum is used whenever there is an urge to smoke. Use is continued for 2 to 4 months.
   b. It is less expensive than the nicotine patch and has similar quit rates.
   c. Many who do not have success with nicotine gum do not use enough of it.
3. Bupropion (Zyban)
   a. Quit rates are similar to that of nicotine replacement therapy (twice that of placebo).
   b. The patient continues treatment for up to 2 months.
   c. The patient can take bupropion in combination with nicotine replacement therapy—combined use may result in higher quit rates than either method alone.
   d. Adverse effects may include dry mouth, insomnia, and headaches.

QUICK HIT

Behavioral modification is crucial for long-term smoking cessation. The patch or gum should be used in conjunction with a smoking withdrawal clinic (behavioral program). Quit rates are higher with this combination.

HEALTH MAINTENANCE

A. Screening for hypertension

1. The United States Preventative Services Task Force (USPSTF) recommends screening all adults 18 years of age and older for HTN. However, other authorities do not recommend screening for HTN until middle age.
2. The recommended interval is 2 years, but this has not been firmly established.

B. Screening for hyperlipidemia

1. Healthy adults ≥20 years of age—**Measure a nonfasting total cholesterol and HDL cholesterol every 5 years.**
   a. If total cholesterol is <200 mg/dL and HDL is >35 mg/dL, repeat screening in 5 years.
   b. If total cholesterol is >240 mg/dL **or** between 200 and 240 with multiple risk factors, get a complete lipoprotein profile (TG levels and calculation of LDL).
   c. Calculating LDL level is not necessary for screening.
   d. Screen more frequently if the patient has increased risk of CAD (e.g., smokers, diabetic patients, family history of CAD, HTN).
2. Adults with CAD—Obtain a complete lipoprotein profile.

C. Colorectal cancer (CRC) screening/surveillance

1. Average-risk patients (patients >50 years of age with no GI symptoms)—**either** of the following:

QUICK HIT

For CRC screening, a colonoscopy is equivalent to flexible sigmoidoscopy plus barium enema but is more expensive.

a. Fecal occult blood test every year **+** flexible sigmoidoscopy every 5 years
b. Fecal occult blood test every year **+** colonoscopy every 10 years

2. Moderate-risk patients
   a. Patients with single or multiple polyps, personal history of CRC—initial colonoscopy; repeat at 3 years—if normal, then colonoscopy every 5 years
   b. Family history of CRC or adenomatous polyps in first-degree relatives—colonoscopy at age 40 or 10 years younger than the youngest case in family; if normal, repeat in 3 to 5 years
3. High-risk patients
   a. Families with familial adenomatous polyposis—genetic testing at age 10; consider colectomy if positive genetic testing or polyposis is confirmed; if not, colonoscopy every 1 to 2 years beginning at puberty
   b. Families with hereditary nonpolyposis colorectal cancer—genetic testing at age 21; if positive, colonoscopy every 2 years until age 40, and then every year thereafter

D. Prostate cancer screening
1. **This is controversial.**
2. The USPSTF has concluded that the evidence is not sufficient to determine whether the benefits of widespread screening (early detection) outweigh the harms (e.g., false-positives, unnecessary treatments, expenses).

E. Women's health
1. Breast cancer
   a. Monthly self-examination for all women ≥20 years of age; physician examination every 3 years until age 40, and yearly thereafter
   b. **Mammogram every 1 to 2 years for women ≥40 years of age** (controversial whether 1 or 2 years) and yearly for women ≥50 years of age
2. Cervical cancer—Pap smear
   a. **Start within 3 years of first sexual activity or at age 21 (whichever comes first).**
   b. If two consecutive smears (at ages 20 and 21) are negative, then repeat every 3 years until age 35, then repeat every 5 years until age 65.
   c. More frequent screening is recommended by some in younger women to due the increasing incidence of cervical cancer in this population, but this is controversial.
3. Sexually transmitted diseases (STDs)
   a. All women at risk should be screened for chlamydia and gonorrhea (pelvic examination with cultures or enzyme immunoassay or DNA probe).
   b. The USPSTF also recommends screening all sexually active women ages 25 and under for chlamydia.
   c. Women (and men) with risk factors should be counseled and screened for HIV on a periodic basis.

F. Miscellaneous
1. The USPSTF recommends screening all adults for depression (and providing appropriate treatment and follow-up). The USPSTF does not recommend for or against screening for dementia.
2. The USPSTF does not recommend routine screening of the general population for glaucoma, but refer any high-risk patients (e.g., family history) to an eye care provider for evaluation. **Remember to refer all diabetic patients to an ophthalmologist for annual funduscopic examination.**
3. Informally test hearing on a periodic basis in elderly patients. Younger adults do not need to be screened unless they are at increased risk (e.g., high occupational noise levels) for hearing impairment.
4. In elderly patients, assess risk factors for PVD, osteoporosis, stroke, and CAD.

TABLE 12-8 Vaccines

Vaccine	Recommended Recipients	Schedule	Contraindications
Influenza	Adults >50 years of age Adults <50 years of age with chronic medical problems (e.g., CHF, DM, lung disease, ESRD) Health care workers Pregnant women in 2nd or 3rd trimester during flu season Anyone wanting to reduce the risk of getting the flu	Given annually Best time to administer vaccine is October to November, but can also be given any time during flu season	Standard contraindications[a] History of severe anaphylaxis to eggs (patients can be tested with dilute vaccine, but vaccine is generally not recommended)
Pneumococcal polysaccharide	Adults >65 years of age Patients with sickle cell disease (usually functionally asplenic) or asplenia Adults with chronic medical problems or immunodeficiencies Women with high-risk pregnancies	Administered as a one-time dose Second dose should be administered 5 years after the first dose for patients at highest risk (e.g., those with asplenia or immunodeficiency, or those requiring dialysis)	Standard contraindications
Tetanus/diphtheria (Td)	Primary series for everyone When indicated in wound management Individuals traveling to countries where risk of diphtheria is high	Primary series: Three doses (1, 1–2, 6–12 mo) After primary series, booster dose q 10 years For the unvaccinated, three doses (0, 1–2 mo, 6–12 mo intervals)	Standard contraindications
Hepatitis B	Given as primary series to infants Patients at risk for HBV[b] Health care workers	Given as three doses (0, 1, 6 mo)	Standard contraindications
Hepatitis A	Travelers to developing countries Patients with chronic liver disease, HCV	Given in two doses Minimum time interval between first and second dose is 6 mo	Safety during pregnancy undetermined
Measles-mumps-rubella (live vaccine) "live"	Given as primary series in children Adults born after 1957 or later who are ≥18 years of age (those born before 1957 are considered immune) if there is no proof of vaccination or immunity All women of childbearing age without proof of rubella immunity or vaccination Health care workers	Given as one or two doses Give the second dose at least 4 weeks after the first dose	Pregnancy Significant immunocompromise[c] (e.g., malignancy, any kind of immunosuppressive medication, radiation therapy) Standard contraindications
Varicella (live vaccine) "live"	Given as primary series in children Adults and adolescents who never had chickenpox (chickenpox confers immunity) Susceptible, close contacts of immunocompromised patients Postexposure prophylaxis in susceptible individuals	Given as two doses, with second dose given 4–8 weeks after first dose	Pregnancy Immunocompromise due to malignancy or cellular immunodeficiency due to HIV or AIDS[d] Standard contraindications
Varicella (shingles) vaccine	Adults >60 years of age (but more data needed)		

(continued)

AMBULATORY MEDICINE

TABLE 12-8	Vaccines *(Continued)*		
Vaccine	**Recommended Recipients**	**Schedule**	**Contraindications**
Polio (inactivated)	Given as primary series in children Not routinely given to unvaccinated adults unless they plan to travel to endemic areas	Refer to ACIP guidelines for schedules and dosing information	Standard contraindications
Meningococcus (serotypes A, C, W-135, and Y)	Asplenic individuals Travelers to area where meningococcal disease is epidemic Military personnel All college students Close contacts of patients with sporadic disease	Administered as single dose	Standard contraindications
Rabies	See Chapter 10 Postexposure prophylaxis Individuals at high risk for exposure to rabies		
HPV vaccine (human papilloma virus)	Recommended for females age 9-26.		

*ᵃStandard contraindications include a history of anaphylactic reaction to the vaccine as well as moderate to severe illness. **Mild illness is not a contraindication.** Unless specified, breastfeeding is not a contraindication to vaccine.*

ᵇPatients at risk for HBV include injectable drug users, practicing male homosexuals, heterosexuals who have had more than one sex partner in the past 6 months, patients recently diagnosed with STDs, sexual partners of HB$_s$Ag-positive patients, and patients on hemodialysis.

ᶜNote that HIV positivity is not a contraindication to the measles-mumps-rubella vaccine unless the patient is severely immunocompromised.

ᵈNote that immunosuppressive therapy is not per se a contraindication to varicella vaccine, but the physician should refer to the ACIP guidelines for delay of vaccine.

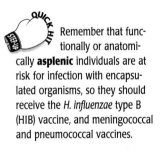

Remember that functionally or anatomically **asplenic** individuals are at risk for infection with encapsulated organisms, so they should receive the *H. influenzae* type B (HIB) vaccine, and meningococcal and pneumococcal vaccines.

G. Vaccinations

1. Vaccination is most commonly associated with children but is very important in adults as well, especially elderly patients and those with chronic medical problems.
2. The most important vaccinations to know are influenza, pneumococcal polysaccharide, hepatitis B, and tetanus; for who should receive them and when, see Table 12-8.
3. There are many misconceptions about contraindications to vaccination. The following are **not** contraindications to vaccination.
   a. Mild illness (e.g., common cold, low-grade fever, mild diarrhea)
   b. Convalescent phase of an illness
   c. Recent exposure to a communicable disease
   d. Breastfeeding
   e. Current antibiotic therapy
   f. History of a nonspecific reaction to penicillin

Appendix

RADIOGRAPHIC INTERPRETATION

Chest Radiograph (CXR)

A. Views: Obtain PA and lateral views for all patients who are well enough to be transported to the radiology department and maintain an upright position. Obtain an AP film (i.e., portable CXR) for all patients who are too ill to be transported and positioned for a PA film.

B. Always try to compare a patient's CXR with a previous film to note any changes in condition and to assess whether changes are new or chronic.

C. Density: The lower the density, the more radiolucent (or transparent) the object will appear on plain radiographs. Following are structures in the body (main composition) listed from most radiolucent to most radiopaque: air (lungs, trachea, gastric bubble), fat (breasts), fluid (most of the structures have high fluid content [e.g., vessels, heart, soft tissues]), bone, metallic foreign bodies (e.g., bullets, orthopedic hardware).

D. Assessment of the film's quality
1. Assess penetration
   a. The intervertebral spaces should be visible on a good-quality film.
   b. The outline of the vertebral bodies should be visible within (or through) the cardiac silhouette.
2. Assess inspiratory effort
   a. A CXR is usually taken at the end of a full, deep inspiration. You should be able to see at least nine posterior ribs on the right side above the diaphragm. In general, if the diaphragm is crossing the tenth rib posteriorly (or the eighth rib anteriorly), inspiratory effort is optimal.
   b. Patients who are ill may not be able to hold a full, deep breath for the CXR, leading to a poor inspiratory effort.
   c. The heart appears larger than it actually is when there is poor inspiratory effort, which can be misleading.
3. Assess for rotation
   a. There should be symmetrical spacing of the clavicles on either side of the sternum, otherwise the patient is probably rotated.
   b. Imagine a horizontal line connecting the clavicular heads and a vertical line down the midline connecting the spinous processes of the vertebrae—these lines should be perpendicular to one another.

E. Examination of the PA/AP CXR (see Figure A-1): No one approach is standard. Be sure to observe the following points:
1. Examine bones: shoulders, clavicles, cervical and thoracic spine, and ribs—on PA films, the horizontal ribs are posterior (anterior ribs are angled downward).

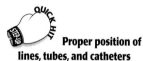

Proper position of lines, tubes, and catheters
- Endotracheal tube—The tip should be approximately 4 to 6 cm above the tracheal carina (this is about the level of the clavicular heads).
- Central line—The tip should be above the right atrium in the superior vena cava.
- Swan-Ganz catheter—The tip should be within the right or left main pulmonary arteries.
- Nasogastric tube—This should be proximal to the gastric pylorus and distal to the esophagogastric junction.

FIGURE
A-1 **A.** PA chest radiograph with diagrammatic overlay: 1. first rib; 2. upper portion of manubrium; 3. trachea; 4. right main bronchus; 5. left main bronchus; 6. main pulmonary artery; 7. left pulmonary artery; 8. right interlobar pulmonary artery; 9. right pulmonary vein; 10. aortic arch. **B.** Chest radiograph of the same subject without diagrammatic overlay. (*continued*)

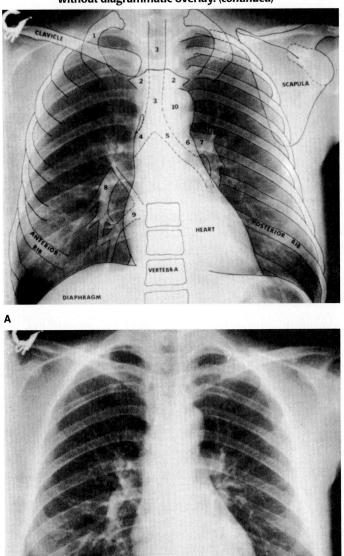

A

B

(**A** and **B** from George RB, Light RW, Matthay MA, et al. Chest Medicine–Essentials of Pulmonary and Critical Care Medicine. 4th Ed. Philadelphia: Lippincott Williams & Wilkins, 2000:69, Figure 5.1A and B.)

FIGURE
A-1 (*Continued*) **C.** Lateral chest radiograph of the same patient as in A: 1. trachea; 2. right upper lobe bronchus; 3. left upper lobe bronchus; 4. right pulmonary artery; 5. left pulmonary artery; 6. inferior vena cava; 7. ascending aorta; 8. descending aorta. **D.** Same lateral chest radiograph without diagrammatic overlay. **E.** Technical adequacy of a chest radiograph: 1. A technically adequate chest radiograph should be labeled with the patient's name, the date, and a side marker; 2. The midportion of the right hemidiaphragm should be below the 10th rib; 3. Vertebral bodies should be visualized throughout the spine; 4. Pulmonary vessels should be visible to the outer third of the lung; 5. The thoracic spinous processes should be midway between the heads of the clavicle.

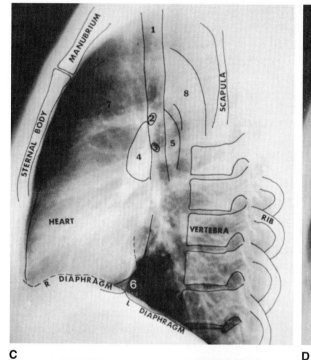

C

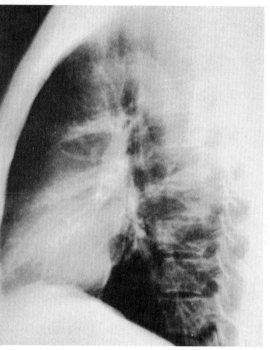

D

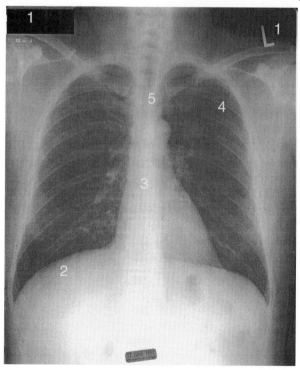

E

(**C** and **D** from George RB, Light RW, Matthay MA, et al. Chest Medicine—Essentials of Pulmonary and Critical Care Medicine. 4th Ed. Philadelphia: Lippincott Williams & Wilkins, 2000:70, Figure 5.2A and B.)

(**E** from Humes DH, DuPont HL, Gardner LB, et al. Kelley's Textbook of Internal Medicine. 4th Ed. Philadelphia: Lippincott Williams & Wilkins, 2000:2570, Figure 386.3.).

2. Evaluate cardiac size—The transverse diameter of the cardiac silhouette should not be more than half the transverse diameter of the thorax; this is the cardiothoracic ratio. (A larger cardiothoracic ratio is acceptable for an AP film because the cardiac silhouette is larger on an AP film.)
3. Check for mediastinal widening, which may be present in aortic dissection, trauma, and lymphoma.
4. Evaluate the position of the trachea; it should be in the midline.
5. Compare right and left lung fields. It is best to divide the lung fields into thirds (horizontally) and compare the two sides.
   a. Look for any infiltrates or consolidation.
   b. Congestion—Look for signs of CHF; large heart without "shape"; pulmonary vessels are more visible and extend further into the lung field than normal.
   c. Pneumothorax—Look for a line demarcating free air (hyperlucent with no pulmonary vascular markings) in the pleural space.
   d. Pleural effusion—Examine the costophrenic angles; they should be sharp and clear without any blunting.
   e. Look at the diaphragms—the right diaphragm is normally slightly higher than the left.

F. Examination of the lateral film (see Figure A-1)
   1. Look at the cardiac silhouette
      a. Anterior border—formed by the right ventricle
      b. Posteroinferior border—formed by the left ventricle
      c. Posterosuperior border—formed by the left atrium
      d. The right atrium cannot be seen.
   2. Look at the trachea.
   3. Examine the retrosternal and retrocardiac spaces for any abnormalities.
   4. Examine the diaphragms—note that the anterior portion of the left hemidiaphragm is not visible because of the cardiac silhouette. The entire right hemidiaphragm should be visible, however.

Abdominal Radiographs

A. The standard abdominal film—KUB—is a supine view, which is ideal for seeing the gas pattern.

B. Order an obstruction series (includes PA CXR, as well as supine and upright abdominal films) to evaluate the gas pattern and to look for the following:
   1. Free intraperitoneal air (see below)—free air is seen under the diaphragm on the CXR. If the patient is too ill to be upright, order a left lateral decubitus film instead (air rises to the nondependent area).
   2. Air-fluid levels—seen on the upright film (see below)

C. Most important things to look for on abdominal films
   1. Air-fluid levels—sign of obstruction; if prominent and multiple, mechanical obstruction is more likely than ileus.
   2. Free air under the diaphragm (perforation of a viscous)—this is a surgical emergency.
   3. Dilated loops of bowel (obstruction, ileus)—It may be difficult to distinguish mechanical obstruction from ileus. The following may help:
      a. If air is in the small intestine, colon, and rectum, ileus is more likely because ileus distention involves the entire GI tract.
      b. In small bowel obstruction, there are distended loops of small bowel proximal to the site of obstruction and multiple air-fluid levels on upright or decubitus films. Colonic gas is usually minimal.

c. In large bowel obstruction, look for haustral markings—they span one-half to two-thirds of the diameter of large bowel—as well as the colonic shadow on the periphery or in the pelvis.

d. In an ileus, the dilated loops are scattered and lack organization (e.g., like a "bag of popcorn"); in mechanical obstruction, dilated loops are stacked on top of one another (e.g., like a "bag of sausages").

e. Too little gas in the abdomen can be due to high obstruction.

ELECTROCARDIOGRAM INTERPRETATION

Electrocardiogram (ECG) Pearls

A. Always look for an old ECG with which to compare the current ECG. This is critical in assessing whether any significant changes have occurred.

B. Determine rate

1. Count the number of large blocks (with five little squares) between each R wave. Divide this number by 300 (the distance between large blocks represents 1/300 minute). Therefore, if there are four blocks between each R wave, there is 4/300 or 1/75 minute between each R wave, which means that the rate is 75. (Note that this is the same as the 300-150-75-60-50 rule.)

2. If the rate is irregular, count the number of beats in 6 seconds and multiply by 10.

3. Each block is 1 mm (0.04 seconds), so 5 boxes equals 0.20 seconds.

4. Tachycardia is defined as a rate >100 beats/min.

5. Bradycardia is defined as a rate of <60 beats/min.

C. Determine rhythm (look at lead II)—Is the rhythm regular or irregular? Note that rhythms may be regularly irregular or irregularly irregular as well. (See Chapter 1, Arrhythmias section.)

D. Determine axis

1. Look at the QRS complex in leads I and aVF.

2. If both are mainly positive, then the axis is normal.

3. If mainly positive in lead I and mainly negative in aVF, the axis is deviated to the left.

4. If mainly negative in lead I and mainly positive in aVF, the axis is deviated to the right.

5. If mainly negative in both I and aVF, then there is extreme right axis deviation.

E. Intervals

1. P-R interval—This should be <0.2 seconds.

   a. In **first-degree heart block**, the P-R interval is >0.2 seconds (one large box).

   b. In **second-degree AV block** (Wenckebach or **Mobitz type I**), there is a progressive lengthening of the P-R interval followed by a dropped QRS complex.

   c. In the **Mobitz type II** form of second-degree heart block, the P-R interval is constant, but not every P wave is followed by a QRS complex. There may be two, three, or even more P waves before a QRS, but the ratio of P waves to QRS complexes (e.g., 2:1, 3:1) is constant.

   d. **In third-degree heart** block, there is no relationship between atrial (P waves) and ventricular (QRS) activity.

2. QRS complex—This should be <0.12 seconds.

   a. Prolongation of the QRS complex is seen in bundle branch block, ventricular rhythms, and paced rhythms.

   b. In **right bundle branch block (RBBB)**, look for a widened QRS complex, an rSR wave in the chest leads, and a wide S wave in lead I.

c. In **left bundle branch block (LBBB)**, look for a widened QRS complex and loss of Q waves with broad, notched R waves in leads I, V_5, or V_6.

3. QT interval—The normal QT interval should be less than half of the R-R interval (<0.42 seconds). Prolongation of the QT interval may be seen in the following.

   a. Medications: tricyclic antidepressants, phenothiazines, nonsedating antihistamines; class IA, IC, and III antiarrhythmics
   b. Electrolyte disturbances: hypocalcemia, hypokalemia
   c. Congenital long QT syndromes
   d. Other: ischemia, significant bradyarrhythmias, and certain CNS lesions

F. Examine waves

1. P waves—There should be one P wave for each QRS complex in a normal sinus rhythm.

   a. **Left atrial enlargement**—wide P wave (>0.12 sec.) in lead II or a diphasic P wave with a deep terminal component in V_1
   b. **Right atrial enlargement**—tall P wave (>2.5 mm) in lead II or a diphasic P wave with a large initial component in V_1
   c. **Multifocal atrial tachycardia**—At least three different P wave morphologies are present.

2. Q waves—indicate myocardial necrosis (acute or old MI)

   a. To be considered significant, they must be >0.04 seconds wide and $>25\%$ of the QRS amplitude.
   b. Isolated Q waves in certain leads may be normal, especially in aVR.

3. QRS complex

   a. Should be narrow (<0.12 sec) with a regular morphology
   b. The following are indicators of **left ventricular hypertrophy** (LVH).
   - S wave in V_1 or $V_2 \geq 30$ mm high
   - R wave in V_5 or $V_6 > 26$ mm high
   - S wave in V_1 + R wave in V_5 or $V_6 > 35$ mm high in adults ($>$age 30)
   - Left axis deviation is often present.
   c. The following are indicators of **right ventricular hypertrophy** (RVH).
   - R wave ≥ 7 mm in V_1
   - R/S ratio in $V_1 \geq 1$
   - Progressive decrease in R wave height across the precordial leads
   - Right axis deviation is often present.

4. ST segments

   a. ST segment depression can occur in the following conditions:
   - Myocardial ischemia
   - Subendocardial MI
   - Digitalis
   - Hypokalemia
   - LBBB
   b. ST segment elevation is a key indicator of myocardial necrosis—It is a hallmark of acute transmural MI, but may persist in an old MI.
   - ST segment elevations in I, aVL, V_5, and V_6 are consistent with a lateral wall MI (circumflex coronary artery).
   - ST segment elevations in V_1 to V_4 are consistent with an anterior wall MI (left anterior descending coronary artery).
   - ST segment elevations in II, III, and aVF are consistent with an inferior wall MI (terminal branches of right or left coronary artery).
   - Diffuse ST segment elevations may be present in pericarditis.
   - Small, concave ST segment elevations may be a normal finding in young people (early repolarization).
   - If LBBB is present, ST segment elevations may be present and are an unreliable indicator of ischemia/infarction.

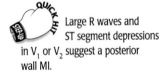

Large R waves and ST segment depressions in V_1 or V_2 suggest a posterior wall MI.

5. T waves
   a. Peaked T waves may be present in the following situations:
      • Very early stages of MI (before true infarction occurs)
      • Hyperkalemia
      • Hypermagnesemia
   b. T wave inversions may be present in the following situations:
      • Myocardial ischemia/infarction
      • Pericarditis
      • Cardiomyopathy
      • Intracranial bleeding
      • Electrolyte disturbances, acidosis
      • LBBB, LVH
      • Small T wave inversions may be normal in the limb leads.

Intravenous (IV) Therapy

A. Forms of IV therapy
1. "IV push"—This is administration of a medication directly into the IV access. It is typically used in emergency situations when a rapid response is needed or when a loading dose of a medication is to be given, followed by a continuous infusion.
2. Continuous administration—Electronic devices deliver fluid or medication at a preset volume per hour.
3. Intermittent administration can be accomplished via a number of methods.
   a. Heparin lock or saline lock—This is used when the patient no longer needs IV fluids and IV medications can be given intermittently. The IV line is kept open with saline or heparin when no medication is being given.
   b. Piggyback—A medication or solution is given through another established primary infusion. The first bag that is hung is the primary infusion. Tubes from both the primary bag and the piggyback bag connect to a common tube that feeds into the patient's vein.
   c. Nontunneled central catheter—The exit site of the catheter is at the skin. Locations include internal jugular (IJ), femoral, and subclavian veins.
   d. Tunneled central catheters (e.g., Hickman)—The catheter is inserted into the subclavian vein, but the end of the catheter is then "tunneled" in the subcutaneous tissue so that it exits the skin away from the site of vein insertion. With both nontunneled and tunneled central catheters, there is easy access but also the risk of infection at the exit site.
   e. Ports—The catheter is inserted into a central vein and is tunneled subcutaneously. There is not an exit site because the catheter attaches to the port (chamber) that is placed subcutaneously as well. To administer medication, an anesthetic agent is used to numb the skin, and the needle is inserted into the chamber. Often used for chemotherapy administration. Port-a-Cath is an example. There is less risk of infection (no exit site), but access is more difficult and must be performed by a medical professional.
   f. Peripherally inserted central catheter (PICC) line—These are often used to administer IV antibiotics at home (or blood products, other medications, or chemotherapy). Locations include cephalic, basilic, or brachial veins. A peripherally inserted central catheter is inserted through the veins of the antecubital fossa, and the tip is advanced into the super vena cava. It can be left in place for weeks to months.

B. Complications of IV therapy
1. Thrombophlebitis—manifested by redness, swelling, and pain at IV site; can be prevented by changing the IV every 2 to 3 days
2. Infiltration—Medication/fluid leaks into the surrounding tissue. If it is significant and involves a large area, it may lead to compartment syndrome.
3. Blockage
4. Air embolus

Central Venous Line

A. Indications

1. Hemodynamic monitoring (e.g., placement of a pulmonary artery catheter)
2. Transvenous pacing
3. Emergent or short-term hemodialysis
4. Emergent delivery of IV medications (particularly in cardiac arrest)—If feasible, it is generally preferable to have a central venous catheter over a peripheral catheter for the administration of drugs in cardiac arrest because the medication is delivered to the heart and the arterial vasculature more rapidly.
5. To administer TPN—The high concentration makes it difficult to administer this through peripheral veins.
6. Administration of medications that can be harmful if given peripherally.
   a. Irritating medications, which can cause thrombophlebitis in peripheral veins (e.g., high-concentration potassium chloride, chemotherapy)
   b. Vasopressors—They cause arterial vasoconstriction and should not be given through peripheral lines, because if infiltration occurs in a peripheral line, it may cause compartment syndrome or skin necrosis.
7. Volume replacement (fluid or blood)—If large volumes of fluid must be given rapidly, large-diameter central catheters are sometimes needed, particularly if the patient does not have adequate peripheral access. (But remember that the flow rate of saline or blood is generally higher in a large-bore peripheral catheter than a central venous catheter because the peripheral catheter is shorter in length.)
8. Although routine or frequent blood draws are not an indication for central venous line placement, an already-existing central line can be used for this purpose.

B. Sites

1. Internal jugular (IJ) vein
2. Subclavian vein
3. Femoral vein

C. Complications

1. Pneumothorax
   a. Can occur with subclavian lines and IJ lines (but more common with subclavian lines); obviously does not occur with femoral lines
   b. Note that patients on PEEP have hyperinflated lungs, and the apex of the lungs is more superior than normal, increasing the chances of an iatrogenic pneumothorax.
2. Venous air embolism—If air is sucked into the vena cava, it can be pumped through the right ventricle into the lungs, leading to pulmonary embolism (PE) of air (instead of clot). This is a potentially life-threatening complication. If the patient has a patent foramen ovale, it can result in a paradoxical air embolism to the brain.
3. Puncture of adjacent artery (carotid, subclavian, or femoral)—Depending on the site, this can lead to complications including hemothorax (subclavian) and hematoma (IJ and femoral). Apply compression if this occurs.
4. Infection—Central lines very commonly cause infections at the site of entry and often lead to sepsis, which can be life-threatening.
5. Thrombosis and thrombophlebitis

Arterial Lines

- Definition—IV catheters (same ones used for peripheral lines) that are inserted into the radial artery (rarely in ulnar or brachial artery)

- Immediately after placing a central line (IJ or subclavian), obtain a CXR to check for pneumothorax and to ensure proper position of the catheter tip. The catheter tip should be in the superior vena cava.
- When removing a line, the patient should be supine and should exhale during removal to prevent an air embolism.

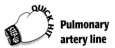

Pulmonary artery line

- A central catheter that is inserted through one of the large veins, threaded through the right ventricle, and into the pulmonary artery
- Sometimes called "Swan-Ganz lines" (after the inventors, Dr. Swan and Dr. Ganz)
- Used to measure various hemodynamic parameters, including central venous pressure, PCWP, cardiac index and output, stroke volume, and systemic vascular resistance

- Uses—Arterial lines have two major uses.
  - BP monitoring is the most important—Arterial lines give more accurate readings than noninvasive blood pressure cuffs. A patient on a pressor or in the ICU generally should have an A-line for proper BP monitoring.
  - Used for frequent blood gas draws

Nutritional Support

A. Enteral nutrition (administered into the GI tract)

1. Enteral nutrition is preferred over parenteral nutrition because the intestine is used in a physiologic manner.
2. There are two methods of administering enteral nutrition.
   a. Nasoenteric tubes (e.g., nasojejunal tubes)—best for short-term nutrition.
   b. Enterostomy tubes (e.g., PEG/G-tubes, J-tubes)—for long-term support.
3. There are many different formulas available for tube feeds—special formulas can be provided for patients with renal disease, liver disease, CHF, and so on.
4. Tube feeds can be delivered intermittently (in boluses) or continuously.
   a. Intermittent feeding (into the stomach) requires close monitoring (by nurses)—gastric residuals should be checked every 4 hours and tube feeds should be held if the residual is >150 mL. Intermittent feeding has a higher risk of aspiration than continuous feeding.
   b. Continuous feeding (into duodenum or jejunum) has a lower risk of aspiration than intermittent feeding and requires less monitoring by nurses.
5. Complications of enteral nutrition
   a. Intolerance to tube feeds—check for diarrhea, constipation, nausea, vomiting, abdominal pain, or distention
   b. Malpositioning of tube (in trachea/bronchus)
   c. Aspiration pneumonia
   d. Overload of solutes—due to high rate of hyperosmolar feedings (can cause diarrhea, electrolyte imbalance, hyperglycemia)

There are two means of providing nutrition for a patient who cannot eat: enteral nutrition and parenteral nutrition.

- PEG tube—The tube is inserted with the help of an endoscope through the mouth. Alternatively, it can also be done through an open abdominal incision, which is called open gastrostomy.
- The J-tube (jejunostomy) is placed in the intestine and can only be done through an open abdominal procedure.

B. Parenteral nutrition (administered into the vasculature)

1. The term TPN is used for a high-concentration solution that can be given alone to meet the body's caloric demands. Parenteral nutrition can also play a supplementary role when enteral feeding alone is inadequate.
2. It is used if the patient cannot eat for prolonged periods or cannot tolerate enteral feedings, and in severely malnourished patients.
3. There are two ways of administration.
   a. Central—via central venous catheter (e.g., subclavian vein)—preferred in patients who require long-term support
   b. Peripheral—via peripheral line—One cannot administer as much protein or calories with this as with a central line. It should only be used for a short-term period. TPN cannot be administered in a peripheral line.
4. Complications of parenteral nutrition
   a. Electrolyte imbalances, volume disturbances
   b. Hyperglycemia
   c. Complications associated with placing a central line (e.g., pneumothorax)
   d. Infection of central (or peripheral) line

Guide to Antibacterial Antibiotic Therapy (see Table A-1)

A. Cell wall inhibitors

1. Penicillins
   a. Mechanism of action
      - Inhibit cross-linkage (transpeptidation step) of bacterial cell walls as they are synthesized
      - Bacterial cell walls lose structural and osmotic integrity.

- Cell lysis ultimately occurs.
- To achieve the desired effect, penicillins must first bind to proteins located inside the bacterial cell wall. These proteins are called penicillin-binding proteins.

b. Antimicrobial coverage (not exhaustive)
- More effective against **gram-positive** than gram-negative organisms
- Acts synergistically with aminoglycosides
- Penicillin G is used to treat syphilis. Because of microbial resistance, it is used less commonly to treat respiratory tract infections caused by streptococcal species, such as pharyngitis secondary to *Streptococcus pyogenes* or pneumococcal pneumonia.
- Penicillin V has some anaerobic activity, so it is more useful for dental infections.
- Ampicillin and amoxicillin have extended gram-negative activity.
- Methicillin and nafcillin are used to treat staphylococcal infections.
- Penicillins are generally ineffective against intracellular bacteria.

c. Adverse reactions
- **Hypersensitivity reactions**—Type I hypersensitivity reaction may present as rash, angioedema, or even anaphylaxis.
- Diarrhea
- Interstitial nephritis

d. Other features
- Penicillin is used as prophylaxis against infection in patients with sickle cell disease.
- Bacteria gain resistance to penicillins through alterations in penicillin-binding proteins—e.g., MRSA.
- Resistance is also conferred by β-lactamases, enzymes that hydrolyze the penicillin's β-lactam ring.

e. Examples (list of examples is not exhaustive)
- Penicillin G
- Penicillin V
- Ampicillin
- Amoxicillin
- Methicillin
- Nafcillin
- Piperacillin

2. **Cephalosporins**
a. Mechanism of action
- Similar mechanism of action to penicillin
- As with penicillin, the β-lactam ring confers **bactericidal** activity.

b. Antimicrobial coverage (not necessarily exhaustive—this applies to the rest of antimicrobial section)
- Cephalosporins are classified according to antimicrobial activity and β-lactamase resistance into "generations."
- First-generation cephalosporins generally serve as substitutes for penicillin, and also have coverage against *Proteus*, *Klebsiella*, and *Escherichia coli*.
- Second-generation cephalosporins have more gram-negative activity and less gram-positive activity. They are used to treat *Haemophilus influenzae* and *Enterobacter* spp.
- Third-generation cephalosporins have even more **gram-negative activity** and are **able to cross the blood-brain barrier.**
- Fourth-generation cephalosporins are the most broad-spectrum, including activity against *Pseudomonas*, *Neisseria*, and methicillin-sensitive *S. aureus*, as well as most of the above-mentioned organisms.

c. Adverse reactions
- **Hypersensitivity reactions**—Allergic cross-reaction with penicillin can occur in 10% of cephalosporins.

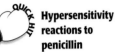

Hypersensitivity reactions to penicillin
- Type I hypersensitivity reaction
- This may present with rash, angioedema, or even anaphylaxis.
- Cross-reactions with other β-lactam antibiotics can occur.
- Nausea, vomiting, and diarrhea are **not** hypersensitivity reactions.
- It may develop at any time, even if past treatments with penicillin were uneventful.

- Certain cephalosporins promote a bleeding diathesis, which is reversible with vitamin K.
- Other cephalosporins cause a disulfiram-like reaction to alcohol.

d. Other features
- First-generation cephalosporins are used for surgical prophylaxis or minor forms of cellulitis.
- Most forms of cephalosporins must be administered intravenously.
- Cefuroxime is sometimes used to treat community-acquired pneumonia.
- Cefoxitin can be used for abdominal infections, such as peritonitis.
- Ceftriaxone can be given as an IM injection to treat gonorrhea. Intravenously it plays an important role in empiric treatment for meningitis.

e. Examples (list of examples is not exhaustive)
- First-generation: cefazolin, cephalexin, cefadroxil
- Second-generation: cefaclor, cefoxitin, cefuroxime, cefotetan
- Third-generation: ceftriaxone, cefixime, cefotaxime, ceftibuten
- Fourth-generation: cefepime

3. **Miscellaneous cell wall inhibitors**

a. Vancomycin
- Inhibits cell wall synthesis by interfering with cross-linkage of peptidoglycan chains (different site of action from penicillin), also damages cell membranes
- Main use is to treat staphylococcal infections resistant to other β-lactams, such as MRSA, or if penicillin allergy is present; not used for gram-negative organisms
- Acts synergistically with aminoglycosides to treat enterococcal infections
- Adverse reactions include fever, nephrotoxicity, ototoxicity, and "**red man syndrome**" (flushing due to infusion-induced histamine release).
- Serum levels must be followed up in prolonged therapy, and doses must be adjusted for renal insufficiency.
- Vancomycin resistance is an emerging, ominous phenomenon.

b. Carbapenems
- Synthetic β-lactams designed to be more resistant to β-lactamases and penicillinases.
- Imipenem and meropenem are the only available carbapenems in the United States.
- They are often combined with cilastatin. This combination results in broad-spectrum antimicrobial coverage, including penicillin-resistant pneumococci, *Pseudomonas*, anaerobes, and *Enterobacter* infections.
- They are used empirically for patients in whom gram-negative sepsis is suspected.
- They may cause nausea, vomiting, and sometimes neutropenia.
- They reduce the seizure threshold.

c. Monobactams
- Aztreonam is currently the only available preparation in the United States.
- Synthetic β-lactam with resistance to β-lactamases
- Narrow spectrum of activity: primarily aerobic gram-negative rods, including *Pseudomonas* and *Serratia*
- Less cross-reactivity with penicillin than other β-lactam antibiotics

d. β-Lactamase inhibitors
- Examples include sulbactam, tazobactam, and clavulanic acid.
- Not used by themselves, but rather combined with penicillins to enhance antimicrobial activity (e.g., amoxicillin + clavulanic acid = Augmentin)

e. Bacitracin
- Inhibits bacterial cell wall synthesis by inhibiting transport of peptidoglycans
- Effective against gram-positive organisms
- Used **topically** only (because it is so nephrotoxic)

B. Protein synthesis inhibitors

1. **Tetracycline**
   a. Mechanism of action
      - Inhibits protein synthesis by binding to 30 S subunit of bacterial ribosome
      - **Bacteriostatic**
   b. Antimicrobial coverage
      - Effective against certain intracellular bacteria: chlamydia, rickettsial diseases (e.g., Rocky Mountain spotted fever), mycoplasma
      - Treats gram-negative *Vibrio cholerae*
      - Also treats spirochete causing Lyme disease (*Borrelia burgdorferi*)
   c. Adverse reactions
      - GI—epigastric pain, nausea, vomiting
      - **Deposits occur in calcified tissues** (e.g., teeth and bones of the fetus if given during pregnancy and potentially in any child <8 years of age). This can result in permanent discoloration of teeth, stunting of growth, and skeletal deformities.
      - Phototoxicity
      - Hepatotoxicity—may occur in pregnant women
   d. Cautions
      - Do not give to pregnant women or children <8 years of age.
      - Do not give to patients with renal insufficiency (except doxycycline).
      - Decreased absorption occurs if taken with milk and antacids.
      - Resistance is common.
   e. Examples
      - Tetracycline
      - Doxycycline
      - Minocycline

2. **Macrolides**
   a. Mechanism of action
      - Inhibit protein synthesis by binding to 50 S subunit of bacterial ribosome
      - **Bacteriostatic** (may be bactericidal at high doses)
   b. Antimicrobial coverage
      - Good at treating intracellular pathogens, such as *Mycoplasma* and *Legionella*
      - Erythromycin and clarithromycin have activity against staphylococci and streptococci.
      - Erythromycin (or clarithromycin) is the treatment of choice for *Mycoplasma* pneumonia ("walking pneumonia") and *Legionella* spp.
      - Erythromycin is also appropriate as an alternative to penicillin G if there is a penicillin allergy (e.g., treatment of chlamydia in pregnancy, to avoid tetracycline).
      - Azithromycin and clarithromycin have activity against *H. influenzae*.
      - Azithromycin also treats *Moraxella catarrhalis*.
   c. Adverse reactions
      - GI side effects are the most common and include epigastric pain, nausea, and vomiting (particularly with erythromycin).
      - Cholestasis
   d. Cautions
      - Erythromycin should not be prescribed to patients with liver failure because it is metabolized in the liver.
      - Erythromycin and clarithromycin interact with many drugs due to their inhibitory effect on the P-450 system.
   e. Examples
      - Azithromycin
      - Clarithromycin
      - Erythromycin

3. **Aminoglycosides**
   a. Mechanism of action
      - Inhibit protein synthesis by binding to 30 S subunit of bacterial ribosome
      - **Bactericidal**
   b. Antimicrobial coverage
      - Treat gram-negative aerobes, such as *E. coli or Klebsiella*
      - Sometimes used in combination with ampicillin for complicated UTIs or certain forms of meningitis
      - Used in conjunction with antipseudomonal penicillin to treat penicillin
   c. Adverse reactions
      - **Ototoxicity—may cause irreversible hearing loss**, especially if infused too quickly
      - **Nephrotoxicity**—may cause renal insufficiency or acute tubular necrosis
   d. Other points
      - Most are given parenterally.
      - Check peak and trough levels to avoid drug toxicities.
   e. Examples
      - Gentamicin
      - Streptomycin
      - Tobramycin
      - Amikacin
      - Neomycin

4. **Miscellaneous protein synthesis inhibitors**
   a. Clindamycin
      - Binds to 50 S subunit of ribosome, inhibiting bacterial protein synthesis
      - Key feature is activity against anaerobic bacteria
      - It can also be used to treat many types of gram-positive cocci. If the patient is allergic to cephalexin (Keflex), clindamycin can be given instead.
      - The most notable adverse effect is its potential to cause **pseudomembranous colitis**, due to overgrowth of toxin producing *Clostridium difficile*.
   b. Chloramphenicol
      - It binds to 50 S bacterial ribosomal subunit, but may also interfere with human ribosomal activity, and so it has the potential to be highly toxic.
      - Broad-spectrum antimicrobial coverage, including anaerobes and rickettsiae; readily penetrates the CSF
      - Adverse effects may be severe and even fatal: **aplastic anemia** and **gray baby syndrome** (cyanosis due to respiratory depression and cardiovascular collapse)
      - Inhibits the P-450 system, potentiating the effect of many important drugs

C. Fluoroquinolones

1. Mechanism of action
   a. Inhibit bacterial DNA gyrase, blocking replication of bacterial DNA
   b. **Bactericidal**
2. Antimicrobial coverage
   a. Fluoroquinolones have excellent activity against gram-negative organisms, including *Pseudomonas*, *Legionella*, and gonorrhea. Gram-positive coverage is variable. Certain fluoroquinolones (e.g., levofloxacin, moxifloxacin) have good gram-positive coverage and are excellent agents for community-acquired pneumonia.
   b. Commonly used to treat UTIs. Ciprofloxacin also treats acute diarrhea due to enteric bacteria (traveler's diarrhea).
3. Adverse reactions
   a. Nausea, vomiting, diarrhea

b. Dizziness, headache, lightheadedness

c. Phototoxicity

d. Nephrotoxicity

e. **May damage cartilage in growing children,** so usage is typically limited to adults

f. Cautions

- Reduced absorption if consumed with divalent cations, such as antacids that contain magnesium
- Must be adjusted for renal insufficiency

g. Examples

- Levofloxacin
- Ciprofloxacin
- Ofloxacin

D. Antituberculosis antibiotics

1. Principles of therapy

   a. **Never treat tuberculosis with only one antibiotic.** Use multidrug therapy because drug resistance is such a problem with *Mycobacterium tuberculosis.*

   b. Treat active tuberculosis with three to four antibiotics (isoniazid [INH], rifampin, pyrazinamide [PZA], and sometimes ethambutol) for 2 months, followed by rifampin and INH for 4 months.

   c. Because *M. tuberculosis* is a slow-growing organism, the required duration of treatment is longer than it is in other bacterial infections.

2. Important first-line antituberculosis agents (many second-line agents also exist).

   a. INH

   - Attacks the enzyme that produces the mycolic acids that comprise the mycobacterial cell walls
   - Resistance to INH develops rapidly if it is used alone.
   - The most important adverse reaction is **drug-induced hepatitis,** which can be fatal.
   - It may cause a relative pyridoxine (vitamin B_6) deficiency, resulting in peripheral neuropathy. This is reversible with pyridoxine administration.

   b. Rifampin

   - Inhibits bacterial RNA synthesis by blocking RNA polymerase
   - In addition to its role as an antituberculosis agent, rifampin is used as prophylaxis for close contacts of patients with meningococcal meningitis.
   - Rifampin is also active against *Mycobacterium leprae,* which causes leprosy.
   - May stain tears or urine an orange-red color; induces hepatic microsomal enzymes and decreases the half-life of many medications

   c. PZA

   - Mechanism of action is unknown
   - Active against tubercle bacilli residing in macrophages
   - May cause hyperuricemia, resulting in a gouty attack
   - Potentially hepatotoxic

   d. Ethambutol

   - Inhibits an essential component of the mycobacterial cell wall
   - It may cause **optic neuritis,** resulting in diminished visual ability as well as red-green color blindness. Periodic visual testing may be necessary.
   - It may also precipitate a gouty attack.

E. Miscellaneous antibiotics

1. Trimethoprim (TMP)

   a. TMP inhibits dihydrofolic acid reductase, blocking bacterial DNA synthesis.

   b. It works synergistically with sulfonamides.

   c. TMP was formerly used alone to treat UTIs but now is most commonly used in combination with sulfamethoxazole (SMX).

   d. It may cause folate deficiency, resulting in megaloblastic anemia.

   e. TMP/SMX is used to treat UTIs, *Pneumocystis carinii* pneumonia, *Shigella,* and *Salmonella,* among other infections.

2. Sulfonamides

   a. Structural analogues of *p*-aminobenzoic acid that inhibit the enzyme dihydropteroate synthase, which is necessary for folic acid, and thus DNA synthesis

   b. Treat both gram-positive and gram-negative bacteria, although resistance to sulfonamides is increasingly common.

   c. Most sulfonamides that were once used alone have been replaced by the combination of TMP/SMX.

   d. Some forms of sulfonamides are still given as monotherapy, such as silver sulfadiazine (topical solution) in burn patients to prevent infection, and sodium sulfacetamide (ophthalmic ointment) for bacterial conjunctivitis.

   e. The most common adverse reactions are rash, photosensitivity, nausea, vomiting, and diarrhea.

   f. A rare but dreaded associated adverse reaction is **Stevens-Johnson syndrome**.

   g. **Do not give to patients with G6PD because they can precipitate a hemolytic response.**

3. Metronidazole

   a. Forms a cytotoxic compound through an oxidation–reduction action

   b. Effective against anaerobic bacteria as well as certain protozoal organisms such as *Entamoeba histolytica, Giardia,* and *Trichomonas*

   c. Results in a **disulfiram-like reaction** if consumed with alcohol

4. Table A-1 lists mechanisms of action, uses, and adverse reactions for important antibiotics.

PHYSICAL EXAMINATION PEARLS

Heart Sounds

- For murmur of mitral stenosis and to hear S_3 and S_4, use the bell of the stethoscope.
- For pericardial friction rubs, aortic/mitral regurgitation murmurs, and to hear S_1 and S_2, use the diaphragm of the stethoscope.
- Ventricular systole takes place between S_1 and S_2, and ventricular diastole between S_2 and S_1. Remember that diastole lasts longer than systole; this distinction makes it easy to identify the two sounds.
- How to differentiate S_3 and S_4 (the lines represent duration of pause between sounds): S_3 comes immediately after S_2, and S_4 comes immediately before S_1.

  - S_1- - - - - -S_2-S_3
  - S_4-S_1- - - - - -S_2

- Splitting of S_2 during inspiration and paradoxical splitting of S_2
  - The second heart sound has two parts: aortic valve closure, then pulmonic valve closure
  - With inspiration, there is increased blood return to the right heart. This increased flow delays pulmonary valve closure, which results in the normal splitting of S_2 during inspiration.
  - Paradoxical splitting of S_2 refers to the **narrowing** of this split during inspiration (instead of the normal widening that occurs). This can occur as a result of delayed aortic closure (as seen in LBBB, aortic stenosis, and hypertension).
- It is easier to hear S_3, S_4, and murmur of mitral stenosis if the patient is lying on his or her left side. Use the bell of the stethoscope and apply light pressure at the apical impulse. S_3 disappears if a lot of pressure is applied.

- S_1 = mitral valve closure
- S_2 = aortic valve closure (pulmonic valve closure contributes)

- Aortic area = right second interspace close to sternum
- Pulmonic area = left second interspace close to sternum
- Tricuspid area = left fourth and fifth interspace
- Mitral area = apex

TABLE A-1 Important Antibiotics

Antibiotic/Antibiotic Category	Mechanism of Action	Most Common Uses	Adverse Reactions Commonly Seen[a]
Penicillins	Cell wall inhibitors (interfere with transpeptidation)	Depends on extension of antimicrobial spectrum Oral and respiratory infections Streptococcal infections Syphilis	Hypersensitivity reactions
Vancomycin	Cell wall inhibitor (see text)	MRSA Enterococcal infections Endocarditis (used with aminoglycoside) Alternative if penicillin allergy present	"Red man" syndrome
Tetracyclines	Inhibit 30 S bacterial ribosomal subunit	Chlamydia Rickettsiae Lyme disease Topical use for acne vulgaris	Deposition in bones and teeth of children >8 years old, fetuses
Macrolides	Inhibit 50 S bacterial ribosomal subunit	Atypical pneumonia Alternative to penicillin (i.e., allergy) Legionella	GI upset
Clindamycin	Inhibits 50 S bacterial ribosomal subunit	Anaerobes	Pseudomembranous colitis
Cephalosporins	Cell wall inhibitors (similar to penicillins)	Depends on generation: First: similar to penicillins, surgical prophylaxis, streptococci and staphylococci infections Second: pneumonia in elderly patients, recurrent pneumonia Third: gonorrhea, meningitis Fourth: broad-spectrum, including streptococci, staphylococci, and pseudomonads	Possible cross-sensitivity with penicillin A few promote bleeding diathesis, correctable with vitamin K.
Fluoroquinolones	Inhibit bacterial DNA-gyrase	UTIs Diarrhea secondary to gram-negative rods Penicillin-resistant pneumonia Some with anti-Pseudomonas activity	Well tolerated Damage to cartilage in children
Aminoglycosides	Inhibit 30 S bacterial ribosomal subunit	Gram-negative sepsis Endocarditis (with vancomycin) Complicated UTIs	Nephrotoxicity Ototoxicity
TMP/SMX	Blocks bacterial DNA synthesis through action on folate pathway (two steps)	*Pneumocystis carinii* pneumonia UTIs	Rash Stevens-Johnson syndrome
Metronidazole	Products of reduction reaction kill susceptible bacteria and protozoans.	Anaerobes *Trichomonas histolytica* and Giardia	Metallic taste Disulfiram-like effect

[a]Note that these are not necessarily the most common side effects.

Murmurs

A. Grade 1—very faint; only a cardiologist can hear it

B. Grade 2—quiet

C. Grade 3—moderately loud

D. Grade 4—loud; associated with a thrill

E. Grade 5—very loud; can hear it with stethoscope partially off the chest

F. Grade 6—heard with stethoscope entirely off the chest

Breath Sounds

A. Vesicular breath sounds
   1. Soft, low-pitched
   2. Audible throughout most lung fields
   3. Heard during all of inspiration and first third of expiration

B. Bronchial breath sounds
   1. Loud, high pitched
   2. Longer expiratory than inspiratory phase (opposite of vesicular sounds)
   3. Hear a gap between inspiration and expiration
   4. Heard in central areas (over trachea)
   5. Bronchial sounds are abnormal if heard over the peripheral lung areas (where only vesicular sounds should be heard). This suggests an area of consolidation.

C. Bronchovesicular sounds
   1. Intermediate pitch
   2. Equal duration of inspiratory and expiratory phases

D. Adventitious breath sounds
   1. Rales (also called crackles)
      a. Can be heard during inspiration or expiration; intermittent (discontinuous) sounds
      b. Usually due to excessive fluid in the lungs or atelectasis
      c. Causes include pneumonia, CHF, interstitial lung disease
      d. Sometimes differentiated based on sound—fine crackles are high-pitched, soft, and brief in duration; coarse crackles are lower-pitched, louder, and longer in duration
   2. Wheezes have a hissing or musical sound caused by air moving through narrowed airways. Asthma is the most common cause.
   3. Rhonchi have a snoring quality and lower pitch, and are due to high mucus production in the large airways (e.g., chronic bronchitis).

> **QUICK HIT**
>
> Remember from MCAT that the speed of sound is fastest in solids. Therefore, if air in the lung has been replaced by fluid or solid, sound is transmitted to that area and bronchial breath sounds are heard.

Abdominal Examination

A. Inspect—Look for scars.

B. Auscultate—Listen to bowel sounds; this is a nonspecific part of the abdominal examination.

C. Palpate—Feel all quadrants, then palpate more deeply in all quadrants.
   1. Is the abdomen soft? A rigid abdomen may be a sign of a perforated viscus or peritoneal inflammation (acute abdomen).

2. Check for tenderness in all quadrants.
3. Check for rebound tenderness—does it hurt when you push down or let go? Pain on withdrawal of the hand is **rebound tenderness** and suggests peritoneal inflammation.
4. Is there guarding? **Guarding** refers to an area of rigidity and is significant when it is involuntary (i.e., not due to voluntary muscular contraction).

Neurologic Examination

A. Evaluate the Following:
1. **Level of consciousness, speech fluency**
2. **Pupillary size and reactivity, extraocular muscle movement**—give information about function of the brainstem, especially CN III and VI.
3. **Complete CN examination**
4. **Muscle strength testing**
5. **Truncal ataxia, pronator drift of arm** (sensitive test of motor weakness)
6. **Sensation**
7. **Cerebellar testing**—finger to nose and heel to shin; test gait on ambulation, heel-to-toe walking is good for detecting mild ataxia.
8. **Deep tendon reflexes**—Asymmetry indicates corticospinal tract dysfunction (upper motor neuron lesion).
9. **Babinski's sign**—Toes should normally flex. If they extend, this is a positive Babinski sign.

B. Upper and Lower Motor Neuron Defects (See Table A-2)
1. Deep Tendon Reflexes
   a. Grading of reflexes
      0 = No reflex
      1 = Diminished reflexes
      2 = Normal
      3 = Increased reflexes
      4 = Hyperactive reflexes
   b. Locations
      1. Biceps (C5)
      2. Brachioradialis (C6)
      3. Triceps (C7)
      4. Patellar (knee jerk) (L4)
      5. Ankle (S1)
2. Muscle Strength
   0 = No contraction
   1 = Flicker of contraction (muscle is "firing")
   2 = Moves limb when gravity is eliminated

> **QUICK HIT**
> If you cannot elicit reflexes, have the patient lock the fingers and pull his or her arms apart as you try again.

TABLE A-2 Upper Versus Lower Motor Neuron Defects	
Upper Motor Neuron Signs	**Lower Motor Neuron Signs**
Spasticity	Flaccid paralysis
Increased deep tendon reflexes (hyperreflexia)	Decreased deep tendon reflexes
Babinski's reflex (plantar response extensor)—toes upward (abnormal)	No Babinski's reflex (plantar response flexor)—toe downward (normal)
No atrophy	Muscle atrophy
No fasciculations	Fasciculations present

FIGURE
A-2 Palpation of the lymph nodes in a physical examination: 1. preauricular; 2. posterior auricular; 3. occipital; 4. tonsillar; 5. submandibular; 6. submental; 7. superficial cervical; 8. posterior cervical; 9. deep cervical chain; 10. supraclavicular.

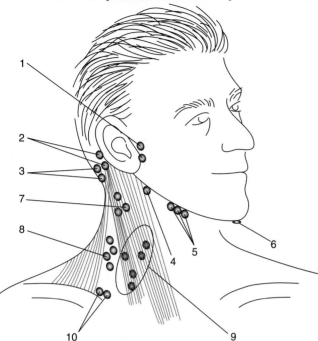

(Adapted from Bickley LS, Szilagyi PG. Bates' Guide to Physical Examination and History Taking. 8th Ed. Philadelphia: Lippincott Williams & Wilkins, 2003:203.)

3 = Moves limb against gravity (but not against any resistance)
4 = Moves limb against gravity and some resistance
5 = Normal muscle strength; moves limb against maximal resistance

C. Palpation of Lymph Nodes (see Figure A-2)

Tumor Markers

Tumor markers and the cancers they differentiate, as well as their usefulness, are covered in Table A-3.

WORKUP AND MANAGEMENT OF COMMON PROBLEMS ON THE WARDS

Refer to respective sections in each chapter for a more thorough discussion.

Hypotension

A. Causes: All causes of shock (sepsis, hypovolemia, cardiogenic, anaphylactic, neurogenic), medication (β-blockers, calcium channel blockers, nitrates, morphine, sedatives, epidural infusion)

B. Management
1. Quickly assess mental status—how symptomatic is the patient?
2. Obtain a full set of vitals, including BP in both arms. Expect a compensatory tachycardia. Bradycardia may result in reduced cardiac output.

APPENDIX

TABLE A-3   Tumor Markers

Tumor Marker	Cancer	Limitations	Uses/Comments
CEA	Colorectal cancer	Lacks sensitivity and specificity—This is not an effective screening test; levels may be elevated in other malignancies and in some nonmalignant diseases.	• Effective for monitoring disease process—A decrease in CEA indicates a favorable response to surgery, and an increase in CEA indicates disease progression. • Prognosis—The risk of recurrence is higher if the CEA level was elevated before surgery.
AFP	HCC and nonseminomatous germ-cell tumors of testis (NSGCT)	Not specific; can be elevated in nonmalignant diseases such as cirrhosis and hepatitis	Highly elevated AFP levels are present almost exclusively in primary HCC and NSGCT of the testis.
CA-125	Ovarian cancer	Neither sensitive nor specific for ovarian cancer, therefore not useful for screening—A normal CA-125 does **not** exclude ovarian cancer.	• Very useful for monitoring the response to therapy (after surgery or chemotherapy)—a decrease in CA-125 after treatment indicates shrinkage of the tumor, and an increase indicates disease progression or recurrence. • From 80% to 90% of women >50 years of age with a pelvic mass and an increased CA-125 will be found to have ovarian cancer.
Prostate-specific antigen (PSA)	See prostate section.		
CA 19-9	Pancreatic cancer	Low specificity—This is elevated in colorectal, pancreatic, and gastric cancer, as well as pancreatitis and ulcerative colitis.	73% of patients with pancreatic cancer have CA 19-9 levels greater than 100 U/mL.
β-hCG	Gestational trophoblastic disease, gonadal germ cell tumor	Elevated in pregnancy	• This has a high sensitivity for diagnosis of choriocarcinoma and trophoblastic neoplasm after evacuation of a molar pregnancy. • Either hCG or AFP is elevated in 90% of patients with NSGCT of the testis. • hCG may be elevated in either seminomatous germ cell tumors or NSGCTs, but AFP is only elevated in NSGCTs. • In testicular cancer, 75% of NSGCTs and 10% of seminomas germ cell tumors are associated with elevated hCG.

3. Determine baseline BP (may not be significantly different)
4. Consider ECG, CXR, arterial blood gas (ABG), blood culture (if febrile), and CBC (if bleeding is suspected).
5. Treatment should be directed toward the cause.
6. If patient is symptomatic, the reverse Trendelenburg position may be helpful.
7. Consider NS bolus (500 mL)—repeat this if BP does not improve (but be careful in patients with CHF or cardiogenic shock).

8. Discontinue or hold antihypertensive medications.
9. Vasopressors may be needed if there is no response to IV fluids.
10. If hypotension is profound or persists despite fluid therapy, consider transferring the patient to the ICU.
11. Put the patient on a cardiac monitor.

Hypertension

A. Causes

1. Failure to administer, order, or take antihypertensive medications
2. Pain, agitation
3. Hypertensive emergencies (manifested by MI, aortic dissection, encephalopathy, hemorrhagic CVA, or CHF)
4. Delirium tremens
5. Eclampsia or preeclampsia
6. Cocaine, amphetamine use

B. Management

1. Always recheck the BP with a properly fitting cuff to confirm HTN. Check other vital signs.
2. Check the patient's medication record to ensure appropriate compliance with therapy.
3. Check for signs of end-organ damage due to HTN, which indicate that a hypertensive emergency is occurring: chest pain/ECG changes, neurologic examination findings/encephalopathy, acute renal insufficiency or failure, papilledema.
4. Consider the following tests as appropriate, given the presentation: ECG, renal function panel, cardiac enzymes, CXR, CT of the head.
5. Treat pain and agitation as needed.
6. If HTN is mild and the patient is asymptomatic, observation with follow-up may be appropriate.
7. Oral antihypertensive medications (e.g., clonidine, ACE inhibitors or oral beta-blockers) can be given for most cases of hypertension. Follow response and repeat medication as needed. Be careful not to overtreat hypertension, especially when long-standing.
8. **Never ignore symptomatic HTN or hypertensive emergencies.** BP must be reduced quickly but carefully. (Reduce mean arterial pressure by no more than 25% in the first 2 hours.) This should be done in the ICU, with IV labetalol, nitroprusside, or enalapril, or additional doses of the patient's current regimen.
9. Reduce or discontinue IV fluids if volume overload is suspected.

 With hypotension or hypertension, treat the patient, not the BP reading. Asymptomatic patients with hypotension often do not require treatment.

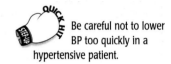 Be careful not to lower BP too quickly in a hypertensive patient.

Chest Pain

A. Causes

1. **Heart/vascular**: angina, MI, pericarditis, aortic dissection
2. **GI**: gastroesophageal reflux disease, diffuse esophageal spasm, peptic ulcer disease, gallbladder disease, acute cholecystitis
3. **Chest wall**: costochondritis, rib fracture, muscle strain, herpes zoster
4. **Psychiatric**: anxiety, somatization
5. **Pulmonary**: PE, pneumothorax, pleuritis
6. **Cocaine use**: can cause angina or MI

B. Management

1. As always, check vital signs. In most cases, obtain an 12-lead ECG. Compare with an old ECG. Get more information about the patient's cardiac history and current history of chest pain.

2. Order cardiac enzymes (creatine kinase; creatine kinase, myocardial bound; troponin) $\times$ 3, every 8 hours, if unstable angina or MI is suspected.
3. Consider CXR (pneumothorax, widened mediastinum, pleural effusion). Consider ABG or CT scan/$\dot{V}/\dot{Q}$ scan if PE is suspected.
4. If myocardial ischemia is suspected:
   a. Oxygen, 2 L by NC, titrate up as needed
   b. Nitroglycerin (sublingual) for pain; if pain continues, can give morphine IV
   c. Keep systolic BP >90 mm Hg.
   d. Aspirin
   e. Heparin—Give a loading dose, then start a drip. Check the PTT in 6 hours. Perform a guaiac stool test **before** starting heparin.
   f. Put the patient on a cardiac monitor, and consider transfer to a cardiac care unit.
2. Treat other suspected conditions appropriately. See discussions of PE, aortic dissection, pneumothorax, GERD, and PUD.

Tachycardia

A. Types: Determine whether the tachycardia is a narrow or wide complex. Obtain an ECG–is it regular? If wide, treat like ventricular tachycardia. If narrow, determine whether the tachycardia is sinus or nonsinus.

B. Sinus tachycardia
   1. HR >100, hardly ever >200 beats/min
   2. Sinus P waves precede each QRS complex
   3. Causes include pain, exercise, anxiety, panic attacks, dehydration, PE, volume loss (bleeding), hyperthyroidism, fever, anemia, albuterol, decongestants, and electrolyte disturbances.
   4. Treat the underlying cause. In older patients with cardiac disease, consider a β-blocker to prevent the increase in myocardial O_2 demand that occurs at a high HR.

C. Nonsinus tachycardia
   1. Either supraventricular (paroxysmal supraventricular tachycardia, atrial flutter, atrial fibrillation, AV nodal tachycardia) or ventricular (VT, ventricular fibrillation) in origin.
   2. Treatments vary according to the arrhythmia.
      a. Paroxysmal supraventricular tachycardia—Treat with vagal maneuvers or IV adenosine.
      b. Atrial fibrillation—Control the rate with a β-blocker, DC cardioversion, anticoagulation.
      c. Atrial flutter—Treat as with atrial fibrillation.
      d. Ventricular tachycardia (VT)—If the patient is stable, give IV amiodarone. If the patient is unstable, perform DC cardioversion.
      e. Ventricular fibrillation—Perform immediate defibrillation and CPR.

Oliguria

A. Typically defined as urine output <400 mL/day or <15 mL/hr.

B. Causes
   1. Prerenal: hypotension, hypovolemia, CHF, renal arterial occlusion
   2. Renal: glomerulonephritis, acute tubular necrosis, acute interstitial nephritis, vascular insult, and so on
   3. Postrenal: obstruction of lower or upper (bilateral) urinary tract

C. Management
   1. Check other vital signs.
   2. Inquire about potential precipitating factors—e.g. recent IV contrast administration, new medications (NSAIDs, ACE inhibitors), surgery, recent intake and output, other comorbid conditions (e.g., sepsis, CHF)

3. Palpate the bladder and insert a Foley catheter. If the patient already has a Foley catheter, flush it with 2 to 30 mL of saline to make sure it is not clogged. If urine flows after the Foley placement or flushing, obstruction was most likely the cause.

4. Order serum and urine chemistries and a renal function panel. Calculate the fractional excretion of sodium (<1% is consistent with prerenal causes).

5. Consider a renal ultrasound to exclude hydronephrosis.

6. If prerenal causes are suspected, give an IV fluid challenge (250 to 500 mL of NS). Repeat boluses and maintenance fluids may be required.

7. If CHF is suspected, consider diuresis (e.g., furosemide 20–60 mg IV).

8. Stop offending agents (nephrotoxic drugs).

9. Give IV fluids if radiocontrast-induced ATN is suspected.

10. Treat electrolyte disturbances and determine if there is an indication for dialysis.

Fever in the Hospitalized Patient

A. Causes

1. Infection: likely sources are central lines, peripheral IV lines, pneumonia, Foley catheter, urinary tract, wounds, heart valves, GI tract (diverticulitis), joints (septic arthritis)

2. Noninfectious causes: PE/DVT, medications, neoplasms, connective tissue disorders, postoperative atelectasis

B. Diagnosis

1. Check vital signs (tachycardia is an expected physiologic response to fever). Hypotension with fever suggests sepsis.

2. Evaluate for signs and symptoms of localizing disease—e.g., cough, abdominal pain, meningeal signs, joint pain, diarrhea, cellulitis

3. Consider CBC, urinalysis, CXR, cultures (blood $\times$ 2, urine, sputum, all ports of all lines, any fluid collections), with sensitivity panels.

4. Lumbar puncture if meningitis is a possible cause; CT of the abdomen if intra-abdominal infection is suspected

C. Therapies

1. Acetaminophen is appropriate in most cases.

2. If the patient is ill-appearing, hemodynamically unstable or neutropenic, start broad-spectrum antimicrobial treatment empirically as soon as cultures are obtained. Transfer to an ICU if patient is in septic shock

3. If the patient is on an antibiotic and the fever spikes again, consider adding another antibiotic or changing the antibiotic altogether. Antifungal agents may be required.

4. Remove or replace IV lines and indwelling catheters. Culture tips of central lines.

5. If no signs of infection and patient is hemodynamically stable, treat underlying etiology or continue diagnostic workup.

Hypoglycemia

• Usually due to excess insulin or oral hypoglycemic administration (relative to dietary intake) in diabetic patients

• If the patient can drink and hypoglycemia is mild, give juice. Consider giving 50 mL of D50W intravenously if the patient is symptomatic.

• If the patient is NPO or hypoglycemia persists, start D5W or D10W at 100 mL/hr.

• If there is no IV access and the patient cannot drink/eat, give glucagon (0.5 to 1.0 mg SC or IM).

• Review and modify insulin and oral hypoglycemic regimens.

Change in Mental Status (Confusion)

A. Causes

1. **Medications and intoxications:** sedatives, narcotics, insulin, oral hypoglycemics, H_2 blockers, TCAs, anticholinergics, corticosteroids, hallucinogens, cocaine, alcohol, methanol, ethylene glycol

2. **Hypoxia**—very common
3. **Postoperative delirium**—compounded by pain medications
4. **Hypotension**—with reduced cerebral perfusion
5. **Substance withdrawal**—e.g., alcohol, benzodiazepines
6. **Hypercapnia**
7. **Infection**: sepsis, meningitis, encephalitis, UTI, intracerebral abscess
8. **Trauma**: head trauma, burns
9. **Metabolic disturbances**: acidosis, hypoglycemia, sodium, calcium, magnesium, hypo/hypernatremia, ammonia (liver failure)
10. **Hyperthyroidism or hypothyroidism, thyroid storm**
11. **Neurologic causes**: CVA, subarachnoid hemorrhage, increased ICP
12. **Dehydration and malnutrition**—deficiencies of thiamine, vitamin B_{12}
13. **ICU psychosis**, sundowning

B. Management

1. Determine if there is a baseline history of dementia—any recent fall?
2. Check vitals; perform a focused examination (including neurologic examination and mental status).
3. Consider pulse oxygen ("pulse ox"), ABG, electrolytes, finger stick, CXR, blood cultures, LFTs, urine toxicology screen.
4. Consider a CT of the head to rule out CVA or intracranial mass or bleed.
5. Correct reversible causes and stop offending medications (if possible).
6. Consider naloxone (2 mg IV), dextrose (D50), and oxygen.
7. If patient is combative or is pulling out IVs, consider haloperidol (Haldol) or possibly restraints if necessary.

Shortness of Breath/Acute Hypoxia

A. Causes

1. Cardiac: PE, CHF exacerbation, MI, arrhythmia
2. Pulmonary: pneumonia, bronchospasm, pleural effusion, pulmonary edema, pneumothorax, upper airway obstruction, hyperventilation
3. Oversedation: narcotics, benzodiazepines (determine exactly how much sedating medication the patient has received)
4. Systemic causes: severe chronic anemia, sepsis, diabetic ketoacidosis
5. Other causes: rib fracture, anxiety, panic attacks

B. Management

1. Perform pulse oximetry immediately. If low, or if the patient appears ill, obtain an ABG and give supplemental oxygen (titrate according to response). Consider biphasic positive airway pressure in cases of COPD.
2. Remember ABCs—intubate if necessary.
3. Consider nebulizer treatments, furosemide, and naloxone as appropriate.
4. Perform portable CXR immediately unless hypoxia is readily resolved (e.g., with naloxone).
5. Consider ECG, CBC (anemia, infection); V̇/Q̇ scan (or spiral CT) if PE suspected
6. Consider anxiolytics if anxiety-related hyperventilation is suspected and the patient is stable.

BASIC STATISTICS AND EVIDENCE-BASED MEDICINE

A. Evidence-based medicine has been defined as "the conscientious, explicit and judicious use of current best evidence in making decisions about the care of individual patients" (Sacket D. BMJ 1996;312:71).

B. Types of research studies
1. Case series—These may describe the results of a specific treatment, determine long-term outcome of a treatment or procedure, or describe the complication rates of a procedure or the natural history of a disease.

- Descriptive study designs (case reports, case series, cross-sectional studies) suggest or generate hypotheses.
- Analytic study designs (observational studies, randomized controlled trials) test hypotheses.

a. Size of a case series can range from two or three patients to thousands of patients. A case report is the description of a rare or interesting case.

b. Major disadvantage is the lack of a comparison group so one cannot reach definitive conclusions about treatment efficacy. Case series are prone to many biases.

c. Very common in surgical research

2. Cross-sectional studies—Subjects are studied at a specific point in time ("snapshot" of a population).

3. Case-control studies

a. Patients are selected because they have a certain outcome, and their history is retrospectively reviewed to identify exposures or risk factors that may be associated with that outcome.

b. By definition, case-control studies can be only retrospective.

c. Good for rare diseases and for diseases with long latent periods

d. Very susceptible to bias because both exposure and disease development occurred prior to initiation of the study

4. Cohort studies

a. Subjects are selected according to exposure (e.g., a new medication, a procedure) and are followed over time to observe the development or progression of disease.

b. Cohort studies can be prospective or retrospective.

c. Prospective cohort studies follow patients over time to observe a certain outcome, but patient assignment into the two treatment groups is not randomized, so confounding variables may be unequally distributed (see below).

5. Randomized controlled trial

a. A type of cohort study involving a control group and an intervention group

b. Patient assignment into either group is left completely to chance (if properly done). Therefore, known and unknown confounders are likely to be equally distributed.

c. Methodologically superior to other study designs because it is least susceptible to bias

6. Meta-analyses

a. Meta-analyses combine data from several individual studies to estimate an overall effect.

b. The strength of a meta-analysis is only as good as the quality of the primary studies it analyzes (e.g., a meta-analysis of 14 flawed, biased studies will produce a biased estimate of effect).

c. A meta-analysis of well-conducted randomized controlled trials is the highest level of evidence.

C. Sensitivity and specificity (see Table A-4)

1. Sensitivity = a/a + c. Tests with high sensitivity are used for screening. They may yield false-positive results but do not miss people with the disease (low false-negative rate).

2. Specificity = d/b + d. Tests with high specificity are used for disease confirmation.

3. Positive predictive value (PPV) = a/a + b

a. If the test is positive, what is the probability that the patient has the disease?

b. PPV depends on the prevalence (the higher the prevalence, the greater the PPV) and the sensitivity/specificity of the test (e.g., an overly sensitive test yields more false-positive results and has a lower PPV).

4. Negative predictive value (NPV) = d/c + d

a. If test is negative, what is the probability that patient does not have the disease? **A high NPV is very important for a screening test.**

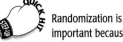 Case-control studies and cohort studies are often referred to as "observational studies."

 Randomization is important because it leaves patient assignment to either experimental or control group completely to **chance**. When any element of human intrusion or judgment enters the process of patient assignment, bias is introduced.

Hierarchy of evidence (from highest to lowest)
1. Meta-analysis of randomized controlled trials
2. Randomized controlled trials
3. Cohort studies
4. Case-control studies
5. Case series
6. Expert opinion

 The basic difference between a randomized controlled trial and a prospective cohort study is the manner in which patients are assigned to either group.
• In a randomized controlled trial, patients are assigned to either the experimental or control group randomly, without input from physician or patient.
• In a cohort study, the treatment decision is not random and is determined by the recommendations of the physician, as well as the wishes of the patient, among other factors.

| **Box** | **A-1** | **Consolidation of Standards for Reporting Trials (CONSORT) Statement** |

- Published in 1996, revised in 2001 (JAMA 2001;285:1987)
- Twenty-one-point checklist of essential items that randomized controlled trial reports should include to facilitate their appraisal and interpretation
- Many journals have endorsed CONSORT, but the rigor of enforcement varies.

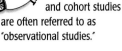
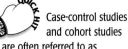

Box **A-2** **Cochrane Library (www.cochrane.org)**

- Regularly updated evidence-based medicine database
- Includes randomized controlled trials and systematic reviews in all specialties of medicine to determine how strong the evidence is for a variety of medical treatments
- Consists of an international network of researchers and physicians who gather and evaluate the evidence in medical research

---

 The null hypothesis postulates that there is no difference between two groups. This hypothesis is either rejected or not rejected by a study.

 Clinical significance is unrelated to statistical significance. A study may obtain statistical significance for differences that have no clinical significance (e.g., 41% vs. 42% infection rate for two groups). With a large enough sample size, any study will obtain statistical significance.

If a study has a power of 80%, this means that if a difference of a particular stated magnitude exists between groups, there is an 80% chance of correctly detecting it.

The lack of statistical power (i.e., sample size too small) invalidates a study because it can lead to statistical insignificance when there actually is a clinically meaningful difference.

b. NPV also depends on prevalence of disease (higher prevalence = lower NPV) and the sensitivity/specificity of the test (the more sensitive the test, the fewer the number of false-negative results, and the higher the NPV).

D. Type 1 and 2 errors

1. Type 1 (alpha) error: null hypothesis is rejected even though it is true (false-positive finding)
   a. *P* value is the chance of a type 1 error occurring.
   b. If the *P* value is ≤0.05, it is unlikely that a type 1 error has been made (i.e., a type 1 error is made five or fewer times out of 100 attempts).
2. Type 2 (beta) error: null hypothesis is not rejected even though it is false (a false-negative finding).
   a. A type 2 error results when the *P* value fails to reach statistical significance **even though the groups being compared are truly different**. A type 2 error usually occurs when sample size is too small.
   b. The likelihood of avoiding a type 2 error is termed the **statistical power** of a study.

E. Statistical power

1. A study with "negative" result (no difference between groups) must have adequate power to detect clinically meaningful differences.
2. Conventionally, a beta error rate of 20% is chosen, which corresponds with a study power of 80%. A study power of less than 80% is believed to have an unacceptably high risk of false negative results (i.e., a study found no difference between two groups, when there actually was a difference).
3. Factors that affect the power of a study
   a. Sample size—When sample size is small, a study is susceptible to type 2 error, which is why sample size calculation is done prior to the study being initiated.
   b. Level of statistical significance—Conventionally, a *P* value of 0.05 is chosen, although this is somewhat arbitrary.
   c. Variability of the sample data—the lower the variability, the fewer subjects are needed to demonstrate significant differences if they do indeed exist.
   d. Effect size chosen by researcher—This is based on pre-existing data and clinical judgment and is beyond the scope of this discussion.

F. Confidence interval (CI)

1. The CI allows the reader to apply the results of a study to the "true" population from which the sample in the study was taken.

TABLE A-4 **Sensitivity and Specificity**

Result of test under investigation	Result of Gold Standard	
	Disease Positive	Disease Negative
Test positive (a + b)	True positive (a)	False positive (b)
Test negative (c + d)	False negative (c)	True negative (d)

2. The most common CI is 95%, which means that the confidence interval (i.e., the range) reported in the study holds true for 95 of 100 samples similar to the one in the study.

3. A "wider" CI increases the certainty of the estimate (i.e., it is more likely that the population from which the sample was selected would fall within the reported interval), but lowers its precision (see Quick Hit). A very wide CI should be interpreted with caution (a larger sample size may be needed to maintain power).

4. The larger the CI, the less power a study has to detect differences between two groups. The width of the CI depends on sample size; the larger the sample size (more likely to have power), the narrower the confidence interval.

Think of the CI as a weather forecast: a vague forecast of "warm with possibility of rain" (this is a "wide" CI) is more likely to hold true but is not very precise. However, a forecast of "70 degrees with 30% chance of rain" (narrow CI) is much more precise but has a lower likelihood of holding true.

G. Association versus correlation

1. Association is used for describing relationships between categorical variables; correlation describes relationships between continuous variables.

2. Neither association nor correlation imply causation. These terms describe only the relationship and strength of this relationship.

3. Correlation is a matter of "degree." It can range from -1.00 (inverse proportionality) to $+1.00$ (proportional relationship). Zero signifies no correlation.

H. Causality—it is very difficult to prove causality. The following factors help assess causality, but none can give indisputable evidence of a cause-and-effect relationship:

1. Strength of association
2. Biological plausibility—does the association make biological sense?
3. Consistency of the association across different studies
4. Dose-response relationship
5. Experimental evidence to support causality—e.g., if you eliminate an exposure, does this reduce the incidence of a particular disease?
6. Temporal sequence (very important)—The causative factor must precede the effect.
7. Experimental evidence—has a randomized controlled trial (highest level of evidence) been performed?

I. Bias

1. A study that is biased lacks internal validity. Bias can be introduced in the design of a study or during the statistical analysis because of the lack of statistical power (inadequate sample size). In addition, conflict of interest can introduce bias and affect the validity of a study. Critical appraisal of medical literature essentially requires the ability to identify bias.

2. There are four main types of bias: selection bias, performance bias, detection bias, and attrition bias (see Box A-3).

Box **A-3** **Types of Bias**

- **Selection bias**—occurs when there are differences in the characteristics of subjects between comparison groups of a study. Unequal distribution of confounding variables among the two groups leads to selection bias.
- **Performance bias**—occurs when subjects in comparison groups are given different care (other than the intervention that is being studied). For example, only one group may receive counseling in addition to the intervention that is being studied (the counseling may affect the outcome in some way). Blinding is important in preventing performance bias (patient and investigators are not aware of the treatment rendered).
- **Detection bias**—refers to inconsistency in outcome assessment. Use of validated outcome measures and blinding of outcome assessors helps prevent detection bias.
- **Attrition bias**—refers to patient drop-outs or exclusion from a study. There is no recognized drop-out rate that is deemed "acceptable." Drop-outs should be kept to a minimum, but if they do occur, **intent-to-treat analysis** is critical to maintain the integrity of randomization (see text).

Selection bias refers to differences in characteristics of subjects included/excluded or differences between selected comparison groups.

Selection bias
Ideally, comparison groups should be identical in all respects other than factor under investigation. In reality, this comparison group does not exist due to confounding variables. Therefore, randomized controlled trials are preferred to minimize confounding.

The only inherent advantage of randomized controlled trials over observational studies is the reduction in confounding.

When evaluating a randomized clinical trial, go through this checklist to assess whether a study is biased:
• Proper randomization
• Concealment of allocation
• Blinding
• Completeness of follow-up and intent-to-treat analysis

Intent-to-treat analysis
Patients are analyzed with the group to which they were randomly assigned, regardless of whether they actually received that treatment or completed the study.

3. A **confounding variable** is a factor other than the intervention under investigation that obscures the primary comparison.
   a. Common confounding variables include age, gender, comorbidities, smoking, and socioeconomic status.
   b. A true confounding variable must meet two criteria: it must be associated with the explanatory (independent) variable, **and** it should be a risk factor for the outcome of interest.
   c. Randomized controlled trials control for both known and **unknown** confounders.
4. Minimizing bias in randomized clinical trials hinges on the following:
   a. **Proper randomization**—Each patient should have an **equal** chance of receiving either treatment.
   b. **Concealment of allocation**—The person enrolling patients into study should be unaware of next "assignment" into either the experimental or control group. This can be done with sealed opaque envelopes, remote allocation (call made to a separate department to determine patient allocation), or computerized allocation.
   c. **Blinding**—The higher the level of blinding, the lower the risk of bias. The following participants can potentially be blinded depending on the nature of the study: patients, physicians, data collectors, assessors of outcome, data analysts. A study should describe precisely which participants were blinded. Terms such as "double" and "triple" blinding, if not defined, are confusing and should be avoided because textbooks and physicians often have varying interpretations of these terms.
   d. **Intent-to-treat analysis**—Drop-outs are analyzed in groups to which they were initially assigned. Excluding drop-outs from analysis threatens the balance that randomization achieves. Drop-outs often do worse than patients who remain, and excluding them creates bias.

J. Glossary of common statistical terms
1. Mean—the average
2. Median—value corresponding to the middle case or middle observation (i.e., 50% of values are less than and 50% of the values are more than the median).
3. Mode—value that occurs most often
4. Standard deviation (SD)—used for normal distributions. An SD of +/− 1 includes about 68% of the observations, an SD of +/− 2 includes about 95% of the observations, and an SD of +/− 3 includes about 99.7% of the observations.
5. Incidence—number of new cases of a disease per year
6. Prevalence—overall proportion of the population who have the disease
7. Relative risk—incidence in exposed group/incidence in unexposed group. Relative risk can be calculated only after a prospective or experimental study,
8. Odds ratio—a method of estimating the relative risk in retrospective studies. It is the probability of an event happening divided by the probability of the event not happening.
9. Reliability—ability of a test or measure to reproduce the same results under the same conditions
10. Validity—extent to which a study correctly represents the relationships being assessed
    a. Internal validity—A study that suffers from bias lacks internal validity.
    b. External validity—A study may have internal validity but its results may not be generalized to a larger population (lacks external validity).

1. A 61-year-old male presents to your office with the chief complaint of "coughing up blood" for the past 3 weeks. He reports at least five to six episodes every 2 to 3 days of coughing of bright red blood, approximately 1 to 2 tablespoons each time. The patient denies any chest pain, fevers, chills, weight loss, or recent travel. He has had a persistent productive cough (clear sputum) for the past month and reports mild dyspnea during this time. PMH is significant for COPD diagnosed 5 years ago and HTN. He has a 30 pack-year smoking history and currently smokes 1 pack per day. On auscultation of his lungs, you note end-expiratory wheezing and a prolonged expiratory phase. Routine laboratory values are all normal. CXR reveals typical changes seen in COPD (flattened diaphragms, hyperinflation) without any localizing abnormalities. What is the appropriate management of this patient?

2. A 67-year-old male presents to the ED with LLQ pain that began a few hours ago. He complains of nausea and loose stools. His PMH is significant for CHF. He reports one episode of blood in his stools a few months ago. Vital signs are as follows: temperature = 101.1, BP = 130/76, pulse = 70. On physical examination, he has guarding and tenderness to palpation in the LLQ. His examination is otherwise unremarkable. His stool is negative for occult blood. Laboratory tests reveal a leukocyte count of 16,000 cells/μL. Plain and upright abdominal films are normal. What is the diagnosis? What tests would you order? What is the next step in managing this patient?

3. A 64-year-old female with a history of HTN presents to the ED with a chief complaint of left-sided chest pain that began 4 to 5 hours ago. She has a history of periodic episodes of chest pain for which she takes sublingual nitroglycerin, but today's episode has been more severe, has lasted longer, and is not relieved by nitroglycerin. She denies nausea/vomiting, any radiation of the pain, or diaphoresis. Temperature = 97.8, BP = 136/76, HR = 80, RR = 20. She seems uncomfortable but physical examination is otherwise unremarkable. What is the diagnosis? How should her chest pain be evaluated? What is the next step in management?

4. A 64-year-old male comes to your office with complaint of a sudden loss of vision, which he likens to "a curtain coming down over my eyes," that occurred 2 days before and lasted 30 minutes. Now he has no visual complaints. Medical history is significant for HTN and DM. He denies headache, loss of consciousness, diplopia, ocular pain, ataxia, and vertigo. Neurologic examination is normal. What is the next step in managing this patient?

5. A 58-year-old male presents to your office with weakness in his legs and a history of frequent falls over the past few months. He also complains of fatigue at the end of the day. He does not drink alcohol or smoke, and his medical history is significant for gastric carcinoma for which he underwent gastrectomy 2 years ago. On physical examination, he is found to have increased deep tendon reflexes and mild weakness of his lower extremities, along with diminished vibratory sense in his toes. His examination is otherwise unremarkable. What is the likely diagnosis and what is the appropriate next step in managing this patient?

6. A 37-year-old female presents to your office complaining of weakness, especially with activities that require muscular force, such as climbing stairs. Her symptoms have developed gradually over the past year or two, and she has largely ignored them. She reports a recent weight gain of 25 lb over the past year and has been feeling melancholy for the past few months. She also has had back pain for the past several months. Her medical history is significant for mild HTN, for which she takes metoprolol, and DM that requires insulin therapy. She takes no other medications. Physical examination reveals mild obesity, with fat deposition mainly around the trunk and the posterior neck. You note some facial hair and scattered purple striae on the abdomen. Radiographs reveal a compressed fracture at the level of T11. Vital signs are as follows: BP = 140/85, pulse = 70. What is the likely diagnosis? What is the appropriate next step in managing this patient?

7. A 56-year-old male with a history of cigarette smoking and hypercholesterolemia is brought to the ED with severe, crushing chest pain that has lasted for 90 minutes. He states that he felt ill all day and then started experiencing pain in his jaw, which progressed to chest pain with radiation to the left arm with nausea. Vital signs are as follows: temperature = 97.4, HR = 100, BP = 150/90, RR = 22, pulse oximetry = 98% on room air. An ECG reveals significant ST elevations in V_1 to V_4. There are ST segment depressions in leads II, III, and aVF. What is the next step in managing this patient?

8. A 34-year-old female presents to the ED with a 2-day history of nausea and vomiting and diffuse abdominal pain. She reports mild diarrhea. She has not been able to keep any food down over the past 36 hours secondary to severe vomiting. Her PMH is unremarkable. Vital signs are as follows: temperature = 99.1, RR = 12, pulse = 110. Her BP is 134/86 when lying down, 112/70 when standing. Abdominal examination reveals mild diffuse tenderness with hyperactive bowel sounds. Her abdomen, soft, and there is no guarding or rebound tenderness. Stool is negative for occult blood. She has poor skin turgor and dry mucous membranes. Laboratory tests reveal the following: WBC = 7.6, Hgb = 11.8, Hct = 34.5, Na^+ = 140, K^+ = 3.2, Cl^- = 95, HCO_3^- = 37, BUN = 40, Cr = 1.5. ABGs are obtained and reveal the following: pH = 7.52, $PaCO_2$ = 46, PaO_2 = 84. What is the acid-base disorder in this patient? What is the appropriate management of this patient?

9. A 64-year-old male presents to your office for a physical examination. His PMH is significant for HTN, for which he takes metoprolol. His stool is positive for occult blood. On examination, there are no palpable masses in the abdomen, no tenderness, and bowel sounds are normal. He denies any change in bowel habits. The remainder of his physical examination is unremarkable. What is the appropriate next step in managing this patient?

10. A 55-year-old male presents to the ED after vomiting several hundred milliliters of blood. His stool was a dark color. His PMH is significant for CAD and HTN. Medications include an ACE inhibitor, a β-blocker, and a daily aspirin tablet. He reports having had "heartburn" for several years but no prior episodes of hematemesis or melena. A nasogastric tube placed in the ED revealed bloody aspirate. Vital signs are as follows: RR = 20, BP = 90/55, pulse = 105. He has a 25-mm Hg orthostatic decrease in BP. His physical examination is unremarkable. Laboratory tests reveal a hemoglobin of 7.3 and hematocrit of 22.0. LFT results are normal. What is the next step in managing this patient?

11. A 74-year-old male presents to the ED with weakness in his right arm, as well as slurred speech that started suddenly that morning during breakfast (6 hours before entering the ED). PMH is significant for MI 10 years ago, HTN, and BPH. He denies chest pain, dizziness, vertigo, ataxia, and a history of arrhythmia. His wife denies that he has had any history of TIAs in the past. Vital signs are as follows: temperature = 97.5, RR = 18, BP = 152/90, pulse = 84. Oxygen saturation is 98% on room air. Physical examination reveals a right facial droop, and muscle strength is diminished in the right arm (2/5 strength) and right leg (3/5 strength). Patient has decreased sensation to light touch and pin prick in the right arm but normal sensation in his right leg. What is the appropriate next step in managing this patient?

12. A 73-year-old female presents to your office with a complaint of lower abdominal pain that began 2 weeks ago. She has been having more frequent bowel movements and has had episodes of loose stools. Her PMH is significant for HTN and hypercholesterolemia. She has mild LLQ pain on abdominal examination, and

bowel sounds are normal. Her stool is negative for occult blood. She is afebrile, WBC count is 7.2, hemoglobin is 12.1, and hematocrit is 36.8. What is the likely diagnosis and the appropriate management of this patient?

13. A 24-year-old female presents to your office for a routine examination. She reports a history of heavy menstrual bleeding since menarche. On further questioning, she states that she has episodes of epistaxis about once every 2 weeks or so and has a tendency to bruise easily. Her physical examination is unremarkable. CBC results are as follows: Hb = 7.9 g/dL, Hct = 23.9%, MCV = 69. Platelet count is 230,000/μL. What is the likely diagnosis? What tests would you order?

14. A 25-year-old female presents to the ED after an episode of numbness in her left leg that lasted for several hours. She has no other complaints. On further questioning, she remembers an episode of transient unilateral loss of vision 2 years ago, which resolved and never recurred. Vital signs are as follows: temperature = 97.4, RR = 18, BP = 128/84, pulse = 76. On examination, she has diminished sensation in her left leg, which she describes as "numb." Her strength is normal, and her examination is otherwise unremarkable. She takes birth control pills but no other medications. What is the likely diagnosis and the appropriate initial workup for this patient?

15. A 59-year-old female presents to the office because she is "sick and tired" of this cough she has had for 5 years, and it is getting worse. The cough is often productive of watery mucus. She is also becoming more and more short of breath and cannot climb a flight of stairs without taking a rest. She denies chest pain, paroxysmal nocturnal dyspnea, fevers, chills, and weight loss. PMH is significant for HTN and a 35 pack-year history of cigarette smoking. Vital signs are as follows: temperature = 99.0, HR = 75, RR = 21, BP = 158/82. Physical examination reveals an obese woman in no acute distress. On lung auscultation, there are coarse breath sounds bilaterally but no wheezes or crackles. Chest radiograph is significant for prominent lung markings at the bases. What is causing this woman's cough and SOB?

16. A 56-year-old male presents to your office for a routine health evaluation. He reports that he is healthy, and his physical examination is unremarkable. However, laboratory tests reveal a PSA level of 5.8 ng/mL. DRE is normal, with no palpable nodule or irregularity in the prostate. What is the appropriate management of this patient?

17. A 67-year-old male presents to your office with complaint of right hip pain for the last week. He denies any history of falls or injury. The pain came on suddenly as he was getting up from a chair. Prior to this episode, he denies any history of hip pain. PMH is significant for HTN, diabetes, and hypothyroidism. He started using a cane a few days ago but due to increasing pain is now in a wheelchair. On physical examination, he has severe pain with any attempted motion of the right hip joint. Pulses are palpable bilaterally, and neurologic examination is normal. Radiographs of the right hip are obtained, and show a displaced fracture of the right femoral neck. In addition to obtaining an orthopaedic surgery referral, what is the appropriate next step in managing this patient?

18. A 38-year-old female presents to your office with chief complaint of fatigue for the past 5 to 6 months. Her fatigue has also affected her performance at work, where she has difficulty concentrating. She feels more tired than usual after work and has difficulty playing with her children in the evening. She did not have any of these symptoms until 6 months ago. PMH is insignificant. The patient smokes five to six cigarettes a day and drinks alcohol socially. She takes birth control pills. Physical examination is normal. What is the appropriate next step in managing this patient?

19. A 45-year-old female presents to your office with a 2-day history of a cough and fever. She states that she has felt tired for the past couple of weeks but is otherwise vague. PMH is unremarkable. On physical examination, she appears ill and has a persistent cough productive of purulent sputum. She has rales in her right posterior chest. BP = 126/74, pulse = 80, RR = 8, temperature = 102.2. WBC count is 14,000/mm^3. You obtain a CXR, which reveals consolidation in the right lower

lobe and a 2.3-cm round opacity in the left lower lobe. What is the appropriate management of this patient?

20. A 75-year-old female with a history of two MIs presents to the ED after fainting. She reports fatigue and dyspnea for 2 months. She denies chest pain, SOB, or orthopnea. A 12-lead ECG reveals a bradycardia with a ventricular rate of 35 bpm. You detect definite, regular P waves and QRS complexes, but notice that there is no relationship between the P waves and the QRS complexes. What type of bradyarrhythmia is this, and how should it be managed?

21. A 40-year-old male presents to your office with a complaint of epigastric abdominal pain for the past 5 to 6 months. The pain is not related to meals and is intermittent. He has tried over-the-counter antacids with minimal relief of pain. He denies any recent weight loss. He is a nonsmoker and does not abuse alcohol. His PMH is significant for HTN, which is controlled with metoprolol. He does not take any other medications. Physical examination is unremarkable. How would you treat this patient?

22. A 32-year-old female presents to your office with a history of diarrhea and intermittent abdominal cramping with flatus. She reports having diarrhea very frequently on and off for several years, but her symptoms have been worse for the past 3 weeks. She also has constipation every once in a while. She has no apparent medical problems. Her physical examination reveals mild LLQ tenderness without guarding or rebound. A stool test for occult blood is negative. She is a college student and is studying for her midterm examinations. What is the likely diagnosis and how would you manage this patient?

23. A 65-year-old female with a history of DM, HTN, and a large anterior wall MI 5 years ago presents to the ED complaining of progressive SOB. Vital signs are: temperature = 98.7, HR = 88, RR = 19, BP = 160/85, oxygen saturation = 90% on room air. She seems short of breath on examination but is able to speak in full sentences. There are bibasilar crackles with scattered expiratory wheezes. There is also 2+ pitting edema of the lower extremities. An ECG reveals left ventricular hypertrophy (LVH), with Q waves and T wave inversions in V_1 to V_4 and diffuse nonspecific ST segment abnormalities. A CXR shows cardiomegaly and considerable congestion of the pulmonary vasculature. What is the most likely diagnosis, and what is the appropriate approach to treatment?

24. A 56-year-old male presents to the ED with complaint of chest pain for the past 3 hours. He has never experienced this pain before, and it started suddenly while he was eating dinner. He describes the pain as "gripping" and radiating into his neck. Physical examination is normal. ECG shows a 1-mm ST segment depression in leads V_4 to V_6. PMH is significant for DM and HTN. Medications include insulin and a β-blocker for the HTN. What is the appropriate next step in managing this patient?

25. A 19-year-old female is brought to the ED reluctantly by her mother because of nausea, vomiting, fever, and flank pain. PMH is otherwise negative. Her only medication is oral contraceptives. Vital signs are: temperature = 103.5, BP = 115/60, pulse = 110, RR = 20. Lungs are clear to auscultation bilaterally. Both heart rate and rhythm are regular, without murmurs. The patient appears ill but is alert and oriented. She has tenderness at the right costovertebral angle. What is the appropriate next step in managing this patient?

26. A 65-year-old female is brought to the ED with a depressed level of consciousness. She was at a wedding reception, had finished dancing with her husband, and was returning to her table when she suddenly collapsed and lost consciousness. She soon regained consciousness, but her speech was not normal and she had an episode of vomiting. She had a severe headache and could not move her right arm and leg. She soon entered a stuporous state and was rushed to the ED. She has a history of HTN but no other medical problems. According to her husband, she takes metoprolol for her HTN, as well as a daily aspirin. In the ED, her vital signs are as follows: temperature = 99.4, RR = 24, BP = 165/98, pulse = 98. On examination, the patient is lethargic and her speech is slurred. She cannot move her

right arm or leg. Sensation is somewhat diminished in her right arm but is normal in her right leg. What are the next steps in managing this patient?

27. A 71-year-old female presents to the ED with a 2-day history of severe abdominal pain. Her symptoms were mild at first, becoming severe in the next 6 to 10 hours. Her PMH is significant for CAD and HTN. Her stool is positive for blood. She is afebrile. Her abdominal examination reveals very mild tenderness in the mid-abdomen. Laboratory studies are normal. What is the appropriate next step in evaluation?

28. A 43-year-old male presents to your office with a 3-day history of chest pain, which is mostly centrally located and radiates to the right side of his neck. The pain worsens with deep breathing and improves when he sits up. He denies nausea, vomiting, sweating, and SOB. He had an upper respiratory infection about 2-weeks ago which resolved without treatment. PMH is significant for hyperlipidemia. He takes lovastatin. He smokes half a pack of cigarettes a day. Vital signs are: temperature = 99.4, BP = 125/80, pulse = 84. Physical examination is significant for a friction rub over the left sternal border heard best when he leans forward. A 12-lead ECG shows ST elevation in leads I, II, III, aVL, V_2, V_3, V_4, V_5, and V_6. What is the diagnosis? How would you manage this patient?

29. A 25-year-old male presents to your office with complaint of chest pain and SOB that started last evening. His chest pain is on the right side of the chest and is stabbing in quality, and the pain increases with inspiration. He is short of breath even at rest. He denies any prior such episodes. He denies any traumatic event or overexertion. PMH is negative. He has a five pack-per-year smoking history. He does not take any medications. Temperature = 98.2, BP = 130/80, HR = 115, RR = 22. Pulse oximetry shows 84% oxygen saturation on room air. He is 6'2" and 175 lb, and he appears healthy. Physical examination reveals decreased breath sounds on the right side. Examination is otherwise unremarkable. What is the appropriate next step in managing this patient?

30. A 53-year-old male with no significant medical history comes to your office. He is doing well, except for some exertional dyspnea over the past few months. He has no history of heart disease. He occasionally feels some palpitations, which are not bothersome to him. On physical examination, you note an irregularly irregular heart rhythm. You obtain an ECG, which confirms the irregularly irregular arrhythmia. The physical examination is otherwise normal. What is the diagnosis? What is the next step in evaluating this patient? Describe the management of this patient.

31. A 73-year-old male with HTN presents to the office with a 3-month history of chest pain induced by lifting weights, shoveling snow, and running on a treadmill. Vital signs are as follows: temperature = 98.3, HR = 85, RR = 17, BP = 165/85. Physical examination reveals a 4/6 crescendo-decrescendo murmur heard at the right upper sternal border with radiation to the carotid arteries, weak and delayed carotid pulses, and an S4 gallop. ECG reveals LVH. What valvular disease is present, and what is the appropriate approach to treatment?

32. A 52-year-old female presents to your office complaining of left knee pain for the past 2 to 3 months. She denies any history of injury. PMH is significant for hypercholesterolemia for which she takes lovastatin. She denies any recent changes in activity level. She describes her pain as primarily "around and under my knee cap." She points to her patella and the anterior aspect of her knee as the site of her pain. She especially has difficulty climbing and descending stairs. Her left knee swells on occasion. On examination, she has a mild effusion and no erythema. She has full range of motion without pain. She has no tenderness along medial or lateral joint lines. Her knee is ligamentously stable. What is appropriate next step in the management of this patient?

33. A 57-year-old male had a fasting plasma glucose level of 160 mg/dL 1 month ago. Today, his fasting glucose level is 140 mg/dL. He has a history of HTN that is controlled with an ACE inhibitor. He has no other medical problems. He is 5' 11" and weighs 215 lb. His deceased father had DM, but the family history is otherwise noncontributory. This patient is asymptomatic, and his physical examination is unremarkable. How would you manage this patient?

34. A 36-year-old African-American female presents to your office with a 4-month history of dry cough, SOB, and fatigue. She has a 10 pack-per-year smoking history. Vital signs are: temperature = 98.2, BP = 132/79, HR = 74, RR = 16. Pulse oximetry shows 96% O_2 saturation on room air and 100% O_2 saturation with supplemental O_2 at 2 L/min via nasal canula. Further history reveals slightly blurred vision over the past few months, as well as occasional pain and swelling in the knees and ankles. Examination reveals crackles bilaterally in the lower lung fields. Heart examination shows regular rate and rhythm, with no murmurs. She has a mild effusion in her left knee but has full range of motion of both knees and ankles. She has two tender erythematous nodules on her left leg measuring approximately 3 × 3 cm. CXR shows bilateral hilar adenopathy. What is the appropriate next step in the management of this patient?

35. A 68-year-old male is brought to the ED by his wife because of headache, nausea, and fatigue. PMH is significant for small cell carcinoma of the lung diagnosed approximately 2 years ago. He also has a history of TIA (6 years ago) and mild CHF. Vital signs are as follows: temperature = 99.8, RR = 18, BP = 140/88, pulse = 76. On examination, he is awake but somewhat lethargic. Physical examination is unremarkable. Laboratory tests reveal the following: WBC = 8.3, Hct and Hgb = 10.2/30.7, glucose = 106, serum Na^+ = 121 mEq/L, K^+ = 4.3, BUN/Cr = 7.0/0.4. What is the likely diagnosis? How would you manage this patient?

36. A 20-year-old male presents for a routine physical evaluation for college football. A required urinalysis reveals macroscopic blood in his urine. This is repeated and remains positive. Microscopic examination is positive for deformed RBCs and RBC casts. He is without complaints and reports that he is in very good health. Where in the renal/genitourinary system is the etiology of this hematuria?

37. A 31-year-old female presents to your office complaining of painful joints for the past 4 to 5 months, affecting her wrists, ankles, and knees. She also reports several outbreaks of a rash over her face over the past few months. Vital signs are as follows: temperature = 99.2, RR = 20, BP = 145/83, pulse = 78. Physical examination reveals three ulcers in her mouth and mild swelling of the left wrist and ankle. She has 1+ pitting edema in her lower extremities bilaterally. Examination is otherwise unremarkable. CBC reveals a WBC count of 2,300/mm³, Hgb = 12.2, Hct = 37, platelets = 82,000/mm³. What is the likely diagnosis? What is the appropriate next step in managing this patient?

38. A 62-year-old male presents to your office accompanied by his wife. He complains of a tremor in his hands that disappears when he uses his hands for writing or handling utensils. His wife thinks he stares often and does not show as much emotion as before. He is slower in moving about than before. On examination you note a mild resting tremor and a fixed expression on his face. Neurologic examination is normal. What is the diagnosis? How would you manage this patient?

39. A 24-year-old male presents to your office having had cramping abdominal pain for the past 2 months. He reports having low-volume diarrhea on and off for the past 1 to 2 years. He also reports occasional pain in the rectal region with defecation. He denies any medical problems and takes no medications. His physical examination reveals mild tenderness in the RLQ with normal bowel sounds. There is a small fissure in the anal region with surrounding erythema. His stool is negative for occult blood. Vital signs are as follows: temperature = 98.7, RR = 15, BP = 122/78, pulse = 65. Laboratory test results (CBC, electrolytes) are within normal limits. How would you further evaluate this patient?

40. A 58-year-old male presents to your office with complaint of left hand numbness and tingling for the past 3 months. He denies any history of injury. He works as a truck driver. PMH is significant for mild HTN. The numbness involves all fingers and occasionally extends up his forearm to his elbow. He denies any weakness. Examination reveals normal sensation throughout bilateral upper extremities. Strength testing is normal. What is the next appropriate step in evaluating this patient?

41. You are a hospitalist called to evaluate a 74-year-old female with dementia for SOB and increasing oxygen requirements. The patient was admitted to the hospital 4 days ago with dehydration. She has not been out of bed since being hospitalized because of her generalized weakness. She denies chest pain or any other symptoms. Temperature = 99.4, BP = 116/74, pulse = 112, RR = 26, oxygen saturation = 91% on 5 L of oxygen via nasal canula. She is moderately tachypneic. Physical examination of heart and lungs is normal. What is the likely diagnosis in this patient? What is the appropriate next step in management?

42. A 63-year-old male collapses suddenly while playing basketball. When the emergency medical technicians arrive, they find the man pulseless and not breathing. After taking over CPR, the emergency medical technicians deliver a 200-joule shock to his chest and he converts to a sinus rhythm. The recorded rhythm strip shows a wide-complex tachycardia (rate, approximately 175 bpm) that is characteristically unresponsive to carotid sinus massage. Which arrhythmia described above induced his cardiac arrest? How would you manage this patient?

43. A 38-year-old female presents to your office with pain in her wrists, ankles, and knees bilaterally. She reports noticing numbness and stiffness in her hands about 1 year ago, mostly in cold weather. This stiffness gradually spread to her wrists, knees, and ankles, with lesser involvement of her shoulders. The stiffness and pain are worse in the morning but improve as the day wears on. Symptoms have gradually worsened. Some days she cannot go outside her house because of the pain. She denies a history of rash or photosensitivity. She often feels tired and "worn out." Medical history is significant for HTN, for which she takes hydrochlorothiazide. On examination, her metacarpal joints and wrists are swollen and tender, as are her knees and ankles bilaterally. Her examination is otherwise unremarkable. What is the likely diagnosis? What is the appropriate next step in management of this patient?

44. A 60-year-old female presents to the ED with a complaint of RUQ abdominal pain that began several hours ago. She felt fine before this episode. Her PMH is significant for HTN and osteoarthritis. On physical examination, she appears ill and has mild RUQ abdominal tenderness. Icterus is noted as well, but her examination is otherwise unremarkable. Vital signs are as follows: temperature = 102.1, RR = 16, BP = 145/90, pulse = 78. Laboratory tests reveal a mild elevation in ALT and AST levels, direct bilirubin 4.5, and WBC count 16,800. What is the next step in managing this patient?

45. A 57-year-old Caucasian female presents to the ED complaining of increasing SOB for the past week. She has a heavy cigarette smoking history and was recently diagnosed with COPD. On examination, her breathing is labored, and she has diffuse wheezing. CXR reveals flattened diaphragms and an enlarged retrosternal space. Spirometry results show that FEV_1 is 40% of predicted value and that FEV_1/FVC is 55% of predicted value. She will be admitted to your team's care, and you need to write the admission orders. What are the appropriate next steps in management?

46. A 64-year-old male presents to your office with left knee pain. He does not recall his history well but does state that the pain is worse when he returns from walking to the store for groceries. He describes the pain as a dull ache that has been present for the past several months, maybe longer. He recalls being in a motor vehicle accident 3 to 4 years ago when he banged his left knee against the dashboard. He had no fractures at the time and the "bruising went away" after a while. He describes some pain in his right knee as well, but it is mild and does not bother him that much. On physical examination, he has a small effusion in his left knee (no effusion in the right knee). He has mild crepitus in both knees, but no erythema or warmth. Strength is normal, and examination does not indicate any ligamentous instability. What is the likely diagnosis? What is the appropriate management of this patient?

47. A 34-year-old male is brought to the ED by EMS after being found unconscious in his apartment by his brother. It is unknown whether he suffered any trauma, but there are no signs of injury on examination. The patient cannot be aroused in the

ED but does respond to pain. Vital signs are as follows: temperature = 100.8, RR = 34, BP = 156/98, pulse = 104. Pupils are round and reactive to light bilaterally. According to his brother, this patient has no known medical problems. Laboratory tests reveal the following: WBC = 8.4, Hgb = 0.3, Hct = 30.9, Na^+ = 42, K^+ = 4.1, Cl^- = 104, HCO_3^- = 11, BUN = 15, Cr = 0.9, glucose = 114. ABGs are obtained and reveal the following: pH = 7.18, Pa_{CO_2} = 23, Pa_{O_2} = 96. What is the acid-base disorder? What is the appropriate management of this patient?

48. A 53-year-old female underwent an uneventful total hip replacement 2 hours ago. In the recovery room, she experiences a sudden onset of SOB, nausea, palpitations, and chest pain. PMH is significant for HTN and hyperthyroidism. She is diaphoretic and agitated. Temperature = 102.4, BP = 155/88, pulse = 134. Oxygen saturation at room air = 96%. Physical examination reveals crackles in bilateral lower lobes. Cardiac examination reveals a regular rhythm with no murmurs. She denies any radiating component to her chest pain. The patient is alert and oriented. What are the appropriate next steps in the management of this patient?

49. A 61-year-old male who has been your patient for several years presents to your office with a complaint of two episodes of bloody urine over the past 24 hours. He denies any pain. PMH is significant for hyperlipidemia, HTN, diabetes, glaucoma, and osteoarthritis. He has smoked one pack of cigarettes per day for the past 35 to 40 years. Physical examination is normal. Urinalysis shows gross hematuria without proteinuria, pyuria, or RBC casts. What is the appropriate next step in managing this patient?

50. A 57-year-old male presents to your office with a 2-week history of cough. He denies fevers or chills. An increased amount of clear sputum is associated with the cough. He typically has a very mild cough daily, but over the past 2 weeks this has significantly worsened. He has experienced chest discomfort due to excessive coughing and sometimes feels short of breath. PMH is negative and he takes no medications. He smokes one pack of cigarettes per day and has a 30 to 35 pack-year history. Temperature is 99.1. Auscultation of lungs reveals clear airway entry. CXR shows mild overexpansion of the lungs without infiltrates. What is the likely diagnosis and how would you approach this problem?

51. A 32-year-old African-American male, who recently moved to the area, presents to your office for the first time for a routine checkup. PMH is significant for type II DM. He is 5'9" and weighs 215 lb. The only medication he takes is metformin. He smokes half a pack of cigarettes a day; does not drink alcohol; and exercises sporadically, approximately once every 2 weeks. His mother died at the age of 62 due to an MI. His father is 73 years of age and is healthy. Physical examination is normal. Vital signs are: BP = 145/95, pulse = 73, RR = 19, temperature = 98.2. Describe the appropriate next steps in the management of this patient.

52. The patient in the previous question returns to your office in 6 weeks for a repeat evaluation. He has no complaints. He states that he has been walking briskly for 30 minutes four times a week, has lost 10 lb., and has been eating a healthier diet. His laboratory results are within normal limits. Hemoglobin A_{1C} is 7.2. CXR, ECG, and urinalysis are normal. His BP today is between 140/90 and 145/95. Physical examination is unchanged from 2 months ago. What is your recommended treatment?

53. A 17-year-old female is referred to the ED by her primary physician; she presents with a 3-day history of fevers, dysuria, and vomiting. She denies vaginal discharge, abdominal pain, or diarrhea. She is sexually active with her boyfriend. Vital signs are as follows: temperature = 103, RR = 20, BP = 98/65, pulse = 100. She appears ill and is unable to tolerate liquids, but she is alert and oriented. Her examination is positive for suprapubic as well as costovertebral angle tenderness bilaterally. Urinalysis reveals numerous WBCs and bacteria, and it is positive for WBC casts. Other laboratory study results are within normal limits. What is the likely diagnosis? Describe the appropriate next steps in management of this patient.

54. A 42-year-old female presents to the ED with a complaint of severe low back pain since last night. She was bending over to pick up a heavy suitcase when she felt

sudden pain in her low back. Ibuprofen does relieve the pain, but not completely. She denies any pain or numbness in the lower extremities. Bowel and bladder function is normal. Physical examination reveals a moderately overweight female in acute distress. She is lying on her side on the examination table holding her back; she cannot lie supine because of severe back pain. She has very minimal tenderness on palpation of her low back. Neurologic examination is normal. What is the appropriate next step in managing this patient?

55. A 29-year-old male with a history of asthma presents to the ED with severe SOB for the past 2 days. He also complains of sore throat, generalized malaise, and a nonproductive cough. He denies chest pain, fever, and chills. Temperature = 98.9, HR = 95, RR = 33, BP = 140/82, and O_2 saturation = 90% on room air. Breathing is labored, and he is speaking in short gasps. Lung auscultation reveals bilateral diffuse expiratory wheezing. ABG is drawn: 7.42/43/70/22. What is the appropriate next step in managing this patient?

56. A 22-year-old female presents to the ED with abrupt onset of a rash, high fever, and vomiting. Vital signs are as follows: temperature = 104, HR = 118, RR = 22, BP = 76/40, and pulse oximetry = 98% on room air. On examination she appears confused and disoriented. Her skin is warm, and there is a diffuse macular rash over her body. She is admitted to the ICU and subsequently develops multisystem organ dysfunction. What is the diagnosis? Describe the appropriate management of this patient.

57. A 33-year-old Caucasian male comes to the clinic with a 4-day history of chest pain. The pain radiates to the right side of the neck and is worsened by deep inspiration and improved by leaning forward. Several weeks ago he had a fever and cough, which have both since improved. He is afebrile, BP is 130/85, and pulse is 88. On examination, there is a scratching sound heard over the left sternal border on expiration. ECG shows ST elevation in leads I, II, III, avL, and V_2 to V_6. What is the etiology of his condition and what medications should be administered?

58. A 20-year-old male presents to your office complaining of low back pain for several months. He reports improvement of the pain with movement and exercise, but that rest worsens the pain. He denies any pain in his legs but does have pain in his right shoulder on occasion. He also feels fatigued much of the time. His low back pain has gradually worsened, and he now has pain when he lies on his back. Medical history is unremarkable. On physical examination, he has limited range of motion in his lumbar spine on flexion and extension, and full extension of the spine is not possible. He has tenderness over the spinous processes of T12-L4 vertebrae. Vital signs are as follows: temperature = 100.9, HR = 68, RR = 16, BP = 124/76. What is the likely diagnosis? What is the appropriate management of this patient?

59. You are paged to come and evaluate a 73-year-old female with SOB and tachycardia. She was admitted 1 week ago for a CVA. For the past 4 days she has been febrile, and her blood cultures are positive for *Escherichia coli*. Her sepsis is being treated with multiple broad-spectrum antibiotics. She had no previous history of cardiovascular or respiratory disease. Her nurse tells you that today she is more confused and appears quite ill. Temperature = 100.4, pulse = 116, BP = 116/56, RR = 36. Oxygen saturation is 87% on room air. Examination shows use of accessory muscles on inspiration. What are the appropriate initial steps to take in the management of this patient?

60. A 20-year-old male hemophiliac patient presents with an intensely painful right knee. His right knee is swollen, warm, and tender to palpation, and the skin is erythematous. His right knee has a very limited range of motion. His examination is otherwise normal, with no other joints affected. What are the appropriate steps to take in this patient?

61. A 20-year-old male presents with a 1-week history of severe sore throat, fever, and malaise. He has other nonspecific complaints such as headache, chills, and nausea. On examination, his lungs are clear to auscultation, but pharyngeal exudates are evident on examination of his throat. His eyes appear swollen, and he has tender posterior cervical lymph nodes. What is the diagnosis? How would you manage this patient?

62. A 21-year-old male presents to your office with chief complaint of cough and a sore throat for 3 days. He also complains of nasal discharge and congestion as well as back pain. He denies any chest pain or shortness of breath. There is no sputum production. Vital signs are: temperature = 100.4, BP = 124/82, pulse = 76, RR = 16. On physical examination, his lungs are clear to auscultation bilaterally, and he has an erythematous oropharynx without pharyngeal exudates. What is the appropriate management of this patient?

63. A 35-year-old male presents with complaint of a 6-month history of fatigue and lethargy. His medical history is unremarkable. He denies melena and recent trauma or surgery. He reports that he does not drink alcohol, smoke, or take any medications. His family history is noncontributory. He appears well nourished. Vital signs are as follows: RR = 16, BP = 130/80, pulse = 70. Laboratory test results are as follows: Hb = 7.6, Hct = 22.8%, and MCV = 68. The remainder of his laboratory test results are normal. What is the likely diagnosis? Describe the appropriate management of this patient.

64. A 56-year-old female presents to the ED with a complaint of severe abdominal pain, primarily in the RUQ and epigastric region. She has had two episodes of vomiting in the past 5 hours. She describes the pain as sharp, without radiation to her back. PMH is significant for DM, HTN, alcoholism, asthma, and chronic low back pain. Her current medications include insulin, atenolol, albuterol inhaler, and oxycodone. She has had abdominal pain several times in the past year, but never this severe and never associated with vomiting. On examination, she has tenderness in the epigastric region. There is no guarding or rebound. Physical examination is otherwise unremarkable. Temperature = 101.3, BP = 136/88, pulse = 116. She is alert and oriented and is in obvious distress. What are the appropriate next steps in the management of this patient?

65. A 37-year-old female presents to your office with a history of fatigue for the past few months. She does not have any other complaints. After a thorough medical history, she admits to mild constipation that is not troublesome for her. She reports a 5-lb weight gain over the past 6 months, which she attributes to living a more sedentary life of late due to her fatigue and lethargy. Her physical examination is unremarkable; her thyroid does not seem enlarged, although her face is slightly puffy. You order thyroid function studies, which show an elevated TSH level. What is the likely diagnosis? How would you manage this patient?

66. A 21-year-old male college student is brought to the ED by his friends after developing fever, neck stiffness, and confusion. Vital signs on admission are as follows: temperature = 105, RR = 20, BP = 120/75, pulse = 92, and pulse oximetry 99% on room air. Examination reveals nuchal rigidity and a diffuse maculopapular rash with petechiae scattered over his trunk and extremities. What organism is responsible for this? How should his college friends and contacts be treated?

67. A 64-year-old male presents with back pain for the past 5 to 6 months. Two days ago he fell while shoveling snow, and he has pain in his right arm as well. Plain films of the spine show several small lytic lesions in the vertebral bodies at the L3-L4 level. Right humerus films reveal lytic areas in the metaphysis and diaphysis of the right humerus. There is a fracture line through the abnormal area on the humerus film. Physical examination reveals tenderness on palpation of the low back and right humerus, but is otherwise unremarkable. There is no splenomegaly or lymphadenopathy. CBC results are as follows: Hb = 9.1 g/dL, Hct = 27.6% MCV = 90, platelet count = 150,000/μL. Serum chemistries are as follows: sodium = 137 mmol/L, potassium = 4.1 mmol/L, chloride = 107 mmol/L, CO_2 = 24 mmol/L, glucose = 89 mg/dL, BUN = 46 mg/dL, Cr = 3.5 mg/dL. What is the likely diagnosis? Describe the appropriate management of this patient.

68. A 47-year-old male presents to your office with severe low back pain for the past 2 days. This morning he had an episode of loss of control of his urine, followed by progressive weakness in bilateral lower extremities. His low back pain is severe and sharp, and it radiates into the right lower extremity. PMH is significant for mild asthma. He has had intermittent low back pain for the past 2 years but never this severe and never associated with weakness or urinary symptoms. On physical examination, he has very limited motion of his lumbar spine secondary to pain. He has 3/5 strength in gastrocnemius muscles bilaterally and 2/5 strength with great toe dorsiflexion bilaterally. He has diminished sensation throughout his lower extremities, and reflexes are diminished. What is the most appropriate next step in the management of this patient?

69. A 67-year-old female presents to the ED after a transient episode of visual loss in her right eye. She reports that she has had right-sided headaches for several months, for which she takes ibuprofen, with some relief. On physical examination, she has tenderness over her scalp in the left temporal region and complains that her jaw "gets tired with chewing." Neurologic examination is normal with no focal deficits. Vital signs are as follows: temperature = 101.1, HR = 72, RR = 16, BP = 140/82. What is the likely diagnosis and the appropriate management of this patient?

70. A 63-year-old female is brought to the ED by the rescue squad after an episode of syncope at home. Her husband witnessed the event. He describes the patient as falling suddenly to the floor from a standing position without any prodromal symptoms and losing consciousness for about 5 seconds, after which she rapidly regained consciousness and was oriented and appropriate. No bowel or bladder incontinence was noted. PMH is significant for DM, HTN, and depression. She denies any chest pain or SOB. Vital signs are: temperature = 100.2, BP = 118/68, pulse = 84, RR = 18. Oxygen saturation on room air is 96%. Physical examination is significant only for bruising of her left wrist and thigh. Heart and lung examination is normal. What are the appropriate next steps in managing this patient?

71. A 63-year-old female presents to your office with complaint of mid to low back pain for the last year, which has become worse over the past 3 months. She denies any weakness or radiating pain in her lower extremities. She currently takes oxycodone for her back pain with inadequate relief. She has difficulty sleeping at night because of the back pain. PMH is significant for HTN, for which she takes a β-blocker. Thoracic and lumbar spine radiographs show multiple compression fractures at T8, T11, L3, and L4, as well as diffuse osteopenia. Laboratory studies are as follows: WBC 8, hemoglobin 9.7, hematocrit 29%, platelets 189, Na$^+$ 142, K$^-$ 4.1, BUN 43, creatinine 2.3, calcium 14.3. Physical examination reveals tenderness on palpation of thoracic and lumbar spine. She has limited lumbar flexion due to pain. Neurological examination is normal. What is the appropriate next step in managing this patient?

72. A 62-year-old female is brought to the ED by EMS for confusion, headache, and vomiting over the past 12 hours. Vital signs are as follows: temperature = 96.9, HR = 100, RR = 22, BP = 220/150. She is disoriented and uncooperative. Examination is otherwise unremarkable. What is the most likely diagnosis, and what is the most appropriate management?

73. A 74-year-old male is brought to your office by his daughter, who is having increasing problems caring for him at home. She states that he behaves inappropriately at times, and on two occasions he has wandered outside the home and has gotten lost. He misplaces items frequently, and his personality has changed to being more belligerent and demanding. He seems to lack judgment in social situations, and he never had this problem in the past. She states that these problems have become worse gradually over the past 4 to 5 years. Physical examination is unremarkable. What is the likely diagnosis? How would you manage this patient?

74. A 73-year-old female is brought to the ED by EMS with a complaint of SOB and mild chest pain that began suddenly a few hours ago. Her medical history is significant for a previous MI 5 years ago and mild CHF. Two weeks ago, the patient fell and fractured her right hip, which was repaired surgically. She was discharged from the hospital 10 days ago and has been resting at home since then. Her chest pain is worse with inspiration. On physical examination, she is in moderate respiratory distress; the examination is otherwise unremarkable. Temperature = 99.1, BP = 138/75, pulse = 96, RR = 28. CXR is normal. Routine laboratory values are all normal. What is the appropriate management?

75. A 39-year-old female presents to your office with a 3-year history of headaches. They occur once or twice per week, lasting several hours. The headaches are throbbing and are usually on her left side. During these episodes, the patient is incapacitated and must lie down in a dark room for several hours. She is sensitive to light during the episodes and cannot move because of the pain. She is often nauseated and has vomited on two occasions. Medical history is significant for hypothyroidism, for which she takes levothyroxine (Synthroid). Her physical examination is unremarkable. What is the appropriate next step in managing this patient?

76. A 55-year-old female presents to your office for a routine follow-up examination. Medical history is significant for poorly controlled DM (20-year history), HTN, and osteoarthritis of bilateral knees. She also has had chronic renal insufficiency for the past 5 years. Her current medications include hydrochlorothiazide, lisinopril, insulin, and metoprolol. She has been taking increasing amounts of NSAIDs for the past several weeks for her painful knees. She is obese with 2+ peripheral pitting edema. Her examination is otherwise unremarkable. Laboratory tests reveal the following: $Na^+ = 135$, $K^+ = 4.9$, $Cl^- = 104$, $HCO_3^- = 27$, $Cr = 3.6$, $WBC = 7.9$, $Hgb = 8.2$, $Hct = 24.6$, $MCV = 75$. On urinalysis, she has 3+ proteinuria. On her last visit 3 months ago, her Cr was 2.3. What is the appropriate next step in managing this patient?

77. A 64-year-old female presents to the ED with sudden onset of severe chest pain. She has a history of angina and takes nitroglycerin, but this time the pain is much worse and is not relieved with nitroglycerin. PMH is significant for HTN. She is afebrile, and $HR = 105$, $BP = 160/105$, $RR = 17$. Cardiac enzymes are negative. CXR shows a widened mediastinum. What is the likely diagnosis?

78. A 17-year-old male presents to the ED with severe pain in his right arm and back that began suddenly a few hours ago. The pain is sharp and throbbing. He has a history of sickle cell disease with frequent painful crises requiring hospitalization once or twice per year. He has no other medical problems. Vital signs are as follows: temperature = 97.6, $HR = 94$, $RR = 20$, $BP = 132/84$. Oxygen saturation is 97% on room air. His right extremity is very tender, as is his low back in the midline. His examination is otherwise unremarkable. CBC results are as follows: $Hb = 7.0$, $Hct = 21\%$, $MCV = 94$. What is the appropriate management of this patient?

79. A 42-year-old male presents to your office because he noticed a "lump" in his neck 1 month ago. He denies any recent weight loss, palpitations, pain, or dysphagia. On physical examination, you note a nontender, firm nodule about 2 cm in size to the left of the midline in the region of the thyroid gland. Vital signs are as follows: $BP = 125/82$, pulse = 75. He does not take any medications and has no significant medical history. He denies any family history of thyroid disease or cancer. His routine serum laboratory values (CBC, electrolytes, BUN, creatinine) are normal. What is the appropriate next step in management of this patient?

80. A 64-year-old female presents to your office with a one month history of intermittent neck and shoulder pain with SOB that normally occurs when she does chores around the house or climbs stairs. She is previously healthy and denies any medical conditions. $BP = 148/86$ and pulse = 88. You order an ECG, CXR, CBC, and electrolytes. What are the next appropriate steps in the management of this patient?

81. A 54-year-old male presents to the ED with severe pain in his right great toe. He says that the pain is extreme and intolerable, and he is in obvious distress. On examination, there is exquisite tenderness, erythema, and swelling of the right great toe as well as the dorsum of the foot, and it feels very warm to the touch. The pain began suddenly a few hours ago. He denies any previous episodes or pain in any other joints. He denies any trauma. Medical history is significant for osteoarthritis of his right knee, for which he takes ibuprofen. He does not take any other medications. Vital signs are as follows: temperature = 98.5, $RR = 16$, $BP = 140/85$, pulse = 78. What is the appropriate next step in managing this patient?

82. A 41-year-old male presents to your office with a complaint of heartburn and epigastric pain for the past several months. He takes over-the-counter antacids, but symptoms have been worse over the past month. He denies any weight loss, vomiting, hematemesis, or melena. The discomfort is worse after eating and when he lies flat in bed. He sometimes gets a horrible taste in his mouth. Medical history is noncontributory. He takes no other medications. He smokes half a pack a day of cigarettes and drinks alcohol socially about once per week. Physical examination is unremarkable except for mild epigastric tenderness. What is the appropriate next step in managing this patient?

83. An 81-year-old female was in a motor vehicle accident 3 days ago and suffered a left femur fracture, for which she had surgery on the same day. She has been hospitalized since the day of surgery and has been taking part in daily physical therapy without difficulty. Her family (husband and daughter) report that she has not been "acting like herself" at times when they come to visit her. She becomes agitated and is belligerent toward them, and she sometimes wonders why she is in the hospital. At other times, the patient is doing very well, and they do not notice these inconsistencies. The patient has a history of borderline HTN. Current medications include a stool softener and morphine for pain control. On examination, the patient is alert and oriented to time/place/person and is appropriately responding to questions. She denies any hallucinations. Neurologic examination is normal. What is the appropriate next step in managing this patient?

84. A 49-year-old female presents to the ED with complaint of severe epigastric and RUQ abdominal pain. Her symptoms started 3 days ago but have progressively worsened over the past 12 hours. Her symptoms are worse with meals. She has had two episodes of vomiting in the past 12 hours and is nauseous currently. PMH is significant for diabetes, osteoarthritis, and HTN. Temperature = 102.3, BP = 146/80, pulse = 110, RR = 16. On physical examination, there is tenderness in the RUQ and rebound tenderness. Bowel sounds are diminished. The patient is lying on her side holding an emesis basin. What is the most appropriate next step in the management of this patient?

85. A 31-year-old female presents to your office with multiple musculoskeletal aches and pains including, but not limited to, her shoulders, elbows, knees, neck, and buttocks. She has had these symptoms for at least the past year. She does not sleep very well when the pain is severe and has no relief with NSAIDs. On palpation, she has marked tenderness over both lateral epicondyles, the anterior aspect of her left shoulder, the medial aspect of her right knee, her posterior neck, and her left greater trochanter. There are no effusions at any of the above sites. Routine laboratory test results are normal. What is the appropriate next step in managing this patient?

86. A 52-year-old male with a long-standing history of alcohol abuse is brought to the ED by his wife for vomiting blood. He vomited bright red blood at least twice this morning. PMH is significant for cirrhosis, HTN, and arthritis. He has never vomited blood before. On examination, the patient is awake but appears nervous and is in moderate distress. You are able to determine that he has vomited approximately 2 liters of blood over the past 6 hours. Vital signs are: temperature = 99.2, BP = 95/60, HR = 134, RR = 20. Pulse oximetry shows 98% oxygenation on room air. Describe the next steps in managing this patient.

87. A 57-year-old female presents to the ED with a complaint of abdominal pain. The pain is diffuse and poorly localized. She has had these symptoms for the past month and has been constipated during this time. She has no significant PMH. Vital signs are: temperature = 99.2, BP = 128/78, HR = 78, RR = 16. On physical examination, there is mild abdominal distention and no guarding or rebound tenderness. The remainder of the examination is normal. What is the next appropriate step in the management of this patient?

88. A 53-year-old male presents to the ED with a 4-hour history of left flank pain radiating to his left groin. The pain was sudden in onset but was mild at first. However, it has been increasing in severity over the past 2 to 3 hours. The pain is now constant and excruciating. It was associated with nausea and vomiting, but the patient denies fevers/chills. He denies seeing any gross blood in his urine. Medical history is insignificant. Vital signs are as follows: temperature = 98.1, RR = 24,

BP = 148/88, pulse = 93. On physical examination, the patient is in obvious distress, writhing in pain. He has marked tenderness along the left flank, but the examination is otherwise unremarkable. Urinalysis reveals 2+ heme. Urine sediment reveals no casts but many RBCs and few WBCs per HPF. Laboratory tests reveal the following: WBC 8.2, Hgb 11.9, Hct 36.1, BUN 14, Cr 0.9. What is the appropriate next step in managing this patient?

89. A 39-year-old female is brought to the ED by her husband with the chief complaint of acute SOB and anxiety that started suddenly 2 to 3 hours ago while she was working around the house. She denies chest pain. Her PMH is unremarkable. She takes oral contraceptives but no other medications. Vital signs are: temperature = 99.1, RR = 34, BP = 148/90, pulse = 100. Oxygen saturation is 94% on room air. On examination, the patient appears healthy although in moderate respiratory distress. Her examination is otherwise unremarkable. Laboratory tests reveal: WBC = 7.1, Hgb = 12.2, Hct = 37.3, Na^+ = 138, K^+ = 4.7, Cl^- = 109, HCO_3^- = 25, BUN = 14, Cr = 0.9, glucose = 106. ABGs are obtained and reveal: pH = 7.52, HCO_3^- = 20, $Paco_2$ = 26, Pao_2 = 70. CXR and ECG are normal. What is the acid-base disorder? What is the appropriate management of this patient?

90. A 63-year-old male is brought to the ED by his wife for altered mental status. The patient regularly drinks alcohol and has a long-standing history of alcohol use. Over the past 24 hours, he has become more confused and is not "acting like himself" according to his wife. She states that he has never acted like this before. On further questioning, the patient had an episode of massive hematemesis last year that required admission to the hospital, necissitating blood transfusion and other treatment that the wife does not recall. On physical examination, the patient is arousable and is alert to person but not to place or time. He is cachectic, with prominent veins over his abdomen. He has a significant ascites. There are several dilated superficial arterioles scattered throughout his body. What is the likely diagnosis? How would you manage this problem?

91. A 65-year-old female presents to your office with a chief complaint of low back pain. She has had this pain for 6 or 7 months. She denies any recent trauma or any event that she recalls precipitating the pain. One year ago she suffered a distal radius fracture when she tripped in her bedroom and landed on her outstretched left arm. Medical history is significant for HTN, for which she takes hydrochlorothiazide. She smokes approximately 12 cigarettes per day and has a 25 pack-per-year history of smoking. She denies any alcohol use. She does not exercise. On physical examination, you note tenderness on palpation of the lower back in the region of L4-L5. She has no radicular symptoms, and the straight-leg test is negative. What is the appropriate next step in managing this patient?

92. A 76-year-old male presents to your office with the complaint of fatigue for the past 2 months. He does not abuse alcohol. His medical history is significant for HTN, for which he takes metoprolol. He denies melena, hematochezia, or any other blood loss. His family history is noncontributory. He has no symptoms other than fatigue. He admits he does not have a good diet. Vital signs are: BP = 135/85, pulse = 70. Physical examination is unremarkable except for mild pallor. Stool is negative for occult blood. Laboratory test results are: Hb = 9.2, Hct = 27.6, MCV = 117. ECG is normal. What is the appropriate next step in managing this patient?

93. A 41-year-old female presents to your office for a routine checkup. Three months ago she had an elevated BP of 155/94. You recommended conservative therapy including weight loss, regular exercise, and a low-sodium diet and had her follow-up in 3 months. On today's visit, her BP is 158/96. She is asymptomatic. Medical history is negative. She smokes one pack of cigarettes per day and has a 20-pack-per-year history. Her father died of an MI at age 54, but she has no other family history of cardiovascular disease. Her total serum cholesterol concentration is 175 mg/dL and HDL is 40 mg/dL. Routine laboratory test results are within normal limits. What is the appropriate next step in managing this patient?

94. A 73-year-old male is brought to the ED in a coma. He was delivered to the ED from a nursing home and was reported by the nursing home staff to have had a seizure that lasted less than 1 minute. He was subsequently confused and soon thereafter entered a comatose state. His medical history is significant for type II DM requiring insulin, HTN, and mild CHF. In the ED, the patient is very lethargic and responds only to pain stimuli. His vital signs are stable, and CBC and electrolyte levels are normal. Serum glucose is 16 mg/dL. What are the **first steps** in the management of this patient? What is the likely cause of this patient's condition?

95. A 78-year-old female presents to your office for a routine checkup. Her only complaint is urinary incontinence that she has had for several years but that has become worse over the past several weeks. She has never sought treatment for this problem. Her medical history is significant for HTN and DM. She has four children, all delivered vaginally. Medications include hydrochlorothiazide for her HTN, insulin, and a daily aspirin. She wears adult pads because she loses large volumes of urine throughout the day and usually cannot reach the bathroom in time. She has the sudden urge to urinate every hour or so and also loses urine during the night. She also reports losing urine when she laughs or coughs. Physical examination is unremarkable. Vital signs are unremarkable. Routine laboratory test results are within normal limits except for a random blood glucose level of 210. Urinalysis shows positive nitrites and bacteria. What is the appropriate next step in managing this patient?

96. A 33-year-old female presents to your office with the complaint of insomnia and difficulty concentrating at work for several weeks. She reports a 20-lb weight loss over the past 2 to 3 months, despite eating more. When questioned, she reports that she frequently feels "hot and sweaty" at work and at home. She denies chest pain or palpitations but does have diarrhea frequently. Vital signs are: temperature = 98.9, RR = 15, BP = 130/80, pulse = 98. She appears worried. On physical examination, she has warm and moist skin. She has a slight hand tremor. On palpation of her thyroid, you note a diffusely enlarged thyroid gland that is nontender. A bruit is auscultated over the thyroid enlargement. What is the appropriate next step in managing this patient?

97. A 72-year-old female is brought to the ED by EMS after suffering smoke inhalation from a house fire. She lives alone, and her son states that she has been leaving the stove on after she cooks. Her son reports that over the past 5 years, she has had a significant decline in her memory. She is scared but is very pleasant and is awake, alert, and fully oriented. Medical history is significant for stroke 5 years ago, and at least three episodes of TIA that the son can recall over the past 8 years. Vital signs are: temperature = 97.8, RR = 22, BP = 164/85, pulse = 88. Pulse oximetry is initially 89% but increases to 95% on 2 L nasal cannula O$_2$. Breath sounds are coarse, but physical examination is otherwise negative. After the patient is stabilized, you perform a mini-mental status examination. You discover that her recent memory is impaired and she cannot carry out simple calculations. Her son asks you if you think she is "going senile." What is your response? What is the appropriate next step in managing this patient?

98. A 71-year-old female is brought to the ED after a fall. Immediately after the fall she was asymptomatic but over the ensuing hours become lethargic and more confused. PMH is significant for HTN. She underwent a right total hip replacement 5 weeks ago and was diagnosed with a DVT 2 weeks after the operation. Medications include hydrochlorothiazide, warfarin, and atorvastatin. Two weeks ago, her INR was 2.7. On examination, patient has slurred speech and appears confused. She is oriented to person but not to place or time. Neurologic examination is normal. The remainder of physical examination is normal. What is the most appropriate initial step that would help guide the management of this patient?

99. A 66-year-old male is brought to your office by his wife with complaint of productive cough, fever, and chills for the past 2 days. The patient lives with his wife and is retired. PMH is significant for DM, for which he takes insulin; CHF, with an ejection fraction of 40%; and a history of renal insufficiency. He is alert and oriented. There is no history of smoking or alcohol use. On physical examination, he has crackles over the left lower lung. Cardiovascular examination is normal. Vital signs are: temperature

= 103.3, BP = 130/64, HR = 128, RR = 24. Oxygen saturation on room air is 97%. CXR shows infiltrates and consolidation in the left lower lobe of the lung. Laboratory test results show WBC 15, hematocrit 36, Na 142, glucose 167, BUN 36, creatinine 1.5. What is the next appropriate step in managing this patient?

100. You are called to see a 69-year-old male with acute SOB. Vital signs are: temperature = 100.1, BP = 166/88, pulse = 130, RR = 33. You rush to see the patient and on your arrival, oxygen saturation is 79% on a 100% oxygen nonrebreather face mask. The nurse informs you that his oxygen saturation was 68% on room air. He currently has heavily labored breathing and appears cyanotic. The nurse informs you that the patient was admitted 2 days ago for cellulitis involving his left leg, which was treated with antibiotics. The cellulitis has not improved, and the plan was to obtain an MRI tomorrow to rule out an abscess. What is the appropriate first step in the management of this patient?

1. **Answer:** In developed countries, bronchogenic carcinoma and bronchitis are the most common causes of hemoptysis, replacing TB and bronchiectasis. Bronchoscopy should be performed in most patients with hemoptysis, although no study has clearly shown whether CT scan or bronchoscopy should be the initial test, especially if the CXR does not reveal any localized lesions. Given this patient's smoking history, lung cancer must be ruled out with bronchoscopy; however, given the acuteness of his illness (last month), bronchitis is also a possibility.

2. **Answer:** This patient likely has diverticulitis (LLQ pain, fever, and leukocytosis are keys to diagnosis). Obtain a CT scan of the abdomen and pelvis to confirm the diagnosis. For the first episode of diverticulitis, surgery is not indicated unless symptoms persist after 3 to 4 days. Broad-spectrum IV antibiotic therapy, bowel rest (NPO), and IV fluids are appropriate next steps.

3. **Answer:** The increased severity and duration of chest pain suggest either unstable angina or acute MI. The only objective means of ruling out an MI is via cardiac enzymes. This patient should be admitted and closely monitored. Initial treatment includes a β-blocker, ACE inhibitor, aspirin, nitroglycerin, oxygen, and consider morphine. Perform a 12-lead ECG when the patient is having chest pain, and again when she is pain-free. Compare with an old ECG if one is available.

4. **Answer:** This is a classic description of **amaurosis fugax**, which is a hallmark symptom of a TIA. By definition, symptoms during a TIA last less than 24 hours. Amaurosis fugax is thought to be caused by emboli to the ophthalmic artery. The first test you should obtain is an ultrasound of the carotid arteries to determine the degree of stenosis. Carotid endarterectomy may be indicated depending on degree of stenosis.

5. **Answer:** This patient likely has vitamin B_{12} deficiency. After gastrectomy, lack of intrinsic factor leads to vitamin B_{12} deficiency. The patient's neurologic deficits are consistent with vitamin B_{12} deficiency. Check routine laboratory values to document anemia and the patient's MCV (should be high). Check the serum vitamin B_{12} level. Serum homocysteine and methylmalonic acid may also be helpful.

6. **Answer:** Based on her history, and particularly on the examination findings, this patient likely has Cushing's syndrome, which can be confirmed by an overnight dexamethasone suppression test. Once the syndrome is diagnosed, your next step is to determine whether the cortisol excess is ACTH-dependent or ACTH-independent, which can be done via the high-dose dexamethasone suppression test.

7. **Answer:** This patient is suffering from an acute anterior-wall MI. Current evidence indicates that revascularization reduces mortality and reinfarction more than thrombolytic therapy in an acute ST segment elevation MI if it can be performed within 2 hours of presentation. Thrombolytic therapy is the treatment of choice in a non-ST segment elevation MI if there are no contraindications.

8. **Answer:** This patient has a metabolic alkalosis (high bicarbonate, high pH) with respiratory compensation (which explains the high $PaCO_2$). Vomiting is the likely cause of her metabolic alkalosis—as HCl is lost during vomiting, the stomach generates bicarbonate, which causes the alkalosis. Examination (and orthostatic BP changes) reveals volume depletion, which is a hallmark finding in saline-sensitive metabolic alkalosis. This patient likely has a viral gastroenteritis. Normal saline plus potassium supplementation will restore the ECF volume. In this patient, an antiemetic agent should be considered.

9. **Answer:** Although the positive predictive value of the Hemoccult test in diagnosing colon cancer is low (20%), all patients with a positive test result should undergo a colonoscopy to rule out colorectal cancer.

10. **Answer:** Based on the history, this patient's upper GI bleeding is most likely due to a bleeding peptic ulcer (NSAIDs) or erosive esophagitis (possible GERD). Based on his vital signs, this patient is in the early stages of hypovolemic shock. Initial management involves hemodynamic stabilization (including transfusion if necessary). An upper endoscopy should follow to identify the cause of the bleeding. Consider starting acid suppression before endoscopy.

11. **Answer:** This presentation suggests an acute CVA. The symptoms are consistent with a lesion involving the left cerebral hemisphere in the MCA distribution. The abrupt onset suggests an embolic source. The first test to obtain is a noncontrast CT of the head to rule out hemorrhage or any mass lesion. The time window (3 hours) for thrombolytic therapy has passed, so management involves aspirin, prevention of aspiration, and cautious control of BP. Ultimately, physical therapy and rehabilitation are the most important therapeutic measures.

12. **Answer:** The most likely diagnosis is diverticulosis, which is usually asymptomatic. Barium enema is the test of choice for diagnosis. The patient should be treated conservatively with high-fiber foods.

13. **Answer:** Hemophilia is unlikely given that her bleeding is so superficial. Given that she has normal platelet counts, this patient may have a defect in platelet function. vWD is the most common inherited bleeding disorder. Tests that may help in diagnosis include a bleeding time, measurement of concentration of vWF antigen, or platelet aggregation tests with ristocetin. It is important that patients with vWD avoid use of NSAIDs and other antiplatelet agents. DDAVP is the treatment of choice.

14. **Answer:** This patient may have multiple sclerosis (MS). Transient sensory deficits are a common presenting feature of MS, as are visual disturbances (due to optic neuritis). First obtain an MRI of the brain to look for any demyelinating lesions in the CNS.

15. **Answer:** This woman has COPD—specifically, she has chronic bronchitis, a form of COPD defined by a cough with sputum production for at least 3 months of the year for at least 2 years. Cigarette smoking is the main risk factor for chronic bronchitis. The degree of dyspnea is reflective of the severity of disease. COPD may also cause pulmonary HTN and cor pulmonale. CXR findings that would suggest left-sided heart failure as the main cause of her dyspnea would be cardiomegaly, pulmonary edema, and possibly pleural effusions.

16. **Answer:** There is much controversy regarding use of PSA for detection of prostate cancer, especially with levels between 4.1 and 10 and a normal DRE. Regardless of the ultimate treatment decision (observation vs. TRUS with biopsy), educate this patient about the role of PSA and its shortcomings as a screening tool, given that TRUS with biopsy is an uncomfortable procedure.

17. **Answer:** The key piece of information in this question is a hip fracture without a history of fall or injury. A hip fracture in the absence of a fall or specific injury should raise the suspicion of a pathologic fracture, and in the elderly patient, metastatic disease must be ruled out. A search for a primary neoplasm should be initiated, with a CT scan of the chest, abdomen, and pelvis, a bone scan, and laboratory studies, including PSA levels.

18. **Answer:** Fatigue is a common complaint among patients, and therefore the physician must ask many questions to determine if the problem is chronic or acute, whether it is clinically significant, and whether there is a clear underlying lifestyle or medical cause. Unexplained, significant fatigue such as that described in this question that has been present for 6 months or more is clearly chronic and warrants further testing. Laboratory studies to consider in the workup of fatigue include CBC (anemia), TSH (hypothyroidism), fasting glucose (diabetes), basic metabolic panel (electrolyte abnormalities), ESR, urinalysis, and renal panel and liver function tests. One must also rule out pregnancy as an underlying cause, although one would expect it to be known to the patient at this point. Chronic fatigue syndrome is a diagnosis of exclusion after medical conditions that could cause fatigue have been ruled out.

19. Answer: This patient has a right lower lobe pneumonia, which should be treated with antibiotics. However, the round opacity in the left lower lobe raises the question of possible malignancy and should be investigated. The first step in investigation of a solitary pulmonary nodule is to obtain a previous CXR for comparison. Malignant nodules tend to grow quickly, and the growth is typically evident within months. The only radiographic findings that are reliable for a benign lesion are lack of growth for at least 2 years and a distinctive central laminated calcification pattern. A CT scan may also be obtained for further evaluation because it is more sensitive in defining the nodule.

20. Answer: This patient has third-degree (complete) AV nodal block. In this rhythm, the atria and ventricles contract independently of each other. This patient's heart block may have been caused by her multiple MIs, which often affect the conduction system. Other causes include digoxin toxicity and a degenerative AV nodal conduction. Third-degree heart block is always an indication for permanent pacemaker placement. If the patient is unstable, then temporary pacing (transvenous or transcutaneous) should be performed until a permanent pacemaker can be placed. This patient is clearly symptomatic, and therefore if only second-degree AV block were present, a pacemaker would still be indicated.

21. Answer: This patient likely has PUD. You can initiate empiric therapy without endoscopy or barium study if there are no signs of complications of the disease, but this is somewhat controversial. Although endoscopy is initially more expensive, its use reduces the number of patients treated inappropriately. Acid suppression with an H$_2$ blocker or PPI is appropriate in this patient. It is acceptable to test or treat empirically for *Helicobacter pylori* because he does not have any other obvious causes of PUD, although this, too, is debatable.

22. Answer: This patient likely has IBS. This is a clinical diagnosis, and extensive testing is unnecessary.

23. Answer: This patient most likely has CHF given the information provided. However, there are multiple other causes of SOB with hypoxia that must be considered. A previous MI and long-standing HTN are both causes of CHF. If a patient has a known history of CHF, it is important to ask him or her about medication compliance (especially diuretics). Other precipitants of CHF exacerbations include high sodium intake, illness or infection, and myocardial ischemia/infarction. Serial cardiac enzyme tests and ECGs should be performed to rule out an MI. She should be given oxygen and diuretics, and urine output should be noted. A transthoracic echocardiogram should be performed to evaluate her chambers, valves, and systolic function.

24. Answer: This patient has pain suggestive of angina. Because his symptoms occurred at rest, this is an example of unstable angina. The patient should be admitted to a floor with continuous cardiac monitoring. The following interventions are indicated: heparin, aspirin, β-blocker, nitrates, and oxygen.

25. Answer: This patient likely has pyelonephritis. If she is not properly treated, sepsis and even septic shock can ensue. Sepsis occurs in 10% to 25% of patients with pyelonephritis. Order the following: CBC, renal panel, urinalysis, and urine and blood cultures. This patient will probably not be able to tolerate oral antibiotics and should be admitted to the hospital, where IV fluids and broad-spectrum IV antibiotics (ciprofloxacin, or ampicillin plus gentamicin) should be started.

26. Answer: The patient's presentation suggests a hemorrhagic stroke. An ischemic stroke is less likely given her loss of consciousness and vomiting/headache. Attention should be directed to the management of ABCs (airway, breathing, and circulation); the patient may need to be intubated given her altered mental status. This patient likely needs to be admitted to the ICU for close monitoring, especially of her intracranial pressure. If she is stable, obtain a CT scan of her head to look for hemorrhage. Her BP is high; lower it cautiously because hypotension can lower cerebral blood flow.

27. Answer: This patient likely has acute mesenteric ischemia (sudden onset of severe abdominal pain disproportional to physical findings is the key to diagnosis). Obtain a mesenteric angiogram emergently; it is critical for definitive diagnosis and therapy. If undiagnosed, the mortality rate is very high due to intestinal infarction.

28. **Answer:** This patient has acute pericarditis. He has a history of recent upper respiratory infection, and the pericarditis is likely postviral. In acute pericarditis, the chest pain is positional and pleuritic. Pericardial friction rub is a classic finding on examination. The diagnosis rests on a combination of history, pericardial friction rub, and typical ECG changes (patient has diffuse ST elevation). Although not present in this patient, PR depression is a specific finding in acute pericarditis. Most cases of acute pericarditis are self-limited. Treatment with an NSAID is mainstay of therapy.

29. **Answer:** The first step is to obtain a CXR and start 100% oxygen via face mask. The patient's history and examination suggest spontaneous pneumothorax, which would be confirmed on CXR (visceral pleural line). Primary spontaneous pneumothorax is more common in tall, lean young males without underlying lung disease. Because he is symptomatic, a chest tube is needed to re-expand the lung.

30. **Answer:** This patient has AFib. The first step in any patient who presents with AFib is to determine whether the patient is stable and to determine HR. If the patient is tachycardic, use a β-blocker (atenolol) to lower the rate. Other options are calcium channel blockers and digoxin. The duration of this patient's AFib is not known, so he would require 3 weeks of anticoagulation before undergoing any cardioversion. Treatment of patients with "lone AFib" who do not have other risk factors for a stroke and are young (<65 years) is somewhat controversial.

31. **Answer:** This man has aortic stenosis (AS), most likely caused by long-standing HTN. AS can also be secondary to rheumatic heart disease, a congenital bicuspid aortic valve, or a calcific aortic valve. The three classic symptoms of AS are angina, syncope, and heart failure (in order of progressing severity). Once symptoms are present, AS is advanced. Classification of severity involves measurement of the aortic valve area, as well as the pressure gradient across the valve. Valve replacement is the only definitive treatment and should be performed if symptoms are present but before overt heart failure is present. Strenuous activity and negative inotropes should be avoided if aortic stenosis is severe. Vasodilators (such as nitrates) should also be avoided.

32. **Answer:** This patient has patellofemoral pain, which is anterior knee pain caused by either chondromalacia of the patella or patellofemoral arthritis. This is a very common cause of knee pain. Classic history is anterior knee pain that is worse with climbing or descending stairs. Patients may describe occasional effusions. Plain radiographs are indicated to evaluate the knee for osteoarthritic changes, especially in the patellofemoral compartment. Physical therapy is indicated and is very effective for patellofemoral pain. A quadriceps/hamstring rehabilitation program aimed at stretching and strengthening these muscles helps unload the patella and shift the load to the thigh muscles.

33. **Answer:** Given two blood glucose measurements of >126 mg/dL, this patient has diabetes. Diet and exercise should be the initial measures taken. If conservative therapy fails, an oral hypoglycemic agent may be initiated (metformin or glipizide). Order an Hb A_{1c} test to get an idea of his average blood glucose over the past few months. Perform a thorough examination (with attention to the feet). Provide teaching on self-monitoring of glucose as well as dietary and exercise education. Screen for microalbuminuria, and refer the patient to an ophthalmologist.

34. **Answer:** This constellation of findings (young African-American female with respiratory complaints, blurred vision, erythema nodosum, and bilateral hilar adenopathy) is suggestive of sarcoidosis. Order the following tests: ACE level, CBC, renal panel, calcium, LFTs. Hypercalcemia is relatively common in sarcoidosis. For definitive diagnosis, a bronchoscopy with transbronchial biopsy is required. The hallmark of sarcoidosis is noncaseating granulomas. Pulmonary function tests should also be ordered, which show reduction in vital capacity, total lung capacity, and diffusion capacity of carbon monoxide, as well as a decreased FEV_1/FVC ratio.

35. **Answer:** This patient has hyponatremia. You need to investigate further to determine the cause of the hyponatremia. Given the history of small cell carcinoma, SIADH is a likely cause, but because SIADH is a diagnosis of exclusion after other causes of hyponatremia have been ruled out, laboratory investigation should begin with a plasma and urine

osmolality, as well as a urine chemistry (urine sodium, osmolality). Consider plasma triglycerides. Note that in SIADH there is no edema or clinical evidence of ECF water expansion or depletion. Also, the urine is concentrated, with a urine osmolality >300 (natriuresis), and BUN and Cr levels are low (as in this case). Neurologic symptoms are **typically** not seen until the sodium level drops below 120. In this patient, water restriction may be enough to reverse the hyponatremia. Consider adding a loop diuretic and giving salt tablets. Do not increase the serum sodium rapidly because central pontine demyelination can occur.

36. **Answer:** The most likely source of the hematuria is the glomerulus. Isolated hematuria is commonly seen in patients with nephrolithiasis, trauma, or neoplasm. Other causes of hematuria include sickle cell anemia, hemophilia, or NSAID abuse. The presence of RBC casts and dysmorphic RBCs suggests glomerular involvement. This patient most likely has IgA nephropathy, which is the most common glomerular cause of recurrent hematuria. It is most commonly diagnosed in young men, and the disease course is variable. Approximately half of patients with IgA nephropathy develop CRF within 20 to 30 years. Patients are often asymptomatic when diagnosed or may have transient flu-like symptoms. Proteinuria may or may not be present.

37. **Answer:** This patient has SLE. Four of the 11 criteria must be fulfilled (see Box 6-1: Useful Criteria for Diagnosing SLE). She has arthritis, malar rash, oral ulcers, and hematologic abnormalities (leukopenia, thrombocytopenia). Order the appropriate serologic tests (e.g., ANA, anti-ds DNA), as well as routine laboratory tests (CBC, BUN, creatinine, urinalysis, serum electrolytes). Refer this patient to a rheumatologist for treatment.

38. **Answer:** Given the history of resting tumor, bradykinesia, and expressionless face, this patient likely has the beginnings of Parkinson's disease. Carbidopa-levodopa (Sinemet) is the agent of choice, although you may wish to delay the use of this drug in favor of one of the dopamine receptor agonists. Refer this patient to a neurologist for pharmacologic treatment.

39. **Answer:** This patient could have IBD. Absence of blood in his stool and RLQ tenderness make Crohn's disease more likely than ulcerative colitis, but a colonoscopy is needed to establish the diagnosis. Other conditions in the differential include diverticulosis (unlikely given his age), viral infection (diarrhea over the past 1 to 2 years makes this unlikely), and IBS (a diagnosis of exclusion). Other initial studies include stool cultures for *Clostridium difficile* and ova and parasites to rule out these diagnoses, as well as a stool culture to determine WBC count.

40. **Answer:** Hand numbness and tingling may be caused by carpal tunnel syndrome, a variety of nerve entrapment syndromes in the upper extremity, and by cervical radiculopathy. Always perform a cervical spine examination in any patient presenting with numbness and tingling in the upper extremities. Although carpal tunnel syndrome is the most common cause of these symptoms, nerve root impingement in the cervical spine can mimic these findings and this should be ruled out. If a patient has normal range of motion of the neck without pain, no history of neck pain, and no radiating pain down the arm, one can reasonably rule out cervical disease. If any doubt exists, electrodiagnostic studies (EMG and nerve conduction studies) can clarify the source of nerve compression. The treatment of carpal tunnel syndrome is initially conservative with wrist splints, NSAIDs. and possibly corticosteroid injections if needed.

41. **Answer:** A sudden increase in oxygen requirement should raise the suspicion of a pulmonary embolus. A history of recent immobilization is a classic risk factor for a DVT with conversion to PE. A $\dot{V}/\dot{Q}$ scan or helical CT scan should be obtained. Iodinated contrast agents are needed for helical CT scans, and therefore one should inquire about a history of allergy to contrast material and know the patient's renal function before ordering this test, because its use may be contraindicated in such cases.

42. **Answer:** Sustained VT is the most likely cause of the cardiac arrest. VT is a tachyarrhythmia often caused by CAD, MI, hypoxia, severe electrolyte disturbances, CHF, or medication toxicity. The QRS complexes are wide (usually >0.14 sec), and the rhythm is characteristically unresponsive to vagal maneuvers. If the patient is hemodynamically unstable (e.g., pulseless or hypotensive), immediate electrical synchronized cardioversion is indicated. If the patient is stable, then IV lidocaine should be administered. Evaluate and treat all potential causes.

43. Answer: Her medical history suggests possible rheumatoid arthritis (RA), with the characteristic morning stiffness and symmetrical polyarthritis. Obtain routine laboratory tests (CBC, chemistry panel) and rheumatoid factor. Plain radiographs of involved joints can aid in diagnosis. Actively search for any extra-articular manifestations of RA. If the diagnosis is established (patient has four of the seven criteria in Box 6-5: Diagnosis of Rheumatoid Arthritis), then refer the patient to a rheumatologist for initiation of disease-modifying therapy. Methotrexate is usually the first-line agent.

44. Answer: This woman has classic findings of cholangitis (RUQ pain, fever, and jaundice are the keys to diagnosis). Administer IV antibiotics and IV fluids and monitor hemodynamics. Early relief of biliary obstruction is important—options include ERCP, PTC, and surgery.

45. Answer: Bronchodilator therapy is the first-line treatment of COPD exacerbations. Beta$_2$ agonists (e.g., albuterol) and anticholinergics (e.g., ipratropium bromide) work synergistically in combination. Systemic steroids (e.g., IV methylprednisolone) are typically given for acute exacerbations requiring hospital admission. Supplemental oxygen and antibiotics also play an important role.

46. Answer: This patient's presentation suggests osteoarthritis. The trauma sustained in the motor vehicle accident is a risk factor for osteoarthritis (macrotrauma). Obtain radiographs for evaluation (look for joint space narrowing and osteophytes). If osteoarthritis is noted on radiographs, treatment includes acetaminophen or NSAIDs, physical therapy, activity modification, and possibly use of a cane if needed. If these modalities fail, depending on severity of disease, a cortisone injection or viscosupplementation may be indicated (see Chapter 12).

47. Answer: This patient has a metabolic acidosis. The first step in evaluation of a patient in metabolic acidosis is calculation of the anion gap (AG). This patient has an increased AG (27) metabolic acidosis. The differential diagnosis includes DKA; alcoholic ketoacidosis; lactic acidosis; starvation; renal failure; and overdose of salicylate, methanol, or ethylene glycol. Given that this patient is not diabetic and has a glucose level of 114, DKA is unlikely. Also, his renal function is not impaired. Because it is unclear what the cause is in this patient, further testing is needed. Initial tests should include serum ketone levels, serum salicylate and lactate levels, blood alcohol levels, and methanol and ethylene glycol levels. The next step is to determine whether this is a primary acid-base disorder or a mixed disorder. Using Winter's formula [1.5 (measured HCO_3^-) $+ 8 \pm 2$], the expected $Paco_2$ level in this patient is in the range of 22.5 to 26.5. With a $Paco_2$ of 23, this patient has an appropriate respiratory compensatory response (RR of 34). In the absence of hyperventilation, $Paco_2$ would be higher, and the pH would be even lower than it is.

48. Answer: The two most likely diagnoses are PE and MI. The first step is to obtain a "stat" CXR and ECG. A $\dot{V}/\dot{Q}$ scan or helical CT scan is indicated to rule out PE. If these two diagnoses are ruled out, one must also consider thyroid storm, which is a life-threatening condition with a mortality rate of up to 20%. There is usually a precipitating factor such as surgery, severe trauma, infection, or DKA. The operation may have triggered a thyroid hormone imbalance. Treatment involves, oxygen, IV fluids, beta-blockers to control heart rate, cooling blankets, and an antithyroid agent (such as propylthiouracil).

49. Answer: Gross painless hematuria is a sign of bladder or kidney malignancy until proven otherwise. Therefore, a cystoscopy is indicated to evaluate the bladder. Blood tests, including CBC, renal panel, and coagulation studies, should also be ordered.

50. Answer: This patient has symptoms and signs of acute bronchitis. The main differential here is pneumonia versus acute bronchitis. CXR is the best way to differentiate these two entities—no infiltrates are seen with acute bronchitis. Acute bronchitis most commonly has a viral etiology, and no antibiotic treatment is necessary. The patient should be advised to quit smoking, because smoking is a contributing factor to development of acute bronchitis.

51. Answer: Because this is the first time you are seeing this patient, a baseline set of laboratory and diagnostic studies, including CXR, ECG, CBC, basic metabolic panel, urinalysis, fasting glucose and lipid profile, and hemoglobin A_{1c} should be obtained. The patient is a diabetic and you should check for microalbuminuria. His HTN needs to be followed closely, and the patient should be scheduled for follow-up within approximately 4 weeks for a repeat BP measurement.

This patient does not have severe HTN or evidence of end-organ damage (target organs are heart, kidneys, eyes, and CNS—the laboratory studies you ordered would identify heart and kidney damage), and therefore one should not diagnose HTN based on one BP reading alone. In the meantime, the patient should be advised on lifestyle changes, such as regular exercise, healthy diet, and weight loss. If on his next visit he is hypertensive, goal is to look for any secondary causes of HTN (order aldosterone, renin, and thyroid function studies). Furthermore, his overall cardiovascular risk should be assessed and treatment based on these factors (see Box 12-1: Risk Factors for Coronary Artery Disease [CAD] in Evaluation of Patients With Hyperlipidemia). A low-sodium diet and antihypertensive medication should be started at that time.

52. **Answer:** This patient has stage 1 HTN. He has multiple cardiovascular risk factors, including male gender, diabetes, HTN, and family history of premature CAD (female first-degree relative died when younger than 65 years of age), but has no evidence of target organ damage; this puts him in risk group B. Lifestyle modification has not achieved the goal of 130/80 mm Hg for this diabetic patient. Thiazide diuretics should be initiated and have been shown to reduce mortality. In addition, an ACE inhibitor should be started; these drugs have been shown to decrease the rate of progression of diabetic nephropathy and retinopathy. At this point, you should also look for secondary causes of HTN (order aldosterone, renin, and thyroid function studies).

53. **Answer:** This patient has acute pyelonephritis, an upper UTI involving the ureter and kidneys. It is most commonly seen in sexually active young females. Complications may include sepsis, renal impairment, and renal abscess. Pyelonephritis in males is less common and usually indicates structural abnormalities such as vesicoureteral reflux or genitourinary obstruction. The presence of fever, chills, and flank pain differentiates pyelonephritis clinically, as does the presence of WBC casts on urinalysis. If patients have no signs of sepsis and are not very ill, they may be treated with 14 days of oral antibiotics (usually a fluoroquinolone or an aminoglycoside). This patient is ill and cannot tolerate PO liquid. She should probably be admitted to the hospital for IV antibiotics (usually ampicillin plus gentamicin or a third-generation cephalosporin) until she improves clinically and can be given oral antibiotics.

54. **Answer:** This patient likely has a muscle strain. Radiographs are not indicated, and treatment involves a very short period of bed rest (no more than 1-2 days), NSAIDs, and reassurance. If symptoms persist for 3 weeks or longer, then further imaging studies are appropriate.

55. **Answer:** This patient is having a severe exacerbation of asthma, most likely triggered by an upper respiratory infection. Do not be misled by the ABG. A patient who is working that hard to breathe is in trouble. For a patient who is this tachypneic, the arterial Pco_2 should be low and the patient should have a respiratory alkalosis. This patient needs oxygen, β-agonists, and IV steroids, and if these measures do not improve his distress, he may require intubation.

56. **Answer:** This woman most likely has TSS, which is most classically associated with menstruating women wearing vaginal tampons. It is caused by an enterotoxin of *Staphylococcus aureus* and is characterized by abrupt onset of fever, hypotension, and rash that eventually desquamates. As in other forms of septic shock, there is diffuse peripheral vasodilation causing the skin to be warm. Cardiac output is high, but because the peripheral vascular resistance is so low, systemic hypotension prevails. There is usually involvement of at least three organ systems in TSS. (TSS is not limited to women, and may occur in patients of both sexes with surgical wounds, burns, and insect bites.) Positive blood cultures are not required for diagnosis; it is the toxin that causes the illness. TSS is a life-threatening condition that should be treated with aggressive fluid resuscitation, IV antibiotics, and removal of the tampon or wound packing.

57. **Answer:** This man has acute pericarditis. Most cases of pericarditis are idiopathic and often are seen in the postviral period. Acute viral and idiopathic forms of pericarditis are usually self-limiting. Aspirin, indomethacin, or NSAIDs are the first-line treatment medications.

58. **Answer:** This patient likely has ankylosing spondylitis. Key diagnostic factors include the limited range of motion in his spine, exacerbation with rest, and improvement with exercise. Sacroiliac joint involvement is a hallmark of this disease, and its presence is required to make the diagnosis. Obtain plain films of the spine and pelvis to visualize the sacroiliac joints. Initial therapy involves NSAIDs and physical therapy.

59. Answer: This patient has developed adult respiratory distress syndrome (ARDS) caused by sepsis. Tachypnea, tachycardia, and hypoxia should raise suspicion for ARDS, especially in the setting of sepsis. High-flow oxygen should be given immediately to prevent further damage to the lungs. However, ARDS characteristically does not respond well to 100% oxygen, and mechanical ventilation is typically required. Other actions should be taken simultaneously, such as ordering a CXR and ABG.

60. Answer: Give analgesics for pain (codeine with or without acetaminophen), immobilize the joint, do not allow him to bear any weight on his right lower extremity, and administer factor VIII concentrate. Needle aspiration of the blood (to relieve swelling) is **not** recommended because of the risk of causing further bleeding and the chance of introducing an infection. Hemophiliacs should also receive factor VIII concentrate before any surgery or dental procedures.

61. Answer: This patient has a classic presentation of infectious mononucleosis. Order the following tests: monospot test, throat culture, CBC, and peripheral blood smear (atypical lymphocytosis is a hallmark of infectious mononucleosis). (The test for EBV-specific antibodies [anti-EA and anti-IgM-VCA titers] is not an appropriate test to order initially because EBV-specific antibodies help in diagnosing cases that are heterophile-negative; however, 90% of cases are heterophile-positive.) Advise the patient to rest and drink plenty of fluids. Antiviral therapy is not indicated in mononucleosis, and antibiotics are needed only if a throat culture reveals group A β-hemolytic streptococci.

62. Answer: This patient has an acute upper respiratory tract infection. His symptoms (nonproductive cough, sore throat, rhinorrhea, nasal congestion, myalgias) are suggestive of a viral infection. Therefore, symptomatic treatment including hydration, rest, and analgesics is appropriate. The main concern with a sore throat is infection with group A β-hemolytic streptococcus (can cause rheumatic fever). Although it is at times difficult to differentiate between a viral and bacterial infection, the presence of a cough, rhinorrhea, nasal congestion, and myalgias is suggestive of a viral infection.

63. Answer: This patient has a microcytic anemia—causes include iron deficiency, thalassemias, ring sideroblastic anemia, and anemia of chronic disease. Draw blood for iron studies (ferritin, TIBC, transferring, serum iron). If iron deficiency anemia is diagnosed, look for a source of bleeding (chronic blood loss is the most common cause of iron deficiency anemia in adults). If iron studies are within normal limits, consider the possibility of thalassemia and perform a hemoglobin electrophoresis.

64. Answer: This patient presents with signs and symptoms of acute pancreatitis. However, gallbladder disease must also be ruled out with a RUQ ultrasound. A full set of laboratory tests is indicated: CBC, renal panel, electrolytes, amylase, lipase, LFTs, and LDH. A CT scan of the abdomen may be obtained; this is the most accurate test for diagnosis of acute pancreatitis. Treatment of acute pancreatitis includes bowel rest (NPO), IV fluids, and pain control.

65. Answer: This patient most likely has Hashimoto's thyroiditis (most common cause of primary hypothyroidism and more common in women). The diagnosis is confirmed by the presence of antithyroglobulin antibodies, antimicrosomal antibodies, or both. Thyroid hormone replacement (with levothyroxine) is appropriate.

66. Answer: *Neisseria meningitidis* is the most likely organism causing acute bacterial meningitis. Although *Streptococcus pneumoniae* is still the most common organism causing meningitis in people over 15 years of age, the rash is characteristic of *N. meningitidis* (meningococcal) meningitis. This organism is commonly associated with epidemics of meningitis in college dormitories and even in high schools. Close contacts should receive chemoprophylaxis, which consists of oral rifampin for 2 days. (The meningococcal vaccine is effective against serotypes A and C, but unfortunately it is serotype B that most commonly causes epidemics of meningitis in the United States.) This patient should be treated with penicillin G; chloramphenicol; or a third-generation cephalosporin, such as ceftriaxone or cefotaxime. If the microbiologic cause is uncertain, treat with ceftriaxone or a cephalosporin. Perform a lumbar puncture and obtain blood cultures to confirm the diagnosis.

67. **Answer:** Bone pain is the most characteristic presenting symptom in multiple myeloma. Lytic lesions are present in this patient, as is a pathologic fracture of the right humerus. Patients with multiple myeloma may have bone pain for several months before diagnosis is made. This patient has a mild anemia and renal insufficiency; both findings that may be present in patients with multiple myeloma. Obtain serum and urine electrophoresis in this patient for detection of monoclonal protein (M-spike). Perform a bone marrow biopsy for confirmation.

68. **Answer:** This patient has a cauda equine syndrome. An emergent MRI of the lumbar spine should be ordered, and the patient needs immediate referral to a spine specialist for surgical decompression. Any patient who presents with low back pain and urinary or bowel dysfunction requires an emergent MRI.

69. **Answer:** This patient's presentation is classic for temporal arteritis, with key diagnostic factors including tenderness over temporal artery, unilateral headaches in the temporal region, visual loss, and low-grade fever. Because there is a history of visual loss, admit the patient to the hospital and start empirical treatment with high-dose IV corticosteroids immediately. Consult ophthalmology, and order an ESR. Although a temporal artery biopsy is required for definitive diagnosis, do not wait for biopsy results to initiate treatment. Patients suspected of having temporal arteritis should be treated with high-dose steroids until an alternate diagnosis is proved or their treatment is complete, because irreversible blindness is a risk.

70. **Answer:** Broadly, syncope can be divided into cardiac and noncardiac causes, and workup should be focused on ruling out life-threatening conditions first (MI, arrhythmias, hemorrhage) and differentiating between cardiac and noncardiac etiologies. The prognosis is poorest for patients with underlying heart disease. Physical examination should focus on cardiovascular examination and the identification of any focal neurologic deficits. Orthostatic vital signs should be obtained. Always check the patient's medications (especially in elderly patients). An ECG is obtained in all patients. Laboratory studies that should be ordered include CBC and metabolic panel. An echocardiogram is useful to screen for any structural heart disease. Additional diagnostic tests are based on the suspected etiology from the history and physical examination.

71. **Answer:** This patient's presentation (multiple compression fractures, back pain, renal failure, hypercalcemia, anemia, and thrombocytopenia) is suggestive of multiple myeloma. Therefore, the next step is to order serum and urine protein electrophoresis. The presence of anemia and thrombocytopenia indicate more advanced disease. Other key findings in multiple myeloma include recurrent infections, lytic bone lesions, rouleaux formation of RBC on the peripheral smear, and Bence Jones proteins in the urine. The other key diagnosis on the differential list is metastatic disease. Therefore, if the protein electrophoresis study is negative, a workup for metastatic disease, including CT scan of chest, abdomen, and pelvis, as well as a bone scan, should be ordered.

72. **Answer:** This patient is probably suffering from hypertensive encephalopathy due to a hypertensive emergency, which is defined as evidence of severe HTN accompanied by evidence of end-organ damage. Any of the following qualify as evidence of end-organ damage: hypertensive encephalopathy, myocardial ischemia or infarction, pulmonary edema, acute CVA (hemorrhagic or ischemic), aortic dissection, acute renal insufficiency, and microangiopathic hemolytic anemia. It is essential to reduce the BP immediately. IV nitroprusside or labetalol are usually the agents of choice. It is important, however, not to achieve a drastic reduction in BP. The initial goal should be to reduce the mean arterial pressure by approximately 25%. Therefore the patient's BP must be monitored acutely. Although the examination is unremarkable, this patient should have a CT scan of the head, ECG, and pertinent laboratory tests performed to rule out some of the abovementioned complications.

73. **Answer:** This clinical presentation is typical of Alzheimer's disease. Initiate donepezil as the first-line agent at this time, but its benefits are marginal.

74. **Answer:** The recent surgery and subsequent immobilization may have caused venous thrombosis. Sudden onset of dyspnea in this clinical scenario suggests PE, and this should be ruled out. A V̇/Q̇ scan should be obtained for diagnosis. However, heparin should be initiated right away, given the high clinical suspicion (one should not wait for study results if there is a high clinical suspicion). Supplemental oxygen is appropriate. An ABG analysis is important to assess oxygenation, ventilation, and acid–base status.

75. Answer: This patient suffers from migraine headaches. A trial of sumatriptan is appropriate. This medication should be taken as soon as symptoms appear. Consider prophylactic treatment, depending on the response.

76. Answer: This patient has chronic renal insufficiency due to diabetic nephropathy with superimposed ARF. Causes of ARF can be grouped into prerenal, renal, and postrenal causes. This patient has been taking increasing amounts of NSAIDs recently, which can cause intrinsic renal damage (especially in combination with ACE inhibitors) and a deterioration of renal function. Further laboratory tests (urine chemistries) may help to elucidate the cause of the ARF. A renal ultrasound may be ordered to rule out obstruction.

77. Answer: Although the history is suggestive of ischemic chest pain, a widened mediastinum suggests an aortic dissection. She should undergo immediate CT or transesophageal echocardiography to diagnose an aortic dissection. It is important to realize that a widened mediastinum may not always be apparent on CXR. A high index of suspicion may be needed to diagnose a dissection because the classic finding of stabbing chest pain radiating to the back may not be present. Cardiac enzyme levels should also be tested.

78. Answer: The patient should be admitted to the hospital. IV morphine is indicated for relief of pain. Other measures include IV fluids for hydration and keeping the patient warm.

79. Answer: Fine needle aspiration should be the initial procedure in this patient. It has a high sensitivity and specificity for malignancy. Cytologic analysis reveals whether the nodule is benign, malignant, or indeterminate. If benign, observation is appropriate. If malignant, surgery is indicated. If indeterminate, a thyroid scan should be obtained.

80. Answer: The patient in this case presents with signs of ischemic heart disease. It is important to have a high suspicion of ischemic heart disease, particularly in women, the elderly, and patients with diabetes, in whom ischemic heart disease may manifest with symptoms other than classic chest pain. Oxygen and sublingual nitroglycerin should be administered. Improvement of symptoms with nitrates points to ischemic heart disease as a likely cause. Nitrates increase the supply of oxygen by reducing ventricular work.

81. Answer: If a patient presents with monoarticular arthritis, septic arthritis is the most worrisome diagnosis and must be excluded. The differential diagnosis in this case includes cellulitis, gout, and pseudogout. Given the location of the pain (great toe) and lack of fever, septic arthritis is less likely, and the presentation is typical for a first acute gouty attack. Order a CBC, ESR, and blood cultures. Also, obtain synovial fluid cultures. For a definitive diagnosis of gout, joint aspirate is necessary to detect needle-shaped, negatively birefringent crystals under polarized light. If the WBC count is not elevated, and the patient is afebrile, make a presumptive diagnosis of gout and treat with indomethacin or colchicine (if renal function is normal).

82. Answer: This patient likely has GERD. He has no alarming symptoms that would suggest serious disease. Recommend lifestyle modifications such as sleeping with the head of the bed elevated, smoking cessation, and not eating before bedtime. Endoscopy is not indicated at this time, and empiric therapy may be initiated. He has already tried antacids; therefore, it would be appropriate to prescribe an H_2 blocker or a PPI.

83. Answer: This patient probably has postoperative delirium, which is common in elderly patients after major surgery. Her presentation is typical of delirium in that her symptoms wax and wane during the course of the day (they are typically worse at night), which is sometimes confusing and frustrating to family members. Because narcotics can worsen the delirium, discontinue them; or, if pain persists, lower the dose as much as possible.

84. Answer: RUQ ultrasound is the study of choice for acute cholecystitis, with high sensitivity and specificity. Initial treatment is bowel rest (NPO), IV fluids, antibiotics, and pain medication. General surgery consult should be obtained for cholecystectomy.

85. Answer: This patient could have fibromyalgia. However, to diagnose fibromyalgia, the patient should have at least 11 of 18 tender points. Rule out the following conditions before considering fibromyalgia: myofascial syndromes, rheumatoid disease, polymyalgia rheumatica, ankylosing spondylitis, spondyloarthropathy, chronic fatigue syndrome, Lyme disease, hypothyroidism, polymyositis, depression, somatization disorder, and hypertrophic osteoarthropathy. This requires ordering the appropriate laboratory tests (ANA, rheumatoid factor, Lyme titers, ESR, TSH level, appropriate radiographs). Once you are able to rule out these conditions, consider fibromyalgia as a diagnosis of exclusion. Patients with fibromyalgia are very difficult to treat, and there are not many therapeutic options.

86. **Answer:** The initial goal in managing a patient with variceal bleeding from cirrhosis is hemodynamic stabilization (ABCs). This patient has unstable vital signs. After assessment of airway and breathing, large-bore IV access is obtained, and IV fluid resuscitation should be started immediately. Blood transfusion (PRBCs) should be ordered and a nasogastric tube placed. Once the patient is hemodynamically stable, an emergent upper GI endoscopy is performed, which is diagnostic and therapeutic. Variceal band ligation is the preferred initial treatment, is usually effective in controlling bleeding, and has a lower rate of rebleeding than sclerotherapy. Also, note that although bleeding varices cause most episodes of GI bleeding in cirrhosis patients, Mallory-Weiss tears or ulcers may be the source of bleeding in a substantial number of patients.

87. **Answer:** Plain radiographs of the abdomen in the supine and upright positions should be obtained. Her presentation is suggestive of bowel obstruction. Colorectal cancer is the most common cause of large bowel obstruction in adults. You should also send a fecal occult blood test.

88. **Answer:** This patient likely has nephrolithiasis. Obtain a KUB for visualization of stones. If it is not diagnostic, a CT scan of the abdomen and pelvis would reveal the stone. The patient should be kept well-hydrated with IV fluids. Pain medication should be given.

89. **Answer:** This patient has respiratory alkalosis. Her hyperventilation may result from pulmonary embolism, or from a number of other conditions, including panic attacks. Given the high clinical suspicion for pulmonary embolism (sudden onset of dyspnea, oral contraceptive use, and hypoxemia), start the patient on heparin and obtain a $\dot{V}/\dot{Q}$ scan or a spiral CT scan.

90. **Answer:** This patient has alcoholic cirrhosis and presents with hepatic encephalopathy. A full set of labs, including CBC, renal panel, electrolytes, PT/PTT, LFT, and ammonia level should be ordered. A paracentesis may be required. The treatment of hepatic encephalopathy is lactulose, which converts ammonia (NH_3) to ammonium (NH_4), which cannot be absorbed in the gut.

91. **Answer:** Obtain plain films of the spine to rule out possible vertebral compression fracture secondary to osteoporosis. Quantitative assessment of bone mass density via DEXA scan is important in confirming a diagnosis of osteoporosis and in determining fracture risk. Calcium and vitamin D supplements are appropriate, as is weight-bearing exercise. If osteoporosis is diagnosed, pharmacologic therapy is appropriate: hormone replacement therapy and either bisphosphonates, raloxifene, or calcitonin.

92. **Answer:** This patient has megaloblastic anemia. It is unclear whether this is due to vitamin B_{12} or folate deficiency. Draw blood for serum vitamin B_{12} and folate levels. Transfusion is probably unnecessary at this time. Once the cause of megaloblastic anemia is known, administer the appropriate vitamin.

93. **Answer:** This patient has stage I (mild) HTN. With her smoking and family history of cardiovascular disease, she falls into risk group B. Lifestyle modification is recommended as the initial therapy in patients in risk group B who have stage I HTN. However, the decision of when to start pharmacologic therapy is often a judgment call. Initiating an antihypertensive agent in this patient, either an ACE inhibitor, hydrochlorothiazide, or a β-blocker, would also be appropriate. Schedule regular follow-up appointments with this patient for BP checks and for monitoring of her serum electrolytes once she begins drug treatment.

94. **Answer:** First, immediately administer thiamine 100 mg, then a bolus of IV D50W. Follow with an infusion of D5W to increase blood glucose levels. This patient is diabetic, and the most likely cause of his hypoglycemia is administration of too much insulin. Once he is stabilized, attempt to find out whether any recent changes have been made to his insulin regimen at the nursing home.

95. Answer: This patient has symptoms of urge incontinence, the most common type of incontinence in elderly patients. However, she likely also has stress incontinence given the loss of urine with laughing/coughing and the history of four vaginal deliveries. Three aspects of her history warrant attention: (1) she takes a diuretic, which exacerbates her condition; (2) she is diabetic; and (3) hyperglycemia can induce osmotic diuresis. Finally, she has a UTI (urinalysis-positive), which can worsen urinary urgency and frequency. All of these issues must be addressed and treated. Behavioral therapy in the form of bladder retraining can be helpful in patients with urge incontinence. Also, Kegel exercises and use of a pessary are conservative options for treating her stress incontinence.

96. Answer: Given the history and examination findings (diffuse enlargement of thyroid with bruit), this patient likely has Graves' disease. Order a serum TSH level for diagnosis. If the diagnosis is established, initiate a β-blocker (e.g., propranolol) for control of symptoms (taper β-blocker after 4 to 8 weeks) along with methimazole, and continue for 1 to 2 years.

97. Answer: This woman is suffering from dementia. Although the most common cause of dementia is Alzheimer's disease, with this woman's medical history (of stroke and TIAs), consider a vascular etiology as well (multi-infarct dementia). CT scan of the head would likely reveal old multi-infarcts and cerebral atrophy. In all cases of dementia, cognitive decline is usually gradual and patients are generally awake and oriented. Attempt to exclude reversible causes and review all medications. If Alzheimer's disease is confirmed, consider pharmacologic therapy and provide a multidisciplinary approach.

98. Answer: The answer is CT scan of the head. Patients on warfarin therapy risk sustaining intracranial bleeding after a fall. A CT scan should be obtained to rule out a subdural or epidural hematoma. If a hematoma is found, the goal is to reverse the acute bleeding that results from warfarin therapy. The quickest method of reversing the effects of warfarin is administration of fresh frozen plasma.

99. Answer: This patient has CAP. The critical decision to make in evaluating a patient with pneumonia is whether to admit the patient or to treat as an outpatient. Factors to consider in making this decision, in addition to clinical judgment, are age, presence of comorbid conditions (liver disease, cancer, CHF, cerebrovascular disease, renal disease), mental status, vital signs and several laboratory markers (see Table 10-1: Pneumonia Severity Index). Using this index, the point total for this patient is 96 (class III), and the recommendation is a brief period of hospitalization. This index is a general guideline, and clinical judgment is more important (and often relied on) in making this decision. Antibiotic treatment with a fluoroquinolone such as levofloxacin is appropriate.

100. Answer: This patient is in acute respiratory failure. Although there are many actions that should be taken to determine the cause of the respiratory failure, the first step must be to stabilize the patient. Given the degree of respiratory distress, hypoxia, and failure to respond to oxygen, mechanical ventilation is indicated, and it should not be delayed for the results of diagnostic testing, including ABGs. This patient should be intubated, and mechanical ventilation should be initiated without further delay.

Anatomic Abbreviations

AP • anteroposterior
LLQ • left lower quadrant
LUQ • left upper quadrant
PA • posteroanterior
RLQ • right lower quadrant
RUQ • right upper quadrant

Dosage Abbreviations

bid • twice per day
/d • per day
IM • intramuscular
IV • intravenous
NPO • nothing by mouth [Latin: *nulla per os*]
PO • by mouth [Latin: *per os*]
q • every
qid • four times per day
SC • subcutaneous
TPN • total parenteral nutrition

Gas/Compound Abbreviations

Ca^{2+} • calcium
$CaPO_4$ • calcium phosphate
Cl^- • chloride (ion)
CO • carbon monoxide
CO_2 • carbon dioxide
H^+ • hydrogen (ion)
HCO_3^- • bicarbonate
H_2O • water
K^+ • potassium (ion)
KCl • potassium chloride
KOH • potassium hydroxide
Mg^{2+} • magnesium (ion)
Na^+ • sodium (ion)
$NaHCO_3$ • sodium bicarbonate
NH_4^+ • ammonium
O_2 • oxygen
PO_4^{3-} • phosphate
SO_4^{2-} • sulfate

General Abbreviations

A-a gradient • alveolar-arterial oxygen difference
Ab • antibody
ABCs • airway, breathing, and circulation
ABG • arterial blood gas
ACAS • Asymptomatic Carotid Atherosclerosis Study

ACE • angiotensin-converting enzyme
AChE • acetylcholinesterase
ACIP • Advisory Committee on Immunization Practices (Centers for Disease Control and Prevention [CDC])
ACTH • adrenocorticotropic hormone
ADA • American Diabetes Association
ADH • antidiuretic hormone
AFB • acid-fast bacilli
AFib • atrial fibrillation
AFP • α-fetoprotein
AG • anion gap
AIDS • acquired immune deficiency syndrome
AIHA • autoimmune hemolytic anemia
AIN • acute interstitial nephritis
ALL • acute lymphocytic or lymphoblastic leukemia
ALT • alanine aminotransferase (formerly serum-glutamic-pyruvic transaminase [SGPT])
AML • acute myelogenous leukemia
ANA • antinuclear antibody
ANC • absolute neutrophil count
anti-HAV • hepatitis A antibody
anti-HBs • anti-hepatitis B surface antigen antibody
anti-Scl-70 • anti-topoisomerase I
anti-Sm • anti-Smith (antibody)
anti-U1-RNP • anti-U1-ribonucleoprotein
ATPase • adenosine triphosphatase
aPTT • activated partial thromboplastin time
ARF • acute renal failure
5-ASA • 5-acetylsalicylic acid
AST • aspartate aminotransferase (formerly serum glutamic-oxaloacetic transaminase [SGOT])
AT III • antithrombin III
ATN • acute tubular necrosis
AV • atrioventricular
aVF • automated volt foot
AVID • Amiodarone Versus Implantable Defibrillators (trial)
BBB • bundle branch block
BIPAP • biphasic positive airway pressure (mechanical ventilation)
BP • blood pressure
BPH • benign prostatic hypertrophy (hyperplasia)
BUN • blood urea nitrogen
CA • cancer antigen (e.g., CA19-9)
cAMP • cyclic adenosine monophosphate
CAP • community-acquired pneumonia
CAPD • chronic ambulatory peritoneal dialysis
CAVD • continuous arteriovenous dialysis
CAST • Cardiac Arrhythmia Suppression Trial

ABBREVIATIONS

CBC • complete blood count
CEA • carcinoembryonic antigen
CFU • colony-forming units
CHF • congestive heart failure
CLL • chronic lymphocytic leukemia
CML • chronic myelogenous leukemia
CMV • cytomegalovirus
CN • cranial nerve
CNS • central nervous system
CONSENSUS • Cooperative North Scandinavian Enalapril Survival Study
CPAP • continuous positive airway pressure (mechanical ventilation)
CPR • cardiopulmonary resuscitation
Cr • creatinine
CREST syndrome • calcinosis, Raynaud's phenomenon, esophageal involvement, sclerodactyly, and telangiectasia
CRF • chronic renal failure
CRH • corticotropin-releasing hormone
CRP • C-reactive protein
CSF • cerebrospinal fluid
CT • computed tomography (scan)
CVA • cerebrovascular accident
DEXA • dual energy x-ray absorptiometry (scan)
DHEA • dehydroepiandrosterone
DIC • disseminated intravascular coagulation
DIP • distal interphalangeal
DKA • diabetic ketoacidosis
DL_{CO} • carbon monoxide diffusion in the lung
DM • diabetes mellitus
DNAse • deoxyribonuclease
ds • double-stranded (DNA)
D5W • 5% dextrose in water
D10W • 10% dextrose in water
D50W • 50% dextrose in water
EBV • Epstein-Barr virus
ECF • extracellular fluid
ECG • electrocardiogram
ED • emergency department
ED&C • electrodesiccation and curettage
EEG • electroencephalogram
EGD • esophagogastroduodenoscopy
EMG • electromyogram
EMS • emergency medical services
ERCP • endoscopic retrograde cholangiopancreatography
ESRD • end-stage renal disease
FDA • U.S. Food and Drug Administration
$FEF_{50\%}$ • forced expiratory flow rate of 50%
FENa • fractional excretion of sodium
FEV_1 • forced expiratory volume in 1 second
FIO_2 • forced inspiratory oxygen
FSGS • focal segmental glomerulosclerosis
FSH • follicle-stimulating hormone
FTA-ABS • fluorescent treponemal antibody absorption (test)
FTI • free thyroxine index
5-FU • 5-fluorouracil (chemotherapy drug)
FUO • fever of unknown origin
FVC • forced vital capacity
GABA • *γ-aminobutyric acid*

GERD • gastroesophageal reflux disease
GFR • glomerular filtration rate
GGT • *γ-glutamyltransferase*
GH • growth hormone
GI • gastrointestinal
G6PD • glucose-6-phosphate dehydrogenase
GN • glomerulonephritis
GnRH • gonadotropin-releasing hormone
HAART • highly active antiretroviral therapy
HAV • hepatitis A virus
Hb • hemoglobin
Hb A • hemoglobin A (adult hemoglobin)
Hb A_{1c} • hemoglobin A_{1c} (the major fraction of glycosylated hemoglobin)
Hb F • hemoglobin F (fetal hemoglobin)
Hb H • homotetramer of Hb
Hb S • hemoglobin S (also known as sickle cell hemoglobin)
HB_cAb • hepatitis B core antibody
HB_eAg • hepatitis B e antigen
HB_sAg • hepatitis B surface antigen
H_2 blocker • histamine blocker
HBV • hepatitis B virus
HCC • hepatocellular carcinoma
hCG • human chorionic gonadotropin
Hct • hematocrit
HDL • high-density lipoprotein
HDV • hepatitis delta (D) virus
HELLP • hemodialysis, elevated liver enzymes, low platelet count
HERS trial • Heart and Estrogen/Progestin Replacement Study trial
HHNS • hyperosmolar hyperglycemic nonketotic syndrome
HIT • heparin-induced thrombocytopenia
HIV • human immunodeficiency virus
HLA • human leukocyte antigen
HMG CoA • 3-hydroxy-3-methylglutaryl coenzyme A
H & P • history and physical examination
HPF • high-power field (microscope)
HPV • human papilloma virus
HR • heart rate
HSV • herpes simplex virus
HTLV-1 • human T-cell lymphoma/leukemia virus, type 1
HTN • hypertension
HUS • hemolytic-uremic syndrome
IBD • inflammatory bowel disease
IBS • irritable bowel syndrome
ICF • intracellular fluid
ICP • intracranial pressure
ICU • intensive care unit
IDDM • insulin-dependent diabetes mellitus
IGF-1 • insulin-like growth factor 1
IJ • internal jugular
INH • isoniazid
INR • international normalized ratio
ITP • idiopathic thrombocytopenic purpura
IVP • intravenous pyelogram
J-tube • jejunostomy tube
KUB • plain film of the kidneys, ureters, and bladder
La • SS-B antigen

LDH • lactate dehydrogenase
LDL • low-density lipoprotein
LE • lupus erythematosus
LES • lower esophageal sphincter
LFTs • liver function tests
LH • luteinizing hormone
LMWH • low-molecular-weight heparin
LP • lumbar puncture
LSD • lysergic acid diethylamide
LV • left ventricle
MAOI • monoamine oxidase inhibitor
MAST • Michigan Alcoholism Screening Test
MCH • mean cell hemoglobin
MCHC • mean cell hemoglobin concentration
MCP • metacarpal phalanges
MEN • multiple endocrine neoplasia
MHA-TP • microhemagglutination–*Treponema pallidum* test
MI • myocardial infarction
MRA • magnetic resonance angiogram/angiography
MRI • magnetic resonance imaging
MRSA • methicillin-resistant *S. aureus*
MTP • metatarsophalangeal joints
NADPH • nicotinamide adenine dinucleotide phosphate (reduced form)
NASCET • North American Symptomatic Carotid Endarterectomy Trial
NASH • nonalcoholic steatohepatitis
NC • nasal canula
NHL • non-Hodgkin's lymphoma
NIDDM • non–insulin-dependent diabetes mellitus
NS • normal saline
NSAIDs • nonsteroidal anti-inflammatory drugs
NSGCT • nonseminomatous germ-cell tumors of the testis
NYHA • New York Heart Association
OA • osteoarthritis
PABA • *p*-aminobenzoic acid
Paco$_2$ • partial pressure of carbon dioxide, arterial
Pao$_2$ • partial pressure of oxygen, arterial
PAN • polyarteritis nodosa
PBC • primary biliary cirrhosis
PBP • penicillin-binding protein
Pco$_2$ • partial pressure of carbon dioxide
PCR • polymerase chain reaction
PCWP • pulmonary capillary wedge pressure
PE • pulmonary embolism
PEEP • positive end-expiratory pressure
PEG • percutaneous endoscopic gastrostomy tube
PET • positron emission tomography
pH • hydrogen ion concentration
PICC • peripherally inserted central catheter
PIP • proximal interphalangeal
PMH • past medical history
PMN • polymorphonucleotide
PNH • paroxysmal nocturnal hemoglobinuria
Po$_2$ • partial pressure of oxygen
PPD • purified protein derivative (test for tuberculosis)
PRBCs • packed red blood cells
PROOF trial • Prevent Recurrence of Osteoporotic Fractures trial
PRTA • percutaneous renal transluminal angioplasty

PSA • prostate-specific antigen
PSC • primary sclerosing cholangitis
PSVT • paroxysmal supraventricular tachycardia
PT • prothrombin time
PTT • partial thromboplastin time
PTC • percutaneous transhepatic cholangiogram
PTH • parathyroid hormone
PTT • partial thromboplastin time
PUD • peptic ulcer disease
PVD • peripheral vascular disease
PZA • pyrazinamide
RA • rheumatoid arthritis
RA • right atrium
RBC • red blood cell
RDW • RBC distribution width
REM • rapid eye movement (state of sleep)
RF • rheumatoid factor
Ro • SS-A antigen
RPR • rapid plasma reagin (test)
RR • respiratory rate
RSV • respiratory syncytial virus
RTA • renal tubular acidosis
RV • right ventricle
SIADH • syndrome of inappropriate secretion of antidiuretic hormone
SLE • systemic lupus erythematosus
SOB • shortness of breath
ss • single-stranded (DNA)
SS-B • Sjögren's syndrome B
SSRI • selective serotonin reuptake inhibitor
STD • sexually transmitted disease
T$_3$ • triiodothyronine
T$_4$ • thyroxine
TBG • thyroid-binding globulin
TBW • total body water
TCA • tricyclic antidepressant
Td • tetanus/diphtheria toxoid
TIA • transient ischemic attack
TIBC • total iron-binding capacity
TIG • tetanus immune globulin
TIPS • transjugular intrahepatic portosystemic shunt
TMP/SMX • trimethoprim/sulfamethoxazole (Bactrim)
TNM • Cancer staging for **T**umor, **N**ode, **M**etastasis
TORCH infections • **T**oxoplasmosis, **O**ther (syphilis, varicella zoster, parvovirus B19), **R**ubella, **C**ytomegalovirus, and **H**erpes infection
TPN • total parenteral nutrition
TRH • thyrotropin-releasing hormone
TSH • thyroid-stimulating hormone
TSS • toxic shock syndrome
TT • thrombin time
TTP • thrombotic thrombocytopenic purpura
UC • ulcerative colitis
UMN • upper motor neuron
USPSTF • U.S. Preventative Services Task Force
UTI • urinary tract infection
UV • ultraviolet
VDRL • Venereal Disease Research Laboratory (serologic test for syphilis)
VFib • ventricular fibrillation
VIP • vasoactive intestinal polypeptide
VLDL • very low density lipoprotein

$\dot{V}/\dot{Q}$ • ventilation/perfusion (scan)
V_T • tidal volume
V_T • ventricular tachycardia
vWD • von Willebrand's disease
vWF • von Willebrand's factor
VZV • varicella zoster virus
WBC • white blood cell

Unit of Measure Abbreviations

bpm • beats per minute
cc • cubic centimeter
cm • centimeter
dB • decibels (hearing)
dL • deciliter
g • gram
hr(s) • hour(s)
IU* • international unit

kg • kilogram
L • liter
μ • micro
μL • microliter
μU • microunit
mEq/L • milliequivalents per liter
mg • milligram
mL • milliliter
mm • millimeter
mm^3 • millimeter, cubic
mm Hg • millimeters of mercury
mmol • millimole
mOsm • milliosmole
ng • nanogram
pg • picogram
lb • pound
sec • second
U§ • unit

‡ JCAHO requires the use of "mL" (for milliliters) instead of "cc" (for cubic centimeters), which can be mistaken for "U" (units) when poorly written.

* JCAHO requires that "International unit" be spelled out so that the abbreviation is not confused with "IV" (for intravenous).

§ JCAHO requires the use of "unit"; can be mistaken for zero, four, or cc.

Index

Page numbers followed by *f, t,* and *b* indicate figures, tables, and boxed material, respectively.

① Restless leg syndrome
 - abnormal sensation in the legs and restlessness relieved by movement.
 - Rx - Dopamine agonist, before initiating Rx check iron levels < 50 ng/mL → give oral iron.
   if < 50 ↳ carbidopa/levodopa
               Ropinirole / pramipexole
② Modafinil - psyostimulant used as a Rx of narcolepsy
   Diagnose OSA using polysomnography.
③ COPD - chronic dyspnea w/ hyperinflated lungs and a prolonged expiratory phase + hx of cigarette smoking
④ Hemothorax - MCC - trauma ; also malignancy, blood dyscrasias, PE, bullous emphysema, necrotizing infections inc. TB (less common endometriosis)
⑤ Irradiation of the mediastim for hodgkins disease → Constrictive pericarditis, CAD, MV-fibrosis, Myocardial fibrosis.
⑥ Pneumothorax - 1° → Needle aspiration - pt. w/ minimal dyspnea < 50 yrs + small pneumothorax (< 2 cm from the lung margin to the chest wall); 2° → tube thoracostomy
                                     ↳ has underlying lung dx.